T0273823

Contents

List of Contributors

Walter Ageno, MD
University of Insubria
Varese
Italy

Elina Armstrong, MD
Coagulation Disorders Unit, Department of
Hematology, Comprehensive Cancer Center
Helsinki University Hospital
Helsinki
Finland

Roopen Arya, MA PhD FRCP FRCPath
Thrombosis and Haemostasis
Department of Haematological Medicine
King's College Hosptial
London
UK

Natalie Aucutt-Walter, MD
Division of Vascular Neurology
Department of Neurology
Penn State Milton S. Hershey Medical Center
Hershey, PA

Catherine N. Bagot, MBBS MD FRCPath
Department of Haematology
Royal Infirmary
Glasgow
UK

Mary Bauman, RN MN NP
Stollery Children's Hospital
University of Alberta Edmonton
Canada

Richard C. Becker, MD
Division of Cardiovascular Health and Disease
University of Cincinnati College of Medicine
Cincinnati
Ohio
USA

Paula HB Bolton-Maggs, DM FRCP FRCPath
Serious Hazards of Transfusion Office
Manchester Blood Centre, Plymouth Grove
Manchester
UK

Aisha Bruce, MD
University of Alberta
Medical Director Pediatric Hematology
Stollery Children's Hospital
Edmonton
Canada

G. Castaman, MD
Center for Bleeding Disorders and Coagulation
Department of oncology
Careggi University Hospital
Florence
Italy

Marco Cattaneo, MD
Medicina III, Ospedale San Paolo
ASST Santi Paolo e Carlo
Dipartimento di Scienze della Salute
Università degli Studi di Milano
Milano, Italy

Adrian Copplestone, MB BS
Plymouth University Peninsula School
of Medicine
UK

B.Cosmi, MD PhD
Dept Angiology and Blood Coagulation
Department of Experimental, Diagnostic and
Specialty Medicine
S.Orsola-Malpighi University Hospital
Bologna, Italy

**Mark Crowther, BSc (Med Sci) MBChB MSc
MRCP FRCPath**
Department of Haematology
Worcestershire Royal Hospital
Worcester
England, UK

Mark A. Crowther, MD
McMaster University
Hamilton
Canada

Vimal K. Derebail, MD MPH
UNC Kidney Center
Division of Nephrology and Hypertension
Department of Medicine
University of North Carolina
North Carolina, USA

Anna Falanga, MD
Department Immunohematology
and Transfusion Medicine
Hospital Papa Giovanni XXIII
Bergamo
Italy

Eti Alessandra Femia, PhD
Medicina 3, Ospedale San Paolo
Dipartimento di Scienze della Salute
Università degli Studi di Milano
Milan
Italy

David A. Garcia, MD
Medicine/Hematology
University of Washington Medical Center
Seattle
USA

Ravi Gill, BM
Southampton University Hospitals Trust
Tremona Road
Southampton
UK

Dr. Paul Harrison, BSc PhD FRCPath
Healing Foundation
Institute of Inflammation and Ageing (IIA)
University of Birmingham Laboratories
New Queen Elizabeth Hospital
Birmingham
UK

David Y. Huang, MD PhD
UNC Health Care Comprehensive Stroke
Center
Division of Stroke and Vascular Neurology
Department of Neurology
University of North Carolina
North Carolina
USA

Beverley J. Hunt, MB ChB FRCP FRCPath MD
Thrombosis & Haemostasis, King's College
Departments of Haematology & Pathology
Guy's & St Thomas' NHS Foundation Trust &
Viapath
London, UK

Dr. Paula James, DM FRCP FRCPath
Department of Medicine
Queen's University
Kingston
Canada

Valerie L. Jewells, DO FACR
Department of Radiology
University of North Carolina at Chapel Hill
Chapel Hill
North Carolina, USA

Walter H.A. Kahr, MD PhD FRCPC
Departments of Pediatrics and Biochemistry
University of Toronto
Division of Hematology/Oncology and
Program in Cell Biology
The Hospital for Sick Children
Toronto
Canada

Raj S. Kasthuri, MB BS
Division of Hematology and Oncology
University of North Carolina
Chapel Hill
North Carolina, USA

David Kavanagh, MB ChB PhD
Institute of Genetic Medicine
Newcastle University
Newcastle upon Tyne
UK

Clive Kearon, MB MRCPI FRCPC PhD
Department of Medicine
Division of Hematology & Thromboembolism
McMaster University
Hamilton, Ontario
Canada

Nigel S. Key, MB ChB FRCP
Division of Hematology and Oncology
University of North Carolina
Chapel Hill, North Carolina
USA

Steve Kitchen, PhD
Sheffield Haemophilia and Thrombosis Centre
Royal Hallamshire Hospital
Sheffield
UK

Riten Kumar, MD MSc
The Ohio State University
The Joan Fellowship in Pediatric
Hemostasis-Thrombosis
Division of Hematology/Oncology/BMT
Nationwide Children's Hospital
Columbus, USA

Sarah Takach Lapner, MD MSc FRCPC
Department of Medicine
Division of Hematology
University of Alberta
Edmonton, Alberta
Canada

Riitta Lassila, MD PhD
University of Helsinki
Haemophilia Center
Department of Hematology
Comprehensive Cancer Center
Helsinki University Hospital
Helsinki
Finland

Dr. David Lillicrap, MD FRCPC
Department of Pathology and Molecular
Medicine
Richardson Laboratory
Queen's University
Kingston
Canada

Lori-Ann Linkins, MD MSc(Clin Epi) FRCPC
Department of Medicine
Division of Hematology & Thromboembolism
McMaster University
Hamilton, Ontario
Canada

Marie Lordkipanidzé, BPharm PhD
Université de Montréal & Research center
Montreal Heart Institute
Canada

Gillian C. Lowe, MRCP FRCPath PhD
University Hospital Birmingham NHS
Foundation Trust and College of Medical
and Dental Sciences
University of Birmingham
UK

Alice Ma, MD
University of North Carolina
Chapel Hill, North Carolina
USA

Rhona M. Maclean, MB ChB
Sheffield Haemophilia and Thrombosis Centre
Royal Hallamshire Hospital
Sheffield
UK

Mike Makris, MD
Sheffield Haemophilia and Thrombosis Centre
Royal Hallamshire Hospital
Sheffield
UK

Marina Marchetti, PhD
Department Immunohematology and
Transfusion Medicine
Hospital Papa Giovanni XXIII
Bergamo
Italy

M. Patricia Massicotte, MD MSc
Director KIDCLOT Program
University of Alberta
Stollery Children's Hospital
Edmonton
Canada

Marshall Mazepa, MD
Department of Pathology and Laboratory
Medicine
University of North Carolina
Chapel Hill, North Carolina
USA

Stephan Moll, MD
University of North Carolina School
of Medicine
Department of Medicine, Division
of Hematology-Oncology
Chapel Hill, North Carolina
USA

Dougald M. Monroe, PhD
Division of Hematology/Oncology
School of Medicine
University of North Carolina
North Carolina
USA

Denise O'Shaughnessy, DPhil
Southampton University Hospitals Trust
Tremona Road
Southampton
UK

Thomas L. Ortel, MD PhD
Division of Hematology
Department of Medicine
Duke University
North Carolina
USA

Gualtiero Palareti, MD
Cardiovascular Diseases
University of Bologna
Italy

Raj K. Patel, MD FRCP FRCPath
Department of Haematological Medicine
King's College Hospital
London
UK

Sue Pavord, MB ChB
Department of Haematology
Oxford University Hospitals
NHS Foundation Trust
UK

Gillian N. Pike, BMedSci MBChB MRCP FRCPath
St. James's University Hospital
Leeds
UK

Gian Marco Podda, PhD MD
Medicina 3, Ospedale San Paolo
Dipartimento di Scienze della Salute
Università degli Studi di Milano
Milan
Italy

Brandi Reeves, MD
Division of Hematology and Oncology
University of North Carolina
Chapel Hill, North Carolina
USA

Lara N. Roberts, MD FRCP FRCPath
Consultant Haematologist
Department of Haematological Medicine
King's College Hospital
London
UK

Francesco Rodeghiero, MD
Hematology Unit
San Bortolo Hospital
Vicenza
Italy

Marie Scully, MD
University College of London Hospitals
London
UK

R. Campbell Tait, MBChB FRCP FRCPath
Department of Haematology
Royal Infirmary
Glasgow
UK

Alberto Tosetto, MD
Hemophilia and Thrombosis Center
Hematology Unit
San Bortolo Hospital
Vicenza
Italy

Sreekanth Vemulapalli, MD
Division of Cardiology, Duke University School
of Medicine
Duke Clinical Research Institute
Durham, North Carolina
USA

Michael J. Wang, MD
UNC Health Care Comprehensive Stroke
Center
Division of Stroke and Vascular Neurology
Department of Neurology
University of North Carolina
North Carolina
USA

Henry G. Watson, MD FRCP FRCPath
Department of Haematology
Aberdeen Royal Infirmary
Aberdeen
Scotland
UK

Amy Webster, MB ChB
Department of Haematology
University Hospitals of Leicester
Leicester
UK

Jonathan Wilde, MB BChir
Department of Haematology
University Hospitals Birmingham NHS
Foundation Trust
Queen Elizabeth Hospital, Queen Elizabeth
Medical Centre
Birmingham
UK

1

Basic Principles Underlying Coagulation

Dougald M. Monroe

Key Points

- This model of hemostasis views the process as having three overlapping phases: initiation, amplification, and propagation.
- Initiation takes place on cells that contain tissue factor when factor VIIa/TF activates factors IX and X; the factor Xa generates a small amount of thrombin.
- Thrombin from the initiation phase contributes to platelet activation and activates factors V and VIII.
- Propagation takes place on the activated platelet when factor IXa from the initiation phase binds to platelet factor VIIIa leading to platelet surface factor Xa, which complexes with factor Va giving a burst of thrombin.
- In clinical assays, the PT assess the initiation phase and the APTT assesses the propagation phase.

This chapter will discuss coagulation in the context of a hemostatic response to a break in the vasculature. *Coagulation* is the process that leads to fibrin formation; this process involves controlled interactions between protein coagulation factors. *Hemostasis* is coagulation that occurs in a physiological (as opposed to pathological) setting and results in sealing a break in the vasculature. This process has a number of components, including adhesion and activation of platelets coupled with ordered reactions of the protein coagulation factors. Hemostasis is essential to protect the integrity of the vascula-

ture. *Thrombosis* is coagulation in a pathological (as opposed to physiological) setting that leads to localized intravascular clotting and potentially occlusion of a vessel. There is an overlap between the components involved in hemostasis and thrombosis, but there is also evidence to suggest that the processes of hemostasis and thrombosis have significant differences. There are also data to suggest that different vascular settings (arterial, venous, tumor microcirculation) may proceed to thrombosis by different mechanisms. Exploitation of these differences could lead to therapeutic agents that selectively target thrombosis without interfering significantly with hemostasis. Other chapters of this book will discuss some of the mechanisms behind thrombosis.

Healthy Vasculature

Intact vasculature has a number of active mechanisms to maintain coagulation in a quiescent state. Healthy endothelium expresses ecto-ADPase (CD39) and produces prostacyclin (PGI$_2$) and nitric oxide (NO); all of these tend to block platelet adhesion to and activation by healthy endothelium [1]. Platelets in turn support a quiescent endothelium, in part through release of platelet granule components [2]. Healthy endothelium also has active anticoagulant mechanisms, some of which will be discussed below. There is evidence that the vasculature is not identical through all parts of the body [3]. Further, it appears that there can be alterations in the vasculature in response to changes in the extracellular environment. These changes can locally alter the ability of endothelium to maintain a quiescent state.

Even though healthy vasculature maintains a quiescent state, there is evidence to support the idea that there is ongoing, low-level activation of coagulation factors [4]. This ongoing activation of coagulation factors is sometimes termed "idling" and may play a role in preparing for a rapid coagulation response to injury. Part of the evidence for idling comes from the observation that the activation peptides of factors IX and X can be detected in the plasma of healthy individuals. Because levels of the factor X activation peptide are significantly reduced in factor VII deficiency but unchanged in hemophilia, the factor VIIa complex with tissue factor is implicated as the key player in this idling process.

Tissue factor is present in a number of tissues throughout the body [5]. Immunohistochemical studies show that tissue factor is present at high levels in the brain, lung, and heart. Only low levels of tissue factor are detected in skeletal muscle, joints, spleen, and liver. In addition to being distributed in tissues, tissue factor is expressed on vascular smooth muscle cells and on the pericytes that surround blood vessels. This concentration of tissue factor around the vasculature has been referred to as a hemostatic envelope [5]. Endothelial cells in vivo do not express tissue factor, except possibly during invasion by cancer cells. Also, there is evidence to suggest that tissue factor may be present on microparticles in the circulation. The information to date suggests that this tissue factor accumulates in pathological thrombi [6]. Further, there is general agreement in these studies that circulating tissue factor levels are extremely low in healthy individuals [7]. Limited data suggest that tissue factor does not incorporate into hemostatic plugs [8], unlike the accumulation of tissue factor seen in thrombosis, and so the model of hemostasis described in this chapter does not include a role for circulating tissue factor in hemostasis.

Given the location of tissue factor, it seems plausible that the processes associated with idling may not be intravascular but may rather occur in the extravascular space. At least two mechanisms are known that can concentrate plasma coagulation factors around the vasculature (Figure 1.1). Coagulation proteins enter the extravascular space in proportion to their size; small proteins readily get into the extravascular space, whereas large proteins do not seem to reach the extravasculature [9]. Because tissue factor binds factor VII so tightly, it can trap factor VII that moves into the extravascular space. This means that blood vessels already have factor VII(a) bound [10]. Also, factor IX binds tightly and specifically to the extracellular matrix protein collagen IV; this results in factor IX being concentrated around blood vessels [11].

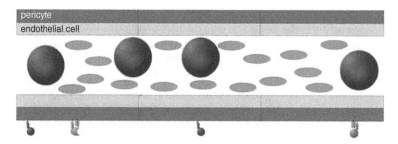

Figure 1.1 *Vessel.* An intact blood vessels is pictured with the endothelial cells (tan) and surrounding pericytes (dark brown). Within the vessel are red blood cells and platelets (blue). Associated with the pericytes, tissue factor complexed with factor VII(a) is shown in green. Factor IX, shown in blue, is associated with collagen IV in the extravascular space. *See Plate section for color representation of this figure.*

A role for this collagen IV-bound factor IX in hemostasis is suggested by the observation that mice expressing a factor IX that cannot bind collagen IV have a mild bleeding tendency [12].

Initiation

A break in the vasculature exposes extracellular matrix to blood and initiates the coagulation process (Figure 1.2). Platelets adhere at the site of injury through a number of specific interactions [13]. The plasma protein von Willebrand factor (VWF) can bind to exposed collagen and, under flow, undergoes a conformational change such that it binds tightly to the abundant platelet receptor glycoprotein Ib. This localization of platelets to the extracellular matrix promotes collagen interaction with platelet glycoprotein VI. Binding of collagen to glycoprotein VI triggers a signaling cascade that results in activation of platelet integrins [14]. Activated integrins

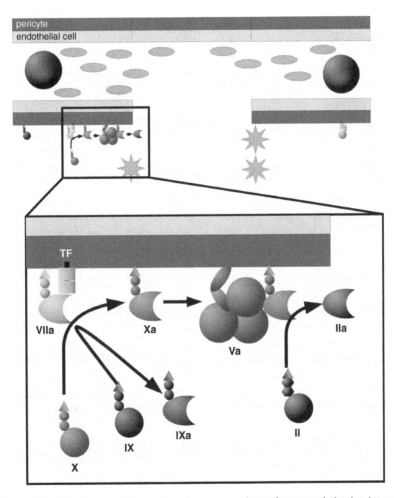

Figure 1.2 *Initiation*. A break in the vasculature brings plasma coagulation factors and platelets into contact with the extravascular space. Unactivated platelets within the vessel are shown as blue disks. Platelets adhering to collagen in the extravascular space are activated and are represented as blue star shapes to indicate cytoskeletal-induced shape change. The expanded view shows the protein reactions in the initiation phase. Factor VIIa–tissue factor activates both factor IX and factor X. Factor Xa, in complex with factor Va released from platelets, can activate a small amount of thrombin (IIa). *See Plate section for color representation of this figure.*

mediate tight binding of platelets to extracellular matrix. This process adheres platelets to the site of injury.

In addition to platelet processes, plasma concentrations of factors IX and X are brought to the preformed factor VIIa/tissue factor complexes at the site of injury. Factor VIIa/tissue factor activates both factor IX and factor X; the activated proteins play distinct roles in the ensuing reactions. Factor IXa moves into association with platelets, where it plays a role in the later stages of hemostasis. Factor Xa forms a complex with factor Va to convert a small amount of prothrombin to thrombin. The source of factor Va for this reaction is likely protein released from the alpha granules of collagen adherent platelets [15]. Platelet factor V is released in a partially active form and does not require further activation to promote thrombin generation [15]. Thrombin formed on pericytes and in the extravascular space can promote local fibrin formation but is not sufficient to provide for hemostasis throughout the wound area [16, 17].

The factor VIIa/ tissue factor complexes are, over time, inhibited by tissue factor pathway inhibitor (TFPI). TFPI participates in a ternary complex with factor Xa and factor VIIa bound to tissue factor.

The initiation process is critical to all subsequent events in the coagulation process. Deficiencies of tissue factor have not been seen in humans, implying that a deficiency is not viable, and a knockout of the tissue factor gene in mouse models leads to embryonic lethality. Factor VII deficiency is associated with a bleeding phenotype, and many patients with <1% factor VII activity have spontaneous, severe bleeding.

Amplification

The thrombin formed in the initiation phase acts as an amplifier by acting on platelets and proteins to facilitate platelet-driven thrombin generation (Figure 1.3). Thrombin has a tight specific interaction with platelet glycoprotein Ib [18]. When bound to glycoprotein Ib, thrombin undergoes a conformational change that alters the activity of the protein and may protect it from inhibition. This conformational change enhances the ability of thrombin to cleave either of the two platelet protease-activated receptors (PARs). PARs are members of the seven transmembrane domain G-coupled family of proteins [19]. Cleavage of a PAR creates a new amino terminal, which can fold back on itself and bind to a receptor site in the transmembrane domain. This intramolecular binding initiates a signaling cascade. In platelets, cleavage of PAR1 leads to signaling that results in platelet activation. This process is initiated after exposure of platelets to very small amounts of thrombin.

Platelet activation leads to numerous significant changes. Platelets undergo cytoskeletal changes leading to a shape change. There are regulated changes in the platelet membrane such that expression of phosphatidylserine on the outer leaflet of the platelets is significantly enhanced [20]. Phosphatidylserine induces allosteric changes in the procoagulant complexes that significantly increase their activity [21]. Platelets degranulate, releasing the contents of both alpha granules and dense granules. Dense granule contents, especially released-ADP, participate in a positive feedback loop either on the same platelet or on nearby platelets to further promote platelet activation. Polyphosphate released from dense granules promotes multiple procoagulant mechanisms [22]. Among the alpha granule contents released when platelets are activated is partially activated factor V.

In addition to its action on platelet receptors, thrombin can also activate procoagulant cofactors. Platelet factor V or plasma factor V bound to platelets is activated by thrombin cleavage to release the B domain; this reaction is significantly enhanced by platelet polyphosphate [22]. VWF, in addition to participating in platelet adhesion, acts as a carrier of factor VIII. It seems reasonable that VWF bound to glycoprotein Ib might bring factor VIII into proximity of thrombin, also bound to glycoprotein Ib. Thrombin cleavage releases factor VIII from VWF as well as activating factor VIII. So the amplification phase results in activated platelets

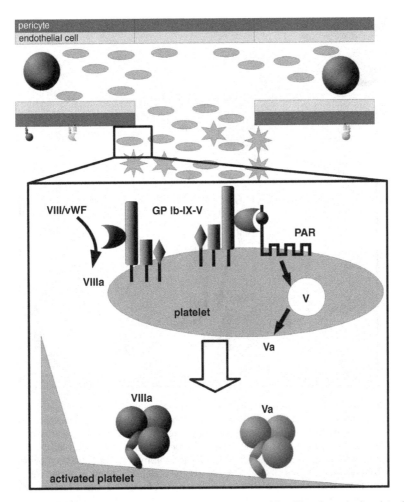

Figure 1.3 *Amplification.* Platelets, shown as blue discs, aggregate to stop blood loss from the break in the vasculature. Activated platelets are shown as star shapes. The expanded view shows thrombin (red) generated during the initiation phase binding to the glycoprotein Ib–IX–V complex (GP Ib–IX–V) on platelets. When bound, thrombin is somewhat protected from inhibition and can cleave protease activated receptor (PAR) 1 at the recognition site (black sphere). When the new amino terminal folds back on the seven transmembrane domain, a signaling cascade is initiated leading to surface exposure of phosphatidylserine as well as degranulation of alpha (white circle) or dense (not shown) granules. Factor Va is released from alpha granules and further activated by thrombin. Also, factor VIII is activated by cleavage and release from von Willebrand factor (vWF). *See Plate section for color representation of this figure.*

that have cofactors Va and VIIIa bound to the surface.

Some schemes of coagulation do not describe amplification as a separate step. But work from the Maastricht group, which was expanded on by Dale and colleagues, shows that platelets can be activated to different levels of procoagulant activity [20, 23]. Platelets activated in different ways appear to play different roles in promoting thrombin generation and stabilizing a clot [24, 25]. This suggests that in vivo the procoagulant activity of platelets may be modulated by local conditions. It also suggests that aspects of platelet activation could be targeted to reduce thrombin generation in pathological settings. So, amplification is included in this model as a discrete step.

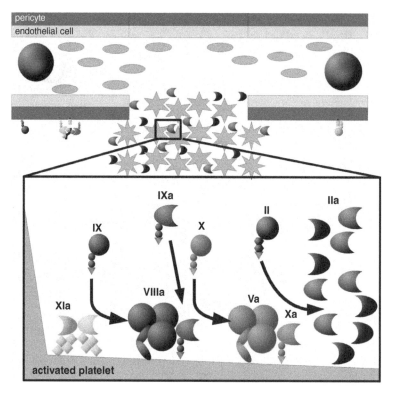

Figure 1.4 *Propagation.* The expanded view shows platelet surface thrombin generation. Factor IXa, formed during the initiation phase, can move into a complex with factor VIIIa formed during the amplification phase. This IXa–VIIIa complex cleaves factor X. Factor Xa, in complex with platelet surface factor Va, generates a burst of thrombin (IIa). This thrombin can feed back and activate platelet surface bound factor XI; the resulting factor XIa can feed more factor IXa into the reaction. This additional factor IXa enhances factor Xa and thrombin generation. As shown in the overview, the burst of thrombin stabilizes the initial platelet plug as all of the platelets are now activated (represented as blue star shapes as opposed to the disc shaped platelets in circulation). The factor VIIa–tissue factor complex with associated factor Xa is inhibited by TFPI. *See Plate section for color representation of this figure.*

Propagation

The activated platelet with activated cofactors is primed for a burst of thrombin generation (Figure 1.4). Factor IXa formed during the initiation phase binds to activated platelets. One component of this binding is a saturable, specific, reversible site independent of factor VIIIa [26], and the other component of this binding is factor VIIIa. The factor IXa/VIIIa complex activates factor X on the platelet surface. This platelet surface-generated factor Xa can move directly into a complex with platelet surface factor Va. In the presence of prothrombin, this factor Xa is protected from inhibition by antithrombin or TFPI

[27]. Data suggest that these factor Xa/Va complexes are very stable for even extended times and, in the presence of a new supply of prothrombin, can immediately act to promote thrombin generation [28]. Platelet surface-generated factor Xa plays a different role than factor X activated by factor VIIa/tissue factor. Because of the rapid inhibition by TFPI of factor Xa that is not in a complex, it is likely that factor X generated by factor VIIa/tissue factor cannot reach the platelet surface. This conclusion is supported by the observation that, in hemophilia, when platelet factor Xa generation is absent or severely defective, the clot is very poor even though factor VIIa/tissue factor activity is normal and fibrin

deposition can be observed at the margins of hemophilic wounds [16, 17].

The burst of thrombin during the propagation phase leads to cleavage of fibrinopeptides from fibrinogen. Cleavage of these fibrinopeptides exposes new binding sites that fit with complementary sites on other fibrin molecules [29]. These interactions lead to fibrin molecules assembling in long, branched chains anchored at the platelet receptor glycoprotein IIb/IIIa. This process stabilizes the initial platelet plug into a consolidated fibrin plug. The nature and stability of the fibrin plug appear to depend on the rate of thrombin generation during the propagation phase [30]. Polyphosphate released from platelet dense granules alters fibrin structure, making the clots more resistant to fibrinolysis [22].

In addition to its role in cleaving fibrinopeptides, thrombin generation participates in a positive feedback loop by activating factor XI on the platelet surface in a reaction that is enhanced by polyphosphate [22, 31]; this factor XIa can activate factor IXa to enhance factor Xa generation. The high levels of thrombin generated during the burst phase can cleave PAR4. Signaling downstream from PAR4 contributes to platelet shape changes and calcium signals that might be important in stabilization of the hemostatic plug [32]. Finally, high levels of thrombin generated during the propagation phase bind to fibrin and, when bound, are protected from inhibition by antithrombin. This fibrin-bound thrombin provides an important role in maintaining hemostasis. Disruption of a plug brings fibrinogen into contact with the bound thrombin, where fibrin formation can be initiated immediately without the need for thrombin generation. One aspect of the bleeding associated with hemophilia may be both the initial poor structure of the fibrin plug and the lack of bound thrombin to stabilize the plug.

Deficiencies of proteins in the propagation phase are associated with bleeding. X chromosome-linked hemophilia in males is associated with deficiencies in factors VIII and IX (hemophilia A and B, respectively). Because both genes are located on the X chromosome, the hemophilic phenotype results from a single-gene defect in males. Bleeding risk in hemophilia A and B is linked to factor level. Factor XI deficiency is also associated with bleeding risk. However, bleeding in factor XI deficiency shows a somewhat weak association with factor level [33]. The proposed model is consistent with this observation in that factor XI is not primary to the pathway leading to thrombin generation, but rather contributes through the positive feedback loop to boost thrombin generation.

Localization

A hemostatic plug should, by definition, seal the break in the vasculature but not continue platelet accumulation and thrombin generation to the point that the entire vessel is occluded. Thrombin released from a platelet plug into flowing blood is swept downstream. At plasma concentrations of antithrombin, the expected half-life of thrombin in blood is well under a minute. Also, factor Xa, either released into the blood or generated on healthy endothelium, is rapidly inhibited by TFPI in solution or TFPIβ, which is associated with the endothelial cell surface through a glycosylphosphatidylinositol linkage [34].

Healthy endothelial cells, in addition to the mechanisms described above for blocking platelet activation, have active mechanisms to downregulate thrombin generation [35]. Thrombin on the platelet surface participates in a positive feedback loop that promotes additional thrombin generation. By contrast, thrombin on healthy endothelium participates in a negative feedback loop that blocks additional thrombin generation (Figure 1.5).

Thrombin that reaches an endothelial cell binds to thrombomodulin. This binding causes a conformational change in thrombin such that it can no longer cleave fibrinogen. Thrombin bound to thrombomodulin is rapidly inhibited by protein C inhibitor [36]. This thrombin–inhibitor complex rapidly dissociates so that thrombomodulin can again bind thrombin, and thrombin bound to thrombomodulin can rapidly activate protein C. The endothelial cell protein C receptor enhances protein C activation by thrombin–

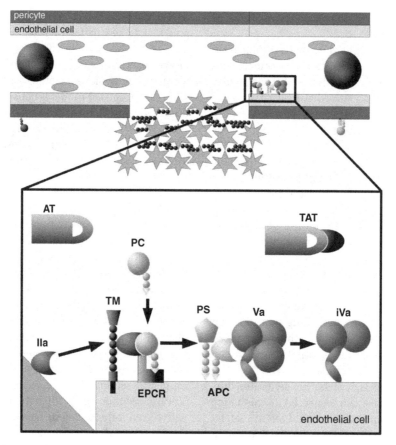

Figure 1.5 *Localization*. Thrombin generated during the propagation phase cleaves fibrinopeptides A and B leading to fibrin assembly (shown as brown distributed among and associated with the blue star shapes that represent activated platelets). The result is a stable platelet plug with fibrin and bound thrombin distributed throughout the plug. The expanded view shows the interface between the platelet plug (blue) and healthy endothelium. Thrombin released into the circulation is inhibited by antithrombin (AT) to form a thrombin–antithrombin complex (TAT). Also, thrombin (IIa) that reaches the endothelial cell surface binds tightly to thrombomodulin (TM). The thrombin–thrombomodulin complex activates protein C (PC) in a reaction enhanced by the endothelial cell protein C receptor (EPCR). Activated protein C (APC) in a reaction enhanced by protein S (PS) can cleave factor Va to inactivated factor Va (iVa). So thrombin on healthy endothelium participates in a negative feedback process that prevents thrombin generation away from the platelet plug that seals an injury. *See Plate section for color representation of this figure.*

thrombomodulin. Activated protein C, in coordination with protein S, inactivates factors Va and VIIIa. The net result is that thrombin generation is confined by healthy endothelium to a site of injury. Deficiencies of protein C or S, or defects that prevent cleavage and inactivation of factor V (factor V Leiden), allow for the spread of thrombi into the vasculature and are associated with venous thrombosis.

Coagulation Assays

The two most common assays in the clinical coagulation laboratory are the prothrombin time (PT) and activated partial thromboplastin time (APTT). In the PT assay, a large excess of thromboplastin (tissue factor) is added to plasma. There is rapid activation of factor X, leading to thrombin generation and clot formation. The assay is sensitive to deficiencies of factors VII, X, V, and prothrombin, but not factors XI, IX, or VIII. Thus, the PT evaluates the factors involved in the initiation phase (Figure 1.2).

Because the PT does not assess factors VIII or IX (the factors that are deficient in hemophilia A and B, respectively), the APTT assay was developed to diagnose hemophilia and monitor therapy. The original APTT used a dilution of thromboplastin, but kaolin was substituted in 1961 [37], resulting in a simple, reproducible, reliable assay (that no longer has a thromboplastin component). The current APTT takes advantage of the ability of factor XII and high molecular weight kininogen to be activated by a negatively charged surface. With this initiator, the clotting reaction proceeds through, and is sensitive to deficiencies of, factors XI, IX, VIII, X, V, and prothrombin. Thus, the APTT assays the factors involved in the platelet surface propagation phase (Figure 1.4).

The APTT uses highly negatively charged surfaces, such as kaolin, to initiate contact factor activation. The extent to which there is a physiologic correlate to such a surface in hemostasis is unclear. Factor XII deficiency is not associated with any bleeding diathesis, suggesting that it is not the dominant mechanism for factor XI activation in normal hemostasis. Platelet polyphosphates, which promote thrombin activation of factor XI, do not promote factor XIIa activation of factor XI [38]. Misfolded proteins can activate the kallikrein–kinin system through activation of factor XII, but this does not promote factor XI activation [39]. It may be that the dominant physiologic role for factor XII is in inflammation through the kallikrein–kinin system and in triggering fibrinolysis.

Summary

This model of hemostasis views the process as having three overlapping phases: initiation, amplification, and propagation. The hemostatic plug is localized to the area of injury by healthy endothelium, which has active processes

to downregulate thrombin generation. It is important to focus on the cellular location of the steps rather than the proteins involved. The protein factors overlap between the steps, but, for example, thrombin bound to platelet surface glycoprotein Ib plays a different role than thrombin bound to endothelial cell thrombomodulin. So, each of the cellular steps must contribute for the overall process to result in a coordinated hemostatic plug. A defect in initiation means that the coagulation reactions will not be started. Tissue factor deficiency is lethal in animals models, and factor VII deficiency is associated with bleeding. Platelet adhesion or activation defects, such as Scott Syndrome, are associated with bleeding. Hemophilia is a defect of factor X activation on the platelet surface during the propagation phase. Factor X activation by factor VIIa–tissue factor during initiation cannot substitute for the platelet surface reactions. Factor Xa is confined to the tissue factor-bearing surface, where it is formed because, when released from the surface, it is rapidly inhibited by TFPI and antithrombin. So, for normal hemostasis, a factor X-activating complex must be formed on activated platelets. The localization process confines platelet deposition and fibrin formation to keep the clot from expanding over healthy endothelium. This is consistent with the observation that defects in antithrombin, TFPI, and proteins C and S are associated with thrombosis. The tie between this model and the standard coagulation assays is that the PT and APTT assess the initiation and propagation phases, respectively.

References

1 Jin RC, Voetsch B, Loscalzo J. Endogenous mechanisms of inhibition of platelet function. *Microcirculation* 2005; 12: 247–258.
2 Ho-Tin-Noé B, Demers M, Wagner DD. How platelets safeguard vascular integrity. *J Thromb Haemost* 2011; 9 Suppl. 1: 56–65.
3 Aird WC. Vascular bed-specific thrombosis. *J Thromb Haemost* 2007; 5 Suppl. 1: 283–291.

4 Bauer KA, Mannucci PM, Gringeri A, *et al.* Factor IXa-factor VIIIa-cell surface complex does not contribute to the basal activation of the coagulation mechanism in vivo. *Blood* 1992; 79: 2039–2047.

5 Drake TA, Morrissey JH, Edgington TS. Selective cellular expression of tissue factor in human tissues. Implications for disorders of hemostasis and thrombosis. *Am J Pathol* 1989; 134: 1087–1097.

6 Balasubramanian V, Grabowski E, Bini A, *et al.* Platelets, circulating tissue factor, and fibrin colocalize in ex vivo thrombi: real-time fluorescence images of thrombus formation and propagation under defined flow conditions. *Blood* 2002; 100: 2787–2792.

7 Butenas S, Bouchard BA, Brummel-Ziedins KE, *et al.* Tissue factor activity in whole blood. *Blood* 2005; 105: 2764–2770.

8 Hoffman M, Whinna HC, Monroe DM. Circulating tissue factor accumulates in thrombi, but not in hemostatic plugs. *J Thromb Haemost* 2006; 4: 2092–2093.

9 Miller GJ, Howarth DJ, Attfield JC, *et al.* Haemostatic factors in human peripheral afferent lymph. *Thromb Haemost* 2000; 83: 427–432.

10 Hoffman M, Colina CM, McDonald AG, *et al.* Tissue factor around dermal vessels has bound factor VII in the absence of injury. *J Thromb Haemost* 2007; 5: 1403–1408.

11 Gui T, Lin H-F, Jin D-Y, *et al.* Circulating and binding characteristics of wild-type factor IX and certain Gla domain mutants in vivo. *Blood* 2002; 100: 153–158.

12 Gui T, Reheman A, Ni H, *et al.* Abnormal hemostasis in a knock-in mouse carrying a variant of factor IX with impaired binding to collagen type IV. *J Thromb Haemost* 2009; 7: 1843–1851.

13 Varga-Szabo D, Pleines I, Nieswandt B. Cell adhesion mechanisms in platelets. *Arterioscler Thromb Vasc Biol* 2008; 28: 403–412.

14 Watson SP, Herbert JMJ, Pollitt AY. GPVI and CLEC-2 in hemostasis and vascular integrity. *J Thromb Haemost* 2010; 8: 1456–1467.

15 Monković DD, Tracy PB. Functional characterization of human platelet-released factor V and its activation by factor Xa and thrombin. *J Biol Chem* 1990; 265: 17132–17140.

16 Sixma JJ, van den Berg A. The haemostatic plug in haemophilia A: a morphological study of haemostatic plug formation in bleeding time skin wounds of patients with severe haemophilia A. *Br J Haematol* 1984; 58: 741–753.

17 Monroe DM, Hoffman M. The clotting system – a major player in wound healing. *Haemophilia* 2012; 18 Suppl. 5: 11–16.

18 De Marco L, Mazzucato M, Masotti A, *et al.* Localization and characterization of an alpha-thrombin-binding site on platelet glycoprotein Ib alpha. *J Biol Chem* 1994; 269: 6478–6484.

19 Coughlin SR. Protease-activated receptors in hemostasis, thrombosis and vascular biology. *J Thromb Haemost* 2005; 3: 1800–1814.

20 Bevers EM, Comfurius P, Zwaal RF. Changes in membrane phospholipid distribution during platelet activation. *Biochim Biophys Acta* 1983; 736: 57–66.

21 Majumder R, Weinreb G, Lentz BR. Efficient thrombin generation requires molecular phosphatidylserine, not a membrane surface. *Biochemistry* 2005; 44: 16998–17006.

22 Morrissey JH, Choi SH, Smith SA. Polyphosphate: an ancient molecule that links platelets, coagulation, and inflammation. *Blood* 2012; 119: 5972–5979.

23 Dale GL. Coated-platelets: an emerging component of the procoagulant response. *J Thromb Haemost* 2005; 3: 2185–2192.

24 Heemskerk JWM, Mattheij NJA, Cosemans JMEM. Platelet-based coagulation: different populations, different functions. *J Thromb Haemost* 2013; 11: 2–16.

25 Mazepa M, Hoffman M, Monroe D. Superactivated platelets: thrombus regulators, thrombin generators, and potential clinical targets. *Arterioscler Thromb Vasc Biol* 2013; 33: 1747–1752.

26 Ahmad SS, Rawala-Sheikh R, Walsh PN. Comparative interactions of factor IX and

factor IXa with human platelets. *J Biol Chem* 1989; 264: 3244–3251.

27 Mast AE, Broze GJ Jr. Physiological concentrations of tissue factor pathway inhibitor do not inhibit prothrombinase. *Blood* 1996; 87: 1845–1850.

28 Orfeo T, Brummel-Ziedins KE, Gissel M, *et al.* The nature of the stable blood clot procoagulant activities. *J Biol Chem* 2008; 283: 9776–9786.

29 Lord ST. Fibrinogen and fibrin: scaffold proteins in hemostasis. *Curr Opin Hematol* 2007; 14: 236–241.

30 Wolberg AS. Thrombin generation and fibrin clot structure. *Blood Rev* 2007; 21: 131–142.

31 Oliver JA, Monroe DM, Roberts HR, *et al.* Thrombin activates factor XI on activated platelets in the absence of factor XII. *Arterioscler Thromb Vasc Biol* 1999; 19: 170–177.

32 Covic L, Gresser AL, Kuliopulos A. Biphasic kinetics of activation and signaling for PAR1 and PAR4 thrombin receptors in platelets. *Biochemistry* 2000; 39: 5458–5467.

33 Seligsohn U. Factor XI in haemostasis and thrombosis: past, present and future. *Thromb Haemost* 2007; 98: 84–89.

34 Piro O, Broze GJ. Comparison of cell-surface TFPIalpha and beta. *J Thromb Haemost* 2005; 3: 2677–2683.

35 Esmon CT. The protein C pathway. *Chest* 2003; 124: 26S–32S.

36 Rezaie AR, Cooper ST, Church FC, *et al.* Protein C inhibitor is a potent inhibitor of the thrombin-thrombomodulin complex. *J Biol Chem* 1995; 270: 25336–25339.

37 Proctor RR, Rapaport SI. The partial thromboplastin time with kaolin. A simple screening test for first stage plasma clotting factor deficiencies. *Am J Clin Pathol* 1961; 36: 212–219.

38 Puy C, Tucker EI, Wong ZC, *et al.* Factor XII promotes blood coagulation independent of factor XI in the presence of long-chain polyphosphates. *J Thromb Haemost* 2013; 11: 1341–1352.

39 Maas C, Govers-Riemslag JWP, Bouma B, *et al.* Misfolded proteins activate factor XII in humans, leading to kallikrein formation without initiating coagulation. *J Clin Invest* 2008; 118: 3208–3218.

2

Laboratory Tests of Hemostasis
Steve Kitchen and Michael Makris

Key Points

- Sample collection and processing has an important impact on the quality of results obtained.
- The sensitivity of any PT or APTT method is highly dependant on the reagents used.
- Clotting factor assays should be performed using several test sample dilutions.
- Specificity of a number of thrombophilia assays may be influenced by interfering substances.
- Oral direct inhibitors have variable effects on coagulation tests and assays, depending on the drug and the laboratory reagents used for testing.

Introduction

In the laboratory investigation of hemostasis, the results of clotting tests can be affected by the collection and processing of blood samples and by the selection, design, quality control, and interpretation of screening tests and specific assays. Such effects can have important diagnostic and therapeutic implications.

Sample Collection and Processing

Collection

For normal screening tests, venous blood should be collected gently but rapidly using a syringe or an evacuated collection system, when possible, from veins in the elbow. Application of a tourniquet to facilitate collection does not normally affect the results of most tests for bleeding disorders, although prolonged application must be avoided and the tourniquet should be applied just before sample collection. If there is any delay between collection and mixing with anticoagulant the blood must be discarded because of possible activation of coagulation. Vigorous shaking should be avoided. Any difficulty in venepuncture may affect the results obtained, particularly for activated partial thromboplastin time (APTT) or tests of platelet function. Prior to analysis, the sample should be assessed and discarded if there is evidence of clotting or hemolysis.

Tests of Fibrinolysis
Minimal stasis should be used because venous stasis causes local release of fibrinolytic components into the vein. The needle should not be more than 21 gauge (for infants, a 22- or 23-gauge needle may be necessary).

Venous Catheters
Collection through peripheral venous catheters or nonheparinized central venous catheters can be successful for prothrombin time (PT) and APTT testing, but is best avoided; if used, sufficient blood must be discarded to prevent contamination or dilution by fluids from the line (typically 5–10 mL of blood from adults).

Practical Hemostasis and Thrombosis, Third Edition. Edited by Nigel S. Key, Michael Makris and David Lillicrap.
© 2017 John Wiley & Sons, Ltd. Published 2017 by John Wiley & Sons, Ltd.

Mixing with Anticoagulant

If there is any delay between collection and mixing with anticoagulant, or delay in filling of the collection system, the blood must be discarded because of possible activation of coagulation. Once blood and anticoagulant are mixed, the container should be sealed and mixed by gentle inversion five times, even for evacuated collection systems. Vigorous shaking should be avoided.

Any difficulty in venepuncture can affect the results obtained, particularly for tests of platelet function. Prior to analysis, the sample should be visually inspected and discarded if there is evidence of clotting or hemolysis. Partially clotted blood is typically associated with a dramatic false shortening of the APTT together with the loss of fibrinogen.

Anticoagulant and Sample Filling

The recommended anticoagulant for collection of blood for investigations of blood clotting is normally trisodium citrate. Different strengths of trisodium citrate have been employed but:

- A strength of 0.105–0.109 mol/L has been recommended for blood used for coagulation testing in general, including factor assays. One volume of anticoagulant is mixed with nine volumes of blood, and the fill volume must be at least 90% of the target volume for some test systems to give accurate results, unless there is evidence that a lower percent fill is acceptable for the sample tube in use [1], either from published studies or local evaluation.
- Although 0.129 mol/L trisodium citrate has been considered acceptable in the past, this is not currently recommended. Samples collected into 0.129 mol/L may be more affected by underfilling than samples collected into the 0.109 mol/L strength.
- If the patient has a hematocrit greater than 55%, results of PT and APTT can be affected, and the volume of anticoagulant should be adjusted to account for the altered plasma volume. Table 2.1 is a guide to the volume of anticoagulant required for a 5-mL sample.

Alternatively, the anticoagulant volume of 0.5 mL can be kept constant and the volume of

Table 2.1 The volume of anticoagulant required for a 5-mL sample.

Hematocrit (%)	Volume of anticoagulant (mL)	Volume of blood (mL)
25–55	0.5	4.5
20	0.7	4.3
60	0.4	4.6
70	0.25	4.75

added blood varied accordingly to the hematocrit. The volume of blood to be added (to 0.5 mL of 0.109 mol/L citrate) is calculated from the formula:

$$\frac{60}{100 - \text{hematocrit}} \times 4.5$$

Container

The inner surface of the sample container employed for blood sample collection can influence the results obtained (particularly for screening tests such as PT and APTT) and should not induce contact activation (nonsiliconized glass is inappropriate). For factor assays there is evidence that results on samples collected in a number of different blood collection tubes are essentially interchangeable.

Processing and Storage of Samples Prior to Analysis

Centrifugation

For preparation of platelet-rich plasma to investigate platelet function, samples should be centrifuged at room temperature (18–25°C) at 150–200 g for 15 minutes, and analyzed within 2 hours of sample collection. For most other tests related to bleeding disorders, samples should be centrifuged at a speed and time that produces samples with residual platelet counts below 10 x 10^9/L; for example, using 2000 g for at least 10 minutes. Centrifugation at a temperature of 18–25°C is acceptable for most clotting tests. Exceptions include labile parameters, such as many tests of fibrinolytic activity. After centrifugation, prolonged storage at 4–8°C should be avoided, as this can cause cold activation, increasing factor VII and XII activity, and shortening of the PT or APTT.

Stability

Factor VIII and Von Willebrand factor are lost from whole blood stored at 4°C so samples should be stored at room temperature prior to processing. Samples for APTT should be analyzed within 4 hours of collection. This is particularly important for samples containing unfractionated heparin, which is progressively lost from samples as a consequence of neutralization by platelet factor 4 released from platelets. The results of some other clotting tests, such as the D-dimer and the PT of samples from warfarinized subjects, are stable for 24 hours or longer. Unless a laboratory has data on the stability of testing plasmas at room temperature for a specific test, the plasmas should be deep frozen within 4 hours of collection for future analysis.

Some clotting factor test results are stable for samples stored at –24°C or lower for up to 3 months and for samples stored at –74°C for up to 18 months (results within 10% of baseline defined as stable). Storage in domestic-grade –20°C freezers is normally unacceptable.

If frozen samples are shipped on dry ice to another laboratory for testing, care must be taken to avoid exposure of the plasma to carbon dioxide, which may affect the pH and the results of screening tests.

Prior to analysis, frozen samples must be thawed rapidly at 37°C for 3–5 minutes. Thawing at lower temperatures is not acceptable because some cryoprecipitation is possible.

The stability of the sample may be affected by the mechanism of transport and pneumatic tube systems should not be used to transport samples prior to tests of platelet function because the agitation associated with passage through some systems may activate platelets, leading to loss of function.

Use of Coagulation Screening Tests

Laboratories usually offer a set of tests (the coagulation screen) that aims to identify most clinically important hemostatic defects. Invariably this includes the PT, APTT, fibrinogen, and usually thrombin time. It is important to perform a full blood count to quantify the platelet count, but assessment of platelet function is not usually offered or performed in the initial tests. The pattern of abnormalities of the coagulation screen, as shown in Table 2.2, suggests possible diagnoses

---

Box 2.1 Recommendations and summary: sample collection and processing

- Avoid prolonged venous stasis.
- Use a 21-gauge or lower gauge needle for adults.
- Avoid indwelling catheters or lines.
- Mix immediately with 0.105–0.109 mol/L trisodium citrate.
- Discard the sample if there was any delay or difficulty in collection.
- Discard if marked hemolysis or evidence of clotting.
- Underfilling (<80–90% of target volume) prolongs some screening tests.
- If the hematocrit is >55%, adjust anticoagulant: blood ratio.

- The sample collection system can affect results by up to 10%.
- For plasma tests, centrifuge at 2000 *g* for at least 10 minutes at room temperature.
- Store at room temperature.
- Only centrifuge and store at 4°C if necessary.
- Test within 4 hours (unless there is evidence for longer stability).
- Freezing may affect results depending on the temperature and time of storage.
- Any deep-frozen plasma should be thawed rapidly at 37°C.

Table 2.2 Interpretation of abnormalities of coagulation screening tests.

PT	APTT	Thrombin time	Fibrinogen	Possible conditions
Prolonged	Normal	Normal	Normal	Factor VII (FVII) deficiency
Normal	Prolonged	Normal	Normal	Deficiency of FVIII, FIX, FXI, FXII, contact factor, or lupus anticoagulant
Prolonged	Prolonged	Normal	Normal	Deficiency of FII, FV, or FX Oral anticoagulant therapy Vitamin K deficiency Combined deficiency of FV and FVIII Combined deficiency of FII, FVII, FIX, and FX Liver disease
Prolonged	Prolonged	Prolonged	Normal or low	Hypo- or dysfibrinogenemia Liver disease Massive transfusion DIC

APTT, activated partial prothrombin time; DIC, disseminated intravascular coagulopathy; PT, prothrombin time .

and allows further tests to be performed to define the abnormality.

Unselected coagulation testing to assess bleeding risk prior to surgery may delay surgery inappropriately, is likely to cause anxiety in patients with "abnormal" test results , and is not cost effective. Coagulation tests are poor predictors of postoperative bleeding so patients with a negative bleeding history do not require routine coagulation screening before surgery. A bleeding history to include details of previous surgery, hemostatic challenges, and family history is much more useful and should be used to identify patients who require further investigation.

Prothrombin Time

Tissue factor (in the form of thromboplastin) and calcium are added to plasma that has been anticoagulated with citrate during collection. Tissue factor reacts with factor VIIa to activate the "extrinsic" pathway and thus form a clot.

Use of the Prothrombin Time Test

The PT is sensitive to deficiencies of factors VII, X, V, and II, and fibrinogen. The PT is particularly useful in monitoring anticoagulation in patients on vitamin K antagonist therapy such as warfarin and should be reported as International Normalized Ratio (INR) in such patients.

Figure 2.1 suggests a pathway for investigation of a patient with a prolonged PT.

Activated Partial Thromboplastin Time

Phospholipid (lacking tissue factor, hence the term "partial" thromboplastin) and particulate matter

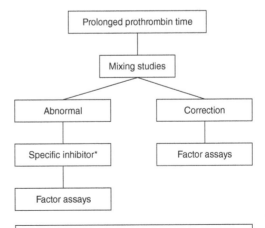

Figure 2.1 Investigation of a prolonged prothrombin time (PT). APTT, activated partial thromboplastin time.

(such as silica or kaolin) or fluid phase activator (such as ellagic acid) are added to plasma to generate a clot. Abnormalities in the "intrinsic" and "common" pathway will result in prolongation of the APTT [1].

Use of the Activated Partial Thromboplastin Time Test

This test is abnormal in patients:

- with deficiencies of prekallikrein (except when ellagic acid is used as activator), high molecular weight kininogen, factors XII, XI, X, IX, VIII, V, II, and fibrinogen;

- on heparin therapy; or
- who have the lupus anticoagulant.

Figure 2.2 suggests a pathway for investigation of patients with prolonged APTT. Prolongation of the APTT, sometimes to a dramatic degree, can be seen in patients without a bleeding diathesis (Table 2.3).

Mixing Studies

These are central in the investigation of a prolonged APTT. The principle is that the test is

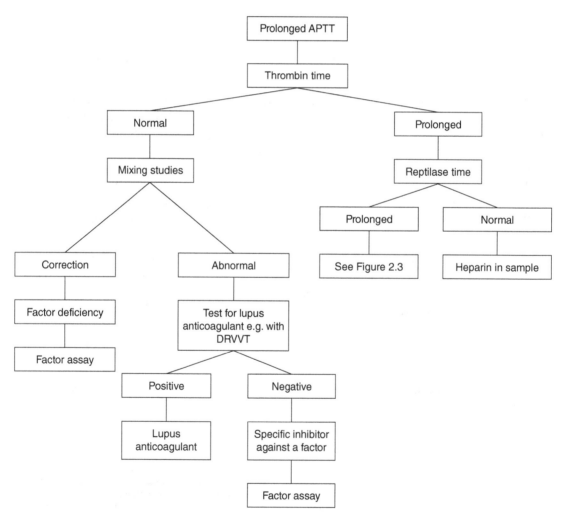

Figure 2.2 Investigation of a prolonged activated partial thromboplastin time (APTT). DRVVT, dilute Russell viper venom time.

Table 2.3 Conditions associated with a prolonged activated partial prothrombin time but without a bleeding diathesis.

Deficiency of:

    Factor XII

    High-molecular-weight kininogen

    Prekallikrein

    Lupus anticoagulant

Excess citrate anticoagulant

repeated, with 50% of the test plasma being replaced by normal plasma (which contains normal amounts of all the clotting factors). The result of the mixing study is that the test will have all the clotting factors to a minimum of 50%, and thus should result in:

- a normal APTT if the cause of the abnormality was a deficiency of a clotting factor; or
- a prolonged APTT if an inhibitor (either to a specific factor or a lupus anticoagulant) is present. Occasionally, the APTT on such a mix may initially be normal in the presence of acquired anti-factor VIII antibodies, but will lengthen on incubation.

Thrombin Time

The thrombin time measures the rate of conversion of fibrinogen to polymerized fibrin after the addition of thrombin to plasma. It is sensitive to and thus prolonged in:

- hypo- and dysfibrinogenemia;
- heparin therapy (or heparin contamination of the sample); and
- the presence of fibrin(ogen) degradation products and factors that influence the fibrin polymerization (e.g., the presence of a paraprotein in myeloma).

Figure 2.3 suggests a pathway for investigation of a prolonged thrombin time. Heparin contamination in a sample can also be confirmed by correction of a prolonged thrombin time after treatment of a sample with heparinase (e.g., hepzyme), testing with reptilase, or

mixing with protamine sulfate or other agent that neutralizes heparin. Thrombin time reagents vary in their sensitivity to heparin. Generally, thrombin times determined using reagents with a lower thrombin concentration will be prolonged at lower heparin levels. Thrombin time may be prolonged in the presence of low molecular weight heparin (LMWH) depending on the molecular weight of the drug. This is more frequent for LMWHs such as tinzaparin, which contain more of the larger polysaccharide chains that support thrombin neutralization.

Fibrinogen

A number of methods are available for measurement of fibrinogen concentration. Most automated coagulation analyzers now provide a measure of fibrinogen concentration, calculated from the degree of change of light scatter or optical density during measurement of the PT (PT-derived fibrinogen). Although this is simple and cheap, it is inaccurate in some patients, such as those with disseminated intravascular coagulopathy, liver disease, renal disease, dysfibrinogenemia, following thrombolytic therapy, and in those with markedly raised or reduced fibrinogen concentrations. The recommended method for measuring fibrinogen concentration as originally described by Clauss is based on the thrombin time and uses a high concentration of thrombin solution [2].

Screening Tests: Assay Issues

The sensitivity of the PT and APTT to the presence of clotting factor deficiencies is dependent on the test system employed. The degree of prolongation in the presence of a clotting factor deficiency can vary dramatically between reagents [3]. There is no clear consensus on what level of clotting factor deficiency is clinically relevant, and therefore the level that should be detected as an abnormal screening test result has not been defined. In relation to the APTT, one important application is the detection of deficiencies associated with bleeding, in particular factors VIII, IX, and XI.

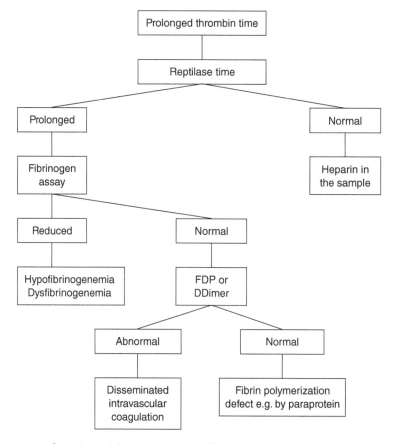

Figure 2.3 Investigation of a prolonged thrombin time. FDP, fibrin(ogen) degradation products.

A number of APTT methods are available for which abnormal results are normally present when the level of clotting factor is below 30 U/dL, and only methods for which this is the case should be used to screen for possible bleeding disorders. In the case of factor VIII, it has been recommended in the past that the APTT technique selected should have a normal reference range that closely corresponds to a factor VIII reference range of 50–200 U/dL. However, it should be noted that, for most methods, normal APTT results will be obtained in at least some patients with factor VIII in the range 30–50 U/dL, and few, if any, reagents will be associated with prolonged results in every patient of this type.

For most techniques, the APTT is less sensitive to the reduction of factor IX levels than for factor VIII, and most, if not all, currently avail-

able techniques will be associated with normal APTT results in at least some cases with factor IX in the range 25–50 IU/dL.

Data from published studies and from external quality assessment programs suggest that most widely used current APTT reagents will have:

- prolonged APTT results in samples from patients with factor IX or XI below 20–25 IU/dL; and
- a more mixed pattern of normal and abnormal results when factor IX or XI is in the range of 25–60 IU/dL.

Finally a subgroup of up to 10% of subjects with mild hemophilia A have a molecular defect that results in reduced activity in two stage and chromogenic factor VIII assays whilst retaining normal activity in one-stage techniques. These subjects have a normal APTT despite the presence of clinically relevant bleeding tendency consistent with mild hemophilia

Lower Limit of Normal Range

The lower limit for factor XI activity is probably between 60 and 70 IU/dL. The lower limit of normal for factor VIII or IX is approximately 50 IU/dL. A normal APTT does not always exclude the presence of a mild deficiency. In plasma from subjects with factor IX or XI deficiency, marked elevation of factor VIII, if present, may normalize the APTT.

Variation with Reagents

There is marked variation between results:

- with different APTT reagents, partly because of the use of different *activators* in the APTT as well as the *phospholipid profile*. Furthermore results are affected by the sample collection tube and its processing and storage. For these reasons, locally determined reference ranges are essential.
- with different PT *thromboplastins* used in the assays of factor VII or X. Sensitive PT techniques will show prolongation of the PT above the upper limit of normal when there is an isolated deficiency of factor VII, X, or V with a level below 30–40 U/dL. In general, the level of factor II (prothrombin) associated with prolongation of the PT is lower than for the other factors. PT results may be different according to the laboratory reagent used for measurement. Some cases of factor VII defi-

ciency, for example, may have a grossly prolonged PT with thromboplastins prepared from rabbit tissue but a normal or near normal PT if a reagent containing human tissue factor is used for analysis. Results obtained with reagents containing human tissue factor are likely to be more clinically relevant.

In the case of both the PT and APTT, it is useful to repeat borderline results on a fresh sample. It should be noted that the within subject variation of the PT and APTT over time may be 6–12%.

For both the PT and APTT, the degree of prolongation may be small in the presence of mild deficiency, and therefore there is a need for adequate quality control procedures and for carefully established accurate normal or reference ranges. In view of the limitations of screening tests, it is important that results are interpreted in conjunction with all relevant personal and family history details when screening for bleeding disorders. *Normal screening tests do not always exclude the presence of mild deficiency states.*

Clotting Factor Assay Design

One-Stage Assays

For many years, the most commonly performed assays for clotting factors have been one-stage clotting assays based on:

- the APTT in the case of factors VIII, IX, or XI; or
- the PT in the case of factors II, V, VII, or X.

Box 2.2 Recommendations and summary: screening tests

- PT and APTT methods vary in sensitivity to factor deficiency.
- Mild deficiency may be associated with normal PT or APTT.
- For bleeding disorders, select a method for which APTT is normally prolonged when factor VIII, IX, or XI is 30 IU/dL or less.

- Elevated factor VIII may normalize APTT in mild factor IX or XI deficiency.
- Assessments of APTT sensitivity should employ samples from patients.

There are a number of general features of the design of one-stage clotting assays that are necessary to ensure accurate, reliable, and valid results. In factor assays, the principle depends on the ability of a sample containing the factor under investigation to correct or shorten the delayed clotting of a plasma completely deficient in that factor. Such deficient plasmas must contain less than 1 U/dL of the clotting factor under investigation and normal levels of all other relevant clotting factors.

It is important that the clotting time measured by the APTT or PT depends directly on the amount of factor present in the mixture of deficient and reference or test plasma. For example, in a factor VIII assay, the level of factor VIII must be rate limiting in relation to the clotting time obtained. This requires dilution of a reference or standard plasma of known concentration. Preparation of several different dilutions of the reference plasma allows construction of a calibration curve in which the clotting time response depends on the dose (concentration) of factor present. At lower plasma dilutions or higher factor concentrations, the factor under investigation may not be rate limiting, and the assay is no longer specific and therefore invalid. It may be necessary to extend the calibration curve by testing additional dilutions when analyzing test plasmas with concentrations below 10 U/dL. At very low concentrations of an individual factor (<1–2 U/dL), the clotting time of the deficient plasma may not be even partially corrected by addition of the test plasma dilution. Dilutions are selected so that there is a linear relationship between concentration (logarithmic scale) and the response in clotting time (logarithmic or linear scale). The reference curve should be prepared using at least three different dilutions, and a calibration curve should be included each time the assay is performed unless there is clear evidence that the responses are so reproducible that a calibration curve can be stored for use on other occasions. The reference plasma should be calibrated by a route traceable back to World Health Organization (WHO) international standards where these are available. Test plasmas should be analyzed by using three dilutions

so that it is possible to confirm that the dose–response curve of the test plasma is linear and parallel to the dose–response curve of the reference plasma. It is not acceptable to test a single test dilution because this reduces the accuracy substantially and may lead to major underestimation of the true concentration when inhibitors are present. If a dose–response curve of a test plasma is not parallel to the reference curve, and the presence of an inhibitor (such as an antiphospholipid antibody) is confirmed or suspected, then the estimate of activity obtained from the highest test plasma dilution is likely to be closest to the real concentration; but it should be noted that the criteria for a valid assay cannot be met and results must be interpreted with caution. In the case of one-stage APTT-based assays the interference by antiphospholipid antibodies is frequently dependent on the APTT reagent used and its phospholipid content. Some APTT reagents, such as Actin FS, contain a high phospholipid concentration, and this type of reagent is much less affected by these antibodies and is particularly suitable for use in factor assays in such cases.

Factor Assays to Monitor Replacement Therapy in Hemophilia

In some clinical settings, replacement of factor VIII and IX in subjects with hemophilia A and B requires laboratory monitoring to be optimal. Both recombinant and plasma derived products are in use in different countries. There are particular issues related to the assay of postinfusion samples if recombinant products are used. Results of chromogenic factor VIII assays may be 20–50% higher than results of one-stage assays when plasma standards are used for assay calibration. Usage of concentrate standards delivers good agreement but, despite this, concentrate standards have not been widely used for monitoring treatment with recombinant factor VIII. Results of chromogenic assay are also higher (by approximately 50%) than one-stage assay results in the presence of Refacto AF/Xyntha, a B domain deleted factor VIII. This has led to the use of product-specific Refacto AF laboratory standard

---

Box 2.3 Recommendations and summary: factor assays

- Assays should be calibrated with reference plasmas traceable back to WHO standards where available.
- Deficient plasmas must have <1 U/dL of the clotting factor being assayed and normal levels of other relevant factors.

- No less than three dilutions of test plasmas should be tested.
- A valid assay requires test and calibration lines to be parallel.
- Interference by antiphospholipid antibodies can be minimized by use of an APTT reagent with a high phospholipid content.

---

in combination with one-stage assay reagents in some countries because this delivers agreement with chromogenic assay, and because the chromogenic assay is used to assign potency to this product. An assessment of assay performance in samples containing N8, a B domain deleted factor VIII from a different manufacturer, reported a difference of around 30% and concluded that a product-specific standard was not required for assay calibration. A number of modified factor VIII and IX molecules are in clinical trials mainly with the aim of extending the half-life of infused clotting factor. This includes pegylated factor VIII and IX proteins. Early data indicate that several chromogenic assays studied so far may be suitable for monitoring with the usual plasma standard to calibrate assays, but that only a few one-stage assay reagent sets will recover values close to those expected from potency labeling. Other one-stage reagent sets grossly underestimate or grossly overestimate the factor VIII or IX activity and are unsuitable for use with conventional plasma standards as assay calibrators. Recent guidance from the International Society on Thrombosis and Haemostasis/Science and Standardization Committee states that the optimal approach to postinfusion testing of such concentrates involves use of product-specific standards but recognizes that this may be difficult to implement [4]. At the time of writing it remains unclear to what extent product-specific standards will become available.

Factor XIII Testing

Factor XIII circulates as a tetramer of two functional/catalytic A subunits carried by two B subunits. Severe factor XIII-A deficiency is associated with severe bleeding events. In severe factor XIII-B deficiency the absence of carrier protein leads to a reduced (but not absent) plasma concentration of the A subunit with milder bleeding symptoms [5]. Subunit A is reduced when the B carrier proteins are deficient. Isolated factor XIII deficiency is associated with normal PT, APTT, thrombin time, and platelet function tests. If the clinical symptoms indicate a bleeding tendency then a full evaluation requires inclusion of a test for factor XIII deficiency in the panel of laboratory investigations. Clot solubility screening tests in which clotted citrated plasma is suspended in urea or acid suffer from poor sensitivity. There is published guidance on diagnosis from the factor XIII subcommittee of the International Society on Thrombosis and Haemostasis [5], which recommends that a functional quantitative factor XIII assay should be used as the first-line screening tests. Some factor XIII concentrates used for replacement therapy contain only the A subunit and are not the treatment of choice in the rare cases of B subunit deficiency. The guideline therefore recommends that factor XIII-A and XIII-B antigen should be measured, and also addresses inhibitor assays in acquired deficiency states.

Thrombophilia Testing

This section addresses some laboratory aspects of testing for heritable thrombophilia: protein C (PC), protein S (PS), antithrombin (AT), activated protein C resistance (APC-R), factor V Leiden (FVL), and the prothrombin 20210A allele [6,7].

Sample Collection, Processing, and Assay

For thrombophilia testing, as for other coagulation tests:

- A citrate concentration of 0.105–0.109 mol/L should be used for sample collection, because citrate strength may affect results, at least for APC-R testing.
- Centrifugation should be as for other coagulation tests described above.
- Residual platelets in plasma following centrifugation can also affect results of APC-R tests, and plasmas should be centrifuged as described above, separated, and recentrifuged a second time to ensure maximum removal of platelets. (Such a procedure is not necessary for AT, PC, or PS testing but can be used for convenience without adverse effects if the same plasma is to be used for these investigations in addition to APC-R.)
- Such double-centrifuged plasma can then be stored deep frozen at −70°C prior to analysis for at least 6 months for clotting PS activity and at least 18 months for PC and AT.
- In general, activity assays are preferable to antigen assays because antigen assays will be normal in some patients with type 2 defects where a normal concentration of a defective protein is present.

In the case of PS, this is complicated by the problems associated with interference by FVL in many different activity assays and can lead to important underestimation of the true level, with misdiagnosis a possibility. At present, the standardization of PS activity assays is poor in that results of different assays may differ substantially, even in normal subjects. For these reasons, PS activity assays must be used with caution.

FVL can also cause underestimation of the true PC level in clotting assays. A chromogenic PC assay may be used to avoid this problem although some type 2 defects give substantially different results in clotting and chromogenic PC assays. Alternatively, the PC clotting assay can be modified to include predilution of test sample 1 in 4 in PC-deficient plasma to restore specificity. A similar procedure can be employed to improve performance of clotting PS assays in the presence of FVL.

Clotting assays of PC and PS may also be influenced adversely by elevated factor VIII, causing underestimation. The presence of the lupus anticoagulant may be associated with falsely high results, with the possibility of a false-normal result in the presence of deficiency.

When assaying PC, PS, and AT, calibration curves should include a minimum of three dilutions and, in general, the most precise test results will be obtained if a calibration curve is prepared with each group of patient samples. As for other tests of hemostasis, it is important to use a reference plasma traceable back to WHO standards, which are available for AT, PC, and PS.

Testing for APC-R is largely based on the APTT in the presence and absence of APC, and therefore many of the variables that affect the APTT will in turn influence APC-R test results. These include the presence of heparin or lupus anticoagulant by prolonging clotting times, or elevated factor VIII, which shortens clotting times and manifest as acquired APC-R. The original APC-R test also requires normal levels of clotting factors, including factor II and X, which are reduced by warfarin therapy. Valid APC-R testing as originally used requires a normal PT and APTT.

There is evidence that standardization of results obtained by the original assay can be improved by calculation of the normalized APC-R ratio (test APC ratio divided by APC ratio of a pooled normal plasma tested in the same batch of tests). The test can be significantly improved by predilution of test plasma in factor V-deficient plasma, making the test 100% sensitive to the presence of FVL. This is typically a 1 in 5 dilution in commercial methods but 1 in 10 dilution may improve separation of results between normal subjects and subjects heterozygous or homozygous for FVL. This modification also makes the test specific for FVL, and will be associated with normal results where APC resistance in the classic assay is not a consequence of FVL. This must be borne in mind when interpreting results. In some versions of the test, there is clear separation between results obtained in heterozygotes and homozygotes but, even for such assays, confirmation by genetic testing may be necessary because it is important to identify homozygotes with certainty.

When genetic testing for the FVL or prothrombin alleles is undertaken, there are fewer relevant preanalytical variables than for phenotypic tests on plasma. Whole blood samples are stable for several weeks, at least for some of the genotyping methods.

Because of the many differences between results of apparently similar assays in thrombophilia testing, it is particularly important to establish locally a reference or normal range (as discussed in Appendix 1).

Clotting Tests in the Presence of Direct Oral Anticoagulants

The effects of apixaban rivaroxaban or dabigatran on some clotting tests are shown in Table 2.4. (see reference [8] for review, references, and UK Guidelines). Many of these data are derived from studies in which drug was added to pooled normal plasma *in vitro* and the findings are better supported where they have been confirmed in samples obtained from patients taking the drug. The expected plasma concentrations in patients taking these drugs are shown in Table 2.5.

Quality Assurance

All laboratory tests of blood coagulation require careful application of quality assurance procedures to ensure reliability of results. Quality assurance is used to describe all the measures that are taken to ensure the reliability of laboratory testing and reporting. This includes the choice of test, the collection of a valid sample from the patient, analysis of the specimen, and the recording of results in a timely and accurate manner, through to interpretation of the results, where appropriate, and communication of these results to the referring clinicians.

Internal quality control (IQC) and external quality assessment (EQA) are complementary components of a laboratory quality assurance program. Quality assurance is required to check that the results of laboratory investigations are reliable enough to be released to assist clinical decision making, monitoring of therapy, and diagnosis of hemostatic abnormalities.

Internal Quality Control

IQC is used to establish whether a series of techniques and procedures are performing consistently over a period of time (precision). It is therefore deployed to ensure day-to-day laboratory consistency. It is important to recognize that a precise technique is not necessarily accurate; accuracy being a measure of the closeness of an estimated value to the true value.

IQC procedures should be applied in a way that ensures immediate and constant control of result generation. Within a laboratory setting, the quality of results obtained is influenced by: maintenance of an up-to-date manual of standard operational procedures; use of reliable reagents

---

Box 2.4 Recommendations and summary: thrombophilia tests

- Double centrifugation is required for APC-R testing.
- Presence of FVL may cause significant underestimation of clotting PC or PS activity.
- Results of PS activity assays are highly dependent on the reagents used.
- Elevated factor VIII or lupus anticoagulant can interfere with PC or PS clotting assays.

- Results of AT assays may depend on the enzyme used in the assay.
- APC-R with factor V-deficient plasma dilution is the most sensitive and specific for FVL.
- Genetic testing for FVL or prothrombin allele may not be error free.

Table 2.4 Effects of direct oral anticoagulants on tests of hemostasis.

Test	Apixaban		Rivaroxaban		Dabigatran	
	peak	Trough	peak	Trough	peak	Trough
PT/INR	Minimal increase	Unaffected	PT ratio 1.3–1.6	Usually normal	INR/PT ratio <1.5	Ratio 1.3–1.4
APTT	Minor increase	Unaffected	Ratio 1.4 –1.6	Normal	Ratio 1.8–2.0	Prolonged
Thrombin time	Unaffected	Unaffected	Unaffected	Unaffected	>10 fold prolonged	Prolonged
Fibrinogen (Clauss)	Unaffected	Unaffected	Unaffected	Unaffected	False low in some assays	Minimal effects
One stage factor assays	Underestimation (higher levels)	Minimal effects	Underestimation	Minimal effects	Underestimation	Minimal effects
DRVVT	False increase	Minimal effects	False prolongation	Minimal effects	False prolongation	Minimal effects
APC-Resistance	Elevated ratio in some methods	Minimal effects	Elevated ratio in some methods	Minimal effects	elevated ratios	Minimal effects
AT	Overestimation in Xa based assays	Minimal effects	Overestimation in Xa based assays	Minimal effects	Overestimation in IIa based assays	Minimal effects
Clot based PC and PS assays	Overestimation	Minimal effects	Overestimation	Minimal effects	Overestimation	Minimal effects

APC, activated protein C; APTT, activated partial prothrombin time; DRVVT, dilute Russell viper venom time; INR, International Normalized Ratio; PT, prothrombin time.

Table 2.5 Expected plasma concentrations of direct oral anticoagulants (DOACs).

Drug	Dose	Peak levels mean and range	Trough levels mean and range
Apixaban	2.5 mg b.i.d.	0.051 mg/L (CV 27%)	0.014 mg/L (CV 53%)
Apixaban	5 mg b.i.d.	0.082 mg/L (CV 18%)	0.025 mg/L (CV 20%)
Dabigatran	150 mg b.i.d.	0.184 mg/L (95% CI 0.064–0.443)	0.090 mg/L (0.031–0.225)
Rivaroxaban	10 mg o.d.	0.125 mg/L (0.091–0.195)	0.009 mg/L (0.001–0.038)
Rivaroxaban	20 mg o.d.	0.223 mg/L (0.16–0.36)	0.022 mg/L (0.004–0.096)

and reference materials; selection of automation and adequate maintenance; adequate records and reporting system for results; and an appropriate complement of suitably trained personnel.

For screening tests, it is important to include regular and frequent testing of quality control material, which should include a normal material and at least one level of abnormal sample. For batch analysis, a quality control sample can be included with each batch. For continuous processing systems, the frequency of quality control testing must be tailored to the work pattern and should be adjusted until the frequency of repeat patient testing resulting from the limits of the quality control studies is at a minimum. For many random access coagulometers performing screening tests, this could typically be every 2 hours of continuous work or every 30–40 samples. For factor assays and parameters typically tested in batches, a quality control sample should be included with each group of tests. Patient results should only be released if quality control results remain within acceptable target limits. It is frequently useful to include IQC material at different critical levels of abnormality and some bodies recommend two levels of control with all tests of hemostasis.

External Quality Assessment

EQA is used to identify the degree of agreement between one laboratory's results and those obtained by other centers, which can be used as a measure of accuracy. The main function of EQA is proficiency testing of individual laboratory testing, but larger programs provide information concerning the relative performance of analytical procedures, including the method principle, reagents, and instruments. As a general principle, all centers undertaking investigations of hemostasis should participate in an accredited EQA program for all tests where available.

Box 2.5 Recommendations and summary: quality control

- Quality control samples should be analyzed regularly and frequently for screening tests and with each group of factor assays.
- Centers should participate in accredited EQA programs for all tests where available.

References

1 Wayne PA. *Collection, Transport, and Processing of Blood Specimens for Testing of Plasma-Based Coagulation Assays and Molecular Hemostasis Assays; Approved Guideline*, 5th edn. CLSI H21-A5. Clinical and Laboratory Standards Institute, 2008:28.

2 Mackie I, Kitchen S, Machin S, Lowe GDO. Guidelines on fibrinogen assays. *Br J Haematol* 2003; 121: 396–400.

3 Marlar RA, Cook JC, Johnston M, *et al. One-Stage Prothrombin Time (PT) Test and Activated Partial Thromboplastin Time (APTT) Test; Approved Guideline*, 2nd edn. CLSI H47-A2. Clinical and Laboratory Standards Institute, 2008.

4 Hubbard AR, Dodt J, Lee T, *et al.* Factor VIII and Factor IX Subcommittee of the Science and Standardisation Committee of the International Society on Thrombosis and Haemostasis. *J Thromb Haem* 2013; 11: 988–989.

5 Kohler HP, Ichinose A, Seitz R, *et al.* on behalf of the FXIII and Fibrinogen SSc Subcommittee of the ISTH. Diagnosis and classification of factor XIII deficiencies. *J Thromb Haem* 2011; 9: 1404–1406.

6 Jennings I, Cooper P. Screening for thrombophilia: a laboratory perspective. *Br J Biomed Sci* 2003; 60: 39–51.

7 Walker ID, Greaves M, Preston FE. Investigation and management of heritable thrombophilia. *Br J Haematol* 2001; 114: 512–518.

8 Kitchen S, Gray E, Mackie I, *et al.* Measurement of non-coumarin anticoagulants and their effects on tests of haemostasis: guidance from the British Committee for Standards in Haematology. *Br J Haem* 2014; 166: 830–841.

3

Molecular Diagnostic Approaches to Hemostasis

Paula James and David Lillicrap

Key Points

- In most instances, the initial diagnosis of disorders of hemostasis and thrombosis will be made using conventional phenotypic tests of coagulation.
- Molecular testing can be used with clear benefits in certain situations such as carrier detection for hemophilia and prenatal diagnosis of inherited bleeding disorders.
- In some instances (e.g., type 2 variants of von Willebrand disease), molecular diagnosis can be used as confirmatory testing where phenotypic analysis has been equivocal.
- Advances in sequencing technologies suggest that in the future there will be increased opportunities for incorporating molecular diagnosis into the clinical management of disorders of hemostasis and thrombosis.

Introduction

The first coagulation factor gene, factor IX (*F9),* was cloned and characterized in 1982 and, since that time, progressive advances have been made in the use of molecular genetic strategies to assist in the diagnosis of coagulation disorders. This chapter summarizes the current state of molecular diagnostics for the more common hemostatic conditions, with a discussion of both hemorrhagic and thrombotic problems for which genetic tests are now available.

It is important to emphasize that, for most hemostatic conditions encountered in clinical practice, the initial diagnostic test of choice will still be one that is performed in a routine hemostasis laboratory. For example, the diagnosis of hemophilia A will still, in the vast majority of cases, be made using a factor VIII clotting assay. The role of molecular genetic testing for this condition will be to assist in genetic counseling and to provide predictive information relating to certain aspects of clinical management. To date, the number of conditions for which the initial diagnostic strategy demands a genetic test is small. One such example is the test for the prothrombin 20210 thrombophilic variant.

A second, general issue that merits brief discussion concerns the appropriate venue for molecular genetic testing for hemostatic disorders. The successful implementation of a molecular diagnostic service for hemostatic conditions requires access to appropriate expertise and technology, and these tests cannot readily be added to the repertoire of a routine clinical coagulation laboratory. Optimal molecular genetic testing approaches incorporate methodologies that require access to equipment that will not be found in a hemostasis laboratory. However, genetic testing for hemostatic problems can easily be incorporated into a general molecular diagnostic facility (that is also providing testing for other inherited and somatic genetic diseases), although the involvement of personnel with an additional interest in the phenotypic aspects of

Practical Hemostasis and Thrombosis, Third Edition. Edited by Nigel S. Key, Michael Makris and David Lillicrap.
© 2017 John Wiley & Sons, Ltd. Published 2017 by John Wiley & Sons, Ltd.

clotting is undoubtedly beneficial for optimizing testing strategies and test interpretation.

Molecular Diagnostics of Bleeding Disorders

Molecular genetic testing for the hemophilias has been available since the cloning of the factor VIII (*F8*) and IX (*F9*) genes in 1984 and 1982, respectively [1,2]. Since then, with the cloning of all the known coagulation factor genes, molecular characterization of the rare inherited bleeding disorders has also been possible. With the completion of the Human Genome Project and the increasing utility of genome-wide strategies for identification of disease-associated loci, progress is also now being made in the discovery of genes involved in conditions such as the rare inherited platelet disorders.

Hemophilia A

To date, all inherited cases of isolated factor VIII deficiency have been linked to mutations of the *F8* gene, located at the telomeric end of the long arm of the X chromosome (Xq28) and encompassing 186 kilobases (kb) of genomic DNA (Figure 3.1). The large size of the gene, which contains 26 exons, was originally a challenge for

the development of molecular diagnostic testing. Initially, linked polymorphisms were used to provide an indirect test of transmission of the hemophilic *F8* gene (polymorphism linkage analysis). However, advances in sequencing technology over the past 15 years have resulted in the application of direct mutation detection for hemophilia in many laboratories worldwide.

Polymorphism Linkage Analysis in Hemophilia A

Linkage analysis is now rarely used for the genetic analysis of hemophilia. However, where there is a family history of the disease and informative intragenic polymorphisms are identified, polymorphism linkage testing can still be a useful and inexpensive strategy for performing carrier diagnosis and prenatal testing. Linkage analysis is nevertheless limited in its utility by a number of factors, the most frequently encountered of which are:

- an isolated case of hemophilia (lack of prior family history);
- the absence of informative polymorphic markers; and
- the problem of nonparticipating family members.

There are highly informative simple sequence repeat polymorphisms in introns 13 and 22 of the

Factor VIII Gene 184 kb: Xq28-qter

Figure 3.1 The *F8* gene and the two additional transcripts originating from the *F8* locus (*F8A* and *F8B*).

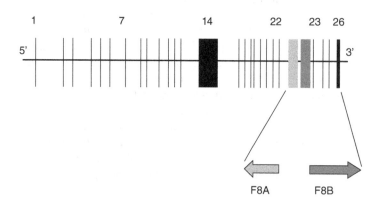

F8 gene and a *Bcl*I dimorphism in intron 18. Together, these polymorphic markers are informative in approximately 90% of families tested, regardless of ethnic background. These studies can produce results for reporting within a few days from the receipt of the test material, an interval that is acceptable for most prenatal testing situations.

Direct Mutation Testing for Hemophilia A

With the rapid advancement of molecular genetic technology that has accompanied the Human Genome Project, even genes as large and complex as *F8* are now readily accessible to direct analysis of the disease-causing mutations. Extensive investigations since the cloning of the *F8* gene have documented mutations at this locus in approximately 95% of patients with hemophilia A. To date, the only other genetic locus that has been associated with isolated factor VIII deficiency is the von Willebrand factor gene in type 2N von Willebrand disease (see below), although two different genes have been implicated in combined inherited factor V and VIII deficiency (*LMAN1* and *MCFD2*).

The current Internet-accessible Hemophilia A Mutation Database (www.factorviii-db.org) lists more than 2100 different *F8* mutations [3]. The majority of these changes represent single-nucleotide substitutions that have now been reported in all 26 exons of the gene. The database also lists many small (<200 nucleotides (nt)) and large deletions and a number of *F8* gene insertions. A single *F8* transcriptional mutation has been reported.

Rationale for Direct Mutation Testing in Hemophilia A

Genetic testing for hemophilia is still performed most frequently to determine the carrier status of potential heterozygous females and for prenatal diagnostic purposes. One of the most frequent groups of subjects for whom direct mutation testing is beneficial are those in whom an isolated report of severe hemophilia precludes the use of linkage analysis to track the mutant *F8* gene. These individuals require direct

mutation analysis to identify the carrier state and for accurate prenatal identification of affected offspring. Direct detection of the hemophilic mutation will also eliminate the uncertainties posed by potential germline mosaicism in the setting of a newly acquired mutation.

The second reason for pursuing the causative mutation in hemophilia A is the evidence that specific *F8* genotypes are more predictive for the risk of acquiring a factor VIII inhibitor [4]. Patients with null genotypes (large deletions, nonsense mutations, and the *F8* inversion mutations) have significantly higher risks for developing an inhibitor (between 20% (inversion mutations) and 70% [large, multidomain deletions]) than those whose hemophilia is caused by missense mutations, small deletions, and gene insertions for whom the risk of inhibitor development is less than 10%. Although the pathogenesis of inhibitor development is complex and multifactorial, given the clinical consequences of inhibitor development and the potential benefit of various forms of immune tolerance protocols, one can reasonably make the case for early mutation testing in all new severe cases of hemophilia A. Furthermore, there is also evidence that the outcome of immune tolerance protocols is also influenced significantly by the *F8* genotype.

Strategies for Direct Mutation Detection in Hemophilia A

Two basic approaches can be taken to identifying the causative mutation in hemophilia A (Figure 3.2) [5]:

1) a mutation screening strategy followed by sequencing of the abnormal region of the gene;
2) direct sequencing of the *F8* gene.

A variety of screening techniques have now been developed for the detection of subtle mutations, including:

- single-strand conformation polymorphism analysis;
- denaturing gradient gel electrophoresis;
- chemical mismatch cleavage;
- conformation-sensitive gel electrophoresis;

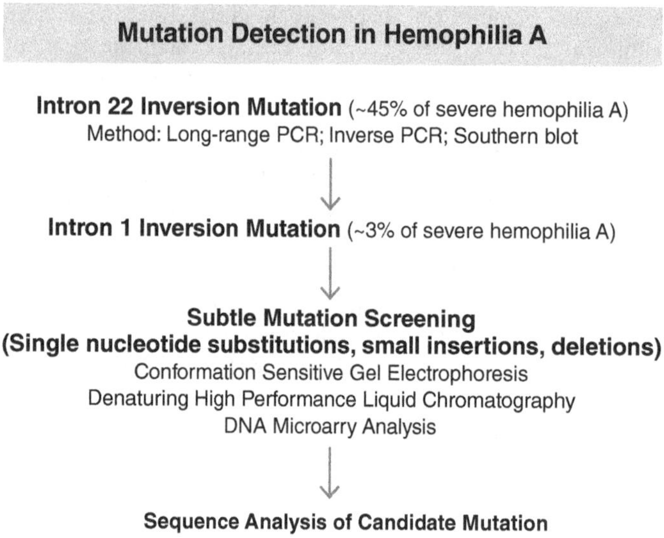

Mutation Detection in Hemophilia A

Figure 3.2 Molecular genetic testing algorithm for severe hemophilia A.

Intron 22 Inversion Mutation (~45% of severe hemophilia A)
Method: Long-range PCR; Inverse PCR; Southern blot

↓

Intron 1 Inversion Mutation (~3% of severe hemophilia A)

↓

Subtle Mutation Screening
(Single nucleotide substitutions, small insertions, deletions)
Conformation Sensitive Gel Electrophoresis
Denaturing High Performance Liquid Chromatography
DNA Microarry Analysis

↓

Sequence Analysis of Candidate Mutation

- denaturing high-performance liquid chromatography; and
- DNA microarray analysis.

In laboratories using any one of these methods on a regular basis, the sensitivity for detecting point mutations is likely to be between 85% and 95%.

Following the identification of an abnormality in one region of the gene, the abnormal fragment can be sequenced (Figure 3.3). With the rapid development of automated sequencing technology, the cost and efficiency of direct sequence analysis of PCR amplicons has now improved to the point where this strategy is now being used routinely for *F8* mutation detection by most molecular diagnostic laboratories. Indeed, the reduced cost and ease of sequencing has now reached a point where initial screening approaches for mutations is rarely justified.

Currently, most genotyping laboratories are sequencing *F8* coding regions and proximal regulatory regions to search for mutations, and in approximately 95% of cases plausible candidate changes are identified. There is now evidence that at least some of the missing mutations involve sequence variants deep within introns, and thus the future application of whole gene analysis, using a next generation sequencing approach may see increasing utility.

Factor VIII Inversion Mutations

There are two significant exceptions to the mutational heterogeneity of hemophilia A:

1) The intron 22 *F8* inversion mutation, found in approximately 45% of patients with a severe hemophilia A phenotype [6]. This inversion involves exons 1–22 of the *F8* gene and is caused by an intrachromosomal recombination event between a copy of the *F8A* gene within intron 22 of *F8* and additional *F8A* copies approximately 400 kb 5′ (telomeric) of *F8*. The inversion is only found in patients with a severe phenotype. In the molecular diagnostic laboratory, testing for the inversion mutation should be the first step in the analysis of any kindred affected by severe hemophilia A. The inversion can be detected with either a Southern blot (Figure 3.4), inverse or a long-range (>10 kb) PCR-based approach. The choice of methodology will depend on a combination of the amount and quality of the sample DNA and the laboratory expertise. In approximately 83% of cases, the recombination event will have been with the distal extragenic copy of *F8A* (type 1 inversions), in approximately 16% with the proximal *F8A* copy (type 2), and in approximately 1% of inversions rare rearrangement patterns are seen.

Figure 3.3 Sequencing chromatogram from a severe hemophilia A patient. In this woman, the *F8* mutation is a single adenine insertion into a run of eight adenine residues in exon 14. The "A" insertion results in a reading frameshift.

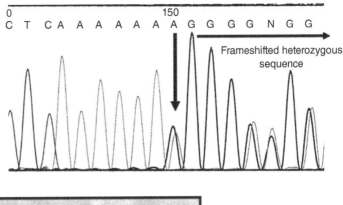

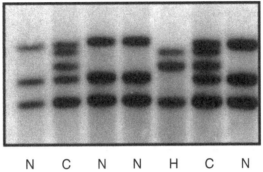

Factor VIII Intron 22 Inversion Mutation Southern Blot

Alternative Methodologies : Long-range PCR or inverse PCR

Figure 3.4 A Southern blot autoradiograph of the intron 22 inversion mutation in *F8*, the cause of ~45% of the cases of severe hemophilia A. N, normal; H, hemophilia A due to the inversion mutation; and C, carrier female for the intron 22 inversion.

2) A second recurring *F8* mutation is seen in ~3% of severe hemophilia A cases and involves an inversion event with sequences in intron 1 [7]. This mutation can readily be detected with a PCR-based approach.

Hemophilia B

All reported cases of hemophilia B have been linked to defects in the *F9* gene, which is centromeric to *F8* on the X chromosome (Xq27). As with hemophilia A, the inherited deficiency of factor IX demonstrates both phenotypic and mutational (allelic) heterogeneity. The molecular diagnostic strategies employed for hemophilia B testing are similar to those discussed for hemophilia A, with the exception that in hemophilia B there is no single predominant mutation equivalent to the *F8* inversions in hemophilia A.

Polymorphism Linkage Analysis in Hemophilia B

Although rarely used nowadays, the *F9* gene contains a number of polymorphisms that can be used for linkage analysis in kindreds in which hemophilia B is known to be segregating. Ethnic variability of several of these polymorphisms is extreme. For instance, in Oriental populations, analysis of the intragenic markers is invariably uninformative.

Direct Mutation Testing for Hemophilia B

In contrast to hemophilia A, where the large size of the gene initially limited direct mutational analysis, direct mutation detection for hemophilia B has been employed for some time (186 kb/26 exons for *F8* vs. 34 kb/8 exons for *F9*). A worldwide Hemophilia B Mutation Database has been in existence since 1990, and the current Internet-accessible registry [8] lists information on more than 1100 different *F9* mutations. As with hemophilia A, most of the mutations resulting in this phenotype are single-nucleotide variations located throughout the *F9* gene. In contrast to hemophilia A, missense mutations are a far more frequent cause of the clotting factor deficit in hemophilia B.

Hemophilia B Mutations of Particular Clinical Significance

Many of the *F9* missense mutations have provided knowledge of the basic structure and function correlates of the factor IX protein. However, several clinically important mutation types are worth highlighting from a molecular diagnostic standpoint.

The first group of mutations of note are a variety of gross *F9* gene deletions and rearrangements that result in severe hemophilia B. These can be complicated by the development of factor IX inhibitors and anaphylactic reactions to factor IX replacement therapy [9]. This constellation of findings has now been reported in a significant number of patients worldwide, and has further emphasized the proposal that all new cases of severe hemophilia B should be screened as soon as possible for gross *F9* deletions or rearrangements.

The second type of *F9* mutation with important clinical consequences involves missense mutations in the propeptide-encoding sequence, resulting in a markedly reduced affinity of the mutant protein for the vitamin K-dependent carboxylase [10]. Two different missense mutations have been described at amino acid residue −10 in the propeptide, and these patients have normal baseline factor IX levels but show marked sensitivity to treatment with vitamin K antagonists, leading to a significantly increased risk of bleeding on oral anticoagulant therapy.

The final group of *F9* mutations that merit recognition are those in the *F9* promoter (18 different point mutations have now been described in the approximately 40 nucleotides adjacent to the transcription start site). These mutations are associated with the hemophilia B Leyden phenotype, where factor IX deficiency undergoes at least a partial spontaneous phenotypic resolution following puberty, as a result of androgen-dependent *F9* gene expression [11]. For some of these mutations (e.g., nt -6 G to A), the phenotype is less severe and patients appear to recover factor IX levels of approximately 30% by age 4 or 5 years. In contrast to the normal hemophilia B Leyden phenotype, four patients have been reported with a mutation at nt -26, in whom no recovery of factor IX levels has been documented. Finally, at least one patient with a mutation at nt +13 in the Leyden-specific region of the promoter and with apparently normal sexual growth and development has failed to recover normal factor IX levels by middle age [12]. This case suggests that caution should be exercised in predicting phenotypic recovery in all instances of Leyden mutations.

von Willebrand Disease

von Willebrand disease (VWD) is the most common inherited bleeding disorder known in humans, and there has been much interest in the genetic pathology of this condition over the past two decades. This is a complex hemostatic disorder and, despite significant advances in our understanding of molecular genetic mechanisms responsible for VWD, the role of molecular diagnostics for disease diagnosis is still somewhat limited and will most often be used to confirm phenotypic testing or in situations such as prenatal diagnosis. Furthermore, with 52 exons encompassing 178 kb of genomic DNA, molecular genetic analysis of the von Willebrand factor (*VWF*) gene has proved to more challenging than testing for the hemophilias (Figure 3.5). This testing is further complicated by the

Figure 3.5 The *VWF* gene with an indication of the region of the gene (exons 23–34) that is duplicated on chromosome 22 in a partial *VWF* pseudogene.

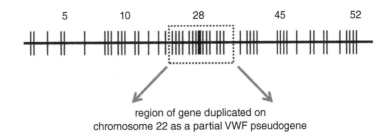

region of gene duplicated on
chromosome 22 as a partial VWF pseudogene

VWF Gene: 178 kb - Chromosome 12 p

presence, on chromosome 22, of a partial pseudogene sequence that replicates exons 23–34 of the chromosome 12 gene with 3% sequence variation [13,14]. Thus, any analysis of this region of the *VWF* gene must ensure that PCR primers and probes are designed for the chromosome 12 sequence. The final major challenge in testing for and interpreting VWF genetic data is the highly polymorphic nature of this gene. The most recent *VWF* mutation database (www.vwf. group.shef.ac.uk) lists 181 polymorphic variants [15], and recent experience indicates that assigning pathogenicity to *VWF* variants, perhaps especially in different ethnic populations, will often be difficult.

Type 3 von Willebrand Disease

Although this disorder is rare (prevalence of ~1 per million population), molecular studies of families with type 3 VWD represent one instance in which molecular diagnostics for VWD can be highly beneficial, as parents with children diagnosed with type 3 VWD may choose prenatal testing in future pregnancies. Given the recessive nature of this condition (at least in the majority of families), the disease incidence is significantly higher in countries in which consanguineous marriages are more frequent.

Highly informative repeat sequence polymorphisms are available for linkage analysis, both within the VWF gene (intron 40) and in the 5′ flanking region of the gene. As with the hemophilias, an Internet-accessible mutation database is also maintained for VWD [15].

A review of this database and the current literature indicates that type 3 VWD can result from a variety of VWF gene mutations, all of which have the consequence of an absence of VWF protein in the plasma. The first group of type 3 mutations to be characterized were complete or partial deletions of the *VWF* gene. Type 3 VWD patients with *VWF* deletion mutations may develop anti-VWF antibodies on exposure to VWF replacement therapy, with the development of anaphylaxis in some patients. Thus, the screening of type 3 VWD patients for complete or partial *VWF* gene deletions with a strategy such as multiplex ligation-dependent probe amplification might be helpful, both for mutation detection and also to evaluate the risk of anti-VWF antibody development. More extensive analysis of type 3 VWD patients has shown that some of these patients synthesize a mutant VWF protein that is presumably grossly misfolded and never leaves the cell of synthesis [16,17]. Many of these missense mutants involve either the loss or gain of cysteine codons, and thus, disruption of dimer and/or multimer assembly is likely.

Type 2 von Willebrand Disease

Type 2 variants of VWD comprise 25–35% of the total VWD patients in most surveys. Although initial investigation of these cases should rely on the use of standard coagulation tests to evaluate the VWF–factor VIII complex, molecular genetic analysis can be used to confirm or refute first diagnostic impressions (Figure 3.6). Type

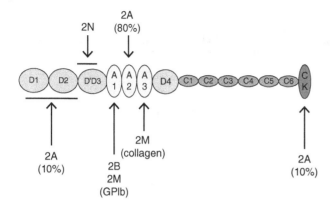

Figure 3.6 Diagram of the VWF protein (propolypeptide and mature subunit) with localization of the molecular defects responsible for type 2 von Willebrand disease (VWD).

2A, 2B, and 2M VWD are transmitted as dominant traits with high penetrance, whereas type 2N disease is recessive in nature.

Type 2A von Willebrand Disease

Type 2A VWD involves loss of high-molecular-weight (HMW) VWF multimers and a resultant decrease in platelet-mediated VWF function.

Two molecular mechanisms have been described for type 2A disease:

1) In group 1, HMW multimers are synthesized ineffectively by the cell.
2) In group 2, HMW multimers secreted into the plasma are more susceptible to proteolysis by ADAMTS13.

Both forms of the disorder are the result of heterozygous missense mutations affecting regions of the VWF protein involved in dimer and multimer formation. Thus, to date, most type 2A VWD mutations have been documented in the VWF propeptide, the A2, and C-terminal domains of the protein. Examination of VWF multimer patterns can, in some instances, predict where the mutations will be found.

In general, molecular diagnostic testing for type 2A VWD should be reserved for those cases in which phenotypic analysis, and particularly VWF:RCo VWF multimer profiles and ristocin-induced platelet agglutination results, are equivocal. No therapeutic benefit is derived from acquiring a molecular genetic diagnosis of type 2A disease.

Type 2B von Willebrand Disease

Type 2B VWD involves dominant gain-of-function changes, enhancing the affinity of mutant VWF for its platelet receptor, glycoprotein (Gp) Ib. These missense mutations are consistently clustered in the region of the gene encoding the A1 protein domain.

Direct sequencing of exon 28 sequences can provide molecular genetic confirmation of the type 2B phenotype. This region of the VWF gene is duplicated, with sequence variation, in the partial pseudogene on chromosome 22, and thus choice of amplification primers should take this fact into consideration. Ninety percent of type 2B VWD cases are caused by the missense mutations R1308C, R1306C, V1316M, and R1341Q.

Given the localized nature of type 2B mutations, molecular genetic confirmation of the phenotypic diagnosis is easily achieved through examination of exon 28 PCR products.

Type 2B VWD demonstrates hemostatic test results that are very similar to those seen in the dominantly inherited platelet disorder, platelet-type VWD. Molecular genetic analysis offers a definitive approach to differentiating between these two conditions (see below).

Type 2M von Willebrand Disease

Type 2M VWD variants exhibit either reduced VWF binding to platelets (GPIb) or reduced binding to collagen. In both instances, a normal VWF multimer profile is present. Here again, as with type 2B disease, the molecular pathology represents a variety of missense mutations localized to the regions of the *VWF* gene encoding the A1 (platelet and/or collagen binding) and A3 (collagen binding) domains of the protein. The platelet binding variant of type 2M disease is essentially the loss-of-function equivalent of type 2B VWD, with the A1 domain missense substitutions resulting in disruption of the interaction with platelet GPIb. As with type 2B disease, genetic confirmation of the type 2M phenotype can be achieved through exon 28 sequencing.

There is a growing appreciation of type 2M collagen binding mutants affecting residues in the VWF A3 and, to a lesser extent, A1 domains. In these cases, the only phenotypic abnormality may be reduced collagen binding and thus diagnostic confirmation through a focused sequencing strategy might prove useful to confirm the phenotypic analysis.

Type 2N von Willebrand Disease

Type 2N VWD is a recessively inherited trait. This condition should be considered in the differential diagnosis of mild–moderate isolated factor VIII deficiency and can easily be confused with mild hemophilia A. Phenotypic testing involves a direct assessment of the factor VIII binding potential of VWF using a microtiter plate-based assay. The most efficient molecular genetic approach to confirm a diagnosis of type 2N disease is to sequence the PCR products amplified from exons 18–25 of the VWF gene, the region encoding the N-terminal D′/D3 factor VIII binding domains of VWF. In patients with type 2N VWD, this analysis will show either homozygous or compound heterozygous missense mutations affecting the factor VIII binding domain of the protein. In addition, coinheritance of a type 2N allele with a severe type 1 or type 3 null allele will also result in this phenotype. The R854Q missense mutation is the most frequent type 2N variant, resulting in factor VIII levels around 20%. Levels of factor VIII of 5–10% are seen with some of the other mutations, such as R816W and T791M.

Type 1 von Willebrand Disease

Despite being the most prevalent form of the disorder, representing 65–75% of all VWD cases, the molecular pathogenesis of type 1 VWD remains the least well understood. Phenotypic diagnosis can often be difficult and is influenced by a variety of factors, including the temporal variability of VWF levels and the ABO blood group of patients, accounting for approximately 30% of the variability in VWF levels, with blood group O subjects having the lowest levels. Another significant complicating factor in attempting to address the genetic basis for type 1 VWD is the marked variability in penetrance and expression of the phenotype within families, which makes the use of classic linkage analysis problematic.

There is now information available from several large population-based studies of the molecular genetic pathology of type 1 VWD [18–20]. The findings from these studies have been similar and demonstrate the following:

- The type 1 VWD phenotype is linked to the *VWF* gene in approximately 60% of families.
- Candidate *VWF* gene mutations can be found in approximately 65% of type 1 VWD patients.
- More than 100 different candidate *VWF* gene mutations have been identified.
- Approximately 65% of the candidate *VWF* mutations are missense substitutions.
- Candidate *VWF* gene mutations are found through out the *VWF* locus from the 5′ flanking region to the C-terminal domain of the protein.
- In approximately 15% of patients, more than a single candidate *VWF* mutation is present.

An analysis of the mutations found in the three population studies has also shown that certain candidate mutations are recurrent. This group of mutations includes Y1584C (found in between 8% and 25% of the type 1 VWD population), R924Q, R1205H, R1315C, R1374H, and R854Q. Suffice it to say that, even with these common variants, the understanding of pathogenic mechanisms is incomplete. Another study of genetic variation at the *VWF* locus has indicated that the assignment of pathogenicity to missense changes is further complicated by the extent of polymorphism exhibited by different ethnic groups [21].

The information derived from these initial molecular surveys of type 1 VWD indicate that, in addition to incomplete penetrance and variable expressivity, the genetics of this complex trait is further complicated by allelic and locus heterogeneity. Whereas most type 1 cases with plasma VWF levels <30% will demonstrate candidate VWF mutations, patients with mild VWF deficiency (30–50%) are more likely to have a phenotype in which contributions from several loci (including the ABO blood group locus) are playing an important pathogenic role. The identity of these additional genetic modifiers is currently under investigation.

Given the size and complexity of the VWF gene and the problems of allelic and locus heterogeneity, the application of molecular genetic analysis to the diagnosis of type 1 VWD is not warranted in the majority of cases. Nevertheless, there may be occasional instances where this approach may provide additional useful information, and this situation may change with further advances in technology and the potential identification of key genetic modifiers of VWF levels.

Less Common Inherited Coagulation Factor Deficiencies

As the genes for all of the procoagulant proteins have been cloned and characterized, molecular genetic testing is feasible for the inherited deficiency of any of these factors. However, the diagnosis of these disorders (factor XI and X deficiencies and others) remains firmly based in the clinical hemostasis laboratory through the performance of biological clotting assays. Nevertheless, with advances in next generation sequencing technologies, the potential application of genetic strategies to the diagnosis of rare inherited bleeding disorders is now under consideration in some laboratories [22].

Although specific research laboratories may be interested in determining the disease-causing mutations in these families, primarily as a means to assist in structure and function analysis, the performance of these tests for diagnostic purposes is not usual. An exception is the documentation of mutations in the *LMAN1* and *MCFD2* genes in patients with inherited combined factor V and VIII deficiencies. Most cases of this rare disorder are caused by one of several recurring point mutations in these intermediate compartment processing proteins; thus, documentation of one of these mutations would definitively establish an otherwise unusual diagnosis.

Inherited Platelet Disorders

As with the less common coagulation factor deficiencies, the diagnosis of inherited platelet disorders is predominantly by phenotypic analysis. Standard morphology, platelet aggregation studies, and an evaluation of platelet receptor density will usually establish or exclude a diagnosis of Bernard–Soulier syndrome or Glanzmann thrombasthenia, the two most frequently encountered, but nevertheless rare, recessive inherited platelet disorders [23].

In unusual instances, knowledge of the causative mutation in these patients could be useful, perhaps for prenatal testing. In the Bernard–Soulier syndrome, a heterogeneous mutational pattern has been documented, with both homozygous and compound heterozygous mutations identified in the genes encoding GPIbα, GPIbβ, and GPIX. A variety of different mutations have been found at these loci, including deletions, frameshifts, and nonsense and missense changes. To date, no Bernard–Soulier mutations have been identified in the *GPV* gene.

In Glanzmann thrombasthenia, a similarly varied pattern of mutations has been documented in the genes for GPIIb and GPIIIa.

As alluded to above, the standard coagulation studies in platelet-type VWD (PT-VWD) are very similar to those encountered in patients with type 2B VWD. Here, clarification of the diagnosis most effectively involves molecular genetic analysis of exon 28 of the VWF gene (for type 2B VWD) and the GPIbα gene (for PT-VWD) [24]. In PT-VWD, heterozygous dominant missense mutations can be found in the GPIbα gene, which have been shown through the analysis of recombinant mutant protein to possess an increased binding affinity for the A1 domain of VWF. One partial deletion mutation in GPIbα has also been identified as being causative for PT-VWD.

Molecular Diagnostics for Thrombotic Disease

Although an inherited tendency for excessive bleeding can often be ascribed to single gene abnormalities, there is ample evidence to suggest that, in contrast, the clinical manifestations of hypercoagulability are usually the result of adverse interactions between multiple genes and the environment [25]. Thus, the use of molecular diagnostics to document markers of thrombotic risk (thrombophilia) will prove to be far more challenging than with the inherited hemorrhagic disorders. To further complicate matters, despite the fact that with appropriate testing, thrombophilic mutations can be identified in approximately 50% of patients following a first clinical episode of venous thromboembolism, interpretation of these results remains problematic in some cases.

After an initial wave of enthusiasm to use molecular testing for the identification of thrombophilic traits, more recent analysis has tended to be far more conservative with the application of this diagnostic approach. In particular, the presence of a strong family history of thrombotic disease is probably, on its own, a significant predictor of risk, and likely represents the combined influences of known and currently unresolved genetic factors responsible for this phenotype.

Inherited Resistance to Activated Protein C: Factor V Leiden

Until 1994, the investigation of patients with clinical evidence of hypercoagulability was usually unproductive. However, with the discovery by Dahlback and Hildebrand of an inherited form of resistance to the proteolytic effects of activated protein C [26], and the subsequent finding of a common missense mutation in the factor V gene by Bertina and colleagues in Leiden [27], a major advance was made in the laboratory assessment of thrombotic risk.

The factor V Leiden mutation substitutes a glutamine for an arginine at amino acid residue 506 in factor V, the initial cleavage site for activated protein C. The mutation is readily detected by a number of PCR-based approaches. Between 2% and 5% of individuals in Western populations have been documented to be heterozygous for factor V Leiden. In contrast, the mutation is extremely rare in subjects of Asian and African descent.

In some laboratories, initial screening for resistance to activated protein C is performed using the prolongation of an activated partial thromboplastin time-based assay as an indicator; patients testing positive (prolongation in the presence of factor V-deficient plasma) are subsequently evaluated by a PCR assay (Figure 3.7).

Increasingly, where access to PCR-based molecular analysis is routine, laboratories will more often choose to proceed directly to the genetic test, as the result is definitive and more than 95% of activated protein C resistance is a result of this single mutation. Rare, alternative factor V mutations have been documented at arginine 306 (Arg to Thr and Arg to Gly), but it seems unlikely that these variants are significant markers of a thrombotic risk.

Persons heterozygous for the factor V Leiden mutation have an approximately fivefold increased relative risk of venous thrombosis. It is found in 15–20% of patients experiencing their first episode of venous thrombosis and in 50–60% of thrombosis patients with a family history of thrombotic disease. The hypercoagulable phenotype associated with factor V Leiden shows incomplete penetrance, and some individuals carrying the Leiden allele may never manifest a clinical thrombotic event. In contrast to the increased relative risk for an initial venous thrombotic event associated

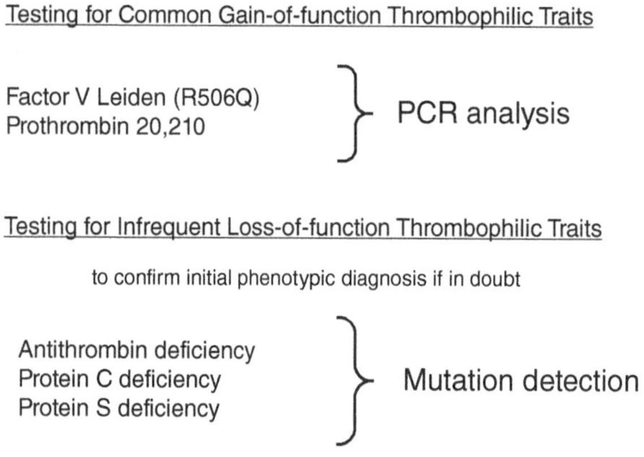

<u>Testing for Common Gain-of-function Thrombophilic Traits</u>

Factor V Leiden (R506Q)
Prothrombin 20,210 ⎱ PCR analysis

<u>Testing for Infrequent Loss-of-function Thrombophilic Traits</u>

to confirm initial phenotypic diagnosis if in doubt

Antithrombin deficiency
Protein C deficiency ⎱ Mutation detection
Protein S deficiency

Figure 3.7 Molecular genetic testing approaches for thrombophilic traits.

with factor V Leiden, this genetic variant is not associated with increased risks for either arterial thrombosis or a recurrence of venous thrombosis. Coinheritance of other inherited thrombotic risk factors or exposure to environmental risk factors (i.e., oral contraceptives) can dramatically enhance the thrombotic risk in carriers of factor V Leiden. Many clinicians test for this disorder in patients with a family history of thrombosis who are about to be exposed to an acquired thrombotic risk factor but, as discussed above, opinions vary about the benefits of this testing approach. Individuals homozygous for the mutation have a 70-fold enhanced relative risk of venous thrombosis, indicating that this phenotype is transmitted as a codominant trait.

Prothrombin 20210 3′ Noncoding Sequence Variant

In 1996, Poort and colleagues described an association between a G to A nucleotide polymorphism at position 20210 in the 3′ untranslated region (UTR) of the prothrombin gene, increased plasma levels of prothrombin, and an enhanced risk for venous thrombosis [28]. This polymorphic nucleotide substitution is at the very end of the 3′ UTR of the prothrombin gene and exerts its effect on prothrombin levels in the heterozygous state. Although the plasma

levels of prothrombin in subjects heterozygous for this polymorphism are higher on average than those in individuals with a normal prothrombin genotype, levels are usually still within the normal range. As a consequence, this polymorphism can only be evaluated by genetic testing, which is achieved by a PCR-based assay, most often involving a form of real-time quantitative assay.

As with the factor V Leiden genotype, the prevalence of the prothrombin 20210 G to A variant in the general population is relatively high at 1–5%. This variant is also rare in persons of Asian and African descent. The heterozygous state is associated with a twofold to fourfold increase in the relative risk for venous thrombosis. There is no influence on venous thrombotic recurrence or arterial thrombosis.

Thermolabile C677T 5,10-Methylene-Tetrahydrofolate Reductase Variant

The third, high-prevalence genetic variant that was initially thought to be associated with an increased thrombotic risk is the C to T variant at nucleotide 677 (an alanine to valine substitution) in the 5,10-methylene-tetrahydrofolate reductase (MTHFR) gene. This genotype results in expression of an enzyme with increased thermolability. Homozygosity for the variant is associated with hyperhomocysteinemia, particularly in the presence of folate deficiency. In many populations (southern Europeans and Hispanic Americans), approximately 10% of subjects are homozygous for the C677T variant, a sequence change that can easily be detected by a PCR-based strategy. After further extended analysis, in contrast to the factor V Leiden and prothrombin 20210 variants, the role of the MTHFR C677T polymorphism as an independent risk factor for venous thromboembolism appears negligible and diagnostic testing for the MTHFR variant is not recommended.

Deficiencies of Antithrombin, Protein C, and Protein S

Deficiencies of the major anticoagulant proteins antithrombin, protein C, and protein S have long been known to represent individual risk factors for the development of venous thromboembolism. The protein deficiencies manifest thrombotic phenotypes in the heterozygous state, but penetrance and expression of the phenotype are extremely variable and relate to both the individual protein deficiency (antithrombin deficiency being the most severe condition) and the specific molecular defect, with all three diseases exhibiting significant allelic heterogeneity. Homozygosity for antithrombin and protein C deficiencies results in the severe neonatal thrombotic condition, purpura fulminans.

Diagnosis of these three disorders relies on standard functional tests or immunoassays that should be performed in the diagnostic hemostasis laboratory. All three of the deficiency states are associated with significant allelic heterogeneity, and routine molecular diagnostic investigation of these mutations is not warranted. However, these are lifelong diagnoses, and if any doubt exists about the phenotypic test results, confirmation of the diagnosis by genetic testing should be considered (Figure 3.7).

The Role of Genetic Testing in the Clinical Management of Oral Anticoagulation

Studies in the past several years have indicated that individual anticoagulant responses to the vitamin K antagonist, Coumadin (warfarin), can be predicted to some extent through the analysis of genotypes for two proteins involved in the metabolism of this drug: cytochrome P-450 2C9 (CYP2C9) and vitamin K epoxide-reductase complex 1 (VKORC1). Analysis of polymorphic haplotypes of the *CYP2C9* and *VKORC1* genes by PCR testing has been shown to be helpful in identifying patients who may be especially sensitive to oral anticoagulant administration [29]. This appears to be particularly the case for *VKORC1* analysis during the initiation phase of oral anticoagulation. Nevertheless, despite an initial endorsement of genetic testing for this purpose by the US Food and Drug Administration, recent studies have failed to confirm the utility of this approach and it is very unlikely that widespread adoption of this strategy will occur [30].

The Future for Diagnostic Molecular Hemostasis

With the completion of the Human Genome Project and the ongoing analysis of complex genetic traits through the performance of genome-wide association studies, additional information pertaining to genetic influences on hemostasis is likely to be derived in the next few years. This fact, along with further advances in genetic methodologies, including more accessible microarray-based testing approaches and next generation sequencing, may well provide further opportunities for the application of molecular diagnostic testing in the area of clinical hemostasis [22]. However, as has already been witnessed with thrombophilia genetic testing and the incorporation of genetic analysis as an adjunct to oral anticoagulant control, initial enthusiasm for test adoption will need to be tempered by formal evidence of clinical benefit deriving from the tests. Indeed, there is a significant possibility that the major genetic influences on most hemostatic phenotypes have already been identified and that any new associations are much less likely to play a clinically important role. An area where this possibility may well be tested in the next decade is that of genetic risk factors for arterial thrombosis. To date, very little benefit can be derived from genetic testing for this phenotype, and it may well be that the combined genetic and environmental background of this condition will be too complex for the useful application of a genetic testing strategy.

References

1 Gitschier J, Wood WI, Goralka TM, *et al*. Characterization of the human factor VIII gene. *Nature* 1984; 312: 326–330.

2 Kurachi K, Davie EW. Isolation and characterization of a cDNA coding for human factor IX. *Proc Natl Acad Sci USA* 1982; 79: 6461–6464.

3 Structural Immunology Group, University College London. *Factor VIII Variant Database*. Available at: www.factorviii-db.org (accessed July 2016).

4 Goodeve AC, Peake IR. The molecular basis of hemophilia A: genotype-phenotype relationships and inhibitor development. *Semin Thromb Hemost* 2003; 29: 23–30.

5 Keeney S, Mitchell M, Goodeve A. The molecular analysis of haemophilia A: a guideline from the UK haemophilia centre doctors' organization haemophilia genetics laboratory network. *Haemophilia* 2005; 11: 387–397.

6 Lakich D, Kazazian HH Jr, Antonarakis SE, *et al*. Inversions disrupting the factor VIII gene are a common cause of severe haemophilia A. *Nat Genet* 1993; 5: 236–241.

7 Bagnall RD, Waseem N, Green PM, *et al*. Recurrent inversion breaking intron 1 of the factor VIII gene is a frequent cause of severe hemophilia A. *Blood* 2002; 99: 168–174.

8 Structural Immunology Group, University College London. *Factor IX Variant Database*. Available at: www.factorix.org (accessed June 2016).

9 Thorland EC, Drost JB, Lusher JM, *et al*. Anaphylactic response to factor IX replacement therapy in haemophilia B patients: complete gene deletions confer the highest risk. *Haemophilia* 1999; 5: 101–105.

10 Oldenburg J, Quenzel EM, Harbrecht U, *et al*. Missense mutations at ALA-10 in the factor IX propeptide: an insignificant variant in normal life but a decisive cause of bleeding during oral anticoagulant therapy. *Br J Haematol* 1997; 98: 240–244.

11 Picketts DJ, Mueller CR, Lillicrap D. Transcriptional control of the factor IX gene: analysis of five cis-acting elements and the deleterious effects of naturally occurring hemophilia B Leyden mutations. *Blood* 1994; 84: 2992–3000.

12 James PD, Stakiw J, Leggo J, *et al*. A case of non-resolving hemophilia B Leyden in a 42-year-old male (F9 promoter + 13 A>G). *J Thromb Haemost* 2008; 6: 885–886.

13 Mancuso DJ, Tuley EA, Westfield LA, *et al*. Structure of the gene for human von Willebrand factor. *J Biol Chem* 1989; 264: 19514–19527.

14 Mancuso DJ, Tuley EA, Westfield LA, *et al*. Human von Willebrand factor gene and pseudogene: structural analysis and differentiation by polymerase chain reaction. *Biochemistry* 1991; 30: 253–269.

15 Hampshire D, International Society on Thrombosis and Haemostasis Scientific and Standardization Committee on von Willebrand factor (ISTH-SSC on VWF). von Willebrand factor Variant Database (VWFdb). Available at: www.vwf.group.shef.ac.uk (accessed June 2016).

16 Baronciani L, Cozzi G, Canciani MT *et al*. Molecular defects in type 3 von Willebrand disease: updated results from 40 multiethnic patients. *Blood Cells Mol Dis* 2003; 30: 264–270.

17 Bowman M, Tuttle A, Notley C, *et al*. The genetics of Canadian type 3 von Willebrand

Disease (VWD): further evidence for co-dominant inheritance of mutant alleles. *J Thromb Haemost* 2013; 11: 512–520.

18 James PD, Notley C, Hegadorn C, *et al*. The mutational spectrum of type 1 von Willebrand disease: Results from a Canadian cohort study. *Blood* 2007; 109: 145–154.

19 Goodeve A, Eikenboom J, Castaman G, *et al*. Phenotype and genotype of a cohort of families historically diagnosed with type 1 von Willebrand disease in the European study, Molecular and clinical markers for the diagnosis and management of type 1 von Willebrand disease (MCMDM-1VWD). *Blood* 2007; 109: 112–121.

20 Cumming A, Grundy P, Keeney S, *et al*. An investigation of the von Willebrand factor genotype in UK patients diagnosed to have type 1 von Willebrand disease. *Thromb Haemost* 2006; 96: 630–641.

21 Bellissimo DB, Christopherson PA, Flood VH, *et al*. Von Willebrand factor mutations and new sequence variations identified in healthy controls are more frequent in the African-American population. *Blood* 2012; 119: 2135–2140.

22 Peyvandi F, Kunicki T, Lillicrap D. Genetic sequence analysis of inherited bleeding diseases. *Blood.* 2013; 122: 3423–3431.

23 Nurden P, Nurden AT. Congenital disorders associated with platelet dysfunctions. *Thromb Haemost* 2008; 99: 253–263.

24 Othman M, Lillicrap D. Distinguishing between non-identical twins: platelet type and type 2B von Willebrand disease. *Br J Haematol* 2007; 138: 665–666.

25 Reitsma PH, Rosendaal FR. Past and future of genetic research in thrombosis. *J Thromb Haemost* 2007; 5 Suppl. 1: 264–269.

26 Dahlback B, Hildebrand B. Inherited resistance to activated protein C is corrected by anticoagulant cofactor activity found to be a property of factor V. *Proc Natl Acad Sci USA* 1994; 91: 1396–1400.

27 Bertina RM, Koeleman BP, Koster T, *et al*. Mutation in blood coagulation factor V associated with resistance to activated protein C. *Nature* 1994; 369: 64–67.

28 Poort SR, Rosendaal FR, Reitsma PH, Bertina RM. A common genetic variation in the 3′-untranslated region of the prothrombin gene is associated with elevated plasma prothrombin levels and an increase in venous thrombosis. *Blood* 1996; 88: 3698–3703.

29 Schwarz UI, Ritchie MD, Bradford Y, *et al*. Genetic determinants of response to warfarin during initial anti-coagulation. *N Engl J Med* 2008; 358: 999–1008.

30 Furie B. Do pharmacogenetics have a role in the dosing of vitamin K antagonists? *Engl J Med* 2013; 369: 2345–2346.

4

Tests of Platelet Function

Marie Lordkipanidzé, Gillian C. Lowe and Paul Harrison

Key Points

- Platelet function tests are used to aid in establishing the diagnosis in patients with a history of excessive bleeding and no abnormalities on initial basic coagulation assays.
- The current gold standard, light transmission aggregometry, allows for investigation of several different platelet activation pathways and is clinically used to diagnose and classify platelet function defects. The diagnostic performance of this assay can be improved by the addition of a real-time luminescent measurement of ATP secretion, as this also detects secretion defects which can be missed when assessing aggregation alone.
- Despite international efforts towards consistency, platelet function testing remains poorly standardized and normal quality control measures are often difficult to implement. In addition, light transmission aggregometry can be time consuming, which limits its use in everyday clinical practice, and restricts testing to specialist centers.
- More in-depth assays, such as electron microscopy and flow cytometry, can also be used to better characterize platelet morphology and function, especially in patients in whom platelet count, size, or granularity appears abnormal on blood films.

Structure of Platelets

Human platelets are small, anucleated cells that circulate in blood and play a critical role in hemostasis and thrombosis. Their lifespan is approximately 10 days [1], and during this time they constantly survey the integrity of the vessel wall. Normal human platelets are small and discoid in shape (0.5 × 3.0 μm), have a mean volume of 7–11 fL, and circulate in relatively high numbers (between 150 and 400 × 10^9/L) [2,3].

A cross-section of a typical discoid platelet is shown in Figure 4.1.

Function

Their small disc shape enables the platelets to be marginated toward the edge of vessels so that the majority circulate adjacent to the vascular endothelial cells that line all blood vessels [5]. Upon detection of vessel wall damage, they undergo rapid and controlled adhesion, activation, and aggregation to form a hemostatic plug and thus rapidly prevent blood loss [2,3]. They also provide a phospholipid surface for initiation of the coagulation cascade [6,7].

Endothelial cells produce a number of potent antiplatelet substances (e.g., nitric oxide, prostacyclin, and CD39) that normally inhibit vessel

Practical Hemostasis and Thrombosis, Third Edition. Edited by Nigel S. Key, Michael Makris and David Lillicrap.
© 2017 John Wiley & Sons, Ltd. Published 2017 by John Wiley & Sons, Ltd.

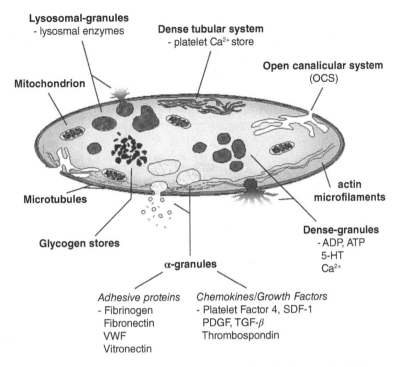

Lysosomal-granules
- lysosmal enzymes

Dense tubular system
- platelet Ca²⁺ store

Open canalicular system
(OCS)

Mitochondrion

Microtubules

actin microfilaments

Glycogen stores

Dense-granules
- ADP, ATP
  5-HT
  Ca²⁺

α-granules

Adhesive proteins
- Fibrinogen
  Fibronectin
  VWF
  Vitronectin

Chemokines/Growth Factors
- Platelet Factor 4, SDF-1
  PDGF, TGF-β
  Thrombospondin

Figure 4.1 Platelet structure and organelles. This diagram summarizes the key structural elements of a platelet, including the open canalicular system (OCS), the dense tubular system, action microfilaments and microtubules, mitochondria, glycogen stores, dense granules, lysosomes, and alpha granules. ADP, adenosine diphosphate; ATP, adenosine triphosphate; PDGF, platelet derived growth factor; SDF, stromal cell derived factor; TGF, transforming growth factor; VWF, von Willebrand factor. *Source:* Watson, 2005 [4]. Reproduced with permission of Wiley-Blackwell.

wall–platelet interactions [8–10]. Vessel wall damage exposes highly adhesive substrates (e.g., P selectin, von Willebrand factor (VWF), collagen, and many other extracellular matrix components), which overcome these inhibitory factors and result in a sequence of stepwise events resulting in the formation of a hemostatic plug (Figure 4.2) [12,13]:

- initial adhesion, transient rolling of platelets along the vessel wall, and slowing of the cells; consequently, platelets are more likely to undergo stable adhesion;
- stable adhesion through additional receptor–ligand interactions;
- platelet activation (if there is more extensive damage or stimuli-promoting platelet activation);
- platelet aggregation;

- generation of platelet procoagulant activity and stabilization of the hemostatic plug via interaction with coagulation factors;
- clot retraction.

The platelets interact with and sense the environment through many types of surface receptors (major receptors and their ligands are summarized in Table 4.1) [13]. The net balance between activating or inhibitory stimuli thus controls whether platelets continue to circulate, begin to reversibly interact with the vessel wall, or become irreversibly adherent to either the vessel wall or each other [2,3].

During adhesion, platelets become activated through signal transduction pathways, which mediate shape change, degranulation, and spreading upon areas of exposed subendothelium [12]. Activated platelets recruit additional

(a) Normal state   **(b) Activation and recruitment**   **(c) Aggregation and clot formation**

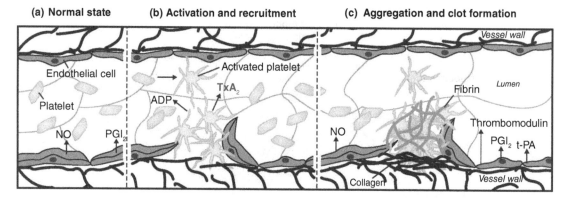

Figure 4.2 Platelet adhesion, activation, and aggregation. (a) Normal endothelium releases antiaggregant molecules promoting hemostasis and nonthrombogenic state. (b) Injured endothelium exposes platelets to thrombogenic subendothelium. Activated platelets release proaggregant molecules. (c) Clot formation at site of injury. Endothelium releases factors that stabilize the clot and limit the haemostatic process to the site of injury. ADP, adenosine diphosphate; NO, nitric oxide; PGI$_2$, prostacyclin; t-PA, tissue plasminogen activator; TxA$_2$, thromboxane A$_2$. *Source:* Lordkipanidzé, 2006 [11]. Reproduced with permission of Elsevier. *See Plate section for color representation of this figure.*

platelets into the growing platelet aggregate or thrombus via a number of positive feedback pathways, including release of dense granular adenosine diphosphate (ADP) and generation of thromboxane [12]. Activated platelets also express negatively charged phospholipids on their surface and release microvesicles, facilitating the local generation of high amounts of thrombin, which not only further activates other platelets, but also stabilizes the platelet plug through fibrin formation via the coagulation cascade [6,7]. In this manner, platelets rapidly seal any areas of vessel wall damage and provide a catalytic surface for coagulation to occur, resulting in the formation of a stable hemostatic plug.

Arterial thrombosis is usually the consequence of inappropriate activation of platelets, especially in regions of abnormal vessel wall lesions or damage (e.g., atherosclerotic plaques) [14]. The high shear stress that often occurs in these regions also significantly contributes to thrombus formation (via promotion of VWF-dependent platelet adhesion and aggregation) along with the events described above.

Antiplatelet drug therapy thus provides an important means to prevent thrombosis in high-risk patients with atherosclerotic disease.

In contrast, there are also many defects in platelet function that can occur in patients, often resulting in an increased risk of bleeding.

Classification of Platelet Defects

Platelet abnormalities can be broadly classified into quantitative (abnormal in number) and qualitative defects (abnormal in function), although in some patients both conditions can coexist [15–17]. Defects in number include many types of thrombocytopenia (e.g., inherited thrombocytopenia resulting in reduced platelet formation or acquired through immune or nonimmune destruction of platelets) and thrombocytosis (increased platelet number, which is mostly acquired and can be secondary to infection, inflammation or iron deficiency, or a result of an acquired bone marrow genetic change leading to myeloproliferative disease, such as JAK2V617F) [15–17]. Defects in platelet function can either be inherited, but more commonly they are acquired (secondary to comorbid disease, such as renal impairment, and medications, such as antiplatelet therapy) [15–17].

Table 4.1 Major platelet agonists and their surface receptors. Platelets express a remarkable number and variety of receptors for a wide range of ligands. For many of these receptor–ligand combinations, however, the effect on platelet activation is weak and of uncertain significance.

Agonist	Receptor	Effect and physiological role
Adhesion molecules		
Collagen	GP VI	Major signaling receptor for collagen
	$\alpha_2\beta_1$	Supports adhesion by collagen
Fibrinogen	$\alpha_{IIb}\beta_3$	Aggregation, spreading and clot retraction
Fibronectin	$\alpha_5\beta_1$, $\alpha_{IIb}\beta_3$	Adhesion through $\alpha_5\beta_1$
Laminin	$\alpha_6\beta_1$	Adhesion
von Willebrand factor	GP Ib-IX-V, $\alpha_{IIb}\beta_3$	Platelet tethering (also fibrinogen)
Amines		
Adrenaline	α_2	Positive feedback agonist
5-HT	5-HT_{2A}	Mediates vasoconstriction, positive feedback agonist
Cytokines		
TPO	c-Mpl	Maturation of megakaryocytes, control of platelet number in circulation
Immune complexes		
Fc portion of antibodies	FcγRIIA	Immune- and bacteria-induced platelet activation
Lipids		
PAF	PAF	Positive feedback agonist
Prostacyclin (PGI_2)	IP	Inhibition of platelet activation
Thromboxanes	TP	Major positive feedback agonist
Prostaglandin E_2 (PGE_2)	EP_3	Inhibition of platelet activation
Nucleotides		
Adenosine	A_{2a}	Inhibition of platelet activation
ADP	$P2Y_1$	Early role in platelet activation
	$P2Y_{12}$	Major positive feedback receptor
ATP	$P2X_1$	Possible early role in platelet activation
Proteases		
Thrombin	PAR_1, PAR_4	Coagulation-dependent platelet activation
Surface molecules		
CD40 ligand	CD40 and $\alpha_{IIb}\beta_3$	Interaction with other blood cells, role in immune response and inflammation
P-selectin glycoprotein ligand 1 (PSGL-1)	P-selectin	Interaction with other blood cells
Tyrosine kinase receptors		
Podoplanin / possible other unknown ligand	CLEC-2	Role in fetal vascular development. Possible role in platelet activation in atherosclerosis and cancer progression?
EphrinB1	EphA4 and EphB1	Late events in platelet activation?

(Continued)

Table 4.1 (Continued)

Agonist	Receptor	Effect and physiological role
Vitamin K-dependent		
Gas6	Sky, Axl, and Mer	Supports platelet activation?

Source: Watson 2004 [4]. Reproduced with permission of Wiley-Blackwell.
5-HT, 5-hydroxytryptamine; ADP, adenosine diphosphate; ATP, adenosine triphosphate; PAF, platelet activating factor; TPO, thrombopoietin.

Inherited platelet disorders include many abnormalities, such as the following:

- defects in various platelet receptors for both adhesive proteins and soluble agonists;
- defects in the storage or release of platelet granules;
- defects in signal transduction pathways;
- defects in exposure of negatively charged phospholipid; or
- inherited thrombocytopenias.

Table 4.2 summarizes the classification of inherited platelet function defects.

Platelet Function Testing

Before platelet function tests are performed, the full clinical history (including family and recent medication history) is obtained and a physical examination of the patient is performed [15–17]. Platelet disorders are usually associated with excessive bruising and bleeding (especially after trauma, surgical and dental procedures, or childbirth), and other features including petechiae, epistaxis, and menorrhagia [15–18]. Coagulation protein defects, in contrast, are traditionally associated with a delayed pattern of bleeding and the presence of hemarthroses and hematomas. In practice, significant overlap exists between the clinical presentation of various categories of bleeding disorders. Several bleeding assessment tools are now used to formally record bleeding and to help standardize history taking, although at present these are mostly research tools and are rarely used in clinical practice [19–22].

As many patients present with a transiently acquired defect of platelet function (e.g., often caused by medications including over-the-counter nonsteroidal anti-inflammatory drugs), repeat testing is often necessary to ensure correct results and diagnosis [23]. If a hemostatic defect is suspected, then laboratories may use a range of testing methods, starting with simple laboratory assays and proceeding to more definitive platelet function testing [24]. These tests include:

- full blood count and blood film;
- coagulation tests (prothrombin time (PT), activated partial thromboplastin time (APTT), thrombin time (TT) and fibrinogen assays, most commonly Clauss fibrinogen assays);
- von Willebrand factor antigen (VWF:Ag) levels and activity (VWF:RCo), and factor VIII:C measurement;
- light transmission platelet aggregation (still considered the gold standard although time consuming); some laboratories use whole blood impedance aggregometry as an alternative;
- measurement of dense granule platelet secretion – can be done by simultaneous measurement with addition of luciferin–luciferase reagent during light transmission aggregation. This method requires use of an aggregometer that can also detect luminescence (chemiluminometer), which is not always available. Alternatives include platelet nucleotide release assays (ATP:ADP ratio), electron microscopy, high-performance liquid chromatography, and the radioactive serotonin release assay.

Table 4.2 Brief reference guide on inherited platelet disorders.

Platelet abnormality	Disease	Inheritance	Defective gene	Laboratory and other findings
Platelet adhesion	Platelet type von Willebrand disease	Autosomal dominant	*GP1BA* (17p13.2)	Thrombocytopenia Diminished or absent large VWF multimers Enhanced ristocetin agglutination (occurs at low concentrations), which corrects when donor platelets and patient plasma are used in mixing studies
	Bernard–Soulier syndrome	Autosomal recessive	*GP9* (3q21.3) *GP1BA* (17p13.2) *GP1BB* (22q11.21)	Thrombocytopenia with increased MPV Anomalies in components of the GPIb-V-IX complex Platelet aggregation: absent ristocetin-induced agglutination
Platelet receptor defects	P2Y$_{12}$ ADP receptor	Autosomal recessive (mild phenotype in heterozygote)	*P2Y12* (3q25.1)	Platelet count normal Platelet aggregation: normal P2Y$_1$ receptor-driven responses: shape change and transient aggregation
	GPVI collagen receptor	Autosomal recessive	*GP6* (19q13.42)	Platelet count normal Platelet aggregation: absent to GPVI-specific agonists, e.g., convluxin and collagen-related peptide; and marked reduction to collagen
	Thromboxane A$_2$ receptor	Autosomal recessive (mild phenotype in heterozygote)	*TBXA2R* (19p13.3)	Platelet count normal Platelet aggregation reduced in heterozygotes to arachidonic acid and U44619 and presumed absent in homozygotes
	GPIIbIIIa (αIIbβ3) (Glanzmann thrombasthenia)	Autosomal recessive	*ITGA2B* (17q21.32) *ITGB3* (17q21.32)	Normal platelet count, size, and morphology Presents with severe bleeding symptoms in early life Absent platelet aggregation with all agonists; agglutination to ristocetin is normal Flow cytometry with CD41 and CD61 antibodies may shows reduced levels of either GPIIb or GPIIIa
Platelet secretion	Hermansky–Pudlak syndrome	Autosomal recessive	*HPS1* (10q24.2), *HPS2/AP3B1* (5q14.1), *HPS3* (3q24), *HPS4* (22q12.1), *HPS5* (11p14), *HPS6* (10q24.32), *HPS7/dysbindin* (6p22.3), *HPS8* (19q13.32), *HPS9* (15q21.1)	Platelet count normal Skin and hair hypopigmentation Reduced/ absent δ-granules on electron microscopy Lumiaggregometry: reduced/ absent ATP release

(Continued)

Table 4.2 (Continued)

Platelet abnormality	Disease	Inheritance	Defective gene	Laboratory and other findings
	Chediak–Higashi syndrome	Autosomal recessive	CHS1/LYST (1q42)	Platelet count normal Skin and hair hypopigmentation Immunodeficiency Giant inclusions in granulocytes and their precursors Reduced or irregular α-granules
	Gray platelet syndrome	Autosomal recessive	NBEAL2 (3p21.31)	Thrombocytopenia Increased MPV with platelet anisocytosis Platelets gray in color on blood film Absent α-granules
	X-linked dyserythropoietic anemia and thrombocytopenia	X-linked	GATA1 (Xp11.23)	Thrombocytopenia with increased MPV Reduced α-granules Anemia
	Arthrogryposis, renal dysfunction and cholestasis (ARC) syndrome	Autosomal recessive	VPS33B (15q26.1) VIPAS39 (14q24.3)	Thrombocytopenia with increased MPV Severe multisystem syndrome, leading to fatal complications very early in life Absent α-granules
	Paris–Trousseau/ Jacobsen syndrome	Autosomal dominant	FLI1 (11q24.1–24.3)	Thrombocytopenia with increased MPV Developmental delay and facial abnormalities
	Quebec platelet disorder	Autosomal dominant	PLAU (10q22.2)	Platelet count at low end of normal range α granule protein degradation Increased urokinase-type plasminogen activator storage in platelets
Platelet cytoskeleton	MYH9-related disorders (May–Hegglin anomaly, also known as Sebastian–Fechtner–Epstein syndrome)	Autosomal dominant	MYH9 (22q12-13)	Thrombocytopenia with increased MPV Döhle-like inclusions in neutrophils Nephritis and hearing loss in some forms

Disorder	Gene	Inheritance	Features
Wiskott–Aldrich syndrome (WAS) / X-linked thrombocytopenia	WAS (Xp11.23)	X-linked	Thrombocytopenia with small platelets; Immune deficiency and eczema (in WAS)
Filamin A disorders (periventricular nodular heretotopia/ otopalatodigital syndrome)	FLNa (Xq28)	X-linked	Thrombocytopenia with raised MPV and abnormal platelet morphology; Abnormal distribution of platelet filamin on confocal microscopy
Actin disorders	ACTN1 (14q24.1)	Autosomal dominant	Thrombocytopenia with raised MCV and platelet anisocytosis; Patients either have moderate bleeding tendency or may be asymptomatic
Platelet procoagulant activity: Scott syndrome	TMEM16F (12q12–13.11)	Autosomal recessive	Platelet count normal; Anomalies in flippases translocating negatively charged phospholipids on the plasma membranes; Impaired annexin A5 binding with flow cytometry
Other thrombocytopenias: Congenital amegakaryocytic thrombocytopenia (CAMT)	MPL (1p34)	Autosomal recessive	Severe thrombocytopenia; Pancytopenia; Absent megakaryocytes in bone marrow; Increased plasma thrombopoietin levels
Thrombocytopenia with absent radius (TAR) syndrome	RBM8A (1q21.1)	Autosomal recessive	Severe thrombocytopenia; Normal platelet morphology; Shortened/ absent radii in forearm
THC2	MASTL, ACBD5, ANKRD26 (all 10p12.1)	Autosomal dominant	Mild to moderate thrombocytopenia with normal MPV; Platelets deficient in GPIa and α-granules; Platelet aggregation normal; Possible dysmegakaryopoiesis
Familial platelet disorder with predisposition to acute myelogenous leukemia (FPD/ AML)	RUNX1 (21q22.12)	Autosomal dominant	Mild thrombocytopenia, with possible raised MPV; Abnormal aggregation to multiple agonists

Source: Watson 2013 [18] Table 1. Reproduced with permission of Wiley.
ADP, adenosine diphosphate; ATP, adenosine triphosphate; GP, glycoprotein; MCV, mean corpuscular volume; MPV, mean platelet volume; THC2, familial thrombocytopenia 2; VWF, von Willebrand factor.

The biggest challenges still present in the laboratory pertain to quality control issues, including type of anticoagulation used, sample quality, sample handling (collection and processing), and lack of standardization of methodologies used to assess platelet function [23]. Several international guidelines are now available in an effort to improve standardization, although their application in clinical laboratories remains scarce [23,25,26].

Platelets are not only prone to artefactual *in vitro* activation but also to desensitization. Most functional tests have to be performed relatively quickly (e.g., less than 4 hours from sampling) [23,25,26]. It is also impossible to use standard quality control material apart from freshly drawn blood from healthy normal volunteers. Healthy volunteers are known to have a wide variation in their responses, although building up data from large cohorts of local healthy volunteers helps to better define normal ranges of response [27,28].

Global Tests of Platelet Function

Bleeding Time

The skin bleeding time was clinically used for over a century and was modified several times in attempts to improve reliability [23]. Briefly, a constant blood pressure of 40 mmHg was applied to the upper arm and a disposable, sterile, automated template device was applied to apply standardized cuts into the skin. Excess blood was then removed with filter paper at regular intervals, and the time for the cessation of bleeding recorded. Whereas bleeding normally stopped within 10 minutes, prolonged bleeding times were encountered in patients with severe platelet defects, and so the test was widely used as a screening tool [29].

The clear advantages of the bleeding time were that it is a simple test of natural hemostasis, including the important contribution of the vessel wall, and it also avoided potential anticoagulation artefacts [29]. The disadvantages are

that bleeding time results are both poorly reproducible and insensitive to milder forms of platelet dysfunction [29,30].

The consensus is that the test does not necessarily correlate well with the bleeding risk and that an accurate clinical history is more valuable [23]. A number of different *in vitro* methods have therefore been devised to try to measure global platelet function within whole blood exposed to conditions that attempt to simulate *in vivo* hemostasis, such as the PFA-100®. Recent guidelines recommend against the use of the bleeding time in contemporaneous practice [23].

Platelet Function Analyzer: PFA-100® / PFA-200®

The PFA-200 is a modern update of the original PFA-100 device first released in the mid 1990s, based on the prototype instrument developed by Kratzer and Born [31]. Widespread experience with the PFA-100/200 is increasing, but how the test should be used within normal laboratory practice remains to be fully defined.

All test components are within disposable cartridges that are loaded into the instrument at the start of the test. Citrated whole blood is pipetted into the cartridge and, after a short incubation period, exposed to high shear (5000–6000/second) through a capillary tube before encountering a membrane with a central aperture of 150 μm diameter. The membrane is coated with collagen and either ADP or epinephrine [31]. A third cartridge (INNOVANCE P2Y®) was developed to increase sensitivity of the test to inhibition of the $P2Y_{12}$ receptor [32,33]; it contains a smaller aperture of 100 μm and the membrane is coated with a combination of collagen, ADP, and PGE_1 supplemented with calcium. The instrument monitors the drop in flow rate as platelets form a hemostatic plug that seals the aperture and stops blood flow. This parameter is recorded as the closure time (CT). The maximal value obtainable is 300 seconds.

To ensure optimal PFA-100/200 performance and data interpretation, there are a number of quality control procedures and good practice guidelines that need to be kept in mind [34]:

- daily instrument checks;
- ensuring the quality of blood sampling;
- ensuring consistency in anticoagulation, 3.8% (0.129 mol/L) or 3.2% (0.105 mol/L) buffered trisodium citrate [35];
- testing within 4 hours of sampling;
- checking for cartridge batch variation;
- always perform a full blood count to help interpret the results;
- a control group within each laboratory setting should be established. These individuals should ideally exhibit CTs within the middle of the established laboratory reference range;
- each laboratory should also ideally establish their own reference ranges on both cartridges using healthy volunteers from their institution.

Typical normal ranges obtained with 3.8% trisodium citrate are 58–151 seconds for collagen/ADP and 94–202 seconds for collagen/epinephrine. With 3.2% trisodium citrate, typical ranges are 55–112 seconds for collagen/ADP and 79–164 seconds for collagen/epinephrine. The INNOVANCE P2Y® cartridge has an upper cutoff of 106 seconds for both concentrations of citrate.

Within-sample coefficients of variation have been reported as approximately 10%, which, although acceptable for a platelet function test, may obviously cause problems with values obtained close to upper normal-range cut-off values.

A number of studies suggest that the PFA-100/200 is a potential *in vitro* replacement of the bleeding time [31]. The disadvantages are that, like the *in vivo* bleeding time, the test is sensitive to both the platelet count and hematocrit, and it is therefore crucial that a full blood count is performed to help interpret abnormal results [36]. The test is usually insensitive to coagulation protein defects, including afibrinogenemia, hemophilia A and B, and other clotting factors [31]. False-negative results are sometimes obtained; for example, in patients with storage pool disease, primary secretion defects, Hermansky–Pudlak syndrome, type 1 VWD, and the Quebec platelet disorder [31]. Diagnosis of these disorders could therefore be missed if relying solely on the PFA-100 as a screening test [23]. In patients with apparently normal platelet function, the instrument has also been shown to occasionally give false-positive results, which then require further detailed testing.

Guidelines on the utility and practice of using the PFA-100/200 for clinical assessment of platelet disorders have been provided by various international and national organizations [23,31,34]. The advantages of the test are that it is simple, rapid, and does not require specialist training (apart from training in the manipulation of blood samples). It is a potential screening tool for assessing patients with many types of platelet abnormalities. Within a typical population of patients tested, the overall negative predictive value of the test can be high (more than 90%), although the test is clearly not sensitive to many mild platelet defects [23,31,34]. Given the high shear conditions to which platelets are exposed during the test, it is not surprising that the test is highly VWF-dependent and is therefore abnormal in patients with von Willebrand disease [37,38]. The instrument thus provides laboratories with a limited but optional screening tool that can give rapid and reliable data with a high negative predictive value [23]. However, further confirmatory testing with light transmission aggregation or a von Willebrand profile would be required, and some clinicians and researchers opt to proceed directly to these assays [23].

Diagnostic Tests

Light Transmission Platelet Aggregometry

In the 1960s, the invention of platelet aggregometry revolutionized the analysis of platelet function within routine laboratory testing [39]. Still regarded as the "gold standard," it is the most widely used platelet function test [24]. Citrated platelet-rich plasma (PRP) is normally stirred under conditions of low shear within an incubated cuvette (37°C) between a light source and a photocell [40].

The addition of different dosages of a panel of agonists triggers platelet activation, shape change, and primary and secondary aggregation events that increase light transmission over time, and this is recorded on the aggregation trace (Figure 4.3). By using a panel of agonists at differing concentrations, it is possible to detect a number of classic platelet defects [25,28]. Modern instruments usually offer multichannel capability and computer analysis and storage of data, although samples and reagents still have to be prepared manually.

The light transmission method is as follows [25]:

- Citrated PRP (prepared by centrifugation at 150–200g for 10–20 minutes; platelet count should not be adjusted within the normal range as this can introduce an artifact) is added to a cuvette at 37°C and preincubated for up to 5 minutes.

- The PRP is stirred at a recommended speed (e.g., 1000–1200 rpm using a magnetic stir bar) to allow platelets to come in contact with each other.
- 100% transmission is set with autologous platelet-poor plasma (PPP) (prepared by centrifugation at 1000g for 10 minutes).
- 0% transmission is set with PRP and a stable baseline established before addition of agonist.
- Agonist is added (up to 10% total volume).
- Aggregation is recorded (5–15 minutes).
- Percentage aggregation (maximum or final) and slope (rate of aggregation) are calculated.
- Hemolyzed or very lipemic samples may interfere with light transmission.
- Thrombocytopenic samples are also unsuitable for analysis.

A typical panel of agonists (stored in frozen aliquots) are [23,25,41]:

- ADP (2.5–20 μmol/L).
- Epinephrine (3–30 μmol/L).
- Collagen (1–5 μg/mL), usually mediates a steep aggregation curve but after a characteristic lag phase of more than 1 minute.

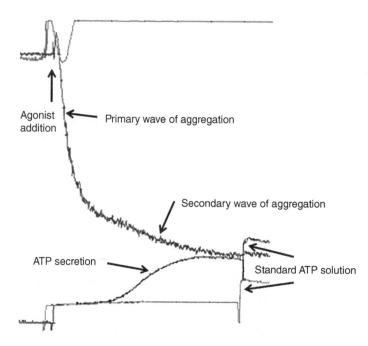

Figure 4.3 Example lumiaggregometry traces from a patient with an ADP P2Y$_{12}$ receptor mutation and from a healthy volunteer (control). The agonist used in this trace was a very high concentration of adenosine diphosphate (ADP) (100 μM). Control aggregation is shown in blue, patient aggregation is shown in red. Control adenosine triphosphate (ATP) secretion is shown in black, patient ATP secretion is shown in green. Secondary wave of aggregation is seen in the healthy volunteer and is labeled, whereas the patient shows no ATP secretion and no secondary wave of aggregation, with deaggregation noted after initial primary wave formation. Addition of the ATP standard to allow calculation of secretion to normalized platelet count is also labeled. *See Plate section for color representation of this figure.*

Agonist addition

Primary wave of aggregation

Secondary wave of aggregation

ATP secretion

Standard ATP solution

- arachidonic acid (0.5–1.5 mmol/L);
- ristocetin (0.5–2 mg/mL) is not strictly an activating agonist but stimulates platelet agglutination through binding of plasma VWF to GPIb and therefore will also give abnormal results in VWD; usually used at a single low (0.5–0.7 mg/mL) and high (1.2–1.5 mg/mL) dose. Low-dose ristocetin only induces agglutination in patients with a gain-in-function of VWF-GP1b interaction (either type 2B VWD with a mutation in the VWF molecule, or platelet type VWD with a mutation in the platelet GP1b glycoprotein);
- thrombin (0.1–0.5 IU/mL) or gamma-thrombin (50–200 ng/mL).

Some laboratories also use an extended panel of agonists, which can include: thrombin receptor-activating peptide (TRAP) with specific amino acid sequence to activate the PAR-1 or the PAR-4 receptor; collagen-related peptide, which contains an amino acid sequence to activate the GPVI receptor; the thromboxane mimetic U46619 to activate the thromboxane receptor; and the calcium ionophore A23187, which induces calcium mobilization and procoagulant activity [23]. Rationalized panels of agonists have recently been developed and validated in diagnosing patients with suspected inherited platelet defects [23,26,28]. It should be noted that it is important to define local reference intervals, and that wide variability in response can be seen at low and intermediate dose concentrations of some agonists in healthy volunteers [27]. For example, a study of 68 healthy volunteers within the UK GAPP study showed a wide range of response to ADP 3μM, with the fifth centile lying at 17% maximal aggregation and the 95th centile lying at 92% maximal aggregation [18].

A typical aggregation curve can often be divided into primary and secondary aggregation responses (see Figure 4.3), the latter being characterized by degranulation and thromboxane generation, which mediate irreversible aggregation. By using a luminescent substrate and ATP standard it is possible to measure dense granule secretion simultaneously and to quantify the amount of released ATP, which is normalized to the platelet count [42]. Thus, any defects in dense granules storage will result in not only a reduced secondary aggregation response to certain agonists but diminished ATP release [42]. Some laboratories prefer to measure stored and released nucleotides (ADP/ATP ratio) (with conversion of ADP to ATP) in standardized platelet preparations using standalone luminometers or HPLC calibrated with ATP standards [42]. There is now evidence suggesting that despite normal aggregation tracings there can be abnormal nucleotide levels in some patients with release defects so these patients may be missed if relying on aggregation tracings alone, although the *in vivo* consequences of these laboratory abnormalities are uncertain [43,44]. There are no commercially available quality control kits for platelet function testing. Aggregometers can be checked by using the PRP and PPP to check percentage aggregation settings, and dilutions (mixes of PRP and PPP) can be performed to check linearity. Normal ranges for each concentration of agonists in healthy volunteers should ideally be established; healthy volunteers can be run in parallel and new batches of reagents should be checked for the same performance as the previous batch. Platelet aggregometry is remarkably poorly standardized (e.g., in the choice and range of concentrations of agonists) as highlighted in many surveys [26,41], but a number of new national and international guidelines are now available with the aim of standardizing the performance of light transmission aggregometry across laboratories worldwide [23,25,26,34]. Typical expected aggregation responses to the more commonly encountered platelet defects are detailed in Table 4.3.

Whole Blood Aggregometry

Whole blood aggregometry measures the change in resistance or impedance between two electrodes as platelets adhere and aggregate in response to classical agonists [24]. The significant advantage of this assay is that anticoagulated blood does not require further

Table 4.3 Typical lumiaggregometry findings in commonly encountered platelet defects.

Disorder	Aggregation findings	Secretion findings
Bernard–Soulier syndrome	Absence of agglutination to high-dose ristocetin with preserved responses to other platelet agonists	Unaffected
Type IIB VWD / Platelet-type von Willebrand disease	Presence of agglutination to low-dose ristocetin with preserved responses to other platelet agonists; exact diagnosis can be established by platelet and plasma mixing studies	Unaffected
Glanzmann thrombasthenia	Absence of sustained aggregation to all agonists except ristocetin Shape change and primary wave of aggregation can be seen	Can be reduced as a result of reduced positive feedback from GPIIbIIIa outside-in signaling
Secretion defects	Commonly, absence of secondary wave aggregation to most agonists used in low concentrations, and epinephrine at all concentrations	Significantly reduced levels of ATP secretion, when normalized for platelet count
Thromboxane pathway defects	Absence/ severe reduction of aggregation in response to arachidonic acid while response to thromboxane mimetics is preserved (for cyclooxygenase defects) or absence of aggregation response to both arachidonic acid and thromboxane mimetics (for thromboxane receptor defects) Commonly, absence of secondary wave aggregation to most agonists used in low concentrations, and epinephrine at all concentrations	Unaffected
Gi-coupled receptor defects	Reduced aggregation to ADP with notable deaggregation even at high concentrations of agonist Reduced primary wave response to epinephrine and absence of secondary wave	Unaffected

processing for analysis. Commercial multi-channel impedance-based aggregometers, such as the Chronolog® or Multiplate® aggregometers, provide the ability to characterize several pathways of platelet activation in parallel. Although the basic methodologies are similar, the way results are reported are different between the Chronolog (in Ω, as the maximal amplitude of impedance achieved) and Multiplate (in arbitrary units, as area under the curve achieved over 6 minutes of aggregation).

The use of these analyzers, especially Multiplate, has seen an important rise in popularity in the last decade. They are better established in the monitoring of antiplatelet therapy with some reported associations between laboratory findings and clinical outcomes, although these are not robust at present and require further investigation [45–47]. At present, clinical guidelines advise against the use of platelet function testing for routine monitoring of antiplatelet therapy [48–50]. The use of whole blood aggregometry analyzers in the diagnosis of inherited platelet defects is limited and is seen in specialized laboratories. Specific guidelines for the use of whole blood aggregometry for the diagnosis of platelet disorders are required before this assay can be widely implemented.

Electron Microscopy

Electron microscopy can be informative of defects in platelet morphology or intracellular contents [51,52]. Various electron microscopy techniques provide detailed analysis of the cytoplasmic organelles and granules of platelets. Most organelles are visualized in thin sections of fixed, plastic embedded platelets (Figure 4.4a). However dense granules can also be easily identified as a single population in unfixed and unstained whole-mount preparations (Figure 4.4b), which makes this technique particularly useful for studying platelets from patients with dense granular defects [51,52].

In general, this technique is scarcely used as it is laborious and requires expertise and expensive microscopy equipment. However, electron microscopy has been shown to be very useful for defining ultrastructural abnormalities associated with a variety of platelet defects, including storage pool disease, Hermansky–Pudlak syndrome, Chédiak–Higashi syndrome, and grey platelet syndrome, as well as macrothrombocytopenia and arthrogryposis, renal dysfunction, and cholestasis (ARC) syndrome [51–56].

Currently, its use is not recommended in routine clinical investigations, but the guidelines also recognize the potential of this assay, especially the simpler whole-mount electron microscopy technique for confirmation of a diagnosis of dense granule defects [23].

Flow Cytometry

Whole-blood flow cytometry offers a very attractive and reliable test for the diagnosis of various platelet receptor, granular, and other defects [57,58]. Platelet responses to various agonists can also be studied by measuring various activation markers. This is potentially useful for measuring platelet function in thrombocytopenia, as flow cytometry responses are independent of platelet count [58,59]. Flow cytometry can rapidly measure the properties and characteristics of a large number of individual platelets.

The method is as follows:

- Diluted whole blood (preferred, minimizing activation) or PRP preparations are labeled with fluorescently conjugated monoclonal antibodies. If required the platelets can be simultaneously stimulated by conventional agonists as used for aggregometry during this step.
- The diluted suspension of platelets is then analyzed at a rate of 1000–100 000 cells/minute through a focused laser beam within the instrument flow cell.
- The cytometer then detects both scattered and fluorescent light emitted by each platelet. The intensity of each signal is directly

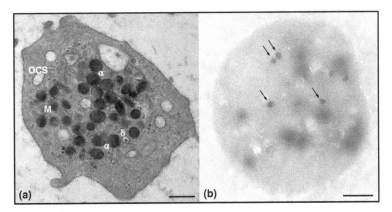

Figure 4.4 Electron microscopy imaging. (a) Transmission electron microscopy (TEM) of a normal platelet. Ultrathin sections (70–90 nm thick) stained with uranyl acetate and lead citrate revealing the different granule populations. M, mitochondria; α, alpha granule; δ, dense granule; OCS, open canalicular system. Scale bar 1 μm. (b) Whole mount electron micrograph of a normal platelet. Platelet-rich plasma was applied directly onto the EM grid and imaged. The dense granules (black arrows) contain calcium, which blocks the electron beam, therefore they appear as black dots. Scale bar 1 μm. *Source:* Reprinted with courtesy of Dr Danai Bem, Postdoctoral Research Fellow, Birmingham Platelet Group, University of Birmingham, United Kingdom. Work performed in the University of Birmingham, United Kingdom, in collaboration with the Electron Microscopy Unit at the Medical Research Council Laboratory for Molecular Cell Biology, University College London, United Kingdom.

proportional to antigen density or the size/granularity of the platelet, and usually 5000–20 000 platelet events are collected in total for each sample.

- Only platelets should be analyzed or gated on by the flow cytometer. This is normally achieved by studying the characteristic light scatter pattern that is obtained with platelets, which normally allows their resolution from red blood cells (RBCs), white blood cells (WBCs), and background "noise" in most samples. However, in some situations where there is an abnormal platelet distribution that overlaps with the RBCs (e.g., macrothrombo-cytopenia and Bernard–Soulier disease), it is often useful to use a specific identifying antibody (e.g., GPIb or IIb/IIIa) to resolve the fluorescent population of platelets from non-fluorescent RBCs/WBCs and debris/noise (Figure 4.5).
- Multiple labeling using a panel of antibodies with different fluorophores is also possible but compensation must be applied to control for overlap of fluorescent signals.

Care needs to be taken that:

- the subject is rested (20–30 minutes);
- the venepuncture is clean (discarding the first few milliliters of blood); and
- there are no time delays between sampling and analysis.

It is recommended that daily quality control procedures be performed with stable, fluorescently labeled bead preparations to ensure optimal instrument and laser performance.

The increasing availability of commercial platelet reagents (e.g., antibodies, ligands, and probes) has facilitated the development of many types of platelet assay, which can be incorporated into a standard protocol (Figure 4.6).

Table 4.4 summarizes the various types of platelet function that can be tested using a flow cytometer. The most commonly used assay is for the diagnosis of the two major platelet glycoprotein abnormalities: Bernard–Soulier syndrome (GPIb deficiency) and Glanzmann thrombasthenia (GPIIb/IIIa deficiency) [57–59]. Diagnostic assays are also available for quantifying copy number of any major glycoprotein, studying granular defects (e.g., storage pool disease), heparin-induced thrombocytopenia, and defects in platelet aggregation, secretion, or procoagulant activity. Popular activation markers include expression of markers (e.g., CD62p, CD63, activated GPIIb/IIIa, CD40L, and phosphatidylserine) not normally present on resting platelets. Some of the flow cytometry

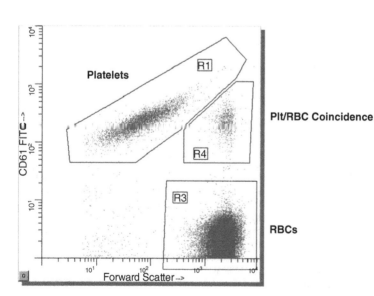

Figure 4.5 A flow cytometry plot using a fluorescent-labeled platelet-identifying antibody (anti-CD61) when triggering on a low value of forward scatter. If the instrument is triggered on this fluorescence, all other nonplatelet events shown (RBCs) will be eliminated from the analysis. Optimization of dilution will also eliminate the coincident events. *Source:* Harrison, 2001 [60]. Reproduced with permission of the American Society of Clinical Pathology.

```
┌─────────────────────────────────────────────────────────────┐
│  Blood collected by atraumatic venepuncture into anticoagulant │
│              and used without time delay                        │
└─────────────────────────────────────────────────────────────┘
```

```
┌─────────────────────────────────────────────────────────────┐
│  Blood (≈ 5 µL) diluted 1:10 in physiological buffer containing directly- │
│  conjugated antibodies, agonists and other reagents. Total volume = 50 µL. │
└─────────────────────────────────────────────────────────────┘
```

```
┌─────────────────────────────────────────────────────────────┐
│         Mix by tapping the tube gently and incubate at          │
│              room temperature for 20 minutes.                   │
└─────────────────────────────────────────────────────────────┘
```

```
┌─────────────────────────────────────────────────────────────┐
│  Samples diluted in buffer or mild fixative. Total volume 1000 – 2000 µL. │
└─────────────────────────────────────────────────────────────┘
```

```
┌─────────────────────────────────────────────────────────────┐
│  Analysis by flow cytometry within 2 hours. Collect > 10 000 events. │
└─────────────────────────────────────────────────────────────┘
```

Figure 4.6 A typical flow cytometry protocol for the testing and analysis of platelets. Small amounts of blood are incubated with test reagents, diluted, and analyzed. New reagents are easily incorporated into this standard procedure.

Table 4.4 Flow cytometric platelet function tests.

Diagnosis of platelet defects	Bernard–Soulier syndrome Glanzmann thrombasthenia Storage pool disease Heparin-induced thrombocytopenia Scott syndrome
Platelet activation markers	Degranulation markers: CD62p, CD63, and CD40L GPIIb/IIIa conformation Platelet–leukocyte conjugates Platelet-derived microvesicles Phosphatidylserine exposure
Measuring platelet production	Reticulated platelets
Accurate platelet counting	Platelet : red blood cell ratio
Blood bank tests	Quality control of concentrates Leukocyte contamination Platelet HPA-1a
Antiplatelet monitoring	Activation markers: CD62p GPIIb/IIIa conformation Vasodilator-associated stimulated phosphoprotein phosphorylation assay

applications listed in Table 4.4, such as use in monitoring antiplatelet therapy, are at present limited to a research context, but may well become part of routine clinical practice in years to come [61–63]. At present, clinical guidelines advise that there is no indication for routine laboratory monitoring of antiplatelet therapy [49,50].

The use of whole blood has several advantages over purified platelet preparations and PRP [57–59]:

- Platelets are analyzed in the presence of erythrocytes and leucocytes.
- Only small quantities of blood are required per tube (2–5 µL).
- There is no loss of subpopulations of cells during separation procedures.
- Providing the venepuncture is well standardized, minimal manipulation of fresh samples results in little artefactual *in vitro* platelet activation.
- It is possible to study platelets from patients with thrombocytopenia and in a pediatric setting.

- Both the *in vivo* resting activation state and dose–response to classical agonists can be measured with high sensitivity.

When diagnosing any platelet function or receptor defect, it is good practice to analyze a sample from a healthy volunteer in parallel to ensure that normal results can be obtained with the test in question and that reagent batches are satisfactory. This will also facilitate the eventual definition of a normal range in healthy volunteers [34]. Results are normally expressed as mean fluorescent intensity (MFI) or as a percentage of the gated platelet population [57–59]. Absolute quantification of receptor density is now possible by using calibrated fluorescent standards, some of which are available in kit form (e.g., Dako, Sigma, Biocytex). The lowest limit of detection by these techniques is quoted as approximately 500 molecules/platelet.

A panel of activation-dependent antibodies (e.g., CD62p, CD63, PAC-1) can be used to assess a patient's platelet response to dose–response curves of agonists that are also used for aggregation (e.g., TRAP, ADP, collagen).

Other Common Assays of Platelet Function

A number of platelet function assays have been developed over the years to be used at the patient's bedside [24]. Most of these assays were specifically developed for monitoring of antiplatelet therapy, and the experience with these assays in identifying platelet defects is limited.

The VerifyNow® device, a fully automated and near patient testing aggregation system, is available solely for the monitoring of the three major classes of antiplatelet drugs (e.g., GPIIb/IIIa inhibitors, aspirin, and P2Y$_{12}$ receptor inhibitors/antagonists) using specific cartridges [64].

Plateletworks®, a standardized platelet counting ratio technique, based upon comparing platelet counts within a control ethylenediamine tetra-acetic acid (EDTA) tube and after aggregation with platelet agonists within citrated tubes, could theoretically also be applied to the diagnosis of platelet disorders, although experience with this assay is limited [65].

Thromboelastography® (TEG) provides various data relating to clot formation and fibrinolysis (the lag time before the clot starts to form, the rate at which clotting occurs, the maximal amplitude of the trace or clot strength, and the extent and rate of amplitude reduction) [66]. With the PlateletMapping™ system, arachidonic acid and ADP can be used as agonists to preactivate platelets within the TEG system, thus making the assay theoretically suitable to monitor antiplatelet drugs, although the test lacks sensitivity to detect moderate changes in platelet function [67]. Its use is currently mostly limited to the monitoring of surgical hemostasis.

Conclusion

Platelet function testing remains challenging in today's hemostasis laboratory. Although efforts have been made to improve standardization, the currently available assays are labor, time and expertise intensive, and require dedicated equipment. This limits the throughput of most platelet function assays and results in platelet function disorders being under-researched; hence the molecular basis of most mild bleeding disorders is poorly characterized. However, several attempts are currently underway to render platelet function testing available outside of specialized laboratories. These include technologies based on microfluidic devices, 96-well plate-based assays, as well as remote platelet function testing on fixed blood samples [63,68–72]. Their validation in large cohorts is needed, but their availability may bring a new era in platelet function testing and research of the molecular basis of platelet defects. Finally, increased availability of rapid-throughput genetic sequencing methodologies (such as second-generation sequencing) may improve the ability, ease, and cost with which specific mutations that alter platelet function can be identified [18]. The molecular characterization of platelet disorders is set to become an expanding clinical and research field in forthcoming years.

References

1 Hartley PS. Platelet senescence and death. *Clin Lab* 2007; 53: 157–166.

2 Gresele P, Fuster V, Lopez H, *et al.* (eds). *Platelets in Hematologic and Cardiovascular Disorders.* Cambridge: Cambridge University Press, 2008.

3 Michelson AD (ed). *Platelets,* 3rd edn. London: Academic Press, 2013.

4 Watson SP, Harrison P. The vascular function of platelets. In: Hoffbrand V, Tuddenham E, Catovsky D, eds. *Postgraduate Haematology,* 5th edn. Oxford: Blackwell, 2004, pp. 819.

5 Watts T, Barigou M, Nash GB. Comparative rheology of the adhesion of platelets and leukocytes from flowing blood: why are platelets so small? *Am J Physiol Heart Circ Physiol* 2013; 304: H1483–1494.

6 Heemskerk JW, Bevers EM, Lindhout T. Platelet activation and blood coagulation. *Thromb Haemost* 2002; 88: 186–193.

7 Kaplan ZS, Jackson SP. The role of platelets in atherothrombosis. *Hematology Am Soc Hematol Educ Program* 2011; 2011: 51–61.

8 Bos CL, Richel DJ, Ritsema T, *et al.* Prostanoids and prostanoid receptors in signal transduction. *Int J Biochem Cell Biol* 2004; 36: 1187–1205.

9 Willoughby S, Holmes A, Loscalzo J. Platelets and cardiovascular disease. *Eur J Cardiovasc Nurs* 2002; 1: 273–288.

10 Freedman JE. Molecular regulation of platelet-dependent thrombosis. *Circulation* 2005; 112: 2725–2734.

11 Lordkipanidzé M, Pharand C, Palisaitis DA, *et al.* Aspirin resistance: truth or dare. *Pharmacol Ther* 2006; 112: 733–743.

12 Jackson SP. The growing complexity of platelet aggregation. *Blood* 2007; 109: 5087–5095.

13 Wei AH, Schoenwaelder SM, Andrews RK, *et al.* New insights into the haemostatic function of platelets. *Br J Haematol* 2009; 147: 415–430.

14 Jackson SP. Arterial thrombosis – insidious, unpredictable and deadly. *Nat Med* 2011; 17: 1423–1436.

15 Bolton-Maggs PH, Chalmers EA, Collins PW, *et al.* A review of inherited platelet disorders with guidelines for their management on behalf of the UKHCDO. *Br J Haematol* 2006; 135: 603–633.

16 Hayward CP, Rao AK, Cattaneo M. Congenital platelet disorders: overview of their mechanisms, diagnostic evaluation and treatment. *Haemophilia* 2006; 12 (Suppl. 3): 128–136.

17 Cox K, Price V, Kahr WH. Inherited platelet disorders: a clinical approach to diagnosis and management. *Expert Rev Hematol* 2011; 4: 455–472.

18 Watson SP, Lowe GC, Lordkipanidzé M, *et al.* Genotyping and phenotyping of platelet function disorders. *J Thromb Haemost* 2013; 11: 351–363.

19 Rydz N, James PD. The evolution and value of bleeding assessment tools. *J Thromb Haemost* 2012; 10: 2223–2229.

20 Rodeghiero F, Tosetto A, Abshire T, *et al.* ISTH/SSC bleeding assessment tool: a standardized questionnaire and a proposal for a new bleeding score for inherited bleeding disorders. *J Thromb Haemost* 2010; 8: 2063–2065.

21 Rodeghiero F, Tosetto A, Castaman G. How to estimate bleeding risk in mild bleeding disorders. *J Thromb Haemost* 2007; 5 (Suppl. 1): 157–166.

22 Lowe GC, Lordkipanidzé M, Watson SP. Utility of the ISTH bleeding assessment tool in predicting platelet defects in participants with suspected inherited platelet function disorders. *J Thromb Haemost* 2013; 11: 1663–1668.

23 Harrison P, Mackie I, Mumford A, *et al.* Guidelines for the laboratory investigation of heritable disorders of platelet function. *Br J Haematol* 2011; 155: 30–44.

24 Harrison P, Lordkipanidzé M. Testing platelet function. *Hematol Oncol Clin North Am* 2013; 27: 411–441.

25 Cattaneo M, Cerletti C, Harrison P, *et al.* Recommendations for the standardization of light transmission aggregometry: a consensus of the working party from the Platelet

Physiology Subcommittee of SSC/ISTH. *J Thromb Haemost* 2013; 11: 1183–1189.

26 Hayward CP, Moffat KA, Raby A, *et al.* Development of North American consensus guidelines for medical laboratories that perform and interpret platelet function testing using light transmission aggregometry. *Am J Clin Pathol* 2010; 134: 955–963.

27 Dawood BB, Wilde J, Watson SP. Reference curves for aggregation and ATP secretion to aid diagnose of platelet-based bleeding disorders: effect of inhibition of ADP and thromboxane A(2) pathways. *Platelets* 2007; 18: 329–345.

28 Dawood BB, Lowe GC, Lordkipanidzé M, *et al.* Evaluation of participants with suspected heritable platelet function disorders including recommendation and validation of a streamlined agonist panel. *Blood* 2012; 120: 5041–5049.

29 Rodgers RP, Levin J. A critical reappraisal of the bleeding time. *Semin Thromb Hemost* 1990; 16: 1–20.

30 Rodgers RP, Levin J. Bleeding time revisited. *Blood* 1992; 79: 2495–2497.

31 Hayward CP, Harrison P, Cattaneo M, *et al.* Platelet function analyzer (PFA)-100 closure time in the evaluation of platelet disorders and platelet function. *J Thromb Haemost* 2006; 4: 312–319.

32 Edwards A, Jakubowski JA, Rechner AR, *et al.* Evaluation of the INNOVANCE PFA P2Y test cartridge: sensitivity to P2Y(12) blockade and influence of anticoagulant. *Platelets* 2012; 23: 106–115.

33 Koessler J, Ehrenschwender M, Kobsar A, *et al.* Evaluation of the new INNOVANCE(R) PFA P2Y cartridge in patients with impaired primary haemostasis. *Platelets* 2012; 23: 571–578.

34 Christie D, Avari T, Carrington L, *et al.* *Platelet Function Testing by Aggregometry: Approved Guideline.* Clinical and Laboratory Standards Institute, 2008; 28: 1–45.

35 von Pape KW, Aland E, Bohner J. Platelet function analysis with PFA-100 in patients medicated with acetylsalicylic acid strongly depends on concentration of sodium citrate used for anticoagulation of blood sample. *Thromb Res* 2000; 98: 295–299.

36 Carcao MD, Blanchette VS, Stephens D, *et al.* Assessment of thrombocytopenic disorders using the Platelet Function Analyzer (PFA-100). *Br J Haematol* 2002; 117: 961–964.

37 Naik S, Teruya J, Dietrich JE, *et al.* Utility of platelet function analyzer as a screening tool for the diagnosis of von Willebrand disease in adolescents with menorrhagia. *Pediatr Blood Cancer* 2013; 60: 1184–1187.

38 Gadisseur A, Hermans C, Berneman Z, *et al.* Laboratory diagnosis and molecular classification of von Willebrand disease. *Acta Haematol* 2009; 121: 71–84.

39 Born GV. Aggregation of blood platelets by adenosine diphosphate and its reversal. *Nature* 1962; 194: 927–929.

40 Born G, Patrono C. Antiplatelet drugs. *Br J Pharmacol* 2006; 147: S241–251.

41 Cattaneo M, Hayward CP, Moffat KA, *et al.* Results of a worldwide survey on the assessment of platelet function by light transmission aggregometry: a report from the platelet physiology subcommittee of the SSC of the ISTH. *J Thromb Haemost* 2009; 7: 1029.

42 Cattaneo M. Light transmission aggregometry and ATP release for the diagnostic assessment of platelet function. *Semin Thromb Hemost* 2009; 35: 158–167.

43 Nieuwenhuis HK, Akkerman JW, Sixma JJ. Patients with a prolonged bleeding time and normal aggregation tests may have storage pool deficiency: studies on one hundred six patients. *Blood* 1987; 70: 620–623.

44 Pai M, Wang G, Moffat KA, *et al.* Diagnostic usefulness of a lumi-aggregometer adenosine triphosphate release assay for the assessment of platelet function disorders. *Am J Clin Pathol* 2011; 136: 350–358.

45 Schimmer C, Hamouda K, Sommer SP, *et al.* The predictive value of multiple electrode platelet aggregometry (multiplate) in adult cardiac surgery. *Thorac Cardiovasc Surg* 2013; 61: 733–743.

46 Siller-Matula JM, Francesconi M, Dechant C, *et al.* Personalized antiplatelet treatment after percutaneous coronary intervention: The

MADONNA study. *Int J Cardiol* 2013; 167: 2018–2023.

47 Sibbing D, Steinhubl SR, Schulz S, *et al.* Platelet aggregation and its association with stent thrombosis and bleeding in clopidogrel-treated patients: initial evidence of a therapeutic window. *J Am Coll Cardiol* 2010; 56: 317–318.

48 Bonello L, Tantry US, Marcucci R, *et al.* Consensus and future directions on the definition of high on-treatment platelet reactivity to adenosine diphosphate. *J Am Coll Cardiol* 2010; 56: 919–933.

49 Wijns W, Kolh P, Danchin N, *et al.* Guidelines on myocardial revascularization: The Task Force on Myocardial Revascularization of the European Society of Cardiology (ESC) and the European Association for Cardio-Thoracic Surgery (EACTS). *Eur Heart J* 2010; 31: 2501–2555.

50 Levine GN, Bates ER, Blankenship JC, *et al.* 2011 ACCF/AHA/SCAI guideline for percutaneous coronary intervention: a report of the American College of Cardiology Foundation/American Heart Association Task Force on Practice Guidelines and the Society for Cardiovascular Angiography and Interventions. *Circulation* 2011; 124: e574–651.

51 White JG. Electron microscopy methods for studying platelet structure and function. *Method Mol Biol* 2004; 272: 47–63.

52 Clauser S, Cramer-Borde E. Role of platelet electron microscopy in the diagnosis of platelet disorders. *Semin Thromb Hemost* 2009; 35: 213–223.

53 Kim SM, Chang HK, Song JW, *et al.* Severance Pediatric Liver Disease Research Group. Agranular platelets as a cardinal feature of ARC syndrome. *J Pediat Hematol Oncol* 2010; 32: 253–258.

54 Pujol-Moix N, Hernandez A, Escolar G, *et al.* Platelet ultrastructural morphometry for diagnosis of partial delta-storage pool disease in patients with mild platelet dysfunction and/or thrombocytopenia of unknown origin. A study of 24 cases. *Haematologica* 2000; 85: 619–626.

55 White JG. Electron opaque structures in human platelets: which are or are not dense bodies? *Platelets* 2008; 19: 455–466.

56 Islam MS, Alamelu J. Morphological and electron microscopic characteristics of grey platelet syndrome. *Br J Haematol* 2011; 152: 1.

57 Michelson AD. Flow cytometry: a clinical test of platelet function. *Blood* 1996; 87: 4925–4936.

58 Schmitz G, Rothe G, Ruf A, *et al.* European Working Group on Clinical Cell Analysis: Consensus protocol for the flow cytometric characterisation of platelet function. *Thromb Haemost* 1998; 79: 885–896.

59 Ault KA. The clinical utility of flow cytometry in the study of platelets. *Semin Hematol* 2001; 38: 160–168.

60 Harrison P, Ault KA, Chapman S, *et al.* An interlaboratory study of a candidate reference method for platelet counting. *Am J Clin Pathol* 2001; 115: 448–459.

61 Michelson AD. Evaluation of platelet function by flow cytometry. *Pathophysiol Haemost Thromb* 2006; 35: 67–82.

62 Frelinger AL 3rd, Li Y, Linden MD, *et al.* Association of cyclooxygenase-1-dependent and -independent platelet function assays with adverse clinical outcomes in aspirin-treated patients presenting for cardiac catheterization. *Circulation* 2009; 120: 2586–2596.

63 Fox SC, May JA, Shah A, *et al.* Measurement of platelet P-selectin for remote testing of platelet function during treatment with clopidogrel and/or aspirin. *Platelets* 2009; 20: 250–259.

64 van Werkum JW, Harmsze AM, Elsenberg EH, *et al.* The use of the VerifyNow system to monitor antiplatelet therapy: a review of the current evidence. *Platelets* 2008; 19: 479–488.

65 Campbell J, Ridgway H, Carville D. Plateletworks®: a novel point of care platelet function screen. *Mol Diagn Ther* 2008; 12: 253–258.

66 Chitlur M, Lusher J. Standardization of thromboelastography: values and challenges. *Semin Thromb Hemost* 2010; 36: 707–711.

67 Scharbert G, Auer A, Kozek-Langenecker S. Evaluation of the platelet mapping assay on rotational thromboelastometry ROTEM. *Platelets* 2009; 20: 125–130.

68 Wurtz M, Hvas AM, Wulff LN, *et al.* Shear-induced platelet aggregation in aspirin-treated patients: initial experience with the novel PlaCor PRT device. *Thromb Res* 2012; 130: 753–758.

69 Westein E, de Witt S, Lamers M, *et al.* Monitoring in vitro thrombus formation with novel microfluidic devices. *Platelets* 2012; 23: 501–509.

70 Conant CG, Schwartz MA, Beecher JE, *et al.* Well plate microfluidic system for investigation of dynamic platelet behavior under variable shear loads. *Biotechnol Bioeng* 2011; 108: 2978–2987.

71 Sun B, Tandon NN, Yamamoto N, *et al.* Luminometric assay of platelet activation in 96-well microplate. *Biotechniques* 2001; 31: 1174, 1176, 1178 passim.

72 De Cuyper IM, Meinders M, van de Vijver E, *et al.* A novel flow cytometry-based platelet aggregation assay. *Blood* 2013; 121: e70–80.

5

Evaluation of the Bleeding Patient

Alice Ma and Marshall Mazepa

Key Points

- A detailed bleeding history should include an orderly evaluation of bleeding starting in infancy, family history of bleeding, and a careful history of medications including over-the-counter drugs.
- Use of a bleeding score may help in distinguishing normal bleeding from pathological bleeding.
- The bleeding history should inform the laboratory evaluation: for example, for patients with a mucosal surface bleeding pattern, tests should include VWF testing and platelet function.
- The PT and APTT tests can be used as screening tests for coagulation factor abnormalities in a patient with a positive bleeding history and abnormal bleeding score.

The Bleeding History

A detailed history of bleeding episodes, including a family history, is critical in elucidating whether a bleeding diathesis is present. To that end, questions are aimed at determining the likelihood of a bleeding disorder being present as well the type of the putative bleeding diathesis (is this a disorder of primary or secondary hemostasis?) and inheritance pattern.

The history should include an orderly description of bleeding during infancy and childhood, including umbilical stump bleeding (characteristic of factor XIII (FXIII) deficiency), bleeding with circumcision (characteristically seen in boys with severe hemophilia A or B), bleeding with loss of deciduous teeth, and bleeding with childhood trauma and surgeries. Bleeding with dental procedures, including wisdom tooth removal, should be explored. Questions such as "Did you have to go back for stitches? Did you awaken with a pillow covered with blood" are more specific than "Did you bleed with tooth removal?" Patients with milder bleeding disorders may only bleed with procedures involving mucosal surfaces, due to the high levels of fibrinolytic activity at these sites. Epistaxis may be a presenting symptom of von Willebrand disease (VWD) or hereditary hemorrhagic telangiectasia, and is especially notable if it does not stop with pressure and requires either cautery or a visit to the emergency department.

Other bleeding episodes, whether spontaneous or provoked, should be elucidated. Bleeding into muscles and joints is characteristic of disorders of humoral clotting factors, whereas mucosal bleeding is seen more in disorders of primary hemostasis. Easy bruisability is a complaint voiced by many patients without underlying bleeding disorders, but certain historical features are worth noting. The new onset of bruising can herald a new thrombocytopenic disorder such as immune thrombocytopenia (ITP) or acute leukemia, or can point to acquired hemophilia. Bruising that only occurs over the hands and forearms suggests the presence of senile purpura.

Practical Hemostasis and Thrombosis, Third Edition. Edited by Nigel S. Key, Michael Makris and David Lillicrap.
© 2017 John Wiley & Sons, Ltd. Published 2017 by John Wiley & Sons, Ltd.

Each individual surgical procedure undergone by the patient should be explored in depth. The details of bleeding, including timing (immediate or delayed), the need for transfusion, comments by the surgeon concerning the characteristics of the bleeding, any known anatomic sources of bleeding, etc., can shed immense light on the bleeding diathesis. Immediate bleeding may be more characteristic of a disorder of primary hemostasis, while delayed bleeding is seen more in patients with deficiencies in humoral clotting factors. Bleeding in patients with an underlying hemorrhagic condition is typically described as "diffuse oozing," without the readily identifiable bleeding source seen with a surgical mishap such as a severed vessel. If a woman has bled with some procedures, but not others, she should be asked if she was on oral contraceptive pills (OCPs) or hormone replacement therapy (HRT) during the procedures in which she had good hemostasis, because OCPs and HRT can increase levels of von Willebrand factor (VWF), leading to normalization of hemostasis.

Women should be carefully questioned about their menstrual history. Duration and severity of flow are more important than the presence or severity of cramping. "How were your periods?" is likely to yield data insufficient to distinguish if a bleeding diathesis is truly present or not. While menorrhagia is medically defined as loss of more than 80 mL of blood per menstrual cycle, few if any women are capable of determining this with any degree of precision. Pad or tampon usage is imprecise as well, because the number of sanitary products used may vary with the degree of fastidiousness of each patient. To that end, pictorial assessments of blood loss (depicting pads or tampons with varying degrees of saturation) have been devised, with scores given for numbers of products used, and their saturation. Scores have been correlated with the likelihood of an underlying bleeding disorder and have been found to have a sensitivity and specificity of approximately 85% [1,2]. An underlying bleeding disorder is found in between 10 and 30% of women who present for evaluation of menorrhagia [3–5]. Historical features correlated with a higher likelihood of an underlying bleeding disorder being found include nighttime "flooding", passage of clots larger than a quarter, duration longer than 8 days, and the development of iron deficiency [6].

While bleeding during pregnancy is less common in women with VWD and other bleeding disorders, postpartum hemorrhage is les rarely seen. This usually occurs 24–48 hours after delivery, and can be markedly prolonged by weeks to months. Endometriosis and hemorrhagic ovarian cysts are seen with increased frequency in women with VWD [7].

A family history of bleeding should be carefully sought out. This may require several visits to fully document, as familial memories are probed. A family history of bleeding with surgical procedures, bleeding requiring transfusions, and menorrhagia leading to hysterectomy at a young age should be queried. However, a negative family history does not rule out a congenital bleeding disorder. Approximately one-third of all cases of hemophilia A arise from spontaneous mutations [8]. Many of the rare coagulation disorders, including deficiency of FII, FV, FVII, FX, Glanzmann thrombasthenia, and VWD type 2N, among others, are inherited in an autosomal recessive fashion, and other family members may be entirely asymptomatic.

Certain medications, herbal, and dietary supplements increase the risk of bleeding. The use of these agents may precipitate a hemorrhage in those with milder bleeding disorders. The use of aspirin and nonsteroidal anti-inflammatory agents impairs primary hemostasis, and their use should be avoided prior to surgery or prior to evaluation of the hemostatic system. Their inclusion in over-the-counter products seems ubiquitous, and careful attention to cold and flu remedy use is warranted. In the Southeast of the USA, aspirin-containing remedies such as Goody powders or BC powders are not viewed as medications, and their use will not be volunteered, but must be specifically queried.

Bleeding Score

An important challenge in assessing the bleeding history is that bleeding is common, even among healthy individuals. Bleeding symptoms in healthy adults were assessed in a study of 500 subjects recruited in advertisements and primary care waiting rooms, where about 1 in 6 subjects reported prolonged bleeding after tooth extraction or easy bruising, 1 in 4 reported epistaxis, and nearly 1 in 2 women reported heavy menstrual bleeding [9]. The goal of the bleeding evaluation is to distinguish between "normal" and "pathological" bleeding for the purpose of determining, first, whether the patient should have further laboratory testing to search for the etiology of the bleeding and, second, evaluate for the risk for future bleeding events (ultimately reducing this future risk with therapeutic interventions). Given the diversity of bleeding symptoms, their range of severity and how common bleeding symptoms are in the healthy population, attempting to make this distinction is challenging. In order to meet this challenge, an objective framework for the evaluation of bleeding symptoms was developed for the research setting, called a bleeding assessment tool (BAT) to allow for a summary of the symptoms and severity to be quantified as a bleeding score [10]. By using the BAT to study VWD, a genotype–phenotype correlation could be more objectively made and the question could be asked as to whether the bleeding score alone could predict the diagnosis. These investigators found that while the BAT was highly specific for a diagnosis of VWD, it was not very sensitive [10]. Several other tools have been developed with refinements of the original "Vicenza bleeding score" with similar formats: in a grid format, specific bleeding symptoms (e.g., epistaxis, dental hemorrhage) are scored in severity from trivial to severe, and then summed to a final bleeding score. Unfortunately, despite these refinements, the shared weakness of these tools of poor sensitivity (as low as 40%) has not been greatly improved upon [11]. Whether these tools are appropriate for use in the clinical setting is still debated [12], but their clinical utility is likely best for excluding patients in whom further testing is not required due to their high negative predictive value [13]. Also, the bleeding scores may be useful in predicting future bleeding: in a large, prospective study of VWD, a higher bleeding score was the strongest predictor of bleeding, even over other laboratory and clinical assessments [14]. Whether the bleeding score's predictive power holds true in other mild bleeding disorders is not yet known. Finally, in response to the variability of bleeding scores utilized in clinical studies that make comparing these studies challenging, the International Society on Thrombosis and Haemostasis (ISTH) has proposed a new consensus BAT with the goal of expanding the understanding of bleeding rates and phenotypes more precisely in congenital bleeding disorders [15].

The Physical Examination

The physical examination is an integral part of any diagnostic evaluation and may provide useful clues to the etiology of the patient's bleeding. Examining the skin may reveal petechiae, indicating thrombocytopenia, or the characteristic ecchymoses and lax skin seen with senile purpura. Patients with scurvy have characteristic perifollicular hemorrhages and "corkscrew hairs." Telangiectasias around the lips or on the fingertips may signal the presence of hereditary hemorrhagic telangiectasia. Bruising should be examined for their pattern and age – if they are they all the same color and lividity, they may have all occurred simultaneously. Is the pattern of distribution indicative of self-infliction, seen sometimes in patients with Munchausen syndrome? Oculocutaneous albinism is associated with several platelet disorders, including the Hermansky–Pudlak syndrome and the Chediak–Higashi syndrome.

Splenomegaly can be associated with thrombocytopenia and may indicate underlying cirrhosis. Other stigmata of liver disease, such as spider angiomata, gynecomastia, asterixis, and jaundice, also suggest that the patient may have liver coagulopathy. Joint hypermobility and skin hyperelasticity may be found in Ehlers–Danlos syndrome, though not all patients with this disorder manifest the skin findings. A harsh systolic murmur may indicate severe aortic stenosis, which can cause an acquired type 2 VWD, with associated GI bleeding from arteriovenous malformations [16]. An enlarged tongue, carpal tunnel syndrome, and periorbital purpura may point to amyloidosis, which is associated with an acquired deficiency of many clotting proteins, including FV and FX, VWF, α2-antiplasmin, and plasminogen activator inhibitor 1 [17,18].

Laboratory Evaluation

Introduction to Coagulation Laboratory Testing

While the history and physical examination can increase suspicion for the presence of a bleeding disorder, laboratory confirmation is required for precise diagnosis and treatment. A negative bleeding history can be seen in individuals with mild bleeding disorders who have never been hemostatically challenged. Moreover, acquired disorders such as acquired hemophilia can present with no prior history of bleeding. On the other hand, laboratory evaluation should be guided by the history and physical examination. When used in this fashion, laboratory studies are most useful. A detailed description of each laboratory test can be found in Chapter 2 of this book.

Clinicians must be aware that laboratory tests are affected by "preanalytic variables." That is, preparation, handling, and sample characteristics will affect test results. The majority of coagulation studies are done on plasma samples isolated from blood anticoagulated with citrate. Tubes that are underfilled will have too much citrate for the plasma volume collected, and results may be erroneous. The ratio of citrate to plasma will also be altered in patients with a hematocrit value that is too high. In this case, too much of the blood volume is occupied by

red cells and the plasma volume is reduced. Samples can be contaminated with heparin when drawn from heparinized lines or from dialysis catheters. Samples should be processed as rapidly as possible to avoid high temperatures which can activate the clotting factors, contact with platelets which can adsorb antiphospholipid antibodies, and prolonged contact with glass tubes which can activate the contact factors. Tests of platelet function are altered by the method of collection. Drawing blood with vacutainer tubes or with needles of too small a gauge will cause shear stress and may activate platelets.

It is also important to note that there is no currently available test that serves as a screening test of global hemostasis. No test can include or exclude the presence of an underlying bleeding disorder. The bleeding time does not predict bleeding, unlike its name would suggest [19]. Screening tests may point to the presence of a factor deficiency or a defect in primary hemostasis, though more precise diagnoses will require more detailed testing. Finally, some patients and families have multiple abnormalities in their hemostatic systems, and fining a single abnormality should not halt the clinical evaluation if the laboratory abnormality fails to explain the entire clinical picture. For example, VWD has been reported in families with classical hemophilia A and B [20].

The Prothrombin Time and the Activated Partial Thromboplastin Time

The prothrombin time (PT) and the activated partial thromboplastin time (APTT) are assays performed on citrated plasma that require enzymatic generation of thrombin on a phospholipid surface. Prolongation of the PT and the APTT can be seen in individuals with either deficiencies of or inhibitors to humoral clotting factors, though not all patients with prolongations of these assays will have bleeding diatheses.

The PT is designed to test components of the extrinsic pathway, including FVII, FV, FX, FII, and fibrinogen. It measures the time needed for formation of an insoluble fibrin clot once citrated plasma has been recalcified and thromboplastin has been added. In general, it is used to follow the efficacy of anticoagulation provided by vitamin K antagonists such as warfarin. Because thromboplastin from various sources and different lots can affect the rates of clotting reactions, the INR measurement was developed to avoid some of this variability in PT measurement. Each batch of thromboplastin reagent has assigned to it a numerical International Sensitivity Index (ISI) value. The INR is determined by the formula:

$$INR = (PT_{patient}/PT_{normal\ mean})^{ISI}$$

The INR is most properly used to measure anticoagulation in patients on vitamin K antagonists and is less predictive of bleeding in patients with liver disease. The INR can be inaccurate in patients with lupus anticoagulants which are strong enough to affect the PT.

The APTT tests the integrity of the intrinsic and the common clotting pathways, including FXII, FXI, FIX, FVIII, FX, FV, FII, fibrinogen, high molecular weight kininogen, and prekallikrein. The reagents are described as a "partial thromboplastin," because hemophilic plasma gave a prolonged clotting, which was not seen in assays such as the PT that used "complete thromboplastins" [21]. Citrated plasma is recalcified, and phospholipids (to provide a scaffold for the clotting reactions) and an activator of the intrinsic system such as kaolin or celite, or silica are added. The reagents used show variable sensitivities to inhibitors such as lupus anticoagulants and heparin, and normal ranges will vary from laboratory to laboratory. APTT values that are vastly different from one laboratory to another should prompt suspicion of a lupus inhibitor.

The Thrombin Clotting Time and Reptilase Time

The thrombin clotting time measures the time needed for clot formation once thrombin is added to citrated plasma. Thrombin enzymatically cleaves fibrinopeptides A and B from the alpha and the beta chains of fibrinogen, allowing for polymerization into fibrin. The thrombin clotting time (TCT or TT) is prolonged in the presence of any thrombin inhibitor such as heparin, lepirudin, or argatroban. Low levels of fibrinogen or structurally abnormal dysfibrinogens also lead to TCT prolongation. Elevated levels of fibrinogen or fibrin degradation products can also prolong the assay by serving as nonspecific inhibitors of the reaction. Patients with paraproteins can have a prolonged TCT because of the inhibitory effect of the paraprotein on fibrin polymerization.

Reptilase is a snake venom from *Bothrops atrox,* which also enzymatically cleaves fibrinogen. Reptilase cleaves only fibrinopeptide A from the alpha chain of fibrinogen but fibrin polymerization still occurs. The reptilase time (RT) is not affected by heparin and may be more sensitive to the presence of a dysfibrinogen.

Mixing Studies

Mixing studies evaluate prolongations of the APTT (less commonly the PT or the TCT) and are useful in making the distinction between an inhibitor and a clotting factor deficiency. The patient's plasma is mixed 1 : 1 with normal control plasma and the assay is repeated (with or without prolonged incubation at 37°C). Correction of the clotting test signifies factor deficiency, because the normal plasma will supply the deficient factor. Incomplete correction of the clotting test after mixing suggests the presence of an inhibitor, because an inhibitor will prolong clotting in normal plasma, just as it does in patient plasma. Incomplete correction can sometimes be seen with other nonspecific inhibitors such as a lupus inhibitor, elevated fibrin split products, or a paraprotein. Additionally, deficiencies of multiple clotting factors can lead to incomplete correction of the mixing study, because the mixing study was designed to correct deficiency of a single factor.

Specific Clotting Factor Assays

Assays measuring the activity of specific clotting factors are done using a variant of the mixing study, in which patient plasma is mixed at different dilutions with reference plasma known to be deficient in the clotting factor of interest. Thus, the only source of the specific clotting factor will be the patient's plasma. The appropriate clotting assay (either PT or APTT) is performed, and the values are plotted on a nomogram to determine the factor activity in the sample. Ordering these assays should be guided by the clinical scenario and the results of screening assays.

The Bethesda Assay

The Bethesda assay quantitates the strength of inhibitors to FVIII and is used to detect, quantify, and follow these inhibitors. Patient plasma is mixed and incubated with serial dilutions of normal control plasma, and the residual activity of FVIII is measured. The assay is controlled for normal decay of FVIII by performing the assay in tandem using control plasma diluted in buffer or in FVIII-deficient plasma (this is the Nijmegen modification). One Bethesda unit is the amount of antibody that inactivates 0.5 U of FVIII in normal plasma after incubation for 2 hours at 37°C. This assay can be adapted to test for inhibitors to other factors such as FIX.

Assays for Fibrinogen

Fibrinogen can be measured in a number of different ways. Clottable fibrinogen is measured using a variant of the thrombin time, in which thrombin is added to citrated plasma. Either the rate at which clotting occurs is measured (Clauss method), or the total degree of clotting is assayed (Ellis method). Immunological methods are used to determine the total amount of fibrinogen protein. Fibrinogen immunoelectrophoresis (IEP) can be used to detect abnormal fibrinogen species.

Factor XIII

Factor XIII is activated by thrombin and serves to crosslink monomeric fibrin strands. Deficiency of FXIII leads to a severe bleeding diathesis but cannot be measured by standard clot-based assays (PT, APTT, or TCT). A simple assay to detect FXIII deficiency is based on the ability of a fibrin clot to resist lysis in a variety of solutions: either 5 M urea, 1% chloracetic acid, or 2% acetic acid. Clots that dissolve in any of these solutions within 24 hours suggest a deficiency of FXIII. More specific functional assays as well as immunological assays are available from reference laboratories.

Testing for von Willebrand Disease

VWF can be assessed using either immunological methods for detection of antigen or functional methods for detection of activity. Activity levels are assayed either by determining the ristocetin cofactor activity or the collagen-binding activity. Multimeric analysis requires electrophoresis on a soft agarose gel, followed by immunoblotting.

Assessment of the Fibrinolytic System

Disorders of the fibrinolytic system, either congenital or acquired, can be associated with increased bleeding. The bleeding may be delayed because a normal clot is formed at the time of injury but breaks down more quickly than normal. Hyperfibrinolysis, as seen in conditions such as envenomations, acute promyelocytic leukemia, overdoses of fibrinolytic agents, prostate cancer, and disseminated intravascular coagulation (DIC).

Fibrinolysis is typically assayed by measuring levels of fibrinogen and levels of breakdown products formed by lysing fibrin clot. Fibrin degradation products (FDPs) or fibrin split products (FSPs) are assayed by latex agglutination using polyclonal antibodies directed against fibrinopeptides D and E. Because this assay does not distinguish between breakdown products of fibrin and those of fibrinogen, it is not specific for DIC versus primary fibrinogenolysis. The D-dimer assay, however, is specific for breakdown products of cross-linked fibrin and uses a variety of immunological techniques. Globally, hyperfibrinolysis can be assayed by use of the euglobulin clot lysis time (ECLT). Citrated plasma is treated to precipitate the euglobulin fraction, which contains fibrinogen and activators of plasminogen as well as a portion of fibrinolytic inhibitors such as plasminogen activator inhibitor-1 (PAI-1). The euglobulin fraction is redissolved and the fibrinogen is clotted. Clot lysis time is then measured. Hyperfibrinolysis produces shortening of the ECLT. There are specific assays for inhibitors of the fibrinolytic system, including PAI-1 and α2-antiplasmin. Deficiencies of these proteins can be either congenital or acquired.

Tests of Platelet Function

This is an area that has been reviewed elsewhere in greater detail and is fraught with controversy [22,23]. Tests are poorly standardized and poorly reproducible. No test definitively assays all aspects of platelet function and normal tests do not exclude a defect in platelet function.

The Bleeding Time
The bleeding time is an assay performed by making a nick of standard size and depth on the forearm with a sphygmomanometer inflated to a pressure of 40 mmHg on the upper arm. Blood is blotted away at standard intervals with a filter paper, and the time for bleeding cessation is measured. By blotting away excess blood, primary hemostasis, rather than fibrin formation, is tested. The bleeding time will be prolonged in cases of platelet dysfunction, VWD, thrombocytopenia and anemia, and disorders of vascular contractility. From a technical standpoint, it is affected by operator experience, cold exposure, vigorous exercise, anxiety, direction of the incision, and excessive wiping of the skin. Mild disorders of primary hemostasis may not, however, produce an abnormal bleeding time, making it less useful as a screening test.

Platelet Function Analyzer-100
The Platelet Function Analyzer-100 (PFA-100) is another screening test for disorders of primary hemostasis and is performed on whole citrated blood, rather than on the skin of the patient. Citrated whole blood is aspirated through an aperture in a cartridge where it contacts a membrane impregnated with either a mixture of collagen and epinephrine (Col/Epi) or collagen and ADP (Col/ADP). Contact with these agonists leads to platelet adhesion, aggregation, and activation, culminating in occlusion of the aperture and cessation of blood flow [24]. The time for aperture closure is known as the closure time (CT) and will be prolonged in patients with hematocrits below 30% and platelet counts below 100×10^9/L. The CTs are reliably prolonged in cases of severe platelet dysfunction and VWD. Milder cases of platelet dysfunction and mild type 1 VWD may not prolong the CT. Prolongation of the CT with Col/Epi but not Col/ADP should lead one to suspect aspirin ingestion or another defect in the thromboxane signaling pathway.

Platelet Aggregation Testing
Platelet-rich plasma is isolated from citrated blood and platelet aggregation tested in a spectrophotometer after exposure to a variety of platelet agonists. Exogenous platelet agonists include (but are not limited to) thrombin, collagen, epinephrine, arachidonic acid, ADP, the thromboxane receptor agonist U46619, and ristocetin. Platelet aggregation tracings in response to weak agonists such as epinephrine and low doses of ADP show a primary wave of aggregation followed by a secondary wave once secretion of ADP within platelet-dense granules has occurred. Stronger agonists, such as thrombin and collagen, generally produce a single deep primary wave of aggregation because they do not require secretion. Platelets must be prepared freshly, and should be drawn with needles no smaller than 19–21 gauge, into a syringe and not a vacutainer, in order to prevent platelet activation before the assay. When preparing platelet-rich plasma, red cell contamination should be avoided, because lysed red cells release ADP and lead to preactivation of platelets [25].

Lumiaggregometry directly measures release of adenine nucleotides via bioluminescence, along with the extent of aggregation. It can be performed on whole blood or platelet rich plasma. ADP released form dense granules is converted to ATP, which then reacts with luciferin, generating adenyl-luciferin, which becomes oxidized and emits light. Whole-blood aggregometry measures the increase in impedance across electrodes placed in anticoagulated blood as they become accreted with activated platelets. Though whole blood aggregometry uses a smaller volume of blood and is therefore better for pediatric patients, it is not sensitive to secretion and therefore does not distinguish between primary and secondary waves of aggregation.

Platelets from patients with Glanzmann thrombasthenia will aggregate to no agonists but will agglutinate to ristocetin, whereas platelets from patients with Bernard–Soulier syndrome show the opposite findings. Patients with storage pool disease (SPD) have deficient secretion and may therefore fail to show a second wave to weaker platelet agonists.

Electron Microscopy

Ultrastructural analysis of platelets can help diagnose mild bleeding disorders due to SPD. Certain patients with mild SPD can have completely negative evaluation, including bleeding time, PFA-100, platelet aggregometry, but show abnormalities in granule number when seen on electron microscopy [26]. Additional disorders that can be diagnosed by electron microscopy include the Hermansky–Pudlak syndrome, May–Hegglin anomaly, Epstein syndrome, Fechtner syndrome, and Sebastian syndrome [27].

Final Integration of Clinical and Laboratory Data

The approach to the bleeding patient differs, depending on the clinical scenario. Patients with active bleeding warrant an immediate, abbreviated evaluation, with clinical history aimed at determining whether the defect is congenital or acquired, and laboratory testing designed to look for gross perturbations of the hemostatic system. Acute bleeding can produce changes in the hemostatic system that make it difficult to detect minor defects. Evaluation of the patient who has had massive bleeding in the past but is now stable can be more detailed and thoughtful. Some patients present for preoperative evaluation because of abnormal laboratory tests, and the clinician must determine if the lab abnormality correlates with an underlying bleeding tendency. Other patients will present because a family member has been diagnosed with a bleeding diathesis and, in this case, the laboratory evaluation may be more truncated. The next section will attempt to provide a useful framework for the patient with a suspected bleeding disorder.

Patients with Bleeding and Prolonged PT and Normal APTT

Prolongation of the PT with a normal APTT should be due to a deficiency in FVII (Figure 5.1). Congenital deficiency of FVII is a rare autosomal recessive disorder with variable manifestations, depending on the FVII activity level. Ten percent FVII activity is generally sufficient to provide hemostasis. Inhibitors to FVII are rare but have been described [28]. Because FVII has the shortest half-life, a systemic defect in coagulation can begin with a prolonged PT out of proportion to the PTT. These include DIC, liver disease, vitamin K deficiency, or warfarin use. Paraproteins and dysfibrinogens can also prolong the PT out of proportion to the APTT. In these latter two cases, the TCT and RT may also be prolonged. Recombinant activated FVII has been approved for treatment of this disorder.

Patients with Bleeding and Normal PT and Prolonged APTT

Congenital Causes

Factor deficiencies in the intrinsic pathway that lead to bleeding include FXI, FIX, and FVIII (Figure 5.2). Congenital deficiency of FXI is autosomal recessive and is seen with increased frequency in Ashkenazi Jews. This generally produces a milder bleeding disorder and, despite being due to a deficiency in a humoral clotting factor, FXI deficiency produces a

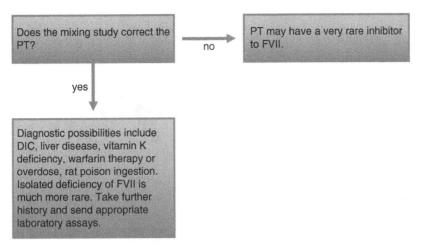

Figure 5.1 Diagnostic evaluation for patient with elevated prothrombin time (PT) and normal activated partial thromboplastin time (APTT). DIC, disseminated intravascular coagulation.

mucocutaneous bleeding pattern; the severity of bleeding is not strictly dependent on the level of FXI activity in plasma. Whether or not FXI-deficient patients bleed may depend upon differences in their ability to generate thrombin, the ability to activate the thrombin activatable fibrinolytic inhibitor (TAFI), and/or the activity of the fibrinolytic system. FXI deficiency is treated with either plasma or a FXI concentrate, depending upon the availability of the latter product.

FVIII and FIX deficiency produce hemophilia A and B, respectively and are the only two soluble clotting factor deficiencies that are inherited as X-linked recessive disorders. More than a thousand distinct mutations in each gene have been reported [29]. These mutations result in mild, moderate, and severe forms of hemophilia, and the clinical manifestations of hemophilia A and B are, for all practical purposes, indistinguishable. In the severe form, both disorders are characterized by recurrent hemarthroses that result in chronic crippling hemarthropathy unless treated by replacing the deficient factor on a prophylactic basis. Bleeding episodes may be "spontaneous" but on close questioning bleeding can usually be related to trauma. Central nervous system hemorrhage is especially hazardous and remains one of the leading causes of death.

Mild hemophilia may present in adulthood with post-traumatic or surgical bleeding. Both plasma-derived and recombinant FVII and FIX concentrates are available. Desmopressin can sometimes be helpful in the treatment of mild hemophilia A.

von Willebrand disease is the most common inherited bleeding disorder, with low levels of VWF found in 1% of the population. It is inherited in an autosomal fashion, with mild disease being codominant and more severe disease being recessive. VWF protects FVIII from degradation and FVIII levels can be low enough in VWD to cause slight prolongation of the APTT. Mild VWD produces mucocutaneous and post-surgical bleeding. Many women with VWD have significant menorrhagia, endometriosis, and postpartum hemorrhage, and may suffer bleeding for more than a decade prior to diagnosis [7]. Type 2N VWD can be confused with mild hemophilia. In this disorder, the site on VWD responsible for binding FVIII is mutated and FVIII levels are usually about 20% of normal, with a normal FVIII gene. Desmopressin can be used for the treatment of mild type 1 VWD, but more severe bleeding and bleeding in patients with type 2 and 3 patients typically requires infusion of VWF-containing FVIII concentrates.

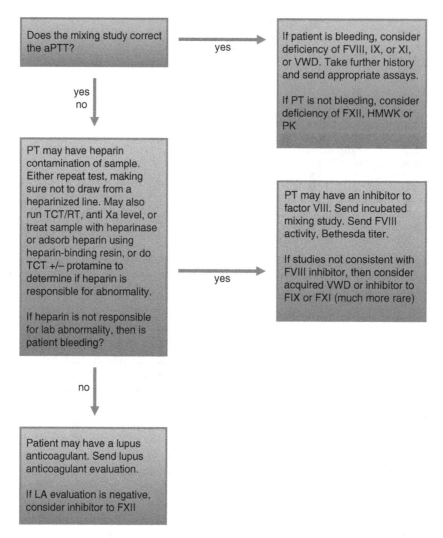

Figure 5.2 Diagnostic algorithm for patient with normal prothrombin time (PT) and prolonged activated partial thromboplastin time (APTT). HMWK, high molecular weight kininogen; LA, lupus anticoagulant; PK, prekallikrein; RT, reptilase time; TCT, thrombin clotting time; VWD, von Willebrand disease.

Acquired Causes

The most common cause of an acquired disorder that causes bleeding with an isolated APTT prolongation is an acquired inhibitor to FVIII. Patients with acquired hemophilia have a bimodal age distribution, with younger patients being female and older patients being male. This condition can be associated with the postpartum state, malignancies, or autoimmune conditions, but 50% of cases will be idiopathic. Patients have no prior history of bleeding but the bleeding at the time of presentation can be severe. Unlike congenital hemophilia, bleeding tends to be mucocutaneous and multifocal, and hemarthroses are rare. The mixing study will fail to correct and will reprolong with incubation. Tests for the lupus inhibitor will be negative, and the Bethesda assay will show the presence of an inhibitor. There may be a small amount of residual FVIII activity in the plasma, but the bleeding will be out of proportion to the FVIII activity [30]. Treatment for acute bleeding episodes will require a bypassing agent if the Bethesda titer is >5, but may be treated with higher doses of FVIII concentrates if the Bethesda titer is below 5. Recombinant porcine FVIII is also available as a therapeutic option for these patients and has the advantage of allowing clinicans to follow measurement of FVIII activity. Patients may require immunosuppression to rid them of their inhibitor.

Acquired VWD is a rare condition that is typically associated with a lymphoproliferative disorder, though it can also be seen in the setting of hypothyroidism, myeloproliferative disorders, and severe aortic stenosis. Patients will have a prolonged APTT along with a prolonged bleeding time and PFA-100. Acquired inhibitors to FXI and FIX are rare and typically seen in association with other autoimmune conditions.

Heparin therapy will cause a prolonged APTT, more commonly with a normal PT, and can cause bleeding. The TCT will be prolonged, and the RT will be normal. Plasma cell dyscrasias can produce a heparin-like substance, which will produce the same pattern of laboratory abnormalities [31].

Patients with Bleeding and Prolongation of both the PT and APTT

Congenital Causes

A deficiency of a factor in the common pathway will prolong both the PT and the APTT. Deficiencies of FII, FV, FX, and fibrinogen are autosomal recessive and are rare (Figure 5.3). FV deficiency produces a bleeding disorder that is less severe than hemophilia A or B, even when FV

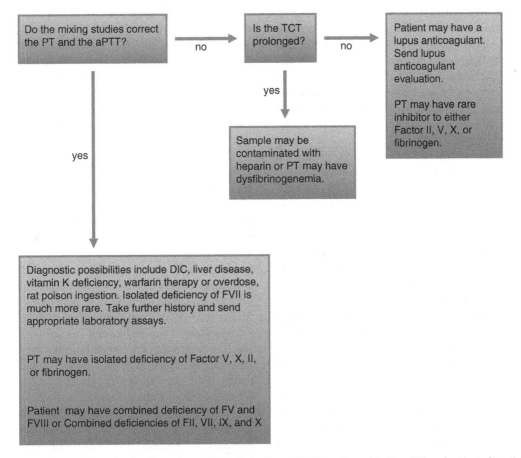

Figure 5.3 Diagnostic evaluation for patient with prolongations of both prothrombin time (PT) and activated partial thromboplastin time (APTT). DIC, disseminated intravascular coagulation; TCT, thrombin clotting time.

levels are <1%. Bleeding times may be prolonged due to lack of platelet FV, which is reported to account for 20% of the FV in the body. It is treated with fresh frozen plasma. FX deficiency can be mild, moderate, or severe, with severe deficiency producing bleeding similar to that seen in classical hemophilia. Patients with bleeding can be treated with prothrombin complex concentrates (PCCs), and FX levels should not be raised above 50% to avoid thromboembolic complications. Inherited prothrombin deficiency is quite rare and can also be treated with PCCs.

Fibrinogen gene mutations lead either to absence of fibrinogen (afibrinogenemia) or to production of a defective molecule (dysfibrinogenemia). Afibrinogenemia is very rare, leading to a severe bleeding disorder manifest by bleeding after trauma into subcutaneous and deeper tissues, which may result in dissection. Bleeding from the umbilical stump is frequent. In addition to prolongation of the PT and the APTT, these patients show a prolonged TCT and RT as well. The bleeding time is also prolonged due to the absence of fibrinogen in the platelet alpha granule. Treatment consists of transfusing cryoprecipitate to raise the fibrinogen level to the range of around 100 mg/dL. Fibrinogen concentrates are now available. The majority of patients with dysfibrinogenemia are heterozygous for the disorder, and ~50% of these patients have neither a hemorrhagic nor thrombotic state. Other dysfibrinogens, however, are associated with bleeding episodes while a few may be associated with venous or arterial thrombosis. Bleeding patients should be treated with infusions of cryoprecipitate.

Combined deficiency of multiple clotting factors can also be inherited, the most common conditions being combined deficiency of FV and FVIII and a combined deficiency of the vitamin K-dependent factors (prothrombin and FVII, FIX, FX, and protein C and S) [32,33]. A combined deficiency of FV and FVIII is inherited in an autosomal recessive fashion and is due to defects in one of two genes: *LMAN1* and *MCFD2* [33]. The products of both genes play an important role in the transport of FV and FVIII from the endoplasmic reticulum to the Golgi apparatus and are necessary for normal secretion of these factors. The disorder results in a mild to moderate bleeding tendency with FV and FVIII levels ranging from 5 to 30% of normal. When both the PT and APTT are prolonged, and either FV or FVIII are found to be decreased, the combined deficiency should be suspected. FVIII is easily replaced using FVIII concentrates, but the only readily available FV replacement is fresh frozen plasma, which is limited in its ability to normalize the FV level. In some cases plasma exchange is necessary to raise the FV to hemostatic levels.

Combined deficiencies of the vitamin K-dependent factors can be due to defects in either the gene for vitamin K-dependent carboxylase or the gene for vitamin K epoxide reductase [34]. This is an autosomal recessive disorder that may be associated with moderate to severe deficiency of prothrombin, FVII, FIX, and FX as well as protein C and S [33]. In this syndrome both the PT and APTT are prolonged, and assays for the individual factors that influence these tests are necessary. Large doses of vitamin K may partially correct the hereditary defect in some but not all cases. Some bleeding episodes will require replacement with PCCs.

Acquired Causes

Inhibitors to FV are typically seen in patients who have undergone redo vascular or cardiac surgery and are provoked by use of bovine thrombin. This hemostatic agent is contaminated with a small amount of bovine FV, and antibodies to bovine FV will cross-react with human FV. This condition may be self-limited, but bleeding can be treated with platelets because platelet FV may be less susceptible to inhibitors in plasma.

Prothrombin antibodies can coexist with the lupus inhibitor and these inhibitors increase clearance of FII, causing an acquired deficiency rather than neutralizing antibodies. Thus, the mixing studies for the PT will be normal.

FX deficiency can be seen in conjunction with amyloidosis because the FX is adsorbed onto the amyloid protein. This can cause a severe hemorrhagic disorder, which has been reported to respond to splenectomy. This condition will also produce a mixing study that normalizes the PT and the APTT.

Combined factor deficiencies can be seen in conditions such as vitamin K deficiency, disseminated intravascular coagulation, and severe liver disease. Severe liver disease can also lead to an acquired dysfibrinogenemia, which can produce a prolonged TCT and RT.

Anticoagulants such as heparin and coumadin can cause prolongation of both the PT and the APTT, especially when given in excess. Direct thrombin inhibitors such as lepirudin and argatroban will prolong the PT, the APTT, and the TCT.

Patients with Bleeding but Normal PT and APTT

Congenital Causes

FXIII deficiency is a rare autosomal disorder that presents with severe bleeding. Prolonged bleeding from the umbilical stump is common, as is spontaneous intracranial hemorrhage. Treatment relies on cryoprecipitate or FXIII concentrates, which have recently been introduced.

Congenital disorders of platelets include thrombocytopenic disorders, disorders of platelet surface glycoproteins, signaling pathway disorders, and secretion disorders. They typically show prolongation of the bleeding time and the PFA-100. Platelet aggregation may show a typical pattern but milder disorders may have normal platelet aggregation tracings. Mild thrombocytopathies may be missed by the bleeding time, the PFA-100, and platelet aggregation testing, and may require more specialized testing such as flow cytometry or electron microscopy.

Congenital deficiencies of fibrinolytic inhibitors such as α2-antiplasmin and plasminogen activator inhibitor-1 have been reported, and bleeding is typically delayed. The euglobulin lysis time can be shortened, and assays for these proteins can be performed, but may not be helpful in the deficiency state, due to assay limitations.

VWD can present with normal APTT values, especially if the FVIII activity level is above 40–50%. Type 1 VWD is a quantitative deficit of

VWF, and all multimeric forms are present. Mild type 1 VWD may be missed by the bleeding time and the PFA-100, making measurement of VWF antigen and activity levels necessary for proper diagnosis. Additionally, levels of VWF fluctuate in response to estrogens, stress, exercise, inflammation, and bleeding, and repeated assays can be required to make the diagnosis.

Hereditary hemorrhagic telangiectasia is an autosomal dominant disorder that is associated with arteriovenous malformations of the small vessels of the skin, oropharynx, lungs, gastrointestinal tract, and other tissues. The syndrome is often suspected by the presence of epistaxis, gastrointestinal bleeding, telangiectasias on the lips and fingertips, and iron deficiency anemia. While bleeding does not occur at birth, it may begin in childhood, and by age 16 the majority of patients will experience hemorrhagic symptoms.

Ehlers–Danlos syndrome is characterized by easy bruising and hemorrhage from ruptured blood vessels and is due to one of several genetic defects [34]. The classic Ehlers–Danlos syndrome (EDS) causing joint hypermotility and hyperextensibility of the skin may be associated with bruising but is not likely to result in massive bleeding. The vascular type IV EDS is the most likely to result in significant bruising and is due to a defect in type III collagen resulting from defects in the COL3A1 gene. In this type of EDS, bruising can be very extensive and vascular rupture can result in death. The skin may be thin and wrinkled, but hyperextensibility of the skin is not common. The bruising is sufficient to make one suspect a platelet disorder but tests of platelet and coagulant function are normal. Diagnosis is dependent upon demonstration of the genetic abnormality or the demonstration of abnormal type III collagen.

Acquired Causes

Many drugs and herbs cause platelet dysfunction and their use needs to be questioned extensively. Uremia, myeloproliferative disorders, and cardiac bypass will also cause a thrombocytopathy.

Amyloidosis has been reported in conjunction with acquired deficiencies of α2-antiplasmin and plasminogen activator inhibitor-1. Inhibitors to FXIII have been reported and are quite rare.

Patients without Bleeding History but with Abnormal Coagulation Testing

When doing preoperative evaluations of these patients, it is important to recognize that many patients with mild bleeding disorders may have no known history of bleeding. Some may recall mild bleeding symptoms when carefully questioned, and some may not have had sufficient challenges to their hemostatic systems. Thus, some evaluation is required, depending on the severity of the surgery that is being planned.

Congenital Causes

Deficiencies of high-molecular-weight kininogen, prekallikrein, and FXII will produce marked prolongation of the APTT without conferring an increased risk of abnormal bleeding. Some patients with FXI deficiency may have no bleeding symptoms, despite low levels of FXI. Patients with mild deficiency of FVII may also have no bleeding symptoms. Additionally, certain mutations in the FVII molecule affect its interaction with bovine but not human thromboplastin, and these mutations are not associated with clinical manifestations. Lastly, most dyfibrinogenemias are also associated with no clinical symptoms.

Acquired Causes

Lupus anticoagulants prolong the APTT and the mixing study fails to correct. Unless associated with hypoprothrombinemia, lupus inhibitors confer no increased risk of bleeding. The majority of acquired FV antibodies are also asymptomatic and are self-limited. Though patients with severe liver disease may have a prolonged PT/INR, their bleeding symptoms may vary. These patients may clot and they are not "autoanticoagulated," because they are deficient in many anticoagulant proteins as well.

Conclusion

Evaluation of the bleeding patient requires a careful history and physical examination. Laboratory workup should be tailored to the clinical presentation and the pretest probability of finding an underlying bleeding diathesis. Many of the laboratory tests are best conducted at a tertiary center with expertise in hemostasis. Accurate diagnosis allows for rational, intelligent treatment and prophylaxis of bleeding.

References

1 Higham JM, O'Brien PM, Shaw RW. Assessment of menstrual blood loss using a pictorial chart. *Br J Obstet Gynaecol* 1990; 97: 734–739.

2 Rodeghiero F, Kadir RA, Tosetto A, *et al.* Relevance of quantitative assessment of bleeding in haemorrhagic disorders. *Haemophilia* 2008; 14 (Suppl. 3): 68–75.

3 Philipp CS, Faiz A, Dowling N, *et al.* Age and the prevalence of bleeding disorders in women with menorrhagia. *Obstet Gynecol* 2005; 1051: 61–66.

4 Trasi SA, Pathare AV, Shetty SD, *et al.* The spectrum of bleeding disorders in women with menorrhagia: a report from Western India. *Ann Hematol* 2005; 845: 339–342.

5 Woo YL, White B, Corbally R, *et al.* von Willebrand's disease: an important cause of dysfunctional uterine bleeding. *Blood Coagul Fibrinolysis* 2002; 132: 89–93.

6 Lee CA. Women and inherited bleeding disorders: menstrual issues. *Semin Hematol* 1999; 36 (3 Suppl. 4): 21–27.

7 James AH. More than menorrhagia: a review of the obstetric and gynaecological manifestations of bleeding disorders. *Haemophilia* 2005; 11: 295–307.

8 Gitschier J. Molecular genetics of hemophilia A. *Schweiz Med Wochenschr* 1989; 119: 1329–1331.

9 Mauer AC, Khazanov NA, Levenkova N, *et al.* Impact of sex, age, race, ethnicity and aspirin use on bleeding symptoms in healthy adults. *J Thromb Haemost* 2011; 9: 100–108.

10 Rodeghiero F, Castaman G, Tosetto A, *et al.* The discriminant power of bleeding history

for the diagnosis of type 1 von Willebrand disease: an international, multicenter study. *J Throm Haemost* 2005; 3: 2619–2626.

11 Tosetto A, Castaman G, Rodeghiero F. Bleeders, bleeding rates, and bleeding score. *J Thromb Haemost* 2013; 11 (Suppl. 1): 142–150.

12 Tosetto A, Castaman G, Rodeghiero F. Bleeding scores in inherited bleeding disorders: clinical or research tools? *Haemophilia* 2008; 14: 415–422.

13 O'Brien SH. Bleeding scores: are they really useful? *ASH Education Program Book* 2012; 2012: 152–156.

14 Castaman G, *et al*. Bleeding tendency and efficacy of anti-haemorrhagic treatments in patients with type 1 von Willebrand disease and increased von Willebrand factor clearance. *Thromb Haemost* 2011; 105: 647–654.

15 Rodeghiero F, Tosetto A, Federici AB, *et al*. ISTH/SSC bleeding assessment tool: a standardized questionnaire and a proposal for a new bleeding score for inherited bleeding disorders. *J Thromb Haemost* 2010; 8: 2063–2065.

16 Sucker C. The Heyde syndrome: proposal for a unifying concept explaining the association of aortic valve stenosis, gastrointestinal angiodysplasia and bleeding. *Int J Cardiol* 2007; 115: 77–78.

17 Sucker C, Hetzel GR, Grabensee B, *et al*. Amyloidosis and bleeding: pathophysiology, diagnosis, and therapy. *Am J Kidney Dis* 2006; 47: 947–955.

18 Mumford AD, O'Donnell J, Gillmore JD, *et al*. Bleeding symptoms and coagulation abnormalities in 337 patients with AL-amyloidosis. *Br J Haematol* 2000; 110: 454–460.

19 Lind SE. The bleeding time does not predict surgical bleeding. *Blood* 1991; 77: 2547–2552.

20 O'Brien SH, Ritchey AK, Ragni MV. Combined clotting factor deficiencies: experience at a single hemophilia treatment center. *Haemophilia* 2007; 13: 26–29.

21 Langdell RD, Wagner RH, Brinkhous KM. Effect of antihemophilic factor on one-stage clotting tests; a presumptive test for hemophilia and a simple one-stage antihemophilic factor assy procedure. *J Lab Clin Med* 1953; 41: 637–647.

22 Shah U, Ma AD. Tests of platelet function. *Curr Opin Hematol* 2007; 14: 432–437.

23 Michelson AD, Frelinger AL 3rd, Furman MI. Current options in platelet function testing. *Am J Cardiol* 2006; 98: 4N–10N.

24 Favaloro EJ. Clinical application of the PFA-100. *Curr Opin Hematol* 2002; 9: 407–415.

25 Zhou L, Schmaier AH. Platelet aggregation testing in platelet-rich plasma: description of procedures with the aim to develop standards in the field. *Am J Clin Pathol* 2005; 123: 172–183.

26 Lorez HP, Richards JG, Da Prada M, *et al*. Storage pool disease: comparative fluorescence microscopical, cytochemical and biochemical studies on amine-storing organelles of human blood platelets. *Br J Haematol* 1979; 43: 297–305.

27 White JG. Use of the electron microscope for diagnosis of platelet disorders. *Semin Thromb Hemost* 1998; 24: 163–168.

28 Mulligan CG, Rischbieth A, Duncan EM, *et al*. Acquired isolated factor VII deficiency associated with severe bleeding and successful treatment with recombinant FVIIa (NovoSeven). *Blood Coagul Fibrinolysis* 2004; 15: 347–351.

29 Stenson PD, Mort M, Ball EV, *et al*. The human gene mutation database: 2008 update. *Genome Med* 2009; 1: 13.

30 Ma AD, Carrizosa D. Acquired factor VIII inhibitors: pathophysiology and treatment. *Hematology Am Soc Hematol Educ Program* 2006; 2006: 432–437.

31 Torjemane L, Guermazi S, Ladeb S, *et al*. Heparin-like anticoagulant associated with multiple myeloma and neutralized with protamine sulfate. *Blood Coagul Fibrinolysis* 2007; 18: 279–281.

32 McMillan CW, Roberts HR. Congenital combined deficiency of coagulation factors II, VII, IX and X. Report of a case. *N Engl J Med* 1966; 274: 1313–1315.

33 Zhang B, Ginsburg D. Familial multiple coagulation factor deficiencies: new biologic insight from rare genetic bleeding disorders. *J Thromb Haemost* 2004; 2: 1564–1572.

34 De Paepe A, Malfait F. Bleeding and bruising in patients with Ehlers-Danlos syndrome and other collagen vascular disorders. *Br J Haematol* 2004; 127: 491–500.

6

Hemophilia A and B
Rhona M. Maclean and Michael Makris

Key Points

- Hemophilia A and B are X-linked disorders due to reduced activity of FVIII and FIX, respectively.
- Joint and muscle hemorrhages are most common in severe hemophilia where they can occur spontaneously.
- Clotting factor concentrates can be used to treat established bleeds or be given regularly prophylactically to prevent them.
- Alloantibodies (inhibitors) develop in a third of severe hemophilia A patients following concentrate treatment rendering FVIII concentrate ineffective.
- Cardiovascular disease is increasingly being recognized in older hemophilic individuals and, although myocardial infarction occurs less frequently, atherosclerosis is found at a similar level as the general population.

Introduction

Hemophilia A and B are inherited X-linked recessive bleeding disorders, caused by deficiencies in factor VIII (FVIII) and factor IX (FIX), respectively. It was initially thought that hemophilia was caused by abnormalities of the vascular system, and it was not until the late 1800s and early 1900s that a deficiency of a component of the blood was thought to be responsible.

All racial groups are equally affected by hemophilia with an incidence of 1 in 5000 live male births for hemophilia A, and 1 in 30 000 for hemophilia B. The clinical symptoms and signs of these two disorders are identical in presentation, and specific clotting factor assays are required to distinguish them. With modern management and the ready availability of clotting factors, children with hemophilia today can look forward to a normal life expectancy [1].

Factor VIII Gene and Protein

In the two decades since the FVIII protein was first purified (1983) and the gene cloned (1982–1984), advances in molecular biology and protein biochemistry have led to a greatly improved understanding of the structure and function of both the FVIII gene and protein. The crystal structure of FVIII has been published [2].

The FVIII gene (*F8*) is located in the most distal band of the long arm of the X chromosome at Xq28, spans 186 000 base pairs (bp) of DNA, contains 26 exons, and is transcribed from the telomeric to centromeric direction to produce a mature mRNA of approximately 9 kb. Recent studies indicate that the precursor protein (2351 amino acids) is predominantly synthesized in sinusoidal and vascular endothelial cells, and has a molecular weight of approximately 293 000 Da.

Practical Hemostasis and Thrombosis, Third Edition. Edited by Nigel S. Key, Michael Makris and David Lillicrap.
© 2017 John Wiley & Sons, Ltd. Published 2017 by John Wiley & Sons, Ltd.

After cleavage of the secretory leader sequence, the FVIII protein has a mature sequence of 2332 amino acids with the domain structure A1-a1-A2-a2-B-a3-A3-C1-C2. The domain structure of FVIII is very similar to that of coagulation FV, and its A domains are homologous with ceruloplasmin. As the FVIII protein is very susceptible to proteolysis after secretion, the majority of circulating FVIII comprises heavy chains (the A1 and A2 domains with variable lengths of the B domain) noncovalently linked to light chains (A3, C1, and C2 domains). The B domain is not required for FVIII procoagulant activity. FVIII exerts its procoagulant activity by accelerating the activation of coagulation FX by FIXa and likely provides cofactor activity as a scaffold for optimal tenase complex assembly. FVIII circulates bound to and is stabilized by von Willebrand factor (VWF), with a ratio of approximately one molecule of FVIII to 50 molecules of VWF.

Mutations in *F8* Gene

There are many *F8* gene defects listed on the online hemophilia A mutation database (www.factorviii-db.org). These can be categorized as: (i) gross gene rearrangements; (ii) insertions or deletions of genetic sequence; or (iii) single base substitutions (leading to missense, nonsense or splicing defects). All types of defects can lead to severe disease, but the most clinically important, responsible for 40–45% of cases of severe hemophilia A, is the *F8* intron 22 inversion. The origin of this inversion mutation is virtually always in male germ cells during spermatogenesis; in more than 95% of hemophiliac patients with the intron 22 inversion, their mothers were demonstrated to be carriers.

The majority of point mutations have been reported only once; however, a number have been reported on several occasions, often with variable clinical phenotype and FVIII activity. This suggests that there are other factors in addition to the *F8* gene defect responsible for the clinical severity of the disease.

Overall, mutations are now identifiable in over 90% of individuals with hemophilia A (see Chapter 3 for further information regarding

molecular defects in hemophilia A and their detection).

Factor IX Gene and Protein

The FIX gene (*F9*) is centromeric to the *F8* gene on the X chromosome at Xq27, and FIX is predominantly synthesized in hepatocytes. It is considerably smaller than the *F8* gene, spanning 34 kb of DNA and containing only eight exons (a–h), which code for an mRNA of 2.8 kb that translates into a protein of 415 amino acids. After secretion, the 18 amino acid prepeptide (encoded by the first exon, a) is cleaved off. The FIX protein is a member of the serine protease family and its domain structure is similar to that of FVII, X, and protein C. As with the other serine proteases, it requires post-translational γ-carboxylation of its glutamyl (Glu) residues by a vitamin-K dependent process.

Mutations in *F9* Gene

There are >1000 different mutations reported in the *F9* gene and a very useful resource is the hemophilia B mutation database (www.factorix.org). The majority of mutations in the FIX gene are point mutations (~80%), with the remainder being splice site, frameshift, or gross deletions/rearrangements (~3–4% each). See Chapter 3 for further information regarding the molecular genetics and diagnostics of hemophilia B.

Severity and Symptoms

Hemophilia is classified as severe, moderate, or mild on the basis of assayed plasma coagulation factor levels. This laboratory classification largely correlates with the clinical bleeding risk (Table 6.1), thus allowing a prediction to be made about individual bleeding risk and outcome. Approximately 50% of patients with hemophilia have severe disease, 10% moderate, and 40% mild hemophilia.

- *Severe disease:* those with severe disease develop spontaneous joint and muscle hematomas, in

Table 6.1 Classification of severity of hemophilia.

Classification of severity	Concentration of coagulation factor
Severe	<0.01 IU/mL or <1% of normal
Moderate	0.01–0.05 IU/mL or 1–5% of normal
Mild	>0.05 IU/mL or >5% of normal

addition to bleeding after minor injuries and surgical procedures. Most patients with severe hemophilia A are diagnosed within the first year of life, either due to testing at birth in those with a family history, or because of abnormal bruising/bleeding. Thereafter in the first 6–9 months of life cutaneous bruising or oral bleeding (due to teething or cuts in the oral cavity) can occur. Once the baby becomes more mobile (rolling, crawling, toddling, cruising) bruising and joint bleeds can occur. Although bruising can be prominent in young children (it resolves once they start prophylaxis), it is not a feature of adult severe hemophilia.

- *Moderate disease:* those with moderate disease do not tend to bleed spontaneously, but develop muscle and joint hematomas after mild trauma. They also bleed excessively after surgery and dental extractions.
- *Mild disease:* individuals with mild hemophilia do not bleed spontaneously. They do, however, bleed after surgery, significant trauma, or dental extractions.

Inheritance

Both hemophilia A and B are X-linked recessive inherited disorders, and therefore affect males almost exclusively. It is not uncommon, however, for carrier females to have reductions in FVIII or FIX levels to the extent that they will require treatment prior to any invasive procedure, or following major trauma.

Where the female is a carrier, there is a 50 : 50 chance that a son will be affected by hemophilia, or that a daughter will be a carrier. When the children are from a hemophilic male and a normal female, all sons will be unaffected, but all daughters will be obligate carriers.

Approximately one-third of cases of hemophilia are "sporadic," that is due to the occurrence of a new mutation, with no family history of the disease.

Mosaicism occurs when a proportion of the cells of the body contain a mutation whereas the majority do not. Gonadal mosaicism, in which the mutation is confined to the gonadal tissue, has been reported in both hemophilia A and B [3]. Should gonadal mosaicism be present, the risk of passing on the disease to any future children will be higher than the risk in the general population. Care must therefore be taken when counseling women who do not appear to be carriers yet have a child with hemophilia.

Females with Markedly Reduced FVIII/IX Levels

This is possible in the following rare circumstances:

- With extreme lyonization of the *F8 or F9* gene in hemophilia carriers – rarely carriers can have levels <10%.
- If there is hemizygosity of the X chromosome (e.g., in Turner (XO) syndrome) in a hemophilia carrier.
- A female can be affected if she is the offspring of a hemophilic male and a carrier female.
- In females with the Normandy variant of von Willebrand disease (VWD) (FVIII deficiency only).
- In females with acquired hemophilia.

Carrier Testing

All females who are obligate or possible carriers of hemophilia should be offered genetic counseling to provide them with the information necessary to make informed reproductive choices, and for the optimal management of their pregnancies. The majority of individuals with hemophilia A and B now have an identifiable genetic defect. If the genetic defect within the family is known, it is usually straightforward to screen the potential carrier and confirm the status of possible carriers. If the mutation is not known, then linkage analysis using informative genetic polymorphisms is usually successful (if sufficient family members are available for testing). All carriers of hemophilia A or B should have their FVIII/FIX levels measured.

Prenatal Diagnosis

Although the treatment of hemophilia has greatly improved over the last 10–20 years, many carriers of hemophilia (often those who have grown up with a family member who had complications of the disease such as inhibitors or viral infections) will request prenatal diagnosis. Chorion villus sampling (CVS) can be performed at 10–12 weeks' gestation, allowing for first trimester termination if desired. Alternatively, amniocentesis can be performed at 16 weeks. The risks of these procedures are low in experienced centers, with a miscarriage rate of 0.5–1%. Fetoscopy to allow for fetal blood sampling is rarely performed as it can only be performed after 20 weeks' gestation and has a higher risk of fetal death (1–6%). Following the discovery of fetal DNA in maternal blood, PCR-based techniques have been developed to detect specific Y-chromosomal sequences in maternal blood samples. Although not yet available in many centers, it is now possible to determine the sex of a fetus from as early as 7 weeks' gestation [4]. Furthermore, it has been shown that as well as identifying the sex in the first trimester, it is possible to determine if a male fetus is affected by hemophilia or not [5].

Embryo Selection: Preimplantation Genetic Diagnosis

Preimplantation genetic diagnosis (PGD) involves the genetic testing of an embryo prior to implantation and before pregnancy occurs. It is used in conjunction with *in vitro* fertilization (IVF), and only embryos found to be free of a specific genetic disorder are transferred into a woman for pregnancy. The advantage of this approach is that the trauma of termination of pregnancy can be avoided [6].

Delivery of an at-Risk Pregnancy

All carriers of hemophilia should have an ultrasound scan at around 20 weeks' gestation to identify the fetal sex (if other prenatal diagnostic tests have not been performed). Should the baby be male, then care should be taken to minimize the risk of bleeding at delivery, for example vacuum (ventouse) extraction, rotational forceps, and invasive monitoring techniques, including placement of scalp electrodes, should be avoided. The mode of delivery should be for obstetric reasons and need not be by caesarean mode. The choice between vaginal and caesarean delivery is a hotly debated issue.

A cord sample should be obtained from all male infants born to known carriers for FVIII/IX estimation. Vitamin K should be given orally until it is definitely known that the baby is not affected by hemophilia.

Making the Diagnosis

Immediately following the birth of a male infant to a known carrier of hemophilia, the following tests should be performed on the cord blood:

- prothrombin time (PT);
- activated partial thromboplastin time (APTT);
- fibrinogen level;
- FVIII or FIX activity;
- where there is no family history, if the FVIII level is low, VWF assays for antigen and activity should be performed.

The APTT of an affected infant will usually be prolonged when compared with a gestation-specific normal range. FVIII levels in infants are comparable with those of adults, allowing for an accurate diagnosis. Although FIX levels in infants are considerably lower than those in adults, if the FIX level is less than 1%, a diagnosis of severe hemophilia B can be made. All neonates given a diagnosis of hemophilia on testing a cord blood sample should have this confirmed on a venous blood sample. Those with equivocal results should have a repeated test at 6 months of age.

Approximately one-third of individuals with hemophilia have no family history of a bleeding disorder. A diagnosis of hemophilia should be suspected if a child has a history of excessive bruising or bleeding, or presents with a swollen painful joint or muscle hematoma.

The majority of children with moderate or severe hemophilia will present by 4–5 years of age. Where there is no family history, it is important to exclude the diagnosis of VWD, as the Normandy variant of VWD is phenotypically identical to mild/moderate hemophilia A (although with autosomal inheritance). If this is suspected, VWF–FVIII binding assay or mutation analysis of exon 18 of *VWF* gene should be undertaken to establish the correct diagnosis (see Chapter 7).

The Neonate with Hemophilia

The neonatal period is defined as the first 28 days after delivery, irrespective of gestation. Most bleeding episodes in neonates with hemophilia are due to birth trauma. It has been estimated that 3.5–4% of neonates with severe hemophilia have intracranial hemorrhage, most associated with the presence of an extracranial hemorrhage, the risk being greater if the delivery was traumatic/vacuum assisted [7]. As yet, there is no consensus as to whether routine cranial ultrasound should be performed after delivery in neonates known to have hemophilia, or whether prophylactic factor concentrate should be given after delivery. Most clinicians would give prophylactic coagulation factor concentrate if the delivery was traumatic, instrumental, or in the presence of prematurity.

Bleeding episodes in the neonate with hemophilia occurring in the first week of birth are usually due to heel pricks performed for blood sampling, intramuscular injections of vitamin K, or after circumcision.

Clinical Manifestations and their Treatment

Bleeding Episodes

General Principles

Bleeding episodes are treated by increasing the appropriate coagulation factor to hemostatic levels. For mild hemophilia, it is often possible to use desmopressin (DDAVP) for this purpose; an infusion of DDAVP 0.3 µg/kg will increase the FVIII levels (and VWF levels) three- to fivefold. For those with moderate or severe hemophilia A or those with hemophilia B, infusions of coagulation factor concentrates are required. Pharmacokinetic studies have shown that 1 U FVIII/kg body weight increases the FVIII level on average 0.02 IU/mL (2%), whereas 1 U FIX/kg body weight increases the FIX level 0.01 IU/mL (1%). Guidelines on the management of patients with hemophilia have been published [8].

Calculating the Quantity of FVIII Required

Units FVIII to be infused = [(desired FVIII level – actual FVIII level) × patient weight]/2

For example, if a 70-kg man with severe hemophilia (FVIII less than 1%) has a muscle hematoma and the desired FVIII level is 50% of normal:

$$\text{Units of FVIII to be infused} = [(50 - 0) \times 70]/2 = 1750\text{U}$$

In practice, dosing is limited by the vial size and usually the lowest vial volume stocked will be 500 U. To avoid wastage the dose given is the nearest whole vial.

Calculating the FIX Required

Units FIX to be infused = (desired level FIX – actual level FIX) × weight in kg

Recombinant FIX has a 30% lower recovery in comparison with plasma-derived FIX. If the product to be used is recombinant FIX, then the result of the above equation should be multiplied by 1.4.

Joint Bleeds

Joints are the most common sites of spontaneous bleeding in those with severe hemophilia A and B (Figure 6.1). The affected joint is painful, warm, swollen, occasionally erythematous, and tends to be held in a flexed position. It must be appreciated that early on there may be no abnormal physical signs of a hemarthrosis, but patients often know if a bleed is starting. If treated promptly, levels of 30–50% will usually suffice to treat a minor bleed, together with paracetamol (acetaminophen) for pain. Occasionally, a second dose (8–12 h after the first) may be required. With severe bleeding, especially where the first dose was delayed, several days of treatment may be required. Table 6.2 shows the distribution of spontaneous bleeds in patients with severe hemophilia.

Table 6.2 Joints most frequently affected by spontaneous bleeds in severe hemophilia.

Joint	Frequency affected (%)
Knee	45
Elbow	25
Ankle	15
Shoulder	5
Hip	5
Other joints	5

Physiotherapy is important from an early stage to ensure muscle atrophy does not occur and to prevent the development of joint flexures. Recurrent joint bleeds usually benefit from regular coagulation factor infusions (secondary prophylaxis) in order to prevent the development of hemophilic arthropathy. In some patients, "target" joints develop (repeated bleeding into a joint, without a return to "normal" between bleeds), with chronic synovitis. Regular coagulation factor prophylaxis, physiotherapy, anti-inflammatory drugs, intra-articular steroids, or synovectomy (whether surgical, radioisotopic, or chemical) may be required to halt the cycle of recurrent bleeds and inflammation [8,9].

Despite the above, a number of patients will need joint replacement surgery; it is expected the need for this should diminish with the increasing use of prophylaxis.

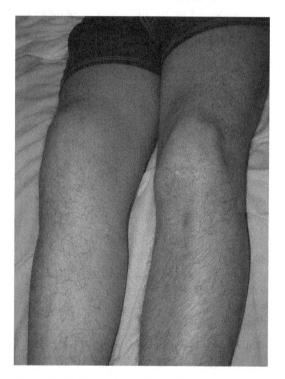

Figure 6.1 Right knee hemarthrosis in a severe hemophilia A patient. Bleeds such as this are unusual in countries where patients have home treatment with clotting factor concentrates. Usually the there are no physical signs and the only symptoms are pain and limitation of joint movement. *See Plate section for color representation of this figure.*

Muscle Bleeds

Muscle bleeds within closed fascial compartments can be limb threatening because of blood vessel and nerve compression. Bleeding into the iliopsoas muscle and retroperitoneum is not uncommon and patients present with:

- groin pain;
- hip flexion; and
- internal rotation of the leg.

Blood loss can be significant and femoral nerve compression can occur, resulting in permanent neurological deficit. Pelvic ultrasound or computed tomography (CT) scanning will confirm the diagnosis and treatment is required to raise the coagulation factor level to 100% for several days [10].

Intracranial Hemorrhage

This is the most common cause of death from bleeding in patients with hemophilia, and can occur spontaneously as well as after trauma (Figure 6.2). If suspected, or if thought to be possible following head trauma, coagulation factor concentrates should be immediately administered to raise the coagulation factor level to 100% prior to any diagnostic tests.

Hematuria

Spontaneous hematuria is relatively common in severe hemophilia. It tends to be painless and is usually self-limiting, unless clots form within the ureters. Management of the hematuria predominantly consists of maintaining adequate hydration and analgesia if required. If the hematuria fails to settle within a few days, it may be necessary to administer clotting factor to raise coagulation factor levels to 50% of normal. Antifibrinolytic drugs should not be given as these increase the likelihood of intraureteric clot formation and clot colic. The etiology of this hematuria is usually unknown, but other causes, such as infection, renal calculi, and neoplastic disease in the older hemophiliac should be considered. One of the HIV protease inhibitor drugs (indinavir) induces crystalluria and calculus formation, which can lead to hematuria.

Gastrointestinal Bleeding

Gastrointestinal bleeding tends to be caused by anatomical lesions rather than coagulation factor deficiency and should be fully investigated. Raising the coagulation factor level to more than 50% is usually sufficient. Antifibrinolytics are helpful in mucosal bleeding.

Pseudotumors

Repeated inadequately treated bleeding episodes at a single site result in the development of an encapsulated hematoma. This progressively enlarges, erodes, and invades surrounding structures, hence the name pseudotumour. Surgical removal is difficult and is associated with a significant morbidity/mortality. These are now rare in countries with ready availability of clotting factor concentrates [11].

Dental Treatment

Minor dental work (scaling and polishing) can be performed without factor replacement but inferior dental nerve blocks or extractions require factor concentrates or desmopressin administration as appropriate. Antifibrinolytic agents (such as tranexamic acid as a mouthwash) should be provided for 3–5 days after any dental extractions.

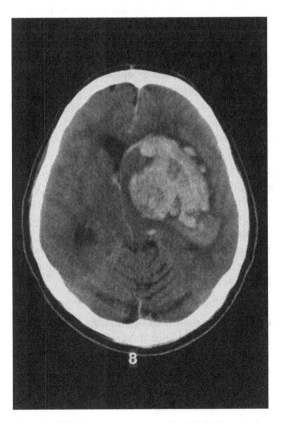

Figure 6.2 Fatal spontaneous cerebral bleed in a hemophilia B patient.

Surgery

For major surgical procedures, coagulation factor levels should be maintained at 50–100% for 7–10 days to ensure adequate hemostasis and wound healing. This can be achieved either by bolus injections, with an initial bolus dose to bring level to 100% followed by once daily FIX or twice daily FVIII injections, or by continuous infusion after the initial bolus dose, as guided by coagulation factor assays.

Continuous infusions have the advantage of:

- eliminating the "peaks and troughs" seen with bolus factor administration;
- less factor concentrate consumption for the same procedure;
- less cost; and
- more convenient for staff to administer.

One disadvantage is that these infusions tend to cause venous irritation, but this can be reduced by an infusion of saline in tandem through the same cannula. Intramuscular injections and non-steroidal anti-inflammatory drugs should be avoided.

Primary Prophylaxis

Primary prophylaxis was first introduced in Sweden by Professor Inga Marie Nilsson in the late 1950s and early 1960s. The rationale was that patients with moderate hemophilia do not develop spontaneous hemarthroses, and they also have significantly less joint arthropathy compared with those with coagulation factor levels of less than 1% [12].

It has since been shown that converting a severe hemophiliac to one with moderate disease by regular infusions of coagulation factor concentrate reduces the number of spontaneous joint bleeds, reduces the resulting joint damage [13], and is now recommended for all children with severe disease.

In the UK, prophylaxis tends to be introduced after one or two spontaneous joint bleeds, and the dose and frequency of administration is titrated to prevent spontaneous bleeding events. FVIII (20–40 IU/kg) is given ideally three times weekly (or alternate days) by intravenous infusion whilst FIX (25–40 IU/kg) usually only needs to be given twice weekly. Traditionally, prophylaxis aimed to always have a trough level over the 1% level but many nonsedentary patients prefer a higher trough level of 3–5% because this allows them to do many activities without getting bleeds.

Initially, prophylaxis is given by staff based at the hemophilia center, while training the parents (and later the child) to take over this role. In many children it is possible to manage with peripheral venous access, but in some it is necessary to use central venous access devices (e.g. Port-A-Cath). Some centers found the use of play therapists significantly increased the proportion of children managing with peripheral venous access. More recently, internal arteriovenous fistulae in the forearm such as those used for hemodialysis have been utilized for venous access because of complications of infection and thrombosis associated with central venous access devices.

Many questions around the optimal use of prophylaxis remain, including when to start, when to stop, as well as optimal dose and frequency of administration.

A significant issue is how adherent patients are to their prophylactic regimen. Whilst in childhood adherence this is very good because the infusions are administered by the parents, the level falls significantly in the teenage years, especially when boys self-administer their prophylaxis. Adherence is the preferred term to use because it implies a persons agreement to a collaborative decision between patient and health professional as opposed to compliance where a patient has to do what is recommended by the doctor.

The benefits of prophylaxis include:

- reduction in number of bleeds;
- preservation of joint structure;
- reduction in intracranial hemorrhage;
- improved quality of life.

Secondary Prophylaxis

Whilst prophylaxis is the gold standard for management of children with severe hemophilia, the issue is less clear cut for adults. A number of studies that randomized adult patients to prophylaxis or on-demand therapy showed as expected that prophylaxis was associated with a dramatic reduction in bleeds suffered by patients [14]. The cost effectiveness of adult prophylaxis remains to be demonstrated in prospective studies.

Secondary prophylaxis with activated prothrombin complex concentrate has also been shown to be effective in patients with inhibitors and this product is licensed for this purpose in several countries, including the USA [15].

Hemophilia and Aging

With improved treatment, the life expectancy of a patient with hemophilia in individuals without HIV/HCV infections is the same as that of the normal population. The result of this is that patients suffer the same comorbidities including cardiac, respiratory, renal, and psychological disease. Whilst in the past, patients with hemophilia received a lot of their nonbleeding management care from their center, it is important to recognize the role of the primary care physician in screening for diabetes, hypertension, hyperlipidemia, cancer, as well as general well being. In very old individuals, particular problems are likely to be encountered including deterioration of vision and manual dexterity, confusion, as well as difficulties that arise after the loss of a spouse.

Treatment

Clotting Factor Replacement

A landmark in the treatment of patients with bleeding disorders was the introduction of fresh frozen plasma in the 1940s which, because it contained all clotting factors, could be used to treat all clotting factor deficiencies. Over the last 70 years, the number of different products – as well as their purity – has increased significantly and in the last 20 years molecular technology has made available FVIII and FIX as recombinant proteins [16].

Table 6.3 Currently available clotting factor concentrates.

Factor concentrate	Type available
Fibrinogen	Plasma derived
Factor VII	Plasma derived and activated recombinant
Factor VIII	Plasma derived and recombinant
von Willebrand factor	Plasma derived and recombinant
Factor IX	Plasma derived and recombinant
Factor XI	Plasma derived
Factor XIII	Plasma derived and recombinant
Prothrombin complex	Plasma derived
Activated prothrombin complex	Plasma derived

Products in development include factor V, and factor X, as well as recombinant porcine FVIII

Plasma-Derived Concentrates

Human plasma-derived concentrates are made from pools with each containing up to 30 000 plasma donations. Table 6.3 lists currently available concentrates.

Transfusion-transmitted infection is the major potential complication of plasma-derived clotting factor concentrates. Because of this, all plasma-derived concentrates undergo viral inactivation by at least one and preferably two different viral inactivation procedures. Table 6.4 lists some of the currently used viral inactivation procedures. Although in the past some of the procedures were not very effective in eliminating all pathogenic viruses, the currently used ones are highly efficient in this respect.

Recombinant Products

Recombinant clotting factors are produced by the insertion of the relevant gene into a mammalian cell line (Chinese hamster ovary (CHO), baby hamster kidney (BHK), or human embryonic

Table 6.4 Viral inactivation and removal techniques.

Heat treatment

    Dry heat at 80°C for 72 hours

    Heat in solution at 60°C for 10 hours (pasteurization)

    Vapor heat at 60°C for 10 hours, 1160 mbar pressure

Solvent detergent treatment

    TNBP and Tween

    Triton X-100

    Cholate

Nanofiltration

Chromatographic purification

    Monoclonal antibody

    Heparin affinity

    Ion exchange

kidney cell (HEK293)). Following cell culture, the clotting factor is secreted into and harvested from the culture medium. Recombinant concentrates are currently available for factors VIII, IX, VII (as activated FVII), and FXIII. Early preparations of recombinant concentrates contained human albumin as a stabilizer and used animal proteins during the manufacturing process (first-generation products). Second-generation recombinant clotting factors are stabilized without the addition of human albumin but have albumin in the cell culture medium. In third-generation products, human and animal proteins have been entirely removed from the culture media. As for plasma-derived products, all recombinant clotting factor concentrates undergo viral inactivation.

Other Hemostatic Agents

Cryoprecipitate and Fresh Frozen Plasma

Hemophilia care should be delivered from hemophilia centers with access to at least plasma-derived, virally inactivated clotting factor concentrates. In resource-poor countries and in developed countries in an emergency (if FVIII concentrate is unavailable), cryoprecipitate can be used as the source of FVIII, but it must be appreciated that each cryoprecipitate unit contains only 80–100 IU of FVIII and it is not virally inactivated. In the absence of FIX concentrates, fresh frozen plasma (preferably virally inactivated) should be used for hemophilia B patients.

Desmopressin

Desmopressin (DDAVP) is a vasopressin analogue that can release stored FVIII and VWF from endothelial cells. It can be given intravenously (0.3 µg/kg as an infusion over 30 min), subcutaneously (0.3 µg/kg), or intranasally. It is useful in the management of mild hemophilia A, type 1 VWD and some patients with platelet function defects. DDAVP administration can be repeated over a short period but efficacy will then decrease because of tachyphylaxis. However, a few days later the endothelial stores are replenished, and original efficacy is re-established.

Common adverse effects include a mild headache, flushing, and fluid retention, so patients should be advised to reduce their fluid intake in the subsequent 12–24 h. Because of the problem with fluid retention, DDAVP should be avoided in children under the age of 2 years.

Tranexamic Acid

Tranexamic acid is an antifibrinolytic agent that can be given orally or intravenously. It is very useful where there is mucosal bleeding and should be routinely administered to patients with hemophilia having dental extractions.

Complications of Treatment

Despite the success of concentrate treatment, a number of complications occur and these are summarized in Table 6.5 [17].

Inhibitor Development

Alloantibodies to FVIII develop in up to 30% of children with severe hemophilia A who receive treatment with FVIII concentrate. In mild or moderate hemophilia A, antibodies to FVIII can develop in approximately 15% of patients who have received repeated treatment with FVIII; in some instances in nonsevere hemophiliacs, these alloantibodies crossreact with autologous FVIII. Anti-FIX antibodies are rare in hemophilia B

Table 6.5 Complications of clotting factor therapy.

Alloantibody formation – inhibitor development

Infections

  HIV

  Hepatitis A, B, C, D

  Parvovirus B19

  ? variant Creutzfeldt–Jakob disease

Immune modulation

Thrombosis

Allergic reactions including anaphylaxis

patients (less than 3%). These antibodies (inhibitors) are more likely to develop:

- before the age of 5 years;
- within the first 50 treatment days;
- in those of African descent;
- where there is a family history of inhibitor development; or
- in patients with FVIII/IX gene deletions.

They are usually suspected when a previously effective treatment is no longer sufficient to achieve hemostasis. The prolonged APTT does not normalize *in vitro* after the addition of normal plasma and confirmation is with the Bethesda assay [18].

The treatment of acute bleeding in patients with inhibitors is difficult and expensive. It depends on the level of the inhibitor and whether it is a low or a high-responding antibody.

High-responding patients develop a rapidly increasing antibody level each time they are exposed to human FVIII. The two main types of treatment of acute bleeding in these patients are:

1) activated prothrombin complex concentrates such as FEIBA; and
2) recombinant FVIIa (NovoSeven).

A comparative study found that the two products are equally effective but some patients respond better to one than the other product [19]. Other than through clinical response, there is currently no reliable widely used method to monitor treatment with these products in the laboratory, although global assays such as thrombin generation and thromboelastometry are showing promise.

Porcine FVIII concentrate is also useful in patients without a crossreacting antibody to porcine FVIII. Although currently not available as a plasma product, a recombinant porcine FVIII product is undergoing clinical trials.

In every patient with an inhibitor, the possibility of elimination through immune tolerance should be considered. There are three immune tolerance protocols available:

1) *high-dose protocol:* administers FVIII daily;
2) *low-dose protocol:* alternate daily administration; or
3) *Malmo protocol:* FVIII is combined with intravenous immunoglobulin, cyclophosphamide, and immunoadsorption or plasmapheresis.

The reported success rates from small series are 30–80%. Once an inhibitor has been eliminated the chance of it recurring is 15%. The International Immune Tolerance Induction Study in patients with severe hemophilia A and inhibitors compared the low and high-dose immune tolerance regimens. Although patients on the high-dose regimen had less bleeds during immune tolerance induction the chance of inhibitor eradication was the same in the two groups [20]. Rituximab (a monoclonal anti-CD20 antibody) treatment has been tried in some hemophilia patients with inhibitors with varying success [21].

Infections

The viral inactivation of concentrates introduced in 1985 was highly effective in eliminating most transfusion-transmitted viruses. The risk of infection in patients treated prior to 1985 was 25–70% for HIV, 100% for hepatitis C, and 50% for hepatitis B.

Human Immunodeficiency Virus (HIV)

The transmission of HIV infections by plasma-derived concentrates in the early 1980s has had a devastating effect in the lives of patients with hemophilia. Approximately two-thirds of the HIV-infected individuals have now died but in those alive, the use of highly active antiretroviral therapy (HAART) has allowed near-normal existence with immune reconstitution and a dramatically reduced mortality.

Hepatitis C

For hepatitis C:

- 15% of patients infected cleared the virus naturally (antibody positive but PCR negative).
- 85% were chronically infected (persistence more than 6 months).
- Approximately 20–30% of infected patients have evidence of cirrhosis.
- 5–10% have developed liver failure or hepatocellular carcinoma.

Factors accelerating liver disease progression include:

- time since infection;
- older age at infection;
- HIV coinfection; and
- higher alcohol consumption.

Treatment with pegylated interferon and ribavirin achieves cure of hepatitis C in 30–40% of those infected with HCV genotype 1 and 70% of those infected with genotype 2 or 3. The addition of boceprevir or telaprevir to the interferon/ribavirin treatment increases the response to 70–80%. A problem with the current therapies, however, are the side-effects associated with the treatment, especially anemia, skin rashes, depression, and flu-like symptoms. Recently new, highly-effective, oral, interferon-free anti-HCV treatments with minimal side-effects and high eradication rates have been introduced [22].

Hepatitis B

Approximately 50% of hemophilic patients treated with pooled plasma products prior to viral inactivation were infected with hepatitis B virus, but most cleared the virus spontaneously – less than 5% of these patients show active chronic hepatitis B virus infection. All nonimmune and noninfected hemophilic patients that could potentially be treated with plasma derived products should be vaccinated against this virus.

Parvoviruses

Parvovirus B19 causes fifth disease in childhood and most adults show evidence of past infection. Although the disease itself is relatively minor, its importance lies in the fact that the virus is resistant to all currently used viral inactivation techniques. The implication of this is that unknown viruses can theoretically be transmitted by all currently available plasma derived clotting factor concentrates, and this is one of the main reasons for the introduction of recombinant concentrates in countries where alternative "safe" plasma-derived concentrates exist. More recently it has been shown that another parvovirus, PERV4, probably can be transmitted by fractionated blood products [23].

Variant Creutzfeldt–Jakob Disease

Variant Creutzfeldt–Jakob disease (vCJD) is a prion disease that is the human equivalent of the bovine spongiform encephalopathy (BSE), which was endemic in the British cow population in the late 1980s and early 1990s. vCJD can be transmitted through transfusion of fresh cellular components. A significant number of UK hemophiliacs have been exposed to plasma from donors who subsequently developed vCJD. A single patient with hemophilia A was found to have prions in his spleen; he was asymptomatic from vCJD and received multiple transfusions of red cell cells as well as FVIII concentrate [24]. The prevalence of prions in lymphoid tissue of asymptomatic UK subjects is 1 in 2000 [25].

Immune Modulation

In vitro it is possible to show that concentrates exert an immunosuppressive effect. This has been observed and reported in patients with hemophilia but this phenomenon could have been a result of the chronic hepatitis C affecting the individuals studied.

Thrombosis

Thrombosis is a rare complication that was well recognized when prothrombin complex concentrates were used to cover surgery in patients with hemophilia B, prior to the addition of antithrombin and heparin to the product. It is still seen in patients treated with activated prothrombin complex concentrates, especially when the daily dosage exceeds 200 IU/kg. Thromboses have been reported with activated FVIIa, especially when used in patients without inherited bleeding disorders.

Anaphylaxis

Allergic reactions to concentrates are now very rare because of the higher purity of the products. Although it used to occur with the administration of porcine plasma-derived FVIII, this is not currently available. Anaphylaxis remains a problem with recombinant FIX concentrate in severe hemophilia B patients, especially those with *F9* gene deletions. The first 20 treatments of newly diagnosed hemophilia B patients should be administered in hospital or at a location with resuscitation facilities.

Acquired Hemophilia A

Acquired hemophilia is a rare bleeding disorder caused by the development of specific autoantibodies that are capable of inhibiting the action of naturally occurring FVIII. Its incidence is 1.5 per million population per year [26]. It is largely a disease of the elderly. Patients with malignancy or autoimmune disorders are more likely to be affected. Less than 10% of all cases occur in the postpartum period [27].

Patients present with prominent subcutaneous hematomas as well as bleeding elsewhere (Figure 6.3). Unlike classic hemophilia, hemarthroses are rare. There is prolongation of the APTT, which does not correct following the *in vitro* addition of normal plasma. The FVIII level is reduced, but rarely to less than 2%. The Bethesda assay demonstrates an inhibitor but the degree of bleeding is often more severe than suggested by the inhibitor or FVIII level.

Treatment is aimed at stopping the acute bleeding and eliminating the inhibitor. Acute bleeds are treated with activated prothrombin

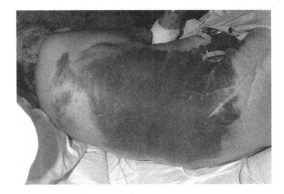

Figure 6.3 Extensive spontaneous subcutaneous hematoma in a patient with acquired hemophilia A. In contrast to congenital hemophilia, these patients often present with extensive subcutaneous bleeds and rarely have hemarthroses. *See Plate section for color representation of this figure.*

complex concentrates or recombinant FVIIa. The efficacy of these two treatments is similar. DDAVP and high doses of FVIII concentrate are rarely helpful in acquired hemophilia. The most common method used to eliminate the inhibitor is immunosuppression with the use of high-dose steroids (prednisolone 1 mg/kg/day) with or without low-dose cytotoxic therapy (cyclophosphamide or azathioprine). Other treatments such as cyclosporine, mycophenolate, and intravenous immunoglobulin (0.4 mg/kg/day for 5 days) may be useful in nonresponsive individuals.

The monoclonal anti-CD20 antibody rituximab has been shown to be effective in the elimination of acquired inhibitors, but its precise role in practice remains to be established. There are no clinical trials comparing its effectiveness prospectively to standard therapy with steroids.

Over 80% of patients achieve remission from the disease but 20% of these relapse. Most patients with acquired hemophilia die within 1–2 years of diagnosis, from comorbid conditions rather than bleeding, which is actually a rare cause of death in this condition, occurring in <10% of patients. In acquired hemophilia more patients die from the complications of immunosuppression than from the disease itself [27].

The Future

Undoubtedly, hemophilia care in the western world is currently the best it has ever been and the clotting factor concentrates have never been safer. As the patents for the first recombinant FVIII and IX run out we are likely to see new biosimilar concentrates from manufacturers new to the hemophilia market.

The major recent development in clotting factor concentrates is the introduction of long acting products. In the case of hemophilia A, the prolongation of FVIII half life by 1.5 times is achieved by pegylation, fusion to the neonatal Fc receptor or albumin, or by producing a single-chain FVIII. The longer half-life is more impressive for FIX, where up to fivefold longer action is achieved by pegylation or fusion of the FIX molecule to the neonatal Fc receptor or albumin [28].

Finally, an exciting new development is likely to be the wider use of gene therapy in clinical trials. Nathwani and colleagues were able to use an AAV8 vector to deliver the FIX gene to the liver by peripheral vein injection in patients with hemophilia B [29]. These individuals were able to produce enough FIX to allow them to stop prophylaxis and dramatically reduce their factor usage for at least 3 years after infusion. Despite this early success it is likely that routine licensed gene therapy is still several years away.

References

1 Mannucci PM, Tuddenham EG. The hemophilias: from royal genes to gene therapy. *N Engl J Med* 2001; 344: 1773–1779.

2 Shen BW, Spiegel PC, Chang CH, *et al.* The tertiary structure and domain organization of coagulation FVIII. *Blood* 2008; 111: 1240–1247.

3 Leuer M, Oldenburg J, Lavergne JM, *et al.* Somatic mosaicism in hemophilia A: a fairly common event. *Am J Hum Genet* 2001; 69: 75–87.

4 Lee CA, Chi C, Pavord SA, *et al.* The obstetric and gynaecological management of women with inherited bleeding disorders – review with guidelines produced by a taskforce of UK Haemophilia Centre Doctors Organization. *Haemophilia* 2006: 12: 301–336.

5 Tsui NBY, Kadir RA, Allen Chan KC, *et al.* Noninvasive prenatal diagnosis of hemophilia by microfluidics digital PCR analysis of maternal plasma DNA. *Blood* 2011; 117: 3684–3691.

6 Michaelides K, Tuddenham EG, Turner C, *et al.* Liver birth following the first mutation specific preimplantation genetic diagnosis for haemophilia A. *Thromb Haemost* 2006; 95: 373–379.

7 Ljung RC. Intracranial haemorrhage in haemophilia A and B. *Br J Haematol* 2008; 140: 378–384.

8 Srivastava A, Brewer AK, Mauser-Bunschoten EP, *et al.* Guidelines for the management of hemophilia. *Haemophilia* 2013; 19: e1–47.

9 Llinas A. The role of synovectomy in the management of a target joint. *Haemophilia* 2008; 14 (Suppl. 3): 177–180.

10 Sorensen B, Benson GM, Bladen M, *et al.* Management of muscle haematomas in paitents with severe haemophilia in an evidence poor world. *Haemophilia* 2012; 18: 598–606.

11 Rodriguez-Merchan EC. Haemophilic cysts (pseudotumours). *Haemophilia* 2002; 8: 393–401.

12 Ljung R. Paediatric care of the child with hemophilia. *Haemophilia* 2002; 8: 178–182.

13 Manco-Johnson MJ, Abshire TC, Shapiro AD, *et al.* Prophylaxis versus episodic treatment to prevent joint disease in boys with severe hemophilia. *N Engl J Med* 2007; 357: 535–544.

14 Manco-Johnson MJ, Kempton CL, Reding MT, *et al.* Randomized, controlled, parallel-group trial of routine prophylaxis vs. On-demand treatment with sucrose formulated recombinant factor VIII in adults with severe hemophilia A (SPINART). *J Thromb Haemost* 2013; 11: 1119–1127.

15 Leissinger C, Gringeri A, Antmen B, *et al.* Anti-inhibitor coagulant complex prophylaxis in hemophilia with inhibitors. *New Engl J Med* 2011; 365: 1684–1692.

16 Keeling D, Tait R, Makris M. Guideline on the selection and use of therapeutic products to treat haemophilia and other hereditary bleeding disorders. *Haemophilia* 2008; 14: 671–684.

17 Mannucci PM. Hemophilia and related bleeding disorders: a story of dismay and success. *Am Soc Hematol Educ Program* 2002; 2002: 1–9.

18 Collins PW, Chalmers E, Hart D, *et al.* Diagnosis and treatment of factor VIII and IX inhibitors in congenital haemophilia: (4th edition). *Br J Haematol* 2013; 160: 153–170.

19 Astermark J, Donfield DM, DiMichele DM, *et al.* A randomised comparison of bypassing agents in hemophilia complicated by an inhibitor: the FEIBA NovoSeven comparative (FENOC) study. *Blood* 2007; 109: 546–557.

20 Hay CRM, DiMichele DM, on behalf of the International Immune Tolerance Study. The principal results of the international immune tolerance study: a randomized dose comparison. *Blood* 2012; 119: 1335–1344.

21 Franchini M, Mengoli C, Lippi G, *et al.* Immune tolerance with rituximab in congenital haemophilia with inhibitors: a systematic literature review based on individual patients' analysis. *Haemophilia* 2008; 14: 903–912.

22 Afdhal NH, Zeuzem S, Schooley RT, *et al.* The new paradigm of hepatitis C therapy: integration of oral therapies into best practices. *J Viral Hepat* 2013; 20: 745–760.

23 Norja P, Lassila R, Makris M. Parvovirus transmission by blood products – a cause for concern? *Br J Haematol* 2012; 159: 385–393.

24 Peden A, McCardle L, Head MW, *et al.* Variant CJD infection in the spleen of a neurologically asymptomatic UK adult patient with haemophilia. *Haemophilia* 2010; 16: 296–304.

25 Gill NO, Spencer Y, Richard-Loendt A, *et al.* Prevalent abnormal prion protein in human appendixes after bovine spongiform encephalopathic epizootic: large scale survey. *BMJ* 2013; 347: f5675.

26 Collins PW, Hirsch S, Baglin TP, *et al.* Acquired haemophilia A in the United Kingdom: a 2 year national surveillance study of the United Kingdom Haemophilia Centre Doctors' Organisation. *Blood* 2007; 109: 1870–1877.

27 Collins PW, Chalmers E, Hart D, *et al.* Diagnosis and management of acquired coagulation inhibitors: a guideline from UKHCDO. *Br J Haematol* 2013; 162: 758–773.

28 Escobar MA. Advances in the treatment of inherited coagulation disorders. *Haemophilia* 2013; 19: 648–659.

29 Nathwani AC, Tuddenham EGD, Rangarajan S, *et al.* Adenovirus-associated virus vector-mediated gene transfer in hemophilia B. *New Engl J Med* 2011; 365: 2357–2365.

7

Von Willebrand Disease

Giancarlo Castaman, Alberto Tosetto and Francesco Rodeghiero

Key Points

- von Willebrand disease is caused by mutation(s) in *VWF* gene and results in variable decrease/abnormality of FVIII and/or VWF.
- The heterogeneity of the laboratory and clinical phenotypes is explained by a complex interplay between a specific mutation and its effect on cellular synthesis, storage, secretion, and clearance of VWF.
- Quantitative estimation of bleeding symptoms is highly desirable during the diagnostic work-up and to predict the severity of bleeding tendency.
- The bleeding risk associated with VWD correlates with the degree of FVIII and VWF levels.
- Desmopressin is the treatment of choice for the majority of type 1 VWD, while VWF/FVIII concentrates are needed when desmopressin is ineffective (mainly type 2 and 3 VWD).

Introduction: The Von Willebrand Factor

von Willebrand disease (VWD) is caused by a deficiency and/or abnormality of von Willebrand factor (VWF) and represents the most frequent inherited bleeding disorder [1]. VWF is synthesized by endothelial cells and megakaryocytes. Its gene includes about 178 kilobases with 52 exons and is located at chromosome 12p13.2. A noncoding homologous pseudogene has been

identified in chromosome 22, which spans the gene sequence from exon 23 to 34 [2]. The primary product of the *VWF* gene is a 2813 amino acid protein comprising a signal peptide of 22 amino acids (also called prepeptide), a large propeptide of 741 amino acids (also called propeptide), and a mature VWF subunit of 2050 amino acids. Four types of repeated molecular domains (D1, D2, D′, D3, A1, A2, A3, D4, B, C1, C2) of cDNA are responsible for the different binding functions of the molecule. A revised annotation of the VWF structure, also using electron microscopy techniques, revealed a globular structure of the A domains, while an intertwined assembly of A3-CK domains occurs where a series of C domains separate the A3-D4 region and the CK domain, thus rendering the protein more flexible [3].

The building block of VWF multimers is a dimer made by two single-chain pro-VWF molecules, joined through disulfide bonds within their C-terminal region. This reaction occurs after the cleavage of the signal peptide and the subsequent translocation and glycosylation of the precursor molecules into the endoplasmic reticulum. The pro-VWF dimers are then transported to the Golgi apparatus, where, after further post-translational modifications, including processing of high mannose oligosaccharides, they are polymerized into very large molecules up to a molecular weight of $20\,000 \times 10^3$ through disulphide bonds connecting the two N-terminal ends of each dimer. After polymerization, pro-VWF multimers move to the trans-Golgi

Practical Hemostasis and Thrombosis, Third Edition. Edited by Nigel S. Key, Michael Makris and David Lillicrap.
© 2017 John Wiley & Sons, Ltd. Published 2017 by John Wiley & Sons, Ltd.

network, where the propeptide, is cleaved off by a paired amino acid-cleaving enzyme (PACE or furin), and remains, at least within the cell, non-covalently associated with VWF [4].

VWF is secreted from the cell via a constitutive and a regulated pathway. The latter is used for a rapid stimuli-induced release (e.g., by desmopressin through its binding to vasopressin V2 receptor of endothelial cells) from specialized storage organelles of endothelial cells known as Weibel–Palade bodies. Only Weibel–Palade bodies or α-granules in platelets contain fully processed and functional VWF with "unusually large" multimers. These large multimers are usually not found in the circulation. Indeed, a specific plasma protease acts on VWF multimers released from the cell, cleaving the VWF subunit at the bond between Tyr 1605 and Met 1606, thus creating the full spectrum of circulating VWF species, ranging from the single dimer to multimers made of up to 20 dimers in each VWF multimer [5].

In addition to endothelial cells, megakaryocytes, and platelets, VWF is present in the subendothelial matrix, where it is bound through specific regions in its A1 and A3 domains to different types of collagen.

Physiological Role of VWF

VWF is essential for platelet–subendothelium adhesion and platelet-to-platelet cohesion and aggregation in vessels with elevated shear stress [6]. Adhesion is promoted by the interaction of a region of the A1 domain of VWF with platelet GpIb. It is thought that high shear stress is able to activate the A1 domain of the collagen-bound VWF by stretching VWF multimers into a filamentous form. The interaction between GPIb and VWF can be mimicked by the addition of the antibiotic ristocetin, which promotes the binding of VWF to GPIb present on fresh or formalin-fixed platelet suspensions. Aggregation of platelets within the growing hemostatic plug is promoted by the interaction with a second receptor on platelets, GPIIb-IIIa (or integrin $a_{II}b\beta_3$), which after activation binds

to VWF and fibrinogen, recruiting more platelets into a stable plug. Both of these binding activities of VWF are highest in the largest VWF multimers.

VWF is the carrier of factor VIII (FVIII) in plasma. VWF protects FVIII from proteolytic degradation, prolonging its half-life in the circulation and efficiently localizing it at the site of vascular injury [7]. Each monomer of VWF has one binding domain, located in the first 272 amino acids of the mature subunit (D′ domain), that is able to bind one FVIII molecule. *In vivo*, however, only 1–2% of available monomers are occupied by FVIII. This explains why high-molecular-weight multimers are not essential for the carrier function of FVIII, although one would expect that molecules of the highest molecular weight should be most effective in localizing FVIII at the site of vascular injury. In any case, any change in plasma VWF level is usually associated with a concordant change in FVIII plasma concentration.

Classification of VWD

The current nomenclature of the FVIII/VWF complex, as recommended by the International Society on Thrombosis and Hemostasis, is summarized in Table 7.1 [8]. The current revised classification of VWD identifies two major categories, characterized by quantitative (type 1 and 3) or qualitative (type 2) VWF defects (Table 7.2). Partial quantitative deficiency of VWF in plasma and/or platelets identifies type 1 VWD, whereas type 3 VWD is characterized by total absence or trace amounts of VWF in plasma and platelets. Type 1 is easily distinguished from type 3 by its milder VWF deficiency (usually in the range of 20–40%), the autosomal dominant inheritance pattern, and the presence of milder bleeding symptoms. Among type 2 variants, four subtypes have been identified reflecting different pathophysiological mechanisms. Classical type 2A is characterized by the absence of high- and intermediate-molecular-weight (HMW) multimers of VWF in plasma. Type 2B is characterized by an increased

Table 7.1 Recommended nomenclature of factor VIII/ von Willebrand factor complex.

Factor VIII	
Protein	VIII
Antigen	VIII: Ag
Function	VIII: C
von Willebrand factor	
Mature protein	VWF
Propeptide	VWFpp
Antigen	VWF: Ag
Ristocetin cofactor activity	VWF: RCo
Collagen binding capacity	VWF: CB
FVIII binding capacity	VWF: FVIIIB

Table 7.2 Classification of von Willebrand disease.

Quantitative deficiency of von Willebrand factor (VWF)

Type 1: Partial quantitative deficiency of VWF (about 70–75% of VWD patients)
Type 3: Virtually complete deficiency of VWF (about 1–2% of VWD patients)

Qualitative deficiency of VWF

Type 2: Qualitative deficiency of VWF (about 25–30% of VWD patients)
Type 2A: Qualitative variants with decreased platelet-dependent function associated with the absence of high- and intermediate-molecular-weight VWF multimers
Type 2B: Qualitative variants with increased affinity for platelet GPIb, with the absence of high-molecular-weight VWF multimers
Type 2M: Qualitative variants with decreased platelet-dependent function not caused by the absence of high-molecular-weight VWF multimers
Type 2N: Qualitative variants with markedly decreased affinity for FVIII

Source: modified from Sadler *et al.* 2006 [8].

affinity of VWF for platelet GpIbα, associated with variable removal of HMW multimers from plasma. As a consequence, ristocetin-induced platelet aggregation (RIPA) in platelet-rich plasma from these patients occurs at low ristocetin concentrations. This type must be differentiated from platelet-type VWD, which shows the same enhanced RIPA. However, in this disorder mutations in the GPIbα gene produce platelets with enhanced affinity for a normal VWF. The identification of variants with decreased platelet-dependent function and the presence of normal multimers on gel electrophoresis have required the addition of a new subtype, called 2M. Type 2N (Normandy) shows a full array of multimers because the defect lies in the N-terminal region of the VWF, where the binding domain for FVIII resides. This subtype is phenotypically identified only by tests exploiting FVIII-VWF binding.

Genetics and Molecular Biology of VWD

The first mutations observed in patients with VWD were detected in exon 28 of the VWF gene, which codes for the A1 and A2 domains of mature VWF, responsible for the interaction with platelet receptor GPIbα. Most type 2A cases are due to missense mutations in the A2 domain. In particular, R1597W or Q or Y and S1506L represent about 60% of cases. Expression experiments have demonstrated two possible mechanisms [9]. Group I mutations show impaired secretion of HMW multimers, due to secondary defective intracellular transport. Group II mutations show normal synthesis and secretion of a VWF that is probably more susceptible to *in vivo* proteolysis. However, studies suggest that type 2A results from the heterogeneous coexistence of various biosynthetic and postbiosynthetic abnormalities influencing production and proteolysis of the protein [10].

The vast majority of type 2B cases are due to missense mutations in the A1 domain causing a gain-of-function of the mutant VWF. About 90% of cases are due to R1306W, R1308C, V1316M, and R1341Q mutations [11]. The identification of the causative mutation in *VWF* allows the clear distinction from platelet-type VWD, which presents similar laboratory features. A peculiar mutation (P1266L) is responsible for the type 2B New York/ Malmö phenotype. These patients show an enhanced RIPA, but HMW multimers are present in plasma and no thrombocytopenia occurs after stress situations. The majority of patients with the P1266L mutation have additional nucleotide substitutions, all matching the VWF pseudogene sequence. This finding has been attributed to a mechanism of gene conversion between the VWF gene and its pseudogene [12]. Usually, type 2A and 2B are autosomal dominant disorders with high penetrance and expressivity.

A few heterogeneous mutations (C1315C, G1324S/A, R1374C/H, etc.) located in the A1 domain are responsible for type 2M [11]. Furthermore, in addition to affecting the interaction with GPIbα, some mutations mainly located in the A3 domain (S1731T, W1745C, S1783A) reduce VWF binding to collagen and may also result in type 2M [13].

Missense mutations in the FVIII-binding domain located at the N terminus of VWF are responsible for type 2N. The R854Q mutation is the most frequent mutation observed, heterozygosity being present in about 2% of the Dutch population. This mutation may cause symptoms only in the homozygous or compound heterozygous state. A type 2N mutation should be considered in the presence of a marked reduction of FVIII in comparison to VWF, and is confirmed by assessing FVIII–VWF binding. Its identification is important for genetic counseling, to exclude mild hemophilia A in males and hemophilia A carriership in affected females [14].

Type 1 VWD is usually an autosomal dominant disorder, with variable expressivity and penetrance [15]. However, three distinct groups pointing to a different genetic background can be identified (Table 7.3). Group A includes cases displaying high penetrance and expressivity: linkage with a *VWF* allele is usually clear [16]. In this group, missense mutations have been described, resulting in a dominant-negative mechanism. In this model, mutant–wild type heterodimers are retained in the endoplasmic reticulum and only wild-type homodimers are released into the circulation [17]. An additional illustrative variant is represented by VWD Vicenza, formerly included among type 2M VWD cases, but now included in type 1 VWD group [8]. These patients are characterized by severely reduced plasma FVIII and VWF levels, the presence of ultralarge VWF multimers in plasma, a normal platelet VWF content, a marked increase of FVIII and VWF after desmopressin, but with a rapid disappearance from the circulation ("increased clearance") [18,19]. *In vivo* studies have demonstrated decreased cellular secretion, and a common genetic background has been identified (R1205H in the D3 domain of VWF) [20]. Group B is characterized by intermediate reduction of VWF, with variable penetrance and expressivity. This heterogeneity may indeed be explained in some cases by the inheritance of two different VWD alleles.

Table 7.3 Type 1 von Willebrand disease: heterogeneity of clinical and laboratory phenotype.

	Group A	Group B	Group C
Symptoms	Manifest bleeding	Intermediate bleeding	Mild or dubious bleeding
Cosegregation (linkage) of symptoms with low VWF/ haplotype	Invariable; VWF gene mutations usually detected	Variable	Inconsistent
VWF level	About 10 U/dL or less	About 30 U/dL	40–50 U/dL
Diagnosis	Easy, often increased VWF clearance	Repeated testing needed	Not always possible; not clinically useful in most cases
Epidemiological ascertainment	Referral-based: appropriate	Referral-based: underestimated	Cross-sectional: overestimated

VWF, von Willebrand factor.

For example, coinheritance of the R854Q mutation with a null mutation increases the severity of bleeding within a given family, so that simple heterozygotes show only minor bleeding symptoms and greater VWF levels [21]. Null alleles may be caused by frameshifts, nonsense mutations, or deletions that overlap with those identified in type 3 VWD. Group C comprises cases with borderline VWF levels and mild symptoms. In some of these families, linkage studies failed to establish a relationship of the phenotype with a given VWF allele. Therefore, it is assumed that gene(s) outside the *VWF* gene, and perhaps other nongenetic factors, contribute to the expression of a bleeding phenotype.

In 2007, the European MCMDM1-VWD and Canadian studies provided illuminating results about the genetic background of type 1 VWD [22,23]. Overall, these studies demonstrated that most of the mutations responsible for type 1 are indeed missense mutations, that the likelihood to detect a mutation was highest in patients with the lowest VWF, and that the linkage to the VWF gene was very high in these patients [24,25]. However, in about 40% of cases, no mutation in the *VWF* gene was evident, suggesting that the phenotype of VWD could be modified by other genes, or by the effect of the ABO blood group. The likelihood of finding a *VWF* gene mutation was clearly related to the plasma levels of VWF. Recently, the UK Haemophilia Centres Doctors' Organization reported similar results through a National study on type 1 VWD [26], with VWF mutations detected in 17/32 index cases (53%), compared to 55% in the MCMDM-1VWD and 63% in the Canadian study. Furthermore, some mutations (e.g., Y1584C or R924Q) shows incomplete penetrance, are strongly influenced by ABO blood group, do not consistently segregate with VWD, and are still questioned as polymorphisms in a particular population. As previously demonstrated in the Canadian study [23], a founder effect is also likely to occur in the UK families. Notwithstanding these grey areas that still require further studies, great progress has been made in elucidating the molecular bases of a large proportion of patients with type 1 VWD.

About 60% of the variation in VWF plasma is due to genetic factors, with VWF level 25–35% lower in type-O subjects than in non-O individuals [27]. Blood group plays a major role in subjects with VWF levels at the lower end of the normal range, in whom heritability is less predictable.

In type 3 VWD, in addition to mechanisms shared with some type 1 cases (see above), partial or total gene deletions have also been reported [28,29]. Notably, homozygosity for gene deletion may be associated with the appearance of neutralizing antibodies against VWF, which may render replacement therapy ineffective and stimulate anaphylactic reaction upon treatment [29]. However, the risk of alloantibody formation in patients with large deletions may not be as high as previously thought at least for some deletions [30]. In general, mutations may be scattered over the entire gene, but some mutations (e.g., 2680delC or R2535X) are particularly recurrent in Northern Europe. Several stop codon mutations, either in homozygotes or compound heterozygotes, have also been reported [28].

Prevalence and Frequency of Subtypes of VWD

Until the late 1980s, estimates of the prevalence of VWD were based on the number of patients registered at specialized centers, with figures ranging from 4 to 10 cases/100 000 inhabitants. It is generally assumed that the number of persons with symptomatic VWD, requiring specific treatment, is at least 100 per million. A few studies estimated the prevalence of VWD by screening small populations using formal, standardized criteria. A prevalence approaching 1% has been demonstrated, without ethnic differences [31]. However, the large majority of cases diagnosed by population studies appear to have a mild disease, and most of these subjects were never referred for detailed hemostatic evaluation. It remains unknown what proportion of these cases is the effect of a gene(s) outside the VWF gene influencing the circulating level of VWF [32].

About 70% of VWD cases appear to have type 1 by center series. These estimates are obviously biased because it is expected that many type 1 cases without major symptoms are not referred for evaluation, whereas almost all severe type 3 cases are followed at a specialized center. Indeed, results from the MCMDM-1 VWD study demonstrated by an accurate VWF multimeric evaluation that many of the patients previously identified as type 1 VWD had subtle multimeric abnormalities that suggested type 2 VWD [33]. However, for most of them, this evidence did not affect their treatment because they showed complete response to desmopressin administration.

In contrast to the above-reported percentages, almost all cases were represented by type 1 in population studies.

Clinical Manifestations

Clinical expression of VWD is usually mild in type 1, with increasing severity in type 2 and type 3. The incidence of bleeding symptoms in VWD has been estimated to vary from 7.5% patient-years in type 1 VWD up to 107% patient-years in type 2A VWD [34,35]. For comparison, this range roughly corresponds to the incidence of bleeding symptoms in patients with mild disorders of platelet function up to that of severe clotting deficiencies.

Mucocutaneous bleeding is the typical manifestation of the disease and may affect the quality of life, the most frequent symptoms being epistaxis, menorrhagia, easy bruising, and bleeding from minor wounds. However, clinical manifestations may be highly variable also within the same family and some VWD patients may have few or no symptoms at diagnosis. Therefore, even a negative bleeding history does not exclude the presence of VWD, particularly in young subjects, and laboratory investigation is required for the diagnosis. VWD may be highly prevalent in patients with isolated menorrhagia. Bleeding after delivery in type 1 is rarely observed because FVIII/VWF levels tend to correct at the end of pregnancy in mild type 1 cases. A few cases, however, fail to have their FVIII/VWF levels normalized and need prophylaxis with DDAVP or FVIII/VWF concentrates before delivery. Type 2A and 2B and type 3 females usually need replacement therapy postpartum to prevent immediate or delayed bleeding. When adequate surgical hemostasis is feasible, postoperative bleeding is very rare, except for type 3 patients in whom prophylactic treatment is always required. Surgery on mucosal tissues is at higher bleeding risk, and postextraction bleeding is common. Because FVIII:C is usually only mildly reduced in type 1 VWD, manifestations of a severe coagulation defect (hemarthrosis, deep muscle hematoma) are rarely observed and are mainly post-traumatic. On the contrary, in type 3 VWD, the severity of bleeding may sometimes be similar to that of hemophilia. Usually, the distribution of different types of bleeding (apart from joint bleeding) is similar among the different subtypes. However, the severity of bleeding manifestations (e.g., menorrhagia or gastrointestinal bleeding) is clearly more prominent in type 3 VWD, often requiring substitution therapy. Heterozygous carriers of type 3 VWD may experience bleeding depending on their circulating FVIII [36].

Diagnosis of VWD

The diagnosis of VWD, and in particular of type 1, may require several clinical and laboratory assessments [11,14]. The diagnostic workup of VWD can be divided into three steps: (i) the identification of patients suspected of having VWD, on the basis of data from personal and family clinical history and results of laboratory screening tests of hemostasis; (ii) diagnosis of VWD with identification of its type; and (iii) characterization of the subtype. Table 7.4 summarizes a practical approach for diagnosing and typing VWD.

Table 7.4 Practical approach to the diagnosis of von Willebrand disease (VWD).

---

1) VWD diagnosis should be considered within the context of an appropriate personal and/or familial bleeding history.

2) Other common hemostatic defects should be excluded by performing PFA or BT, platelet count, APTT, PT.

3) If personal and/or familial bleeding history is significant, VWF:RCo assay should be carried out at this stage. If not possible, VWF:Ag assay or VWF:CB assay should be performed. VWF: Ag <3 U/dL suggests type 3 VWD.

4) If any of these tests is below 40 U/dL, the diagnosis of VWD should be considered.

5) Other family members with possible bleeding history should be evaluated. Finding another member with bleeding and reduced VWF strongly confirms the diagnosis.

6) VWF:Ag and VWF:RCo and FVIII:C should be measured to assess the presence of reduced ratio VWF:RCo/VWF:Ag (a ratio <0.6 suggests type 2 VWD) or FVIII:C/VWF:Ag (a ratio <0.6 suggests type 2N VWD, to be confirmed by binding study of FVIII:C to patient's VWF).

7) Aggregation of patient platelet-rich plasma in presence of increasing concentration of ristocetin (0.25, 0.5, 1.0 mg/mL, final concentration) should be assessed. Aggregation at low concentration (≤0.5 mg) suggests type 2B VWD.

8) Multimeric pattern using a low-resolution gel should be evaluated. Lack of HMW multimers suggests type 2A and/or 2B. Presence of full complement of multimers suggests type 1 (or 2N, 2M). Absence of multimers in type 3.

9) If bleeding history is clinically significant, carry out a test infusion with desmopressin. FVIII/VWF measurements should be evaluated at least at baseline, 60 and 240 minutes from the start of intravenous infusion or subcutaneous injection. Bleeding time (or PFA-100 if available) should be measured at 60 and 240 minutes.

10) VWF genetic analysis could be advisable for differential diagnosis of mild hemophilia A vs. 2N VWD in males, hemophilia A carriership vs. 2N VWD in females, and for type 2B VWD vs. platelet type-VWD.

11) VWF genetic analysis may be required for prenatal diagnosis in type 3.

Ag, antigen; APTT, activated partial thromboplastin time; BT, bleeding time; CB, collagen binding; HMW, high molecular weight; PT, prothrombin time; PFA-100, Platelet Function Analyzer; RCo, ristocetin cofactor; VWF, von Willebrand factor.

Bleeding History

A history of mucocutaneous bleeding symptoms may be considered the hallmark of VWD, and it could therefore be considered a necessary requirement before a full laboratory assessment is initiated. It is recommended that a thorough clinical investigation on type and frequency of bleeding symptoms is collected in all prospective patients. A bleeding history could, however, be absent in those patients without any prior hemostatic challenges, as in very young subjects; in these patients, screening for VWD is recommended only when there is a strong clinical suspicion (e.g., one ore more relatives with a diagnosis of VWD). Studies on large cohorts of VWD patients have shown that a positive bleeding history is highly specific (>95%) but not completely sensitive (50–60%) for the presence of VWD. A bleeding history may be considered to be suggestive for VWD when the patient has at least three different hemorrhagic symptoms or when the bleeding score is greater than 3 in males or greater than 5 in females [37,38]. The bleeding score is a summative index accounting for both the number and the severity of bleeding symptoms that is generated by summing the severity of all bleeding symptoms reported by a subject, and graded according to an arbitrary scale (Table 7.5). Laboratory investigation for VWD should be considered only in patients fulfilling the criteria for a positive bleeding history, or in young patients with a single severe bleeding manifestation (e.g., isolated menorrhagia causing anemia) or in siblings of VWD families.

Laboratory Evaluation

In VWD patients, the platelet count is usually normal, but mild thrombocytopenia may occur in patients with type 2B. The bleeding time (BT) is usually prolonged but may be normal in patients with mild forms of VWD, especially when platelet VWF content is normal. The prothrombin time (PT) is normal, whereas the partial thromboplastin time (PTT) may be prolonged to a variable degree, depending on the plasma FVIII levels and the sensitivity of the

Table 7.5 Grades of bleeding severity used to compute the bleeding score in the ISTH Consensus Bleeding Assessment Tool.

Symptoms (up to the time of diagnosis)	SCORE				
	0[a]	1[a]	2	3	4
Epistaxis	No/trivial	>5/year or more than 10 minutes	Consultation only[b]	Packing or cauterization or antifibrinolytic	Blood transfusion or replacement therapy (use of hemostatic blood components and rFVIIa) or desmopressin
Cutaneous	No/trivial	For bruises 5 or more (>1 cm) in exposed areas	Consultation only[b]	Extensive	Spontaneous hematoma requiring blood transfusion
Bleeding from minor wounds	No/trivial	>5/year or more than 10 minutes	Consultation only[b]	Surgical hemostasis	Blood transfusion, replacement therapy, or desmopressin
Oral cavity	No/trivial	Present	Consultation only[b]	Surgical hemostasis or antifibrinolytic	Blood transfusion, replacement therapy or desmopressin
GI bleeding	No/trivial	Present (not associated with ulcer, portal hypertension, hemorrhoids, angiodysplasia)	Consultation only[b]	Surgical hemostasis, antifibrinolytic	Blood transfusion, replacement therapy or desmopressin
Hematuria	No/trivial	Present (macroscopic)	Consultation only[b]	Surgical hemostasis, iron therapy	Blood transfusion, replacement therapy or desmopressin
Tooth extraction	No/trivial or none done	Reported in ≤25% of all procedures, no intervention[c]	Reported in >25% of all procedures, no intervention[c]	Resuturing or packing	Blood transfusion, replacement therapy or desmopressin
Surgery	No/trivial or none done	Reported in ≤25% of all procedures, no intervention[c]	Reported in >25% of all procedures, no intervention[c]	Surgical hemostasis or antifibrinolytic	Blood transfusion, replacement therapy or desmopressin
Menorrhagia	No/trivial	Consultation only[b] or Changing pads more frequently than every 2 hours or Clot and flooding or PBAC score>100[d]	Time off work/school > 2/year or Requiring antifibrinolytics or hormonal or iron therapy	Requiring combined treatment with antifibrinolytics and hormonal therapy or Present since menarche and > 12 months	Acute menorrhagia requiring hospital admission and emergency treatment or Requiring blood transfusion, replacement therapy, desmopressin, or Requiring dilatation and curettage or endometrial ablation or hysterectomy

(Continued)

Table 7.5 (Continued)

Symptoms (up to the time of diagnosis)	SCORE				
	0[a]	1[a]	2	3	4
Postpartum hemorrhage	No/trivial or no deliveries	Consultation only[b] or - Use of syntocin or Lochia >6 weeks	Iron therapy or Antifibrinolytics	Requiring blood transfusion, replacement therapy, desmopressin or Requiring examination under anesthesia and/or the use of uterin balloon/package to tamponade the uterus	Any procedure requiring critical care or surgical intervention (e.g., hysterectomy, internal iliac artery legation, uterine artery embolization, uterine brace sutures)
Muscle hematomas	Never	Post trauma, no therapy	Spontaneous, no therapy	Spontaneous or traumatic, requiring desmopressin or replacement therapy	Spontaneous or traumatic, requiring surgical intervention or blood transfusion
Hemarthrosis	Never	Post trauma, no therapy	Spontaneous, no therapy	Spontaneous or traumatic, requiring desmopressin or replacement therapy	Spontaneous or traumatic, requiring surgical intervention or blood transfusion
CNS bleeding	Never	—	—	Subdural, any intervention	Intracerebral, any intervention
Other bleedings[e]	No/trivial	Present	Consultation only[b]	Surgical hemostasis, antifibrinolytics	Blood transfusion or replacement therapy or desmopressin

Source: www.ISTH.org.

a) Distinction between 0 and 1 is of critical importance. Score 1 means that the symptom is judged as present in the patient's history by the interviewer but does not qualify for a score 2 or more.

b) Consultation only: the patient sought medical evaluation and was either referred to a specialist or offered detailed laboratory investigation.

c) Example: 1 extraction/ surgery resulting in bleeding (100%): the score to be assigned is 2; 2 extractions/surgeries, 1 resulting in bleeding (50%): the score to be assigned is 2; 3 extractions/ surgeries, 1 resulting in bleeding (33%): the score to be assigned is 2; 4 extractions/surgeries, 1 resulting in bleeding (25%): the score to be assigned is 1.

d) If already available at the time of collection.

e) Include: umbilical stump bleeding, cephalohematoma, cheek hematoma caused by sucking during breast/bottle feeding, conjunctival hemorrhage or excessive bleeding following circumcision or venipuncture. Their presence in infancy requires detailed investigation independently from the overall score. PBAC, pictorial blood loss assessment chart.

PTT reagent to FVIII reduction. Whatever the results of these screening tests, VWD diagnosis always requires the demonstration of reduced VWF antigen and/or activity. The diagnosis of VWD has been greatly facilitated in the recent years by several technical developments that have made possible the measurement of VWF antigen and function in automated coagulometers. Because type 2 VWD variants are relatively common, it is recommended that laboratories measure VWF both with an antigenic and a functional assay.

VWF antigen (VWF:Ag) is measured using the enzyme-linked immunosorbent assay (ELISA) or latex-based methods. These latter methods are automatable, fast, and have a high analytical precision. The ristocetin cofactor assay (VWF:RCo) explores the interaction of VWF with the platelet glycoprotein Ib/IX/V complex, based on the property of the antibiotic ristocetin to agglutinate formalin-fixed normal platelets in the presence of VWF. Preparation of formalin-fixed platelets is cumbersome, however, and the method has been superseded by measuring the binding of patient VWF to latex microparticles coated with recombinant platelet glycoprotein Ib in the presence of ristocetin.

Both VWF:Ag and VWF:RCo have wide variation in normal subjects. VWD should be suspected when VWF:Ag and VWF:RCo are below 40 U/dL, and the likelihood of VWD is particularly high for values below 30 U/dL [14,39,40]. In type 1 VWD patients, concomitantly reduced levels of VWF:RCo and VWF:Ag are observed, because in these patients circulating VWF has a normal structure. A VWF:RCo/VWF:Ag ratio below 0.6 is considered diagnostic for the presence of type 2 VWD. Type 3 is diagnosed when VWF:Ag levels are below 3 U/dL.

ELISA for VWF:CB are also commercially available as an alternative functional test for VWF. VWF:CB activity is reduced in type 1, type 3, and type 2A defects, but not in patients with type 2M affecting platelet binding. Therefore, the use of VWF:CB is suggested mainly to differentiate type 2A from type 2M in selected laboratories.

FVIII:C plasma levels are very low (1–5%) in patients with type 3 VWD. In patients with type 1 or type 2 VWD, FVIII may be decreased to a variable extent but sometimes is normal.

Additional tests used in VWD diagnosis include the closure time (CT) The evaluation of CT with PFA-100 (Platelet Function Analyzer) allows rapid and simple determination of VWF-dependent platelet function at high-shear stress. This system was demonstrated to be sensitive and reproducible when screening for severe VWD, even though the CT is normal in type 2N VWD. Its use in the clinical setting, however, remains to be demonstrated, because it may potentially miss milder forms of VWD [41].

The VWF Scientific and Standardization Subcommittee of the International Society on Thrombosis and Haemostasis has derived recommendations for diagnostic testing that are summarized in Tables 7.6 and 7.7.

Characterization of the Subtype

For a more precise diagnosis, other assays are necessary to define specific subtypes of VWD [11,14].

RIPA is performed by mixing increasing concentrations of ristocetin and patient platelet-rich plasma in the aggregometer. Results are expressed as the concentration of ristocetin (mg/mL) that induces 30% of maximal agglutination. Most VWD types and subtypes are characterized by hyporesponsiveness to ristocetin, at variance with type 2B, which is characterized by hyper-responsiveness to ristocetin, due to a higher than normal affinity of VWF for the platelet GP Ib/IX/V complex. According to the RIPA method, type 2B VWD can be diagnosed by an enhanced RIPA (<0.8 mg/mL), whereas type 2A and 2M are characterized by reduced RIPA (>1.2 mg/mL).

VWF multimeric analysis with low-resolution agarose gels distinguishes VWF multimers, which are conventionally indicated as high, intermediate, and low molecular weight. In type 1 VWD, all multimers are present, whereas in types 2A and 2B, high and intermediate or high

Table 7.6 Basic and discriminating laboratory assays for the diagnosis of von Willebrand disease.

Test	Pathophysiological significance	Diagnostic significance
Ristocetin cofactor (VWF: RCo), using formalin-fixed platelets and fixed ristocetin concentration (1 mg/mL)	VWF-Gp Ib interaction as mediated by ristocetin *in vitro* (ristocetin, normal platelets, patient's plasma)	"Functional test"; most sensitive screening test Sensitivity low for levels <10 U/dL, difficulties in standardization
Immunological assay with polyclonal antibody (VWF:Ag)	Antigen concentration	Correlates with VWF:RCo in type 1; reduced VWF:RCo/VWF: Ag (<0.6) suggests type 2 VWD; level <3 U/dL suggests type 3 VWD
FVIII:C level (one-stage assay)	FVIII–VWF interaction	Not specific, but useful for patient management; disproportionately reduced compared with VWF in type 2N VWD
Bleeding time (Ivy method)	Platelet–vessel wall VWF-mediated interaction	Not specific; correlates with platelet VWF content in type 1 VWD
RIPA using patient platelets	Threshold ristocetin concentration inducing patient's platelet-rich plasma aggregation	Allows the discrimination of type 2B, characterized by reduced threshold; absent in type 3 at every ristocetin concentration
Multimeric analysis (low-resolution gel)	Multimeric composition of VWF	Presence of full range of multimers in type 1; high- and intermediate-molecular-weight multimers absent in type 2A and high in type 2B; multimers absent in type 3
Platelet VWF	Reflects endothelial stores	Useful to predict responsiveness to desmopressin in type 1
Binding of VIII: C to VWF	Interaction of normal FVIII with patient plasma VWF	Allows the identification of type 2N, characterized by low binding values

RIPA, ristocetin-induced platelet aggregation; VWF, von Willebrand factor.

multimers, respectively, are missing. Multimeric analysis with high-resolution agarose gels can allow better identification of type 1 and type 2A (lack of the largest and intermediate multimers) and 2M (all multimers present as in normal plasma). VWF:CB can also be used to distinguish between type 2A and type 2M if multimeric analysis is not available.

Platelet VWF plays an important role in primary hemostasis, because it can be released from alpha granules directly at the site of vascular injury. On the basis of its measurement, type 1 VWD may be classified into three subtypes: type 1 "platelet normal," with a normal content of functionally normal VWF; type 1 "platelet low," with low concentrations of functionally

normal VWF; and type 1 "platelet discordant," containing dysfunctional VWF in platelets.

Factor VIII binding assay measures the affinity of VWF for FVIII. This assay allows type 2N VWD to be distinguished from mild to moderate hemophilia A.

Type 2N VWD can be suspected in cases with discrepant values between FVIII and VWF:Ag (ratio <0.6), and the diagnosis is confirmed by a specific test of VWF:FVIII binding capacity (VWF:FVIIIB)

The level of VWF in plasma is the result of the ratio between its production and clearance. The VWF propeptide (VWFpp) dimers noncovalently associate with mature VWF multimers from which they dissociate after secretion into

Table 7.7 Other tests proposed for von Willebrand disease diagnosis.

Test	Pathophysiological significance	Diagnostic significance
Binding of VWF to collagen (VWF:CB)	VWF–collagen interaction	Correlates with VWF:RCo in type 1 VWD; some collagen preparations more sensitive to HMW multimers; not yet well standardized
Closure time PFA-100	Simulates primary hemostasis after injury to a small vessel	More sensitive than BT in screening for VWD; specificity unknown; more data needed before recommending for clinical laboratory
Monoclonal antibody-based ELISA	moAb against an epitope of VWF involved in the interaction with GpIb	Correlation with VWF:RCo not confirmed; not to be used in place of VWF:RCo
ELISA-based "VWF:RCo"	Measures interaction between VWF and captured rGpIbα fragment in the presence of ristocetin	Promising new test proposed as a substitute for VWF:RCo; validation on larger patient series required
Propeptide assay (VWFpp)	Measures the amount of VWFpp released in plasma	Increased VWFpp/VWF:Ag ratio identifies patients with shortened VWF survival after desmopressin; still for research purposes

Ag, antigen; BT, bleeding time; CB, collagen binding; ELISA, enzyme-linked immunosorbent assay; HMW, high molecular weight; moAb, monoclonal antibody; PFA-100, Platelet Function Analyzer; RCo, ristocetin cofactor; VWFpp, von Willebrand factor propeptide.

plasma. The half-life of VWFpp is around 2–3 hours, whereas normal VWF has a half-life of 8–12 hours. An increased clearance of VWF from plasma has been reported as a novel mechanism for type 1 VWD. Patients with R1205H (VWD Vicenza) show a shortened VWF survival after desmopressin (1–2 hours only), in contrast to the VWFpp half-life, which is normal [19]. Thus, an increased ratio of steady-state plasma VWFpp to VWF:Ag (ratio >3) has been demonstrated to identify patients with increased VWF clearance. Typically, they show a severe VWF reduction at baseline and a marked but short-lived VWF increase after desmopressin. In addition to R1205H, other mutations have been convincingly associated with increased clearance (C1130F, W1144G, S2179F) [42,43]. Thus, the measurement of VWFpp in plasma by an ELISA could help to identify the pathophysiological mechanism responsible for low VWF in a given patient, predicting his/her response to desmopressin. The assay is still used for research purposes, but it is

likely that it could soon be widely available to all labs dealing with the diagnosis of VWD [44].

Management of Patients with VWD

Desmopressin and transfusional therapy with blood products represent the two treatments of choice in VWD [14,45]. Other forms of treatment can be considered as adjunctive or alternative to these two modalities.

Desmopressin

Desmopressin (1-deamino-8-D-arginine vasopressin; DDAVP) is a synthetic analog of vasopressin originally designed for the treatment of diabetes insipidus. DDAVP increases FVIII and VWF plasma concentrations without relevant side-effects when administered to healthy volunteers or patients with mild hemophilia A and VWD. DDAVP has become widely used for the treatment of these diseases. It is relatively inexpensive and carries no risk of transmitting blood-borne viruses. DDAVP is usually administered intravenously at a dose of 0.3 μg/kg diluted in 50–100 mL saline infused over 30 minutes. The drug is also available in concentrated form for subcutaneous or intranasal administration, which can be convenient for home treatment. This treatment increases plasma FVIII/VWF three to five times above basal levels within 30–60 minutes. In general, high FVIII/VWF concentrations last for 6–8 hours. Because the responses in a given patient and within his/her family are consistent on different occasions, a test dose of DDAVP administered at the time of diagnosis helps to establish the individual response pattern and will permit planning of future treatment. Infusions can be repeated every 12–24 hours depending on the type and severity of the bleeding episode. However, most patients treated repeatedly with DDAVP become less responsive to therapy.

Side-effects of DDAVP may include mild tachycardia, headache, and flushing. These symptoms are attributed to the vasomotor effects of the drug and can often be attenuated by slowing the rate of infusion. Hyponatremia (with rare hyponatremic seizures) and volume overload due to the antidiuretic effects of DDAVP are relatively infrequent complications. A few cases have been described, mostly in young children who received closely repeated infusions. Even though no thrombotic episodes have been reported in VWD patients treated with DDAVP, this drug should be used with caution in elderly patients with atherosclerotic disease, because a few cases of myocardial infarction and stroke have occurred in hemophiliacs and uremic patients given DDAVP.

Patients with type 1 VWD are the best candidates for DDAVP treatment. In these patients, FVIII, VWF, and the BT are usually corrected within 30 minutes and remain normal for 6–8 hours. Response to DDAVP is assessed at least after 1 hour (peak) following the infusion and is defined as an increase of at least threefold over baseline levels of FVIII:C and VWF:RCo,

reaching plasma levels of at least 30 U/dL. FVIII:C and VWF:RCo plasma levels should also be assessed at 4 hours post-DDAVP infusion to assess the pattern of clearance of these moieties and to identify patients with increased clearance who are possible candidates for alternative or adjunctive treatments [42,43].

In other VWD subtypes, responsiveness to DDAVP is variable. In type 2A, FVIII levels are usually increased by DDAVP, but the BT is shortened in only a minority of cases. Desmopressin is best avoided in type 2B, because of the transient appearance of thrombocytopenia, although there have been reports on the clinical usefulness of DDAVP in some 2B cases. In any case, platelet count should be checked during test infusion to unravel possible nonclassical type 2B cases with thrombocytopenia occurring after infusion. In type 2N, relatively high levels of FVIII are observed following DDAVP, but released FVIII circulates for a shorter time period in patient plasma because the stabilizing effect of VWF is impaired. Patients with type 3 VWD are usually unresponsive to DDAVP, although in some patients, an increase of FVIII:C to effective hemostatic levels may occur, despite no change in the BT [45,46].

Other nontransfusional Therapies for VWD

Two other types of nontransfusional therapies are used in the management of VWD: antifibrinolytic amino acids and estrogens. Antifibrinolytic amino acids are synthetic drugs that interfere with the lysis of newly formed clots by saturating the binding sites on plasminogen, thereby preventing its attachment to fibrin and making plasminogen unavailable within the forming clot. Epsilon aminocaproic acid (50 mg/kg four times a day) and tranexamic acid (15–25 mg/kg three times a day) are the most frequently used antifibrinolytic amino acids. Both medications can be administered orally, intravenously, or topically and are useful alone or as adjuncts in the management of oral cavity bleeding, epistaxis, gastrointestinal bleeding, and menorrhagia. They carry a potential risk of thrombosis in patients with an underlying prothrombotic state. They are also contraindicated in the management of urinary tract bleeding. Estrogens increase plasma VWF levels, but the response is quite variable and unpredictable, so they are not widely used for therapeutic purposes. It is common clinical experience that the continued use of oral contraceptives is very useful in reducing the severity of menorrhagia in women with VWD, even in those with type 3, although FVIII/VWF levels are not modified.

Transfusional Therapies

Transfusional therapy with blood products containing FVIII/VWF is currently the treatment of choice in patients who are unresponsive to DDAVP [14,45]. Cryoprecipitate has been the mainstay of VWD therapy for many years. However, at present, its role remains significant only in the emerging countries, and it should preferably be prepared from virus-inactivated plasma using simple physical methods, such as methylene blue inactivation. In Western countries, virus-inactivated concentrates, originally developed for the treatment of hemophilia A, are the treatment of choice for VWD patients unresponsive to DDAVP. Several intermediate and high-purity products containing both VWF and FVIII are licensed in Europe for treatment of VWD [14]. After infusion, the half-life of FVIII:C is usually approximately twice that of VWF:Ag (~20–24 hours versus ~10–14 hours), because of the endogenous production of FVIII. A chromatography-purified concentrate particularly rich in VWF and with a very low content of FVIII has also been produced (very-high-purity VWF concentrate). The very low content in FVIII requires the infusion of a single supplemental dose of purified FVIII concentrate for the treatment of acute bleeding episodes and for emergency surgeries to ensure hemostasis. Thereafter, infused VWF stabilizes endogenously synthesized FVIII with normalization of FVIII levels after 6–8 hours, so that no further infusion of FVIII containing concentrates is necessary.

The dosages of concentrates recommended for the control of bleeding episodes are summarized in Table 7.8. Because commercially available intermediate and high-purity FVIII/VWF concentrates contain large amounts of FVIII and VWF, high postinfusion levels of these moieties are consistently obtained. Theoretically, products labeled for VWF content and with a VWF/FVIII ratio around 1 should be preferred, since the expected rise postinfusion can be easily predicted. Moreover, there is a sustained rise in FVIII lasting for up to 24 hours, higher than predicted from the doses infused. The addition of exogenous FVIII infused with the concentrates

Table 7.8 Doses of FVIII–VWF concentrates recommended in von Willebrand disease patients unresponsive to desmopressin.

Type of bleeding	Dose VWF (IU/kg)	Number of infusions	Objective
Major surgery	50–60	Once a day or every other day	Maintain FVIII >50 U/dL for at least 7 days
Minor surgery	30–60	Once a day or every other day	FVIII >30 U/dL for at least 2–4 days
Dental extractions	20–40	Single	FVIII >30 U/dL for up to 12 hours
Spontaneous or post-traumatic bleeding	20–40	Single	
Delivery and puerperium	50	Once a day	Maintain FVIII >50 U/dL for 3–4 days

to that endogenously synthesized and stabilized by infused VWF causes very high FVIII levels when multiple infusions are given for severe bleeding episodes or to cover major surgery. Episodes of deep vein thrombosis have been reported in patients with VWD receiving repeated infusions of FVIII/VWF concentrates for maintaining clinical hemostasis, especially following surgery.

These FVIII/VWF products are not always effective in correcting the BT [47]. No concentrate contains a completely functional VWF, as tested *in vitro* by evaluating the multimeric pattern, because VWF proteolysis occurs during purification due to the action of platelet and leukocyte proteases contaminating the plasma used for fractionation. Despite their limited and inconsistent effect on the BT, FVIII/VWF concentrates are successfully used for the treatment of VWD patients unresponsive to DDAVP, especially for soft-tissue and postoperative bleeding. A prospective study evaluated the choice of doses in the management of surgical patients through a careful PK analysis of 29 cases with VWD undergoing elective surgery and showed that serial dosing decisions based on preoperative median values were efficacious and safe [48]. This study demonstrated for the first time that the incremental recovery is constant over a wide range of doses of VWF/FVIII concentrate (dose linearity relationship) and that the pretreatment PK results can be used to decide the plan of treatment in these patients.

A recombinant VWF concentrate has recently completed successful clinical trials, but at present no indications on its clinical use are available.

When BT remains prolonged and bleeding persists despite replacement therapy, other therapeutic options are available. DDAVP, given after cryoprecipitate, further shortened or normalized the BT in patients with type 3 VWD in whom cryoprecipitate failed to correct the BT. Platelet concentrates (given before or after cryoprecipitate, at doses of 4–5 × 10^{11} platelets) achieved similar effects in patients unresponsive to cryoprecipitate alone, both in terms of BT correction and bleeding control. These data emphasize the important role of platelet VWF in establishing and maintaining primary hemostasis. For the rare patients with type 3 VWD who develop anti-VWF alloantibodies after multiple transfusions, the infusion of VWF concentrates may not only be ineffective, but may also cause postinfusion life-threatening anaphylaxis due to the formation of immune complexes.

Figure 7.1 summarizes a practical approach to VWD treatment.

Secondary Long-term Prophylaxis

Patients with severe forms of VWD (i.e., FVIII:C levels <5 U/dL) may suffer from recurrent hemarthroses or gastrointestinal bleeding, which may also affect patients with type 2 and the loss of HMW multimers, and may therefore benefit from secondary long-term prophylaxis. Even children with frequent epistaxis could represent

Figure 7.1 Flow-chart of a practical approach to the treatment of von Willebrand disease. Platelet count drops in type 2B after desmopressin; exclusion of type 2B with RIPA desirable. *Urine output and serum electrolytes control; caution in young children.

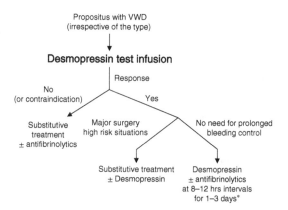

ideal candidates. The largest experience on secondary prophylaxis in VWD has been collected in Sweden in 35 patients with severe VWD, with excellent results [49]. Secondary prophylaxis was also retrospectively evaluated in a cohort of 12 Italian VWD patients, who underwent 17 long-term secondary prophylaxis periods to prevent recurrent gastrointestinal or joint bleeding, with clinical responses rated as excellent or good in 100% of cases [50].

However, prospective trials are needed to better evaluate the cost-effectiveness of this approach and the impact on patient's quality of life in comparison with on-demand therapy.

Treatment of Women with VWD

Women with VWD in childbearing age may suffer from special therapeutic problems related to physiological events, such as pregnancy and parturition [51]. Furthermore, they may undergo hysterectomy more frequently than normal women. Pregnant women with VWD are at increased risk of postpartum hemorrhage if untreated (16–29% in the first 24 hours and 22–29% after 24 hours compared with 3–5% in the general population). In patients with VWD types 1 or 2, the levels of VWF and FVIII rise two- to threefold during the second and third trimester but fall to baseline levels after delivery. Patients with the frequent VWD Vicenza and C1130F mutations show only a slight increase of these moieties during pregnancy, so that treatment with desmopressin is required at delivery [52,53]. Patients with type 2N associated with the common R854Q mutation show a complete normalization of FVIII:C, and no treatment is usually required [54]. In VWD type 2B, the increase of the abnormal VWF can cause or worsen thrombocytopenia.

In general, VWD patients should be monitored for VWF:RCo and FVIII:C levels once during the third trimester of pregnancy and within 10 days of the expected delivery date [55]. The risk of bleeding is minimal when FVIII:C and VWF:RCo levels are around or higher than 50 U/dL and these levels should be achieved prior to epidural anesthesia. In type 1

VWD pregnant women with FVIII:C levels <30 U/dL, desmopressin on the day of villocentesis, amniocentesis, and parturition, and for a couple of days there after, is advisable. In order to prevent late bleeding, VWF:RCo and FVIII:C levels should be checked and women monitored clinically for at least 2 weeks postpartum. In type 3 VWD women, VWF and FVIII do not increase during pregnancy, and thus VWF/FVIII concentrates are required to cover delivery or cesarean section. The latter should be reserved only for the usual obstetric indications. There is no apparent increased bleeding risk for neonates with VWD.

Conclusions

VWD is the most frequent inherited bleeding disorder. Definite diagnosis and characterization usually requires an array of tests and should be reserved for patients with a significant bleeding history. For subjects belonging to Group C (Table 7.3), the benefit of a definite diagnosis of VWD versus the social burden of receiving the stigmata of a congenital disorder and the related anxiety should be carefully weighed. For these cases, simply reassuring the patient that she/he does not have a severe bleeding disorder, and offering the possibility of consultation in case of need, is the preferred choice. Today, several safe and effective therapeutic options are easily available to prevent or control bleeding episodes, which rarely persistently affect the quality of life.

References

1 Rodeghiero F, Castaman G, Dini E. Epidemiological investigation of the prevalence of von Willebrand's disease. *Blood* 1987; 69: 454–459.

2 Mancuso DJ, Tuley EA, Westfield LA, *et al.* Human von Willebrand factor gene and pseudogene: structural analysis and differentiation by polymerase chain reaction. *Biochemistry* 1991; 30: 253–269.

3 Zhou Y-F, Eng ET, Zhu J, *et al.* Sequence and structure relationships within von Willebrand factor. *Blood* 2012; 120: 449–458.

4 Wagner DD. Cell biology of von Willebrand factor. *Annu Rev Cell Biol* 1990; 6: 217–246.

5 Furlan M, Robles R, Lammle B. Partial purification and characterization of a protease from human plasma cleaving von Willebrand factor to fragments produced by in vivo proteolysis. *Blood* 1996; 87: 4223–4234.

6 Ruggeri ZM. Structure of von Willebrand factor and its function in platelet adhesion and thrombus formation. *Clin Haematol* 2001; 14: 257–279.

7 Vlot AJ, Koppelman SJ, Bouma BN, *et al.* Factor VIII and von Willebrand Factor. *Thromb Haemost* 1998; 79: 456–465.

8 Sadler JE, Budde U, Eikenboom JC, *et al.* Update on the pathophysiology and classification of von Willebrand disease: a report of the Subcommittee on von Willebrand Factor. *J Thromb Haemost* 2006; 4: 2103–2114.

9 Lyons SE, Bruck ME, Bowie EJW, *et al.* Impaired cellular transport produced by a subset of type IIA von Willebrand disease mutations. *J Biol Chem* 1992; 267: 4424–4430.

10 Jacobi PM, Gill JC, Flood VH, *et al.* Intersection of mechanisms of type 2A VWD through defects in VWF multimerization, secretion, ADAMTS13 susceptibility, and regulated storage. *Blood* 2012; 119: 4543–4553.

11 Castaman G, Federici AB, Rodeghiero F, *et al.* Von Willebrand's disease in the year 2003: towards the complete identification of gene defects for correct diagnosis and treatment. *Haematologica* 2003; 88: 94–108.

12 Baronciani L, Federici AB, Castaman G, *et al.* Prevalence of type 2b 'Malmo¨'/New York' von Willebrand disease in Italy: the role of von Willebrand factor gene conversion. *J Thromb Haemost* 2008; 6: 887–890.

13 Riddell A, Gomez K, Millar C, *et al.* Characterisation of W1745C and S1783A, two novel collagen binding defects in the A3 domain of von Willebrand factor. *Blood* 2009; 114: 3489–3496.

14 Castaman G, Goodeve A, Eikenboom J. Principle of care for the diagnosis and treatment of von Willebrand disease. *Haematologica* 2013; 98: 667–674.

15 Rodeghiero F, Castaman G. Congenital von Wille-brand disease type I: definition, phenotypes, clinical and laboratory assessment. *Best Pract Res Clin Haematol* 2001; 14: 321–335.

16 Castaman G, Eikenboom JCJ, Missiaglia E, *et al.* Autosomal dominant type 1 von Willebrand disease due to G3639T mutation (C1130F) in exon 26 of von Willebrand factor gene: description of five Italian families and evidence for a founder effect. *Br J Haematol* 2000; 108: 876–879.

17 Eikenboom JC, Matsushita T, Reitsma PH, *et al.* Dominant type 1 von Willebrand disease caused by mutated cysteine residues in the D3 domain of von Willebrand factor. *Blood* 1996; 88: 2433–2441.

18 Mannucci PM, Lombardi R, Castaman G, *et al.* von Willebrand disease "Vicenza" with larger-than-normal (supranormal) von Willebrand factor multimers. *Blood* 1988; 71: 65–70.

19 Casonato A, Pontara E, Sartorello F, *et al.* Reduced von Willebrand factor survival in type Vicenza von Wille-brand disease. *Blood* 2002; 99: 180–184.

20 Schneppenheim R, Federici AB, Budde U, *et al.* Von Willebrand disease type 2 M "Vicenza" in Italian and German patients: identification of the first candidate mutation (G3864A; R1205H) in 8 families. *Thromb Haemost* 2000; 83: 136–140.

21 Eikenboom JCJ, Reitsma PH, Peerlinck KMJ, *et al.* Recessive inheritance of von Willebrand's disease type I. *Lancet* 1993; 341: 982–986.

22 Goodeve A, Eikenboom J, Castaman G, *et al.* Pheno-type and genotype of a cohort of families historically diagnosed with type 1 von Willebrand disease in the European study, Molecular and Clinical Markers for the Diagnosis and Management of Type 1 von Willebrand Disease (MCMDM-1VWD). *Blood* 2007; 109: 112–121.

23 James PD, Notley C, Hegadorn C, *et al.* The mutational spectrum of type 1 von Willebrand disease: Results from a Canadian cohort study. *Blood* 2007; 109: 145–154.

24 Eikenboom J, Van Marion V, Putter H, *et al.* Linkage analysis in families diagnosed with type 1 von Wille-brand disease in the European study, molecular and clinical markers for the diagnosis and management of type 1 VWD. *J Thromb Haemost* 2006; 4: 774–782.

25 James PD, Paterson AD, Notley C, *et al.* Genetic linkage and association analysis in type 1 von Willebrand disease: results from the Canadian type 1 VWD study. *J Thromb Haemost* 2006; 4: 783–792.

26 Cumming A, Grundy P, Keeney S, *et al.* An investigation of the von Willebrand factor genotype in UK patients diagnosed to have type 1 von Willebrand disease. *Thromb Haemost* 2006; 96: 630–641.

27 Mohlke KL, Ginsburg D. von Willebrand disease and quantitative variation in von Willebrand factor. *J Lab Clin Med* 1997; 130: 252–261.

28 Eikenboom JCJ. Congenital von Willebrand disease type 3: clinical manifestations, pathophysiology and molecular biology. *Clin Haematol* 2001; 14: 365–379.

29 James PD, Lillicrap D, Mannucci PM. Alloantibodies in von Willebrand disease. *Blood* 2013; 122: 636–640.

30 Mohl A, Boda Z, Jager R, *et al.* Common large partial VWF gene deletion does not cause alloantibody formation in the Hungarian type 3 von Willebrand disease population. *J Thromb Haemost* 2011; 9: 945–952.

31 Castaman G, Rodeghiero F. The epidemiology of von Willebrand disease. In: Federici AB, Lee CA, Lillicrap D, Montgomery RR, eds. *Von Willebrand Disease.* Oxford: Blackwell, 2011, pp. 86–90.

32 Castaman G, Eikenboom JCJ, Bertina R, *et al.* Inconsistency of association between type 1 von Willebrand disease phenotype and genotype in families identified in an epidemiologic investigation. *Thromb Haemostas* 1999; 82: 1065–1070.

33 Budde U, Schneppenheim R, Eikenboom J, *et al.* Detailed von Willebrand factor multimer analysis in patients with von Willebrand disease in the European study, molecular and clinical markers for the diagnosis and management of type 1 von Willebrand disease (MCMDM-1VWD). *J Thromb Haemost* 2008; 6: 762–771.

34 Castaman G, Tosetto A, Federici AB, *et al.* Bleeding tendency and efficacy of anti-haemorrhagic treatments in patients with type 1 von Willebrand disease and increased von Willebrand factor clearance. *Thromb Haemost* 2011; 105: 647–654.

35 Castaman G, Federici AB, Tosetto A, *et al.* Different bleeding risk in type 2 A and 2 M Von Willebrand disease: a two-year prospective study in 107 patients. *J Thromb Haemost* 2012; 10: 632–638.

36 Castaman G, Rodeghiero F, Tosetto A, *et al.* Hemorrhagic symptoms and bleeding risk in obligatory carriers of type 3 von Willebrand disease: an International, multicenter study. *J Thromb Haemost* 2006; 4: 2164–2169.

37 Rodeghiero F, Castaman G, Tosetto A, *et al.* The discriminant power of bleeding history for the diagnosis of type 1 von Willebrand disease: an international, multi-center study. *J Thromb Haemost* 2005; 3: 2619–2626.

38 Tosetto A, Rodeghiero F, Castaman G, *et al.* Impact of plasma von Willebrand factor levels in the diagnosis of type 1 von Willebrand disease: results from a multicenter European study (MCMDM-1VWD). *J Thromb Haemost* 2007; 5: 715–721.

39 Tosetto A, Castaman G, Rodeghiero F. Evidence-based diagnosis of type 1 von Willebrand disease: a Bayes theorem approach. *Blood* 2008; 111: 3998–4003.

40 Nichols WL, Hultin MB, James AH, *et al.* Montgomery RR, Ortel TL, et al von Willebrand disease (VWD): evidence-based diagnosis and management guidelines, the National Heart, Lung, and Blood Institute (NHLBI) Expert Panel report (USA). *Haemophilia* 2008; 14: 171–232.

41 Castaman G, Tosetto A, Goodeve A, *et al.* The impact of bleeding history, von Willebrand factor and PFA-100(®) on the diagnosis of

type 1 von Willebrand disease: results from the European study MCMDM-1VWD. *Br J Haematol* 2010; 151: 245–251.

42 Castaman G, Lethagen S, Federici AB, *et al.* Response to desmopressin is influenced by the genotype and phenotype in type 1 von Willebrand disease (VWD): results from the European Study MCMDM-1VWD. *Blood* 2008; 111: 3531–3539.

43 Haberichter SL, Castaman G, Budde U, *et al.* Identification of type 1 von Willebrand disease patients with reduced von Willebrand factor survival by assay of the VWF propeptide in the European study: molecular and clinical markers for the diagnosis and management of type 1 VWD (MCMDM-1VWD). *Blood* 2008; 111: 4979–4985.

44 Eikenboom J, Federici AB, Dirven RJ, *et al.* MCMDM-1VWD Study Group. VWF propeptide and ratios between VWF, VWF propeptide, and FVIII in the characterization of type 1 von Willebrand disease. *Blood* 2013; 121: 2336–2339.

45 Rodeghiero F, Castaman G, Tosetto A. How I treat von Willebrand disease. *Blood* 2009; 114: 1158–1165.

46 Castaman G, Lattuada A, Mannucci PM, *et al.* Factor VIII: C increases after desmopressin in a subgroup of patients with autosomal recessive von Willebrand disease. *Br J Haematol* 1995; 89: 147–151.

47 Mannucci PM, Tenconi PM, Castaman G, *et al.* Comparison of four virus-inactivated plasma concentrates for treatment of severe von Willebrand disease: a cross-over randomized trial. *Blood* 1992; 79: 3130–3137.

48 Lethagen S, Kyrle PA, Castaman G, *et al.* von Wille-brand factor/factor VIII concentrate (Haemate P) dosing based on pharmacokinetics: a prospective multicenter trial in elective surgery. *J Thromb Haemost* 2007; 5: 1420–1430.

49 Berntorp E, Petrini P. Long-term prophylaxis in von Willebrand disease. *Blood Coagul Fibrinolysis* 2005; 16: S23–26.

50 Federici AB, Castaman G, Franchini M, *et al.* Clinical use of Haemate P in inherited von Willebrand disease: a cohort study on 100 Italian patients. *Haematologica* 2007; 92: 944–951.

51 Kouides PA. Females with von Willebrand disease: 72 years as the silent majority. *Haemophilia* 1998; 4: 665–676.

52 Castaman G, Eikenboom JCJ, Contri A, *et al.* Pregnancy in women with type 1 von Willebrand disease caused by heterozygosity for von Willebrand factor mutation C1130F. *Thromb Haemostas* 2000; 84: 351–352.

53 Castaman G, Federici AB, Bernardi M, *et al.* Factor VIII and von Wille-brand factor changes after desmopressin and during pregnancy in type 2M von Willebrand disease Vicenza: a prospective study comparing patients with single (R1205H) and double (R1205H-M740I) defect. *J Thromb Haemost* 2006; 4: 357–360.

54 Castaman G, Bertoncello K, Bernardi M, *et al.* Pregnancy and delivery in patients with homozygous or heterozygous R854Q type 2N von Willebrand disease. *J Thromb Haemost* 2005; 3: 391–392.

55 Castaman G, Tosetto A, Rodeghiero F. Pregnancy and delivery in women with von Willebrand's disease and different von Willebrand factor mutations. *Haematologica* 2010; 95: 963–969.

8

The Rarer Inherited Coagulation Disorders

Paula H.B. Bolton-Maggs, Jonathan Wilde and Gillian N. Pike

Key Points

- The rarer inherited coagulation disorders (fibrinogen, factors II, V, VII, X, XI, XIII, and some combined deficiencies) are more variable in their bleeding symptoms than hemophilia A and B.
- Factor levels are not clearly predictive for bleeding, particularly in factor VII and XI deficiencies.
- Many of these deficiencies are not truly recessive as symptoms may occur in heterozygotes, notably in factor XI deficiency.
- These factor deficiencies are more common in communities where consanguineous marriage is common and severe cases may present with intracranial hemorrhage at or soon after birth.

Introduction

The inherited coagulation disorders hemophilia A and B (described in Chapter 6) and von Willebrand disease (described in Chapter 7) are well characterized. However, inherited abnormalities of all the other coagulation factors have been recognized but are not so well known. All are inherited autosomally and generally, with the exception of factor XI (FXI), are associated with few or no symptoms in heterozygote individuals. Most of the factor deficiencies are caused by abnormalities in the gene encoding for the particular factor. There are three interesting exceptions.

1) Combined FV and FVIII deficiency is caused by a defect in one of two genes that encode for proteins involved in the intracellular transport of FV and FVIII within the hepatic cells.
2) Combined deficiency of the vitamin K-dependent factors is a disorder caused by mutations in genes encoding enzymes involved in vitamin K-dependent carboxylation.
3) A third syndrome has been described in which production of FVII and FX are both affected by abnormalities (deletions or translocations) in chromosome 13, where both genes are located, and usually associated with other abnormalities, such as mental retardation, microcephaly, and cleft palate [1].

As all these disorders are rare (Table 8.1), most hematologists and pediatricians will have limited experience, and it is essential that the affected individuals are registered with a hemophilia center.

The annual report from the UKHCDO national database [2] shows that FXI deficiency (9% of reported patients) is more common than hemophilia B (5%), demonstrating that this should perhaps no longer be considered a "rare" bleeding disorder. The other disorders to be considered in this chapter are all rare, making up a total of 6% of patients in the UK register. The World Federation of Hemophilia (WFH) performs annual global surveys via the national patient organizations in about 100 countries.

Practical Hemostasis and Thrombosis, Third Edition. Edited by Nigel S. Key, Michael Makris and David Lillicrap.
© 2017 John Wiley & Sons, Ltd. Published 2017 by John Wiley & Sons, Ltd.

Table 8.1 Prevalence and chromosomal location of affected gene in the rare inherited coagulation disorders.

Deficiency	Estimated prevalence of severe deficiency (factor level <10%)	Chromosome
Factor VIII	133 : 1 000 000 males[a]	X
Factor IX	133 : 1 000 000 males[a]	
Fibrinogen	1 : 1 000 000	4
Prothrombin	1 : 2 000 000	11
Factor V	1 : 1 000 000	1
Combined V and VIII	1 : 1 000 000	18 (*LMAN1*), 2 (*MCFD2*)
Factor VII	1 : 500 000	13
Factor X	1 : 1 000 000	13
Factor XI	1 : 1 000 000[b]	4
Factor XIII	1 : 2 000 000	6 (subunit A) 1 (subunit B)

Source: modified from Peyvandi *et al.* 2002 [33].
a) Data from World Federation of Hemophilia, combined factor VIII and IX, all severity.
b) Higher in Ashkenazy Jews, where the prevalence of severe deficiency is estimated to be 1 in 190, and 8.1% of the population are heterozygotes [34].

Since 2004, the survey has reported some information about the rare disorders and confirms the variation in distribution in different parts of the world, with higher prevalence of these disorders in countries where consanguineous marriage is common. The global surveys can be viewed on the WFH web site (www.wfh.org).

Rare bleeding disorders have certain features in common that can be considered together.

Genetics

Most of these disorders are autosomal recessive conditions and most commonly occur in individuals whose parents are related, so therefore are much more common in ethnic groups in which consanguineous marriage is customary, such as in many Asian and Arabic communities. FXI deficiency is particularly common in Ashkenazi Jews. Heterozygous individuals have partial deficiency, which may be associated with some bleeding symptoms certainly in FXI deficiency. Only two of the disorders described below are truly recessive, with normal factor levels in heterozygotes. These are combined FV plus FVIII deficiency, and the combined vitamin K-dependent factors deficiency.

Clinical Features

As autosomal disorders, both males and females are affected. Menorrhagia is a common feature of all these disorders and many are associated with hemorrhage related to childbirth [3]. Bleeding at ovulation or from corpus luteum cysts is also reported and can be very severe [4].

Severely deficient infants with these disorders (except FXI) are particularly at risk for intracranial hemorrhage (ICH) and need to be identified quickly so that appropriate treatment is rapidly available for serious bleeding.

In general, bleeding manifestations in these disorders tend to be more variable and less predictable than in hemophilia A and B and the classification by factor level used for mild, moderate, and severe hemophilia is not applicable to these other disorders. Some of the deficiencies (FVII, fibrinogen) are associated with thrombosis, probably as a consequence of particular molecular defects, although in some instances this may be due to coinheritance of a prothrombotic disorder.

Treatment products for most of these conditions are generally not licensed and are not stocked in most hospitals. If fresh frozen plasma (FFP) is used, either because it is the only treatment option or in an emergency while awaiting a specific concentrate, it should preferably be virally inactivated (either by solvent–detergent or methylene blue treatment). As plasma products are used for treatment in most of these disorders, affected individuals should be vaccinated against both hepatitis A and B, using the subcutaneous route in order to avoid the risk of muscle hematoma associated with the intramuscular route [5].

Antifibrinolytic therapy, such as tranexamic acid, is a useful adjunct to blood products, particularly for mucous membrane bleeding, but must be used with caution in those disorders with an associated risk of thrombosis.

Guidelines covering treatment products have been published. These guidelines should be consulted for further information [6]. The WFH updated its registry of clotting factor concentrates in 2012 [7].

Pregnancy

Pregnancy and delivery should be carried out in an obstetric unit with an associated hemophilia center, or at least in close liaison with a hemophilia center specialist. Women with severe deficiency of fibrinogen and FXIII are at risk of miscarriage if not treated prophylactically during pregnancy. Good communication is essential between obstetric, hemophilia unit, and pediatric staff in order to optimize treatment for the mother and to rapidly identify and plan replacement therapy for an affected neonate [3].

Investigation

Accurate laboratory testing is important in the identification of these disorders. Sampling of neonates and young infants can be particularly difficult. It is vital to establish that a sample has been properly obtained in order to interpret the results. The use of appropriate normal ranges for infants is also essential [8]. Vitamin K deficiency will affect the levels of FII, FVII, FIX, and FX. This may need to be taken into account in interpretation of results, especially in newborn infants due to the physiological deficiency of vitamin K. Normal adult population ranges should be defined for each assay by the local laboratory. The lower limit of normal for many of these factors is higher than the frequently quoted 50 IU/dL.

Individual Deficiencies

Fibrinogen

Hereditary defects of the fibrinogen gene result in three phenotypes [9]:

1) impaired production: hypofibrinogenemia or afibrinogenemia, depending on severity;
2) synthesis of abnormally structured molecules, dysfibrinogenemia;
3) reduced production of an abnormal molecule, hypodysfibrinogenemia (rare).

Afibrinogenemia

This defect is associated with a bleeding tendency, although variable, and people with severe deficiency may have infrequent bleeding, whereas others have marked mucosal and intramuscular bleeding. Neonates may present with umbilical cord bleeding, and they may have ICH. Wound healing may be impaired. Women are at risk of recurrent miscarriage and both ante- and postpartum hemorrhage. Paradoxically, thrombosis has also been reported in severe deficiency not in relation to therapy or other provoking events. Fibrinogen replacement therapy may also induce thrombosis. Individuals with hypofibrinogenemia are also at risk of bleeding with less severe manifestations, such as bleeding after surgery rather than spontaneous events. The diagnosis of afibrinogenemia depends on demonstrating absence of fibrinogen by both functional and antigenic assays.

Dysfibrinogenemia

This is a collection of disorders with variable clinical features. Over 300 variants have been described. About 25% of patients have a mild bleeding disorder. In roughly another 25%, the specific molecular defects are associated with thrombosis [10]. The diagnosis may be difficult, although generally there is a significant discordance between fibrinogen antigen and activity values. Family studies may be extremely informative, as many dysfibrinogenemias are inherited in an autosomal dominant manner [9]. The personal and family history of bleeding and thrombosis will help guide management.

Treatment

Fibrinogen concentrates are available in some countries [7]. These are preferred to cryoprecipitate as they are treated to reduce risks of viral transmission. The half-life of fibrinogen is 3–5 days, and a level of more than 0.5 g/L is associated with a reduced risk of bleeding.

Prothrombin

Prothrombin deficiency is extremely rare [11,12]. Complete deficiency is not recorded and is probably incompatible with life (analogous to the situation in prothrombin "knockout" mice). The two phenotypes are:

- quantitative (hypoprothrombinemia); and
- qualitative (dysprothrombinemia).

Individuals with homozygous hypoprothrombinemia usually have prothrombin levels of less than 10 IU/dL and may suffer from joint and muscle bleeds and also mucosal bleeding. Heterozygotes may be missed as the prothrombin time may be normal. They are usually asymptomatic but may have excessive bleeding after surgery. Individuals with dysprothrombinemia have both variable bleeding symptoms and prothrombin activity levels (1–50 IU/dL). It is notable that about 70% of patients with prothrombin disorders are of Latin American country origin.

Treatment can be given with three-factor (II, IX, X) or four-factor (II, VII, IX, X) concentrates (prothrombin complex concentrates, originally developed for FIX deficiency). Prothrombin has a long half-life, so that treatment may be given every 2–3 days.

Factor V Deficiency

Factor V deficiency presents in childhood with bruising and mucous membrane bleeding. Infants with severe deficiency are at risk of ICH, which may occur antenatally. Reported cases appear to have a high risk of inhibitor development associated with replacement therapy. Affected children should also have a FVIII assay performed to exclude combined deficiency (see below).

Treatment is with FFP. Large volumes may be required, leading to a risk of fluid overload. The minimum level of FV required for hemostasis is at least 15 U/dL. Platelets contain approximately 20% of circulating FV and may be given, particularly in patients with inhibitors or in patients with severe bleeding not responding to FFP.

Combined Deficiency of Factors V and VIII

This interesting disorder is caused by mutations in either the *LMAN1* (70% of cases) or *MCFD2* genes, which encode for proteins involved in the intracellular transport of FV and FVIII within hepatocytes [13,14]. These gene defects result in the impaired release of these coagulation factors into the circulation. Levels of both factors are most commonly between 5 and 20 IU/dL. Severe spontaneous bleeding is relatively uncommon; bleeding after surgery is a risk. Parents have normal levels of both factors.

Treatment is with both FVIII concentrate (principles as for hemophilia A) and FFP (as for FV deficiency).

Factor VII Deficiency

This is the most common of the rare disorders (excluding FXI). People with mild deficiency (heterozygotes) do not usually have a bleeding problem. Generally, bleeding is confined to individuals with very low levels (<2 IU/dL), but the correlation of level with bleeding is not close [15]; that is, some individuals with very low levels do not bleed, whereas those with higher levels do.

Mucous membrane bleeding is particularly common. Menorrhagia is common in women. Thrombosis has also been reported. Neonates with severe deficiency are at risk of ICH [16], particularly with promoter region mutations [17]. The molecular defects are heterogeneous. Girolami has reported that different mutations may give similar phenotypes and conversely patients with the same mutation may have different phenotypes, illustrating the complexity of the genotype–phenotype relationship [11]. It is also important to note that the FVII level can vary depending on the source of the thromboplastin used in the laboratory assay and may be related to particular molecular abnormalities (e.g., FVII Padua). For example, people formerly diagnosed as FVII-deficient using rabbit brain thromboplastin have been shown to have normal FVIIC levels with recombinant human thromboplastin [18].

The recommended treatment is with recombinant activated FVII (rFVIIa) at a low dosage (10–20 μg/kg) or with plasma-derived FVII concentrate. The half-life of FVII is particularly short (6 hours) but, despite this, prophylaxis (where indicated) one to three times a week may be sufficient.

Factor X Deficiency

Severe FX deficiency (FX <1 IU/dL) is associated with a significant risk of ICH in the first weeks of life. Umbilical stump bleeding also occurs. Mucosal hemorrhage is a particular feature, with severe epistaxis being common at any level of deficiency. Menorrhagia occurs in half of affected females. Severe arthropathy may occur as a result of recurrent joint bleeds. Patients with moderate deficiency (1–5 IU/dL) have fewer spontaneous bleeds but bleed after surgery. Mild deficiency is defined by FX levels of 6–10 IU/dL; these individuals are often

diagnosed incidentally but may experience easy bruising or menorrhagia. Heterozygotes may have significant bleeding or may be asymptomatic. A number of clinical variants have been described, and FX assay by more than one method is recommended in order not to miss some variants [19].

Antifibrinolytic medication is particularly useful for mucous membrane bleeding. FX is present in prothrombin complex concentrates, which are therefore the recommended treatment. The half-life of FX is 20–40 hours. Caution is required because of the known prothrombotic properties of these concentrates. Therefore, FX levels should be monitored.

In those children with recurrent joint bleeds, prophylaxis has been successful if administered either every third day or once a week. Experience with FFP suggests that, in severe deficiency, an FX level of 20–35 IU/dL is sufficient for hemostasis postoperatively in severe deficiency, but it is likely that levels lower than this (e.g., down to 5 IU/dL) may be sufficient.

Factor XI Deficiency

The role of FXI in the coagulation mechanism is debated. FXI is physiologically activated by traces of thrombin and serves to potentiate the propagatory pathway once coagulation has been initiated via the tissue factor pathway [20]. Polyphosphates secreted by activated platelets enhance thrombin activation of FXI [21]. FXI is a serine protease that is unique in being a dimer. Although FXI deficiency is particularly common in Ashkenazi Jews, it is found in all ethnic groups. The mutations in Jewish patients are restricted, with two mutations being particularly common [22]. Overall, the prevalence of severe deficiency is 1 in 1 million, but mild deficiency is much more common. In the UK, mild FXI deficiency is reported more often than hemophilia B. This is partly because activated partial thromboplastin time (APTT) reagents are sensitive to mild FXI deficiency and there is a greater readiness to investigate these mildly prolonged APTT levels.

FXI deficiency is unlike most of the other rare coagulation disorders in that heterozygotes may have a significant bleeding tendency that is poorly predicted by the FXI level [15,20]. Spontaneous bleeding is extremely rare, even in those with undetectable FXI levels; bleeding is provoked by injury and surgery, particularly in areas of high fibrinolytic activity (mouth, nose, and genitourinary tract). Women with both severe and mild deficiency may suffer menorrhagia and bleeding in relation to childbirth. The bleeding tendency varies within both a family and an individual at different times. This may be related to mild variation in other factors, such as von Willebrand factor. These factors make the management of surgery in FXI deficiency more complicated. Babies with severe deficiency do not bleed spontaneously (ICH and other serious bleeding is not reported). Male babies are at risk of excessive bleeding at circumcision. UK guidelines recommend that the FXI level should be checked and, if less than 10 IU/dL at birth, circumcision should be delayed and the level checked at 6 months. If still less than 10 IU/dL, the procedure should be performed in hospital with FFP or concentrate cover (see below), and the religious requirements discussed with the family. If the level is more than 10 IU/dL, tranexamic acid alone can be given.

Oral antifibrinolytic therapy is very useful for the management of mucosal bleeding, especially menorrhagia, and is sufficient for the management of dental extractions, even in people with severe deficiency. The management of other types of surgery depends, to some extent, on whether it is in an area of high fibrinolytic activity (such as tonsillectomy) where FXI replacement is indicated, as opposed to other types of surgery (e.g., herniorrhaphy) where replacement therapy may be more parsimonious [23].

Two FXI concentrates are available in certain countries, but both have been associated with thrombotic events in some individuals, particularly those with additional risk factors, such as older age, the presence of cardiovascular disease, or malignancy. Because of this, antifibrinolytic drugs should not accompany them,

and peak levels of more than 70 IU/dL should be avoided. FFP can be used, but in people with severe deficiency it is difficult to produce a sufficient rise to hemostatic levels (about 20–30 IU/dL) without the risk of fluid overload.

The management of subjects with heterozygous deficiency and a bleeding history (FXI of about 20–60 IU/dL) is more difficult and is dependent on the bleeding history of the individual patient, the presence or absence of associated factor deficiencies, and the nature of the hemostatic challenge.

Inhibitors can develop in severe deficiency [24]. Low dose activated recombinant FVII (rFVIIa) has been used successfully in these individuals [25]. It may also be useful in patients without inhibitors but in standard dose has been associated with thrombosis in this setting.

Factor XIII Deficiency

Factor XIII cross-links and stabilizes fibrin and is also important in wound healing and placental attachment [26]. Severe deficiency, with undetectable FXIII, is associated with:

- a serious bleeding disorder, usually presenting in infancy;
- bleeding from the umbilical stump in 80%;
- ICH;
- joint and muscle bleeds;
- miscarriages and bleeding after delivery or surgery; and
- delayed wound healing.

For these reasons, usually, once severe deficiency is detected, an individual is treated with prophylaxis for life. Individuals with levels of 1–4 U/dL are also likely to have bleeding symptoms, and rarely bleeding is reported in people with levels above 5 U/dL. There are some data emerging suggesting a bleeding diathesis in some heterozygous individuals.

The diagnosis is suspected when the coagulation screen is normal in the presence of a significant bleeding history. Clot solubility has been used as a screening test but is unreliable, and the defect should be confirmed by a FXIII assay [27]. Because this is not a routine test in most laboratories, it is advisable to send the sample to a specialist center.

A FXIII concentrate is the treatment of choice and a recombinant FXIII concentrate has completed successful clinical trials [28]. FXIII has a long half-life of 7–10 days and, in practice, prophylactic dosing at 4 to 6-weekly intervals has proved effective. It is suggested that levels of 4–10 U/dL are sufficient to prevent hemorrhage. During pregnancy prophylactic replacement of FXIII should be given to prevent miscarriage, aiming for a FXIII level of greater than 10 U/dL.

In the emergency situation, for example when presented with an infant with a serious bleeding diathesis, once blood has been taken for testing, either FFP or cryoprecipitate is effective treatment.

Combined Deficiencies of the Vitamin K-dependent Factors: II, VII, IX, and X

Vitamin K-dependent clotting factors deficiency (VKCFD) is a rare but important bleeding disorder to recognize. The inheritance is autosomal recessive and is caused by two clinically similar subtypes of the disorder: VKCFD1 due to point mutations in the gamma- glutamyl carboxylase gene (*GGCX*) and VKCFD2 resulting from defects in the vitamin K 2-3 epoxide reductase gene (*VKORC1*). The bleeding risk correlates with factor levels, with severe bleeding symptoms occurring when factor levels are less than 5 IU/dL. Mucocutaneous and postsurgery-related bleeding has been reported. Severe cases may present with ICH or umbilical cord bleeding in infancy [29,30]. The clinical picture and response to vitamin K is variable, some responding to low-dose oral vitamin K and others nonresponsive even to high-dose intravenous replacement. In those nonresponsive to vitamin K, prothrombin complex concentrates are the product of choice. Levels of the factors range from less than 1–50 IU/dL. Some individuals have associated skeletal abnormalities as a result of reduced carboxylation of bone Gla proteins and central nervous system defects have also been reported in a few cases.

Illustrative Case Histories

Case 1

A 13-month-old infant presented with a 2-cm diameter swelling on his head and a swollen thigh caused by running into a door 2 weeks previously. He was thought to be suffering from nonaccidental injury and was admitted. Ultrasound examination confirmed a muscle hematoma. Coagulation screening demonstrated a prolonged prothrombin time (PT) of 25.4 seconds (NR 11.5–15) and APTT of 80 seconds (NR 27–39). His FX level was <1 U/dL. Both parents (who were unrelated) had prolonged coagulation tests and low FX levels. Both were asymptomatic. He was treated for the acute bleed with a prothrombin complex concentrate with monitoring of FX levels. Over the next 3 years, he had repeated muscle and joint bleeds and is now being treated with once-weekly prophylaxis. His concentrate dose is determined by regular dose–response and half-life analysis.

Comment: This case illustrates a picture similar to severe hemophilia A. Nonaccidental injury is unfortunately more common than bleeding disorders, so that, unless appropriate investigations are undertaken, diagnosis may be delayed or missed.

Case 2

A baby boy developed massive bilateral cephalhematomas 24 hours after spontaneous vaginal delivery. He was otherwise well with normal, unrelated parents. Blood tests showed a profound anemia (Hb 7.0 g/dL) and incoagulable blood with undetectable fibrinogen. Liver disease was excluded and he was not septic. Cranial ultrasound confirmed that there was no evidence of ICH. Both parents and both maternal grandmothers were noted to have low fibrinogen levels and prolonged thrombin times. He was transfused with red cells and treated with regular cryoprecipitate until fibrinogen concentrate could be obtained. He was treated prophylactically, requiring a central venous access device, but by 9 months of age, was noted to have subclavian vein thrombosis related to this. Magnetic resonance scanning demonstrated extensive thrombosis of the upper body venous system. It was not possible to determine whether therapy had contributed to the thrombotic risk. Prophylaxis was stopped for 5 months, during which time he had several bruises and was treated for minor bumps to the head, but had no serious bleeding. When he began to walk and fall, his mother was anxious for regular prophylaxis to be resumed. It is unclear whether this is necessary in the long term.

Comment: In the absence of mutation detection, it was impossible to be sure that this child did not have compound heterozygosity for hypo- and dysfibrinogenemia, which might have increased his risk of thrombosis. Mutation detection can be helpful in predicting the clinical picture in fibrinogen disorders, and will probably also prove useful in FVII and FX deficiency where the clinical picture can be variable.

Case 3

A 12-year-old girl was admitted after a heavy third menstrual period. She had been bleeding for 10 days, fainted at school, and on admission was found to have severe anemia with Hb 6.0 g/dL. Coagulation testing demonstrated a normal APTT and a PT of 41 seconds. Her FVII level was 2.2 IU/dL (2.2%). She had been adopted and had no other bleeding problems; she had not bled excessively after being bitten by a dog, requiring open reduction of a fracture of the forearm, nor after being knocked down by a car. Once her periods had become established and controlled with hormone therapy, she did not have any other bleeding problems. She defaulted from follow-up, but was seen in her 20s when she gave birth to two children. She had no further bleeding symptoms since previous review but was treated at delivery as a precaution with recombinant activated FVII concentrate.

Comment: This case illustrates that individuals with severe FVII deficiency may have very few problems and contrasts with the next case.

Case 4

An Asian baby with parents who were first cousins was delivered by cesarean section. He was noted to have nasal bleeds twice on day 3 and a bloodstained discharge from the umbilical cord on day 5. He was admitted with irritability on day 18 and collapsed on admission with Hb 8 g/dL, PT 32 seconds, APTT 39 seconds. CT scanning of the head showed ICH in the posterior fossa. His FVII level was 4 IU/dL. He was treated initially with FFP (which did not shorten the PT) until a FVII concentrate was available. He was treated symptomatically over this acute event. However, further episodes of ICH occurred over the next 2 months, leading to cerebral atrophy and predictable developmental delay. He was started on prophylaxis twice a week at the age of 6 months via a venous access device. At 4.5 years, he had a mental age of 2.5, epilepsy, no speech, and no vision on the right side as a consequence of his previous ICHs. At the age of 5.5 years, he was noted to have severe iron deficiency (Hb 6.9 g/dL, MCV 59), common in children of Asian origin (dietary), compounded by developmental problems and his bleeding disorder.

Comment: Where ICH occurs in relation to a severe congenital factor deficiency, it needs to be recognized and treated early and intensively to try to avoid long-term developmental problems. Iron deficiency is very common in the Asian community due to dietary deficiency.

Case 5

A Pakistani child with related parents was referred at the age of 1 year. She had easy bruising and bleeding from minor cuts, which lasted several hours. Her PT was 45 seconds and the APTT was 92 seconds. FV was <1 U/dL. At the age of 15 and 18 months, she had recurrent mouth bleeds from trauma associated with walking and was treated prophylactically twice-weekly with FFP. At 2 years, she had a retroperitoneal hemorrhage. At 3 years, there were concerns about her neurological development, and at 5.5 years, imaging supported the occurrence of a possible ICH in the past. At 3 years, there was evidence of a FV inhibitor and regular FFP infusions were stopped. She had recurrent muscle bleeds leading to shortening and wasting, and the necessity for tendon-lengthening surgery at the age of 7 years, by which time her inhibitor had disappeared. She continued to have recurrent muscle and joint bleeds treated symptomatically with FFP infusions (the inhibitor having resolved). Menarche occurred at age 13, and although her periods were initially not unduly heavy, they have become troublesome and required active management with antifibrinolytics and hormone therapy.

Comment: FV deficiency is difficult to manage and may be associated with the development of inhibitors, as in this case.

Conclusion

The rare coagulation disorders may present with serious and life-threatening bleeding. Prompt investigation and recognition of these disorders is essential so that the appropriate treatment can be instigated. ICH is a serious risk in many of these disorders and may have catastrophic consequences. Hematologists need to work closely with pediatricians to recognize these disorders. In communities where consanguinity is common, there needs to be a heightened awareness of the risk of these potentially serious bleeding disorders. Mutation analysis can be very helpful, as it offers the potential for subsequent antenatal diagnosis in families with severe bleeding disorders.

Acknowledgments

This chapter is based on guidelines published by members of the Rare Haemostatic Disorders Working Party of the United Kingdom Haemophilia Centre Doctors' Organization [31,32].

References

Please note that in addition to these listed below, a series of articles on the rare bleeding disorders can be found in specific issues of each of the following journals:
Haemophilia **2008: 14; 1151–1280.**
Semin Thromb Haemostas **2009: 35; 345–447.**

1 Girolami A, Ruzzon E, Tezza F, *et al*. Congenital FX deficiency combined with other clotting defects or with other abnormalities: a critical evaluation of the literature. *Haemophilia* 2008; 14: 323–328.

2 United Kingdon Haemophilia Centre Doctors' Organisation (UKHCDO). Bleeding Disorder Statistics for April 2011 to March 2012, 2012. Available at: www.ukhcdo.org/docs/AnnualReports/2012/1UK%20National%20Haemophilia%20Database%20Bleeding%20Disorder%20Statistics%202011-2012%20for%20website.pdf (accessed July 2016).

3 Pike GN, Bolton-Maggs PH. Factor deficiencies in pregnancy. *Hematol Oncol Clin North Am* 2011; 25: 359–378, viii–ix.

4 Gupta N, Dadhwal V, Deka D, *et al*. Corpus luteum hemorrhage: rare complication of congenital and acquired coagulation abnormalities. *J Obstet Gynaecol Res* 2007; 33: 376–380.

5 Watson HG, Wilde JT, Dolan G, *et al*. Update to UKHCDO guidance on vaccination against hepatitis A and B viruses in patients with inherited coagulation factor deficiencies and von Willebrand disease. *Haemophilia* 2013; 19: e191.

6 Keeling D, Tait C, Makris M. Guideline on the selection and use of therapeutic products to treat haemophilia and other hereditary bleeding disorders. A United Kingdom Haemophilia Center Doctors' Organisation (UKHCDO) guideline approved by the British Committee for Standards in Haematology. *Haemophilia* 2008; 14: 671–684.

7 Brooker M. Registry of clotting factor concentrates. In: *World Federation of Hemophilia. Facts and Figures*, 9th edn. Montreal: WFH, 2012.

8 Williams MD, Chalmers EA, Gibson BE. The investigation and management of neonatal haemostasis and thrombosis. *Br J Haematol* 2002; 119: 295–309.

9 Acharya SS, Dimichele DM. Rare inherited disorders of fibrinogen. *Haemophilia* 2008; 14: 1151–1158.

10 Haverkate F, Samama M. Familial dysfibrinogenemia and thrombophilia. Report on a study of the SSC Subcommittee on Fibrinogen. *Thromb Haemost* 1995; 73: 151–161.

11 Girolami A, Scandellari R, Scapin M, *et al*. Congenital bleeding disorders of the vitamin K-dependent clotting factors. *Vitam Horm* 2008; 78: 281–374.

12 Meeks SL, Abshire TC. Abnormalities of prothrombin: a review of the pathophysiology, diagnosis, and treatment. *Haemophilia* 2008; 14: 1159–1163.

13 Nichols WC, Seligsohn U, Zivelin A, *et al*. Mutations in the ER-Golgi intermediate compartment protein ERGIC-53 cause combined deficiency of coagulation factors V and VIII. *Cell* 1998; 93: 61–70.

14 Zhang B, McGee B, Yamaoka JS, *et al*. Combined deficiency of factor V and factor VIII is due to mutations in either LMAN1 or MCFD2. *Blood* 2006; 107: 1903–1907.

15 Peyvandi F, Di Michele D, Bolton-Maggs PH, *et al*. Project on Consensus Definitions in Rare Bleeding Disorders of the Factor VIII/FIXScientific and Standardisation Committee of the International Society on Thrombosis and Haemostasis: Classification of rare bleeding disorders (RBDs) based on the association between coagulant factor activity and clinical bleeding severity. *J Thromb Haemost* 2012; 10: 1938–1943.

16 Perry DJ. Factor VII deficiency. *Br J Haematol* 2002; 118: 689–700.

17 Giansily-Blaizot M, Lopez E, Viart V, *et al*. Lethal factor VII deficiency due to novel mutations in the F7 promoter: functional analysis reveals disruption of HNF4 binding site. *Thromb Haemost* 2012; 108: 277–283.

18 Bolton-Maggs PH, Hay CR, Shanks D, *et al*. The importance of tissue factor source in the management of Factor VII deficiency. *Thromb Haemost* 2007; 97: 151–152.

19 Brown DL, Kouides PA. Diagnosis and treatment of inherited factor X deficiency. *Haemophilia* 2008; 14: 1176–1182.

20 Bolton-Maggs P. Factor XI deficiency-resolving the enigma? *American Society of Hematology Education Program Book* 2009: 97–105.

21 Choi SH, Smith SA, Morrissey JH. Polyphosphate is a cofactor for the activation of factor XI by thrombin. *Blood* 2011; 118: 6963–6970.

22 Hancock JF, Wieland K, Pugh RE, *et al*. A molecular genetic study of factor XI deficiency. *Blood* 1991; 77: 1942–1948.

23 Salomon O, Steinberg DM, Seligshon U. Variable bleeding manifestations characterize different types of surgery in patients with severe factor XI deficiency enabling parsimonious use of replacement therapy. *Haemophilia* 2006; 12: 490–493.

24 Salomon O, Zivelin A, Livnat T, *et al*. Prevalence, causes, and characterization of factor XI inhibitors in patients with inherited factor XI deficiency. *Blood* 2003; 101: 4783–4788.

25 Livnat T, Tamarin I, Mor Y, *et al*. Recombinant activated factor VII and tranexamic acid are haemostatically effective during major surgery in factor XI-deficient patients with inhibitor antibodies. *Thromb Haemost* 2009; 102: 487–492.

26 Hsieh L, Nugent D. Factor XIII deficiency. *Haemophilia* 2008; 14: 1190–1200.

27 Kohler HP, Ichinose A, Seitz R, *et al*. Factor X, Fibrinogen SSCSOTI: Diagnosis and classification of factor XIII deficiencies. *J Thromb Haemost* 2011; 9: 1404–1406.

28 Lovejoy AE, Reynolds TC, Visich JE, *et al*. Safety and pharmacokinetics of recombinant factor XIII-A2 administration in patients with congenital factor XIII deficiency. *Blood* 2006; 108: 57–62.

29 Brenner B. Hereditary deficiency of vitamin K-dependent coagulation factors. *Thromb Haemost* 2000; 84: 935–936.

30 Oldenburg J, von Brederlow B, Fregin A, *et al*. Congenital deficiency of vitamin K dependent

coagulation factors in two families presents as a genetic defect of the vitamin K-epoxide-reductase-complex. *Thromb Haemost* 2000; 84: 937–941.

31 Bolton-Maggs PH, Perry DJ, Chalmers EA, *et al.* The rare coagulation disorders--review with guidelines for management from the United Kingdom Haemophilia Centre Doctors' Organisation. *Haemophilia* 2004; 10: 593–628.

32 Mumford AD, Ackroyd S, Alikhan R, Grainger J, Mainwaring J, Mathias M, *et al.* Guideline for the diagnosis and management of the rare coagulation disorders: a United Kingdom Haemophilia Centre Doctors' Organization guideline on behalf of the British Committee for Standards in Haematology. Br J *Haematol* 2014; 167: 304–26.

33 Peyvandi F, Duga S, Akhavan S, *et al.* Rare coagulation deficiencies. *Haemophilia* 2002; 8: 308–321.

34 Seligsohn U, Peretz H. Molecular genetics aspects of factor XI deficiency and Glanzmann thrombasthenia. *Haemostasis* 1994; 24: 81–85.

9

Acquired Inhibitors of Coagulation

Riitta Lassila and Elina Armstrong

Key Points

- Acquired bleeding disorders are very rare, and their clinical and laboratory diagnosis is usually significantly delayed.
- Laboratory evaluation of specific coagulation factor analysis is needed for diagnosis. When an inhibitor against a coagulation factor is detected, whether linked to clinical bleeding symptoms or not, the patient should always be referred to a comprehensive care center with appropriate clinical and laboratory expertise.
- Management includes: (i) rapid and accurate diagnosis; (ii) control of bleeding; (iii) investigation for an underlying cause; and (iv) eradication of the inhibitor by immunomodulation.
- Immunosuppression with steroids combined with cytotoxic agents should be started as soon as the diagnosis is made and continued for several weeks or months until the factor levels resume normal reference values.

Introduction

Acquired bleeding disorders are rare (yearly incidence being about $1-15:10^6$ inhabitants, increasing in older populations), and accordingly their diagnosis is often delayed. Despite the frequent severity and atypical features of the bleeding phenotype, with multiple large and deep soft tissue hematomas and a generalized bleeding tendency, patients are often referred to hematologists after a significant time (several days to weeks) has elapsed from the initial symptoms. The responsible autoantibodies show a striking target specificity to a certain coagulation factor, either inactivating the target by interfering with key functional activity or enhancing clearance of the factor. Immunological triggers include surgery or other challenges, such as pregnancy or malignancy, but about 50% do not have an established risk factor. Recognized syndromes include acquired hemophilia A (lack of FVIII), von Willebrand syndrome (AVWS), and other even rarer disorders, caused by autoantibodies directed to specific coagulation factors, such as FII, FV, FVII, FIX, FX, and FXIII. This article focuses exclusively on the bleeding disorders that are associated with significantly reduced coagulation factor levels (below 40%) and the presence of autoantibodies in patients without a previous history of bleeds.

Pathophysiology of Acquired Hemophilia, Acquired Von Willebrand Syndrome, and Other Acquired Coagulation Factor Deficiencies

Acquired inhibitors are autoantibodies that neutralize the target coagulation activity, often by interfering with binding to phospholipid surfaces. The responsible immunoglobulin is usually

Practical Hemostasis and Thrombosis, Third Edition. Edited by Nigel S. Key, Michael Makris and David Lillicrap.
© 2017 John Wiley & Sons, Ltd. Published 2017 by John Wiley & Sons, Ltd.

subclass IgG4 or IgG1, which binds to and delivers the coagulation factor to the specific cellular Fc receptor, Fcγ. Three classes (I, II, and III) of Fcγ receptors have been identified. FcγRI, a high-affinity receptor, is able to bind monomeric IgG. This is in contrast to the low-affinity receptors which bind to dimeric IgG. FcγRII (subclasses a, an activating receptor, and b, an inhibitory receptor) and FcγRIII bind exclusively aggregated immunoglobulins or antigen–antibody complexes [1]. FcγRI is expressed on monocytes/macrophages, neutrophils, eosinophils, and dendritic cells, while FcγRIIa is expressed also on platelets and Langerhans cells, whereas FcγRIIb is expressed on B-lymphocytes and mast cells. The FcγRIIb is the only inhibitory receptor, while all the others activate cells [2]. FcγRIII is subdivided into FcγRIIIa present on natural killer cells and macrophages, and FcγRIIIb, expressed on eosinophils, neutrophils, macrophages, mast cells, and follicular dendritic cells. If mast cell activation occurs, heparin is released, which may further unexpectedly impair coagulation at the tissue level.

Chronic lymphocytic leukemia and other lymphoproliferative diseases may be associated with rapid disappearance of von Willebrand factor (VWF, both antigen and activity) and FVIII, leading to a severe bleeding phenotype. The most common solid tumors associated with acquired hemophilia include prostate and lung cancer, but underlying hematological malignancy is also frequently present. The presence of a paraprotein may result in binding of the coagulation factor thereby impairing its availability for hemostasis.

The antibodies causing acquired hemophilia generally belong to the IgG class and do not bind complement. Certain gene polymorphisms have been associated with FVIII antibody formation, including HLA and CTLA4 and autoreactive CD4+ T lymphocytes. Most often, the antibodies bind to the C2 domain of FVIII, thus interfering with its phospholipid binding on activated platelets and endothelial cells. Analogously to FVIII, FV can be inhibited by antibodies that bind to its structurally similar C2 domain. Exposure to non-human plasma material has been shown to induce FV antibody formation. Acquired fibrinogen deficiency can be seen in syndromes of hemophagocytosis, and FX deficiency can result from adsorption to amyloid plaques. Also, some specific coagulation factor defects may evolve in immunocompromised patients with severe infections, including hepatitis B and C, as well as HIV.

Epidemiology

Acquired disorders of coagulation are significantly rarer than the congenital forms of the disease. The diagnosis is often delayed when disorders are not recognized and appropriate coagulation testing is not requested. Therefore, the overall incidence of these conditions is likely underestimated.

Acquired Hemophilia

Acquired hemophilia is typically a disease of middle age and the elderly, occurs in all ethnic groups worldwide, and in both genders about equally. The overall incidence has been calculated at 1–2/million [3,4]. It is not typically seen in childhood. In an analysis of pooled data from 20 surveys and 249 patients the median age was 64 years, with a range of 8–93 years, and 55% of patients were women [5]. In the UK study data, the median age at diagnosis was 78 years, with only 15% being less than 65 years, and a yearly incidence of only 0.045/million for those younger than 16 years, but 14.7/million for age older than 85 years [3]. The age distribution is biphasic with a minor peak between 20 and 30 years due to postpartum inhibitors and female preponderance, and a major peak between ages 68 and 80 years (Figure 9.1).

An associated underlying condition can be identified in approximately 50% of cases. These include pregnancy, autoimmune conditions, malignancy, and certain drugs (Table 9.1). Mortality has been reported in the range of 8–22%, with the highest risk during the first weeks of presentation and in the presence of comorbidities [3]. Association with pregnancy was present in about 8% according to the EACH2

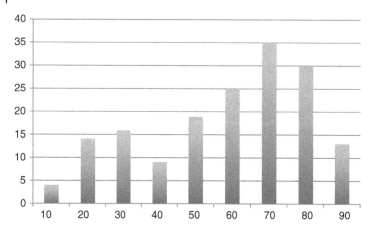

Figure 9.1 Age-related incidence of acquired hemophilia A. Data are shown for the percentage of patients presenting with acquired hemophilia A in each decade of life in two large cohorts, a treatment study and a combined analysis of 20 cohorts. *Source:* data from Green and Lechner 1981, Collins *et al.* 2007 [3,6]; Morrison *et al.* 1993, Delgado *et al.* 2003 [5,7]; and EACH2 registry Levesque *et al.* 2009 [8].

Table 9.1 Underlying conditions in acquired hemophilia.

Condition	Examples
Pregnancy	
Autoimmune disorders	SLE, rheumatoid arthritis, multiple sclerosis, Sjögren syndrome, AIHA, Goodpasture syndrome, myasthenia gravis, Graves disease, autoimmune hypothyroidism
Solid malignancies	Cancers of the prostate, lung, colon, pancreas, stomach, biliary tract, head and neck, cervix, breast, kidney, seminoma, melanoma
Hematological malignancies	CLL, NHL, MM, Waldenström macroglobulinemia, MDS, MF, erythroleukemia
Inflammatory bowel disease	Ulcerative colitis
Dermatological disorders	Psoriasis, pemphigus
Respiratory diseases	Asthma, COPD
Diabetes	
Acute hepatitis	HCV, HBV
Drugs	Penicillin, sulfa and their derivatives, phenytoin, chloramphenicol, methyldopa, depot thioxanthene, interpheron-alpha, fludarabine, levodopa, clopidogrel

Source: Franchini and Lippi, 2008 [11].
AIHA, autoimmune hemolytic anemia; CLL, chronic lymphatic leukemia; COPD, chronic obstructive pulmonary disease; HBV, hepatitis B virus; HCV, hepatitis C virus; NHL, non-Hodgkin lymphoma; MM, multiple myeloma; MDS, myelodysplastic syndrome; MF, myelofibrosis; SLE, systemic lupus erythematosus.

registry [4]. The diagnosis was usually made about 3 months after delivery, and most cases were encountered during the first pregnancy. The prognosis was good, as survival was reported to be nearly 100% [9,10], without major clinical consequences.

Acquired von Willebrand Syndrome

Acquired von Willebrand syndrome (AVWS) is a rare acquired bleeding disorder presenting in adulthood. Underlying disease entities include lympho- and myeloproliferative disorders, such as monoclonal gammopathy of undetermined significance (MGUS), polycythemia vera, essential thrombocythemia, myelodysplastic syndrome, and certain types of malignancy and autoimmune diseases [12]. Cardiovascular conditions, such as aortic valve stenosis, account for one-fifth of cases.

Other Acquired Coagulation Inhibitors

Acquired inhibitors to other coagulation factors are exceedingly rare. Inhibitors directed against FV, FVII, FIX, FX, FXI, and FXIII have been described. Underlying causes include autoimmune conditions, the postpartum state, and malignancies. Differential diagnosis for the traditional coagulation inhibitors is presented in Table 9.2.

Autoantibodies to thrombin and FV have been described following exposure to fibrin glues or bovine thrombin preparations contaminated with bovine FV [13,14]. These situations are now practically abolished with the use of modern recombinant or human-derived local hemostatic agents. Also, FV inhibitors have been described in association with underlying conditions such as malignancy, autoimmune disease, and the postpartum state [15,16].

Acquired FX deficiency can be due to underlying amyloidosis, where the protein is bound to tissue amyloid fibrils [17]. FXIII antibodies are even rarer than the congenital form of the disease [18]. Fibrinogen can be consumed in syndromes of hemophagocytosis, leading to disproportional hemostatic disturbances.

Signs and Symptoms

Bleeding is the main presenting symptom of acquired disorders of coagulation, and is often severe or life threatening, constituting a medical emergency. Unlike the congenital deficiency state, in acquired hemophilia the bleeds are subcutane-

Table 9.2 Laboratory findings and differential diagnosis for acquired hemophilia, AVWS and other acquired coagulation inhibitors.

Laboratory deficiency or other findings	Differential diagnosis
APTT and/or PT and thrombin time prolonged and fibrinogen unmeasurable (Clauss assay), ferritin elevated	Hemophagocytosis; histiocytosis, lymphoproliferative disorders, listeriosis, strepto- or staphylococcal disease, large dose of fibrinolytic therapy, sepsis, DIC, cancer
PT prolonged FV deficiency FIX deficiency	Vitamin K deficiency (measure FIX separately), malabsorption, alcoholism, anticoagulants (VKA, severe accumulation of dabigatran, rivaroxaban, apixaban, edoxaban), liver disease (FV low, FVIII high)
APTT and PT variously prolonged, serum protein electrophoresis, paraprotein FX deficiency	Amyloidosis, Waldenström macroglobulinemia, MGUS, cancer, severe accumulation of dabigatran, rivaroxaban, apixaban, edoxaban
PT prolonged, thrombocytopenia, D-dimer elevation, antithrombin low	DIC
Acute hepatitis, viral expression, thrombocytopenia	HCV, HBV and HIV
Autoimmune disorders with various antibodies: cardiolipin, beta2-glycoprotein-I, antinuclear, ANCA, MPO, PR3, basement membrane antibodies, antithyroideal antibodies	SLE, rheumatoid arthritis, multiple sclerosis, Sjögren's syndrome, AIHA, Goodpasture's syndrome, myasthenia gravis, Graves disease, autoimmune hypothyroidism; may link to acquired coagulation inhibitors as well

AIHA, autoimmune hemolytic anemia; ANCA, antineutrophil cytoplasmic antibodies; APTT, activate partial thromboplastin time; DIC, disseminated intravascular coagulation; HBV, hepatitis B virus; HCV, hepatitis C virus; HIV, human immunodeficiency virus; MGUS, monoclonal gammopathy of undetermined significance; MPO, myeloperoxidase; PR3, proteinase 3; PT, prothrombin time; SLE, systemic lupus erythematosus; VKA, vitamin K antagonist.

ous or large soft-tissue hematomas, suggestive of involvement of defects engaging tissue hemostasis. In AVWS the bleeds resemble the congenital form of type 3 von Willebrand disease, with mucosal and cutaneous lesions and difficult to manage gastrointestinal bleeds. Clinical manifestations include large spontaneous hematomas, soft-tissue bleeds that occur spontaneously or after mild pressure, such as sleeping on the side, and oozing and rebleeding after invasive procedures (Figure 9.2).

Life-threatening situations can result from intracranial bleeds or bleeds in the head and neck area that threaten the airway. The superficial hematomas usually resolve spontaneously, while other bleeds need active management with bypassing agents. About one-third of the bleeds do not need any hemostatic treatment. Not only is hemostasis impaired, but so too is wound healing in all forms of acquired coagulation inhibitors, and also therefore – in addition to immediate hemostatic problems and further immunological activation – surgery should be avoided whenever possible.

Acquired Hemophilia

Acquired hemophilia typically presents in a distinct way compared with congenital hemophilia, where joint bleeding is the hallmark of the severe forms of the disease. Hemarthrosis is unusual, however, in the acquired disorder. The principal manifestation is bleeding into skin and soft tissues (Figure 9.2). Purpura and hematomas can be extensive causing anemia, further impairing primary hemostasis, and may progress to a compartment syndrome.

In a single-center survey that included 24 cases [19], skin and soft tissue were the bleeding sites in the majority of patients. Other sites included hematuria, gastrointestinal, and prolonged postpartum hemorrhage. Excessive bleeds may also result from trauma or surgery without an appropriate hemostatic treatment. Bleeds are reported to be a direct or contributing cause of death in 8–22% of cases of acquired hemophilia [3,6].

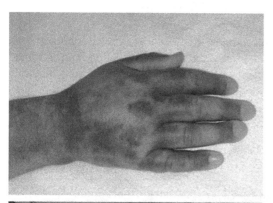
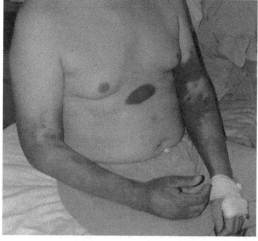

Figure 9.2 Patient presenting with acquired hemophilia having typical large soft tissue bleeds, after sleeping on his left side and exerting his left arm. The photograph is from the time of diagnosis, which was delayed for several days. *Source:* With permission from Duodecim Medical Journal, Finland, 2003. *See Plate section for color representation of this figure. See also figure 6.3, page 91.*

Acquired von Willebrand Syndrome

Symptoms of AVWS are often similar to the congenital form of von Willebrand disease. Recurring gastrointestinal bleeds are difficult to manage, and involve small angiodysplasias, which may not be visible with enteroscopic techniques. Bleeds from various mucocutaneous sites are typical, and some similarity to acquired hemophilia is encountered if the FVIII levels are very low.

Other Coagulation Factor Deficiencies

Bleeds associated with other coagulation defects are usually disproportional to the clinical challenge, with prolonged rebleeding. FV-associated bleeds affect primary hemostasis in mucosal tissues. Spontaneous bleeds may occur in soft tissues. Deficiency of FXIII is a risk factor for intracranial bleeds and prolongation of hemorrhage after trivial trauma.

Diagnosis – Laboratory Measures to be Complemented with Clinical Findings

The diagnosis should be suspected in a patient with a suggestive clinical presentation and prolongation of the activated partial prothrombin time (APTT) or another suggestive coagulation abnormality. Prothrombin time (PT) is normal, unless the antibody affects FII, FVII, FX, or FV. A deficiency of FV is picked up by the PT Quick reagent, but not with the Owren reagent, which is mainly used in Northern Europe. The laboratory work-up and differential diagnosis are illustrated in Table 9.2.

The prolongation of the APTT always needs explanation, however small the prolongation. Any contamination with heparin has to be excluded, usually with a thrombin time or anti-FXa activity. However, when fibrinogen is dysfunctional or deficient, or in the case of a rare thrombin inhibitor (associated with older preparations of topical thrombin), the thrombin time will be prolonged. In cases of lupoid autoimmune diseases (e.g., systemic lupus erythematosus) or antiphospholipid antibody syndrome, the APTT may also be prolonged. Some APTT reagents are less sensitive to lupus anticoagulants, and are thus more suitable to bleeding disorder diagnostics. Knowledge of the reagent in use is therefore crucial in the interpretation of a prolonged APTT. Mixing tests may show a time-dependent inhibitor of FVIII. The measured plasma levels of FVIII are mostly compatible with moderate (1–5%) or mild (5–40%) hemophilia, but severely reduced levels (<1%) may also be observed.

FVIII autoantibodies are usually polyclonal and of the IG4 subtype. Depending on the epitope recognized by the antibody, a chromogenic or clotting-based assay may indicate a lower or higher level of FVIII. The antibody exerts type II kinetics, with some residual activity of FVIII despite the presence of a high-titer inhibitor. This is in contrast to inhibitors occurring in congenital hemophilia, when FVIII or IX levels are undetectable (<1%), almost without an exception. The Nijmegen modified- Bethesda inhibitor assay typically detects acquired antibodies at 5–30 BU/mL, which (by definition) are high titer, but generally lower compared to inhibitor titers in congenital hemophilia. However, the bleeding tendency correlates poorly with the FVIII level and the inhibitor titer.

In AVWS, the APTT may be normal or somewhat prolonged, but von Willebrand factor activity or ristocetin cofactor activity is reduced, and antigen is either normal or reduced. Also, VWF binding to collagen may be impaired. If VWF antigen is normal or reduced with a discrepant activity to antigen ratio, the phenotype resembles VWD type 2A, which is the most common variant of the AVWS. FVIII activity may be normal or somewhat reduced. In the PFA-100/PFA-200 (Platelet Function Analyzer), prolongation of occlusion times is usual in both collagen-coated cartridges, that is with ADP and adrenaline. The autoantibodies may recognize both VWF and FVIII or VWF alone.

Differential Diagnosis

The causes of bleeding need to be considered in terms of liver and kidney disease, cancer, and infection, as well as use of drugs affecting hemostasis (e.g., selective serotonin or noradrenaline reuptake inhibitors, nonsteroidal anti-inflammatory drugs, and tyrosine kinase inhibitors).

Hemophagocytosis may be associated with pancytopenia, and very high levels of serum ferritin. Therein a nonmeasureable fibrinogen is a hallmark, due to macrophage-mediated digestion of cellular and integrin ligand material, including fibrinogen, important for platelet aggregation and clot formation.

The diagnosis of acquired FX deficiency due to amyloidosis requires tissue detection of

Congo-positive discoloration of the plaques. Serum electrophoresis may reveal a paraprotein, which is generally a manifestation of MGUS. Paraproteins may bind to the coagulation proteins, including VWF, removing them from the circulation.

Many infective agents utilize the coagulation system in their tissue invasion and may cause nonspecific coagulation abnormalities, including enhanced fibrinolytic activity, with disproportionately high D-dimer levels and dys- or afibrinogenemia. These bacteria include streptococci (streptokinase), staphylococci (staphylokinase), and Listeria. Also, some hemorrhagic fevers, for example caused by Dengue and Hantaviruses, may be associated with low levels of procoagulant proteins and thrombocytopenia, usually manifest by microthrombosis and consumption coagulopathy or disseminated intravascular coagulation (DIC).

Management of Coagulation Inhibitors

When an inhibitor against a coagulation factor is detected, whether linked to clinical bleeding symptoms or not, the patient should be referred to an specialized center with clinical and laboratory expertise in hemostatic disorders. A thorough medical history, physical examination with blood tests, and imaging studies are indicated to investigate the possible underlying etiology.

Management includes: (i) rapid and accurate diagnosis, (ii) control of bleeding, (iii) investigation and treatment for an underlying cause, and (iv) eradication of the inhibitor by immunomodulation.

Diagnosis is based on clinical suspicion of a systemic bleeding diathesis and abnormal coagulation screening tests. In acquired hemophilia, the APTT is prolonged and even a minor abnormality should trigger further investigations. In AVWS, depending on the severity, the APTT may be within the normal range but, as in other factor deficiencies, clinical suspicion should direct further coagulation testing.

Poor prognostic factors are related to the nature of the underlying condition, especially malignancy, achievement of a complete remission, and older age (>65 years). Other comorbidities may also be important in this regard. Surgery needs to be discouraged unless it is urgent or unavoidable.

Control of Bleeding Episodes

Acquired bleeding disorders may present as an acute medical emergency or as subtle and gradually progressing symptoms. Superficial hematomas resolve spontaneously in most cases, while other bleeds need active management, generally with bypassing agents. Other causes of impaired hemostasis need to be eliminated and treated concurrently. Anemia may impair thrombin generation and primary hemostasis, and needs appropriate management. Recombinant FVIIa (NovoSeven®) and activated prothrombin complex concentrate (aPCC, FEIBA®) are traditionally the first lines of therapy in acquired hemophilia. APCC, a plasma-derived coagulation factor product, contains activated FII, FVII, FIX, and FX.

Recently, recombinant B-domain deleted porcine sequence FVIII (r-pFVIII; Obizur®) has been licensed in several countries for the treatment of bleeding in acquired hemophilia. r-pFVIII is sufficiently similar to human FVIII to be hemostatically active, but sufficiently dissimilar to render it less susceptible to inactivation by inhibitory autoantibodies. The choice of product is determined by the clinical scenario, feasibility of administration, and product availability (Table 9.3). The possibility of thromboembolic complications with the bypassing agents needs to be taken into consideration.

FEIBA® is dosed at 50–100 IU/kg every 8–12 hours (maximum dose 200 IU/kg/day). Antifibrinolytic agents, tranexamic acid or ε-aminocaproic acid (EACA), are not recommended with aPCCs due to the potential thrombotic risk. At least 6 hours should elapse after a dose of tranexamic acid before FEIBA is given. Special caution should be used in the elderly, patients with advanced atherosclerosis, vascular disease, and with signs of abnormal proteolysis, as

Table 9.3 Rates of control for the first bleeding episodes by first-line therapy.

Hemostatic agent	First-line bleeding control	
	n	%
Bypassing agent	219	91.8
FVIIa	159	91.2
aPCC	60	93.3
Replacement therapy	69	69.6
FVIII	55	70.1
DDAVP	14	64.3

FVIIa, aktivated factor VII; aPCC, activated prothrombin complex concentrate; FVIII, factor VIII; DDAVP, 1-deamino-8-D-arginine vasopressin (desmopressin) *Source:* Collins and Percy, 2010 [20]. Reproduced with permission of Wiley.

in sepsis. Antifibrinolytics may be used topically, for example, for oral or nasal mucosal bleeding.

NovoSeven is typically administered at a dose of 90–120 μg/kg every 2–4 hours. Antifibrinolytic treatment is recommended to be used together with rFVIIa to enhance its hemostatic effect. If switching from FEIBA to NovoSeven is planned, at least 6 hours should pass before NovoSeven is administered, while vice versa, 2 hours is recommended. In patients with uncontrolled bleeding, sequential therapy with aPCC and rFVIIa has been used, keeping the recommended dose frequency according to that of aPCCs.

In the absence of specific information on the antiporcine FVIII titer at presentation – which is generally significantly lower than the antihuman FVIII titer – a starting dose of 200 IU/kg of r-pFVIII is recommended [21]. Subsequent doses are individualized according to the measured plasma FVIII recovery and half-life.

However, as there are no validated laboratory methods to monitor the treatment effect with the bypassing agents, it is important to closely monitor the patients clinically. Changes in the routine coagulation test times do not correlate with clinical effect. Some experience has been gained with whole-blood rotational thromboelastometry, but more controlled data are needed before it can be routinely recommended.

Experience with desmopressin (DDAVP, 1-deamino-8-D-arginine vasopressin) is limited to a few case reports [22]. It can be used in the treatment of minor bleeding episodes or prophylaxis of minor surgical/invasive procedures in patients with acquired hemophilia and mild AVWS with a low inhibitor titer and measurable baseline levels (and responsive postinfusion levels) of circulating plasma FVIII.

Inhibition of fibrinolysis is often beneficial. Tranexamic acid is most effective when administered repeatedly, as its tissue concentration rises. In an emergency, intravenous administration of tranexamic acid is preferable to reach the desired concentrations, usually at a dose of 10 mg/kg three times daily. A potential concern with tranexamic acid or EACA is their use in upper urinary tract bleeds, when a stable fibrin clot may occlude the upper urinary tract and result in hydronephrosis. In other bleeds, such as at mucosal sites, the administration of tranexamic acid for several days is useful to control fibrinolysis. Also, the additive effect of tranexamic acid with DDAVP may be due to the simultaneous liberation of von Willebrand factor and tissue plasminogen activator (t-PA) – which is then functionally neutralized – from endothelial stores.

Immunomodulation

Immunosuppression should be started as soon as the diagnosis is made. Commonly used regimens are steroids alone or in combination with cytotoxic agents. The best evidence for these agents in the management of acquired hemophilia A is from the EACH2 registry of 501 patients [4,23]. The likelihood of achieving stable remission was not affected by the underlying etiology, but was influenced by the presenting inhibitor titer and FVIII level.

Treatment options include steroids alone, steroids combined with cyclophosphamide, or less frequently with azathioprine [24]. Usually, prednisone (or prednisolone) at a dose of 1 mg/kg/day is started as soon as the diagnosis is made. Remission is more likely with steroids and cyclophosphamide at 50–100 mg/day than steroids alone. Also, rituximab has been used in these combinations, but the current evidence does not show improved outcome or reduced side-effects. Rituximab may be used as the second-line treatment if traditional immunomodulation has failed.

Second-line immunosuppressants, including mycophenolate and cyclosporin A, have been reported beneficial and well tolerated in small case series of acquired hemophilia [25].

Intravenous immunoglobulin (IVIg) has not been proven to be helpful in acquired hemophilia, but may have a role in AVWS, both acutely and for the maintenance of hemostatic VWF and FVIII levels. When IVIg is infused followed by VWF concentrate, factor levels may rise to hemostatic levels, at least for some time.

Treatment side-effects need to be considered on an individual basis. Steroids may cause serious side-effects, including diabetes mellitus, psychosis, electrolyte changes, osteoporosis, and development of cataracts. All of these adverse effects may limit their use, as patients are often elderly and frail. Azathioprine may be better tolerated than cyclophosphamide in elderly patients [24]. Furthermore, this often elderly population – with or without malignancy – may develop thrombosis when subjected to bypassing agents. The frequency of this complication is reported at about 5% during the first weeks of treatment.

Ethical issues, such as how far to pursue investigation and treatment of possible underlying conditions or the duration of efforts to treat prolonged bleeding symptoms in the case of poor response to immunomodulative regimens, may become important considerations.

Clinical Follow up

Immunosuppression should be continued for several weeks to months, because of a 10–20% rate of relapse at 6 months after discontinuation of immunosuppression. A higher rate of relapse is seen in patients with a high inhibitor titer and/or low FVIII level; in addition, surgical and other immunological challenges may reactivate the inhibitor. In AVWS, IVIg administration at regular intervals may prolong the half-life of VWF and thereby also FVIII. Follow up of these patients in collaboration with an expert hemophilia center is recommended.

References

1 Hullett MD, Hogarth PM. Molecular basis of Fc receptor function. *Adv Immunol* 1994; 57: 1–127.

2 Ravetch JV, Bolland S. IgG Fc receptors. *Annu Rev Immunol* 2001; 19: 275–290.

3 Collins PW, Hirsch S, Baglin T, *et al.* Acquired haemophilia A in the United Kingdom: a 2-year national surveillance study by the United Kingdom Haemophilia Centre Doctors' Organization. *Blood* 2007; 109: 1870–1877.

4 Collins P, Baudo F, Knoebl P, *et al.* on behalf of the EACH2 registry collaborators. Immunosuppression for acquired hemophilia A: results from the European Acquired Haemophilia Registry (EACH2). *Blood* 2012; 120: 47–55.

5 Delgado J, Jimenez-Yuste V, Hernandez-Navarro F, *et al.* Acquired haemophilia: review and meta-analysis focused on therapy and prognostic factors. *Br J Haematol* 2003; 12: 21–35.

6 Green D, Lechner K. A survey of 215 non-hemophilic patients with inhibitors to Factor VIII. *Thromb Haemost* 1981; 45: 200–203.

7 Morrison AE, Ludlam, CA, Kessler C. Use of porcine factor VIII in the treatment of patients with acquired hemophilia. *Blood* 1993; 81: 1513–1520.

8 Levesque H, Tengborg L, Marco P, *et al.* Acquired haemophilia: descriptive data of the European acquired haemophilia registry (EACH2). *J Thromb Haemost 2009*; 7: Abstr We 604.

9 Franchini M. Postpartum acquired factor VIII inhibitors. *Am J Hematol* 2006; 81: 768–773.

10 Tengborn L, Baudo F, Huth-Kühne A, *et al.* EACH2 registry contributors. Pregnancy-associated acquired haemophilia A: results from the European Acquired Haemophilia (EACH2) registry. *BJOG* 2012; 119: 1529–1537.

11 Franchini M, Lippi G. Acquired factor VIII inhibitors. *Blood* 2008; 112: 250–255.

12 Federici AB, Budde U, Castaman G, *et al.* Current diagnostic and therapeutic approaches to patients with acquired von Willebrand syndrome: a 2013 update. *Semin Thromb Hemost* 2013; 39: 191–201.

13 Flaherty MJ, Henderson R, Wener MH. Iatrogenic immunization with bovine thrombin: a mechanism for prolonged thrombin times after surgery. *Ann Intern Med* 1989; 111: 631–634.

14 Ortel TL, Charles LA, Keller FG, *et al.* Topical thrombin and acquired coagulation factor inhibitors: clinical spectrum and laboratory diagnosis. *Am J Hematol* 1994; 45: 128–135.

15 Knöbl P, Lechner K. Acquired factor V inhibitors. *Baillieres Clin Haematol* 1998; 11: 305–318.

16 Franchini M, Lippi G. Acquired factor V inhibitors: a systematic review. *J Thromb Thrombolysis* 2011; 31: 449–457.

17 Choufani EB, Sanchorawala V, Ernst T, *et al.* Acquired factor X deficiency in patients with amyloid light-chain amyloidosis: incidence, bleeding manifestations, and response to high-dose chamotherapy. *Blood* 2001; 97: 1885–1887.

18 Boehlen F, Casini A, Chizzolini C, *et al.* Acquired factor XIII deficiency: a therapeutic challenge. *Thromb Haemost* 2013; 109: 479–487.

19 Yee TT, Taher A, Pasi KJ, *et al.* A survey of patients with acquired haemophilia centre over a 28-year period. *Clin Lab Haematol* 2000; 22: 275–278.

20 Collins PW, Percy CL. Advances of the understanding of acquired haemophilia: implications for clinical practice. *Br J Haematol* 2010; 148: 183–194.

21 Kruse-Jarres R, St-Louis J, Greist A, *et al.* Efficacy and safety of OBI-1, and antihaemophilic factor VIII (recombinant), porcine sequence, in subjects with acquired haemophilia A. *Haemophilia* 2015; 21: 162–170.

22 Franchini M, Lippi G. The use of desmopressin in acquired haemophilia A: a systematic review. *Blood Transfus* 2011; 9: 377–382.

23 Knoebl P, Marco P, Baudo F, *et al.* EACH2 Registry Contributors. Demographic and clinical data in acquired hemophilia A: results from the European Acquired Haemophilia Registry (EACH2). *J Thromb Haemost* 2012; 10: 622–631.

24 Tay L, Duncan E, Singhal D, *et al.* Twelve years of experience of acquired hemophilia A: trials and tribulations in South Australia. *Semin Thromb Hemost* 2009; 35: 769–777.

25 Lee YS, Ng HJ. Mycophenolate in the remission induction of patients with acquired haemophilia A. *Haemophilia* 2010; 16: 179–189.

10

Quantitative Platelet Disorders

Riten Kumar and Walter H.A. Kahr

Key Points

- Thrombocytopenia, defined as a platelet count less that $150 \times 10^9/L$, may be acquired or congenital.
- Evaluating a thrombocytopenic patient includes obtaining a thorough personal and family history, medication history, physical examination, complete blood count with review of blood film, and appropriate second-line laboratory investigations.
- Immune thrombocytopenia (ITP) occurs secondary to autoantibodies that accelerate platelet destruction and additionally impair megakaryo-cytopoiesis.
- Neonatal thrombocytopenia, one of the most common hematological abnormalities observed in the neonatal period, may be classified based on the timing of the thrombocytopenia.
- Congenital thrombocytopenias are a heterogeneous group of disorders associated with thrombocytopenia that may or may not be apparent at birth, and associated phenotypic abnormalities depending on the specific defect.

hemostasis, and increased bleeding due to thrombocytopenia alone rarely occurs until the count drops below $50 \times 10^9/L$. Historically, platelet counts of less than $20 \times 10^9/L$ were thought to increase the risk of spontaneous life-threatening bleeding (e.g., central nervous system or gastrointestinal). However, several prospective studies have revealed that the hemorrhagic risk was similar using a $10 \times 10^9/L$ or $20 \times 10^9/L$ threshold for prophylactic platelet transfusions, suggesting that the risk of life-threatening bleeding increases significantly only when the platelet count drops below $10 \times 10^9/L$ [1].

The differential diagnosis of thrombocytopenia varies with age of onset, severity, clinical features, and presence or absence of other hematological abnormalities. For example, the most likely cause of thrombocytopenia in a newborn infant is different from that of an older child or adult, or that of a pregnant woman. This chapter focuses on a practical approach to the assessment and management of congenital and acquired quantitative platelet disorders. Qualitative platelet disorders are covered in Chapter 11.

Introduction

Thrombocytopenia, defined as a platelet count of less than $150 \times 10^9/L$, may be congenital or acquired. The normal platelet count in a healthy individual ($150 - 450 \times 10^9/L$) far exceeds the number of platelets actually required for

Platelet Production

Platelet production is the final stage in a developmental process that begins with hematopoietic stem cells that grow and differentiate into mature megakaryocytes, each of which sheds hundreds of platelets into the bloodstream [2].

Practical Hemostasis and Thrombosis, Third Edition. Edited by Nigel S. Key, Michael Makris and David Lillicrap.
© 2017 John Wiley & Sons, Ltd. Published 2017 by John Wiley & Sons, Ltd.

The growth factor thrombopoietin (TPO) is the primary physiological cytokine responsible for all stages of megakaryopoiesis, which is also influenced by interleukin-3 (IL-3), IL-11, and granulocyte colony stimulating factor (G-CSF) [3]. TPO is synthesized predominantly in the liver and is released at a constant rate into the circulation, where it is largely cleared by binding to a specific cell-surface receptor (c-Mpl, TPO-R) present on platelets, megakaryocytes, and hematopoetic stem cells. The TPO-R mediates its action via a signal transduction pathway similar to that of erythropoietin [4]. Thrombopoietin levels are increased up to 20-fold in bone marrow failure states, only slightly elevated in immune thrombocytopenia (ITP), and low in liver failure.

The average life span of human platelets is 7–10 days. Older platelets are removed from the circulation by reticuloendothelial cells, although little is known about how senescent platelets are identified. A daily turnover of approximately 40×10^9 platelets/L blood is required to maintain a constant platelet count.

Mechanisms of Thrombocytopenia in Children and Adults

Thrombocytopenia may be classified according to increased platelet sequestration, decreased platelet production or accelerated platelet destruction (Table 10.1). In addition, dilutional thrombocytopenia following massive transfusion is a common iatrogenic mechanism whereby platelet concentration is reduced but total platelet mass is preserved [5]. Artefactual thrombocytopenia is another important consideration in the initial diagnostic evaluation, particularly when an asymptomatic individual is unexpectedly found to have a severely reduced platelet count. This often results from the anticoagulant ethylenediaminetetraacetic acid (EDTA) causing *ex vivo* platelet clumping (pseudothrombocytopenia), or the formation of small clots in the specimen tube following a traumatic collection

(e.g., heelprick collection in neonates). A diagnostic strategy for evaluating thrombocytopenia in a child or adult is shown in Figure 10.1.

Platelet Sequestration

In healthy individuals, splenic pooling (sequestration) accounts for approximately one-third of the total platelet mass, but may be as high as 90% in individuals with massive splenomegaly. The platelet count does not always correlate directly with spleen size, and the underlying mechanisms of platelet trapping within the extravascular splenic pool remain poorly understood. Preferential diversion of platelets through the splenic cords (by virtue of their small size) as well as binding to receptors on splenic macrophages may play a role in pathophysiology.

Decreased Platelet Production

Platelets originate from megakaryocytes in the bone marrow that protrude extensions (proplatelets) into blood vessels, where the shear force of flowing blood facilitates platelet shedding into the circulation [2,6]. Reduction of total megakaryocyte mass or functional impairment results in underproduction of platelets and subsequent thrombocytopenia. Drug-associated marrow suppression resulting in pancytopenia is the most common cause, although some agents are thought to preferentially affect megakaryocytes (see below). Excess alcohol is also directly toxic to megakaryocytes, and thrombocytopenia in this setting may be exacerbated by other factors such as nutritional deficiencies and chronic liver disease. A number of viruses also cause thrombocytopenia by inhibition of megakaryopoiesis, including measles, human immunodeficiency virus (HIV), varicella, mumps, Epstein–Barr virus (EBV), rubella, cytomegalovirus (CMV), parvovirus, and dengue infection. Thrombocytopenia resulting from marrow suppression usually recovers once the offending agent has been removed.

Marrow infiltration (myelophthisis) by leukemia, solid tumors, and storage diseases causes

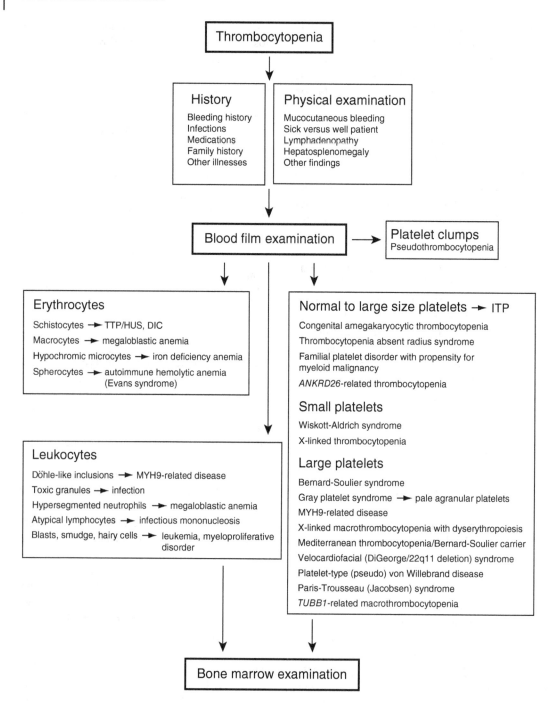

Figure 10.1 Diagnostic strategy for evaluating thrombocytopenia. DIC, disseminated intravascular coagulation; HUS, hemolytic uremic syndrome; ITP, immune thrombocytopenia; TTP, thrombotic thrombocytopenic purpura.

Table 10.1 Causes of thrombocytopenia in children and adults.

Increased platelet sequestration

Hypersplenism

Decreased platelet production

Aplastic anemia (idiopathic or drug-induced)

Myelodysplastic syndrome

Marrow infiltrative process

Infection (bacterial; viral: HIV, CMV, HCV)

Osteopetrosis

Nutritional deficiencies (iron, folate, vitamin B_{12})

Drug or radiation-induced (see Table 10.3)

Congenital platelet disorders (see Table 10.2)

Increased platelet destruction

Immune mediated thrombocytopenias

Acute and chronic ITP

Autoimmune diseases with ITP (SLE, Evans syndrome, autoimmune lymphoproliferative disorders, lymphoma, antiphospholipid antibody syndrome)

Infection-related (viral, bacterial, fungal, protozoan)

Alloimmune (e.g., NAIT)

Post-transfusion purpura

Drug-induced (immune or non-immune)

Non-immune-mediated thrombocytopenias

Disseminated intravascular coagulation

Kasabach–Merritt syndrome

Thrombotic thrombocytopenic purpura

Hemolytic uremic syndrome

Catheters, prostheses, cardiopulmonary bypass

Familial hemophagocytic lymphohistiocytosis

Hereditary platelet disorders (see Table 10.2)

Miscellaneous

Liver disease, renal disease, thyroid disease

Massive transfusions, exchange transfusions, extracorporeal circulation

Allogeneic bone marrow transplantation, graft-versus-host disease

Heat or cold injury

HIV, human immunodeficiency virus; CMV, cytomegalovirus; HCV, hepatitis C virus; SLE, systemic lupus erythematosus.

thrombocytopenia through displacement of normal hematopoietic cells, including megakaryocytes. Pancytopenia is more common than isolated thrombocytopenia in this context. Acquired or inherited bone marrow failure (e.g., aplastic anemia, Fanconi anemia) is characterized by progressive pancytopenia in association with a hypocellular marrow. However, isolated thrombocytopenia with megakaryocytic hypoplasia can occur early in the course of some of these disorders (e.g., congenital amegakaryocytic thrombocytopenia). Ineffective megakaryocytopoiesis results in thrombocytopenia despite normal or increased megakaryocyte mass. This typically accompanies megaloblastic anemia (vitamin B_{12} or folate deficiency), but may also be a prominent feature of some myelodysplastic syndromes.

Increased Platelet Destruction

Accelerated platelet destruction is the most common cause of thrombocytopenia. It is usually immune-mediated, although nonimmune (consumptive) mechanisms are well characterized (Table 10.1). Antibodies against epitopes on the platelet surface are frequently implicated, although T-cell and dendritic cell mediated immunological mechanisms are also thought to play a role [7]. The bone marrow in destructive thrombocytopenias typically reveals megakaryocytic hyperplasia; however, ITP may be associated with suboptimal megakaryopoiesis.

Evaluating a Thrombocytopenic Patient

Patient History

Immediate (rather than delayed) bleeding is typical of thrombocytopenia, similar to other disorders of primary hemostasis, including platelet function defects and von Willebrand disease (VWD). Distinctive features include:

- petechiae;
- mucocutaneous bleeding;
- epistaxis;
- menorrhagia.

Conversely, hemarthroses and intramuscular hematomas are rare, in contrast to defects of secondary hemostasis such as hemophilia. A careful history assessing the response to trauma, surgical challenges (including circumcision, dental extraction, tonsillectomy), menses, and postpartum hemorrhage can be useful in defining the presence of a primary hemostatic defect. Bleeding since birth or early childhood is suggestive of an inherited condition, whereas symptoms in older patients are more likely to be caused by an acquired defect. Use of a standardized bleeding questionnaire in this setting may help identify patients who warrant further investigation [8,9].

Family History

A family history of bleeding and thrombocytopenia suggests an inherited condition. Table 10.2 lists some congenital thrombocytopenias and their mode of inheritance. A diagnosis of neonatal alloimmune thrombocytopenia (NAIT) may be foreshadowed by a history of a previous child (sibling or cousin) affected by intracranial hemorrhage (ICH) or thrombocytopenia during the neonatal period.

Medication History

A careful medication history is important, because many drugs can cause thrombocytopenia, as shown in Table 10.3. Platelet-inhibiting drugs such as aspirin (acetylsalicylic acid, ASA) and other nonsteroidal anti-inflammatory drugs (NSAIDs), ticlopidine, clopidogrel, dipyridamole, and GPIIb/IIIa antagonists (abciximab, tirofiban, eptifibatide), should also be identified when evaluating a thrombocytopenic patient, as these agents may exacerbate the bleeding. Particular attention should be paid to whether the patient is receiving heparin (including exposure to heparin in line flushes) because heparin-induced thrombocytopenia (HIT; see below) needs to be excluded. Nonprescription (e.g., herbal) medications should also be documented, as they may contribute to thrombocytopenia and/or platelet dysfunction.

Medical History

Infection

One of the most common causes of thrombocytopenia is infection. Infectious causes of thrombocytopenia include HIV, hepatitis C virus (HCV), influenza, varicella zoster virus, rubella virus, EBV, CMV, hantavirus, mycoplasma, mycobacteria, malaria, trypanosomiasis, *Rickettsiae*, and *Ehrlichiae*. Transient thrombocytopenia may be observed in children receiving live viral vaccines, although a direct causative role has not been established. *Helicobacter pylori* infection can be associated with ITP, and antimicrobial therapy is recommended for such patients [10].

Infection-associated hemolytic uremic syndrome (HUS) caused by *Escherichia coli* (serotype O157:H7), *Shigella*, *Salmonella*, and *Campylobacter jejuni* typically follows an acute diarrheal illness and is characterized by the classic triad of thrombocytopenia, microangiopathic hemolytic anemia and renal dysfunction. Meningococcemia should always be considered in any unwell child found to have thrombocytopenia. Severe sepsis resulting from bacterial infection leading to disseminated intravascular coagulation (DIC) results in thrombocytopenia and associated coagulopathy (see below). It should also be highlighted that numerous infections may be associated with petechiae and/or purpura in the absence of thrombocytopenia.

Systemic Diseases

Systemic diseases involving the bone marrow, such as aplastic anemia, myelofibrosis, leukemia, lymphoma, or metastatic cancers infiltrating the bone marrow, may result in thrombocytopenia, though the classic presentation is often pancytopenia involving all three cell lines. Other systemic illnesses such as renal and liver disease not only affect platelet function, but also are often accompanied by mild to moderate thrombocytopenia.

Other Causes

Poor nutritional intake, such as can occur in the elderly or alcoholics, may result in decreased intake of vitamin B_{12} and folate resulting in

Table 10.2 Congenital thrombocytopenias characterized according to inheritance pattern, genetic mutations and associated findings.

Syndrome (OMIM Entry)	Inheritance pattern	Gene involved	Chromosomal location	Associated findings
MYH9- RD (multiple)	Autosomal dominant	*MYH9*	22q12-13	Döhle like leukocyte inclusion bodies, nephritis, sensorineural hearing loss and pre-senile cataracts
Paris-Trousseau (Jacobsen) syndrome (188025; 147791)	Autosomal dominant	*FLI1*	11q23.3-24	Cognitive and facial abnormalities
Platelet-type von Willebrand disease (PT-VWD) (177820)	Autosomal dominant	*GP1BA*	17p13	Low VWF:RCo assay, decrease in HMWVW multimers, increased low-dose RIPA. Needs to be differentiated from type IIb VWD
Radioulnar synostosis with amegakaryocytic Thrombocytopenia (605432)	Autosomal dominant	*HOXA11*	17p15.2	Radio-ulnar synostosis, clinodactyly, syndactyly, hip dysplasia, sensorineural hearing loss and progression to pancytopenia
Familial Platelet disorder with propensity for myeloid malignancy (FPD/AML) (601399)	Autosomal dominant	*RUNX1*	22q22	Platelet aggregations shows impaired aggregation to collagen and epinephrine, 35% of the cohort may go on to develop AML
ANKRD26-related thrombocytopenia (610855)	Autosomal dominant	*ANKRD26*	10p2	Normal sized platelets with bone marrow shows dysmegakaryopoiesis. Possible increased risk of leukemia
CYCS-related thrombocytopenia (612004)	Autosomal dominant	*CYCS*	7p15.3	None
TUBB1-related macrothrombocytopenia (613112)	Autosomal dominant	*TUBB1*	6p21.3	None
Bernard-Soulier syndrome (231200)	Autosomal recessive	*GP1BA, GP1BB, GP9*	17p13, 22q11, 3q21	Platelet aggregation studies show absent ristocetin induced response
Gray Platelet syndrome (139090)	Autosomal recessive (mostly)	*NBEAL2*	3p21	None
Congenital Amegakaryocytic Thrombocytopenia (CAMT) (604498)	Autosomal recessive	*MPL*	1p34	Progression to pancytopenia

(Continued)

Table 10.2 (Continued)

Syndrome (OMIM Entry)	Inheritance pattern	Gene involved	Chromosomal location	Associated findings
Thrombocytopenia with absent radii (TAR) syndrome (274000)	Autosomal recessive	*RBM8A*	1q21.1	Bilateral absent radii with thumb present. Lower limb, cardiac, gastro-intestinal and renal anomalies
Thrombocytopenia associated with sitosterolemia (210250)	Autosomal recessive	*ABCG5, ABCG8*	2p21	Stomatocytosis, tendon xanthomas and premature atherosclerosis
Wiskott-Aldrich syndrome (X-linked thrombocytopenia) (301000)	X-linked	*WAS*	Xp11.22	Recurrent infections, eczema, with a risk of auto-immunity and lymphoid malignancy
X-linked thrombocytopenia with dyserythropoiesis (300367; 314050)	X-linked	*GATA1*	Xp11.23	Dyserythropoietic anemia
FLNA-related thrombocytopenia (nd)	X-linked	FLNA	Xq28	Possible association with periventricular nodular heterotopia

Source: Kumar and Kahr 2013 [12]. Reproduced with permission of Elseiver.

Table 10.3 Drugs causing thrombocytopenia.

Drug	Mechanism
Immune-mediated	
Acetaminophen	
Aminoglutethimide	
Aminosalicylic acid	
Amiodarone	
Amphotericin B	
Carbamazepine	May also induce marrow aplasia
Cimetidine	
Chlorothiazide/hydrochlorothiazide	
Danazol	
Diatrizoate meglumine (Hypaque)	
Diclofenac	
Digoxin	
Gold/gold salts	May also induce marrow aplasia
IFN-a	May also inhibit megakaryocyte proliferation
Levamisole	
Meclofenamate	
Methyldopa	
Nalidixic acid	
Oxprenolol	
Procainamide	
Quinidine and quinine	May also produce a TTP-like picture
Ranitidine	
Rifampin	
Simvastatin	
Sulfasalazine	
Sulfisoxazole	
Trimethoprim-sulfamethoxazole	
Vancomycin	
Unique antibody-mediated process	
Heparin	PF4-heparin-antibody causes HIT by platelet activation
Abciximab, eptifibatide and tirofiban	GP IIb/IIIa (αIIbβ3 integrin) antagonist; or peptide derivative
Suppression of platelet production	
Anagrelide	Inhibits megakaryocyte maturation
Imatinib	
Thiazide diuretics	

(Continued)

Table 10.3 (Continued)

Drug	Mechanism
Valproic acid	Inhibits megakaryocyte maturation; dose-related; may also induce marrow aplasia
Suppression of all hematopoietic cells	
Chemotherapeutic agents	Some also cause immune-mediated destruction
Thrombotic thrombocytopenic purpura	
Ticlopidine	May also induce marrow aplasia
Clopidogrel	
Cyclosporine and FK506 (tacrolimus)	
Mitomycin C	Dose-related
Unknown mechanism	
Monoclonal antibodies	

Source: Modified from Dlott *et al.* 2004 [37] and Aster and Bougie 2007 [38].

megaloblastic anemia and thrombocytopenia. In addition, excessive alcohol intake has direct inhibitory effects on platelet production. Pregnancy is commonly associated with thrombocytopenia (approximately 6–10% of pregnant women), usually appearing during the third trimester; in this situation, multiple etiologies need to be considered (see below).

Transfusion History

Previous transfusions may place an individual at risk of developing post-transfusion purpura, in which severe thrombocytopenia can appear 7–14 days after the transfusion of a blood product. Transfusion-associated infection, such as HIV, HCV, CMV, West Nile virus, or malaria may be complicated by thrombocytopenia.

Physical Examination

The clinical appearance is of paramount importance in the assessment of the thrombocytopenic patient, and provides the first clue as to the likely etiology. A sick patient in the intensive care unit may have a number of possible contributing factors, including severe sepsis, DIC, drug-induced, post-transfusion purpura, massive blood transfusion, and systemic illness. In contrast, a well patient with newly diagnosed isolated thrombocytopenia may have congenital

thrombocytopenia, ITP, or, in a neonate, auto- or alloimmune thrombocytopenia.

Petechiae consisting of small (<2 mm), red, flat, discrete lesions, occurring most frequently in the dependent areas on the ankles and feet, represent extravasated red cells from capillaries and are the hallmark of a primary hemostatic disorder. They are nontender and do not blanch under pressure. Purpura (<1 cm) and ecchymoses (>1 cm) represent larger areas of bleeding, and when observed in mucous membranes such as the oropharynx are described as "wet purpura". These findings are in contrast to delayed bleeding into joints or muscle, which suggest a coagulation disorder rather than a platelet or von Willebrand factor (VWF) problem.

Laboratory Evaluation

Laboratory tests are discussed in detail elsewhere, so only selected points are emphasized here. Modern technology has greatly facilitated laboratory evaluation and reporting of clinical tests.

Blood Film

The importance of examining a blood film in a patient with newly diagnosed thrombocytopenia cannot be overemphasized. For example:

- Visualization of schistocytes (red blood cell (RBC) fragments) could be indicative of thrombotic thrombocytopenic purpura/ hemolytic uremic syndrome (TTP/HUS), or DIC (Figure 10.2).

- Evidence of platelet clumps may suggest pseudothrombocytopenia.
- Megathrombocytes with Döhle-like inclusions in neutrophils could be indicative of MYH9-related diseases (MYH9-RD) (Figure 10.3).
- Pale agranular-appearing platelets could represent gray platelet syndrome (Figure 10.4).
- Blasts suggest the diagnosis of leukemia or a myeloproliferative disorder.
- Macrocytes with hypersegmented neutrophils suggests megaloblastic anemia.
- Toxic granulation suggests infection.
- Spherocytes and polychromasia may be observed in Evan syndrome (coexisting autoimmune hemolytic anemia and ITP).

Pseudothrombocytopenia resulting from EDTA-induced platelet clumping may be overcome by obtaining a film from a drop of blood smeared directly onto a slide, or by collection of blood into citrate or heparin anticoagulants.

Mean Platelet Volume and Reticulated Platelets

For inherited causes of thrombocytopenia, diagnostic algorithms based on the platelet size

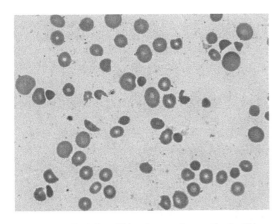

Figure 10.2 Peripheral blood smear in a patient with microangiopathic hemolytic anemia showing helmet cells, schistocytes, and microspherocytes. *Source*: Kumar *et al*. 2013 [47]. Reproduced with permission of Karger Medical and Scientific Publishers. *See Plate section for color representation of this figure.*

or mean platelet volume (MPV) have been suggested [11]. Furthermore, it has been demonstrated that diagnostic criteria that combine MPV and mean platelet diameter (MPD) may help distinguish congenital thrombocytopenia from ITP [12]. In a prospective study of 35 patients with congenital thrombocytopenia MYH9-RD and Bernard–Soulier Syndrome (BSS)) and 50 with ITP, MPV and MPD were significantly higher in patients with congenital thrombocytopenia. Receiver operating characteristic curves (ROC curves) identified that an MPV >12.4 fL had an 83% sensitivity and 89% specificity whereas a MPD >3.3 μm had an 89% sensitivity and 88% specificity in differentiating congenital thrombocytopenia from ITP [13]. One caveat of this approach is that not all automated counters are able detect very small platelets (e.g., Wiskott–Aldrich syndrome) or very large platelets (e.g., BSS), resulting in underestimation of the platelet count [14]. This emphasizes the importance of examining the blood film.

Platelets with a higher RNA content are believed to represent younger ("immature") cells, and it has been postulated that an increase in the relative proportion of young platelets is indicative of increased platelet turnover, akin to the reticulocytosis that occurs during marrow recovery or hemolytic anemia. Many modern hematology analyzers utilize a flow cytometer in combination with a dye that binds to RNA within cells to provide a direct estimate of the immature platelet fraction ("reticulated platelets"). The utility of this technology has not yet been clearly defined; however, the parameter may be useful in predicting platelet recovery following chemotherapy, and also in the initial diagnostic evaluation of the thrombocytopenic patient [15].

Bone Marrow Examination

For a typical presentation of ITP, a bone marrow examination is not required in patients. However, a bone marrow aspirate and biopsy is recommended in:

- those with additional cytopenias;

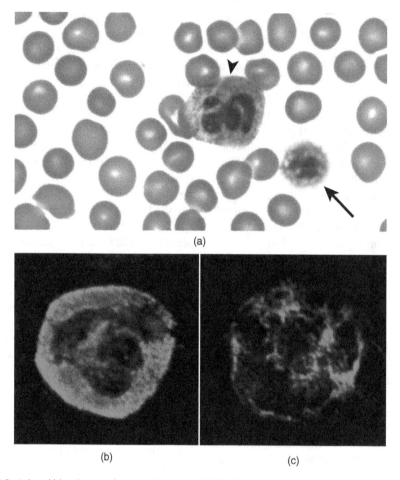

Figure 10.3 (a) Peripheral blood smear from a patient with MYH9-RD demonstrating giant platelet (arrow) and neutrophil inclusion (arrowhead). Immunofluorescent visualization of nonmuscle myosin heavy chain IIA aggregates: (b) normal homogenous cytoplasmic staining (lower left) and (c) abnormal variable speckled cytoplasmic staining. *See Plate section for color representation of this figure.*

- patients with lassitude, protracted fever, bone, or joint pain;
- patients with lymphadenopathy and/or organomegaly;
- those with unexplained macrocytosis or dysplastic features on blood film.

Specialized Platelet Function Tests

Specialized tests (see Chapter 4) that may be indicated in the evaluation of specific congenital thrombocytopenias include:

- platelet aggregation;

- flow cytometry using antibodies labeling GPIb (for BSS);
- platelet electron microscopy (for gray platelet syndrome; Figure 10.4);
- specialized immunocytochemistry (for MYH9-RD; Figure 10.3);
- western blot for protein analyses (for Quebec platelet disorder); and
- given the emerging data showing a genotype–phenotype correlation for several congenital thrombocytopenias, effort should be made to refer samples to specialized laboratories which can perform DNA analysis.

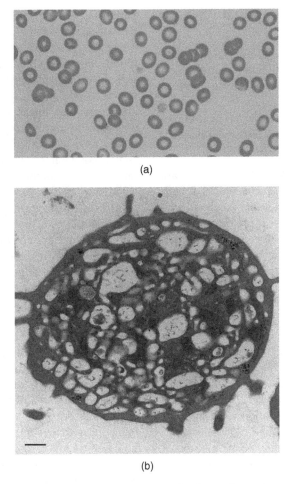

(a)

(b)

Figure 10.4 (a) Peripheral blood smear from a patient with gray platelet syndrome demonstrating large gray-appearing platelets. (b) Platelet transmission electron micrograph from a patient with gray platelet syndrome showing complete absence of alpha granules with increased vacuoles. Scale bar represents 5 nanometers. *Source:* Kumar and Kahr 2013 [12]. Reproduced with permission of Elsevier. *See Plate section for color representation of this figure.*

Specific Conditions

Immune Thrombocytopenia

Historically called immune thrombocytopenic purpura, an international working group (IWG) has recently recommended that the condition be renamed "immune thrombocytopenia" (though retaining the abbreviation ITP), emphasizing the fact that "purpura" and bleeding symptoms are either absent or rarely seen in a large proportion of the patients with ITP [16, 17]. ITP is an

autoimmune syndrome that occurs secondary to autoantibodies that accelerate platelet destruction and additionally impair megakaryocytopoiesis [18]. It has an estimated incidence of 2.2–5.3 per 10^5 children/year and 3.3 per 10^5 adults/year [19]. There is a modest female predominance in adults, while young boys and girls are affected equally. In children the condition is typically acute and spontaneous resolution is common, while in adults it is frequently a chronic disorder with an insidious onset, often diagnosed incidentally when a blood count is performed for other reasons [20]. The IWG has classified ITP into:

1) primary ITP: autoimmune condition characterized by platelet count $< 100 \times 10^9/L$, in the absence of other causes know to be associated with ITP;

2) secondary ITP: all other forms of immune mediated thrombocytopenia except primary ITP [17].

It is estimated that 80% of all cases of ITP are primary whereas 20% occur associated with underlying comorbid conditions such as systemic lupus erythematosus (SLE) (5%), antiphospholipid antibody syndrome (2%), common variable immune deficiency (CVID) (1%), chronic lymphocytic leukemia (CLL) (2%), Evan syndrome (2%), acquired lymphoproliferative syndrome (ALPS) (1%), HCV infection (2%), HIV (1%), *Helicobacter pylori* infection (1%), and postvaccination (3%) [21]. Of note, 5–10% of adult patients initially diagnosed with primary ITP will subsequently develop an underlying systemic autoimmune disease, resulting in a change in their classification. ITP may also be classified based on the duration of symptoms: newly diagnosed ITP (within 3 months of diagnosis), persistent ITP (within 3–12 months of diagnosis), and chronic ITP (lasting for more than 12 months) [17].

While the exact pathophysiology of ITP remains unclear, it has been postulated that the immune tolerance defects resulting in thrombocytopenia may be classified into three categories: peripheral tolerance defects which occur in the setting of immune stimulation (e.g., postvaccination or infection associated ITP); differentiation blocks with skewed peripheral B-cell subsets (e.g., CVID and CLL-associated ITP); and central tolerance defects arising during development or in the bone marrow (e.g., Evan syndrome, ALPS).

Diagnosis

The diagnosis of primary ITP is predominantly one of exclusion, and is suggested by the presence of isolated thrombocytopenia (platelet count $< 100 \times 10^9/L$) in an otherwise healthy patient in the absence of other causes. The patient may present with evidence of mucocutaneous bleeding, or after a routine complete blood count (CBC) in an asymptomatic individual. A thorough history and physical examination, combined with careful review of a CBC and peripheral smear, is usually sufficient for diagnosis in most cases. Underlying systemic diseases, drug-induced thrombocytopenias, as well as congenital thrombocytopenias (positive family history, abnormal blood film) should be ruled out. In the absence of atypical clinical features (weight loss, persistent fever, bone pain, night sweats, lymphadenopathy, recurrent infections, and dysmorphic features), and when additional abnormalities are not noted on the peripheral smear, bone marrow aspiration and biopsy are no longer recommended, irrespective of the age of the patients [10,22].

Platelet autoantibody measurements are neither sensitive nor specific enough to be clinically useful, and should not be relied upon for diagnosis. Interestingly, plasma TPO levels are usually normal or mildly elevated in ITP, but are greatly elevated in amegakaryocytic states (e.g., congenital amegakaryocytic thrombocytopenia, bone marrow suppression, and aplastic anemia) and therefore may be diagnostically useful if available. Currently, measurement of TPO is largely limited to the research setting. Testing for antinuclear antibodies, lupus anticoagulant, and anticardiolipin antibodies, or for abnormal serum immunoglobulin levels is not recommended in the acute setting, though testing may be indicated for patients with persistent or chronic thrombocytopenia. Of note, the American Society of Hematology recommends testing for HIV and hepatitis C in all adults with acute ITP, given that treatment of the underlying disease may alter the course of secondary ITP [10].

Prognosis

Most children with ITP (80%) have complete recovery of counts by 1 year, though in a minority the low counts persist beyond a year, thereby resulting in a classification of chronic ITP. Several studies have evaluated both clinical and laboratory markers that might predict a chronic course. In general, older age at onset of symptoms, higher platelet counts at presentation, higher levels of inflammatory cytokines (IL-6), and lack of mucosal bleeding symptoms at diagnosis are thought to herald a chronic course [23–25].

Principles of Management

The therapeutic goal is to attain a safe platelet count that prevents major bleeding and allows a patient to lead a relatively normal life, rather than correcting the platelet counts to normal levels [17]. In adults, treatment is generally indicated if the platelet count is below 30×10^9/L [10]. Those with higher counts can be observed, as the bleeding risk is low and early treatment does not modify the course of the disease. Platelet-inhibiting drugs such as ASA and other NSAIDs should be avoided. First-line management of ITP consists of glucocorticoids (prednisone 1 mg/kg/day po), IV immunoglobulin (IVIG 1 g/kg) or IV anti-D ($50 - 75\,\mu g\,/\,kg$) in Rh(D)-positive patients with intact spleens. With major bleeding episodes, or if the platelet count is less than 10×10^9/L, glucocorticoids can be given together with either IVIG or IV anti-D [10,22]. In the presence of intracranial hemorrhage (ICH) platelet transfusions are also indicated.

There has been a paradigm shift in the management guidelines for pediatric ITP. Historically, treatment was recommended for all children with bleeding symptoms and those with platelet counts $< 20 \times 10^9$/L. The current guidelines, however, indicate that observation is sufficient for children with no symptoms, or skin manifestations (petechiae, purpura, or ecchymosis) alone, regardless of the platelet count [10]. However, treatment may be considered when the family is geographically isolated and compliance to close follow up is difficult. Oral prednisone (3–4 mg/kg/day for 3–4 days), IVIG ($0.8 - 1\,g\,/\,kg \times 1\,dose$), or IV anti-D ($50 - 75\,\mu g\,/\,kg \times 1\,dose$) in Rh(D)-positive, non-splenectomized children are all efficacious regimens, although the response to IVIG is generally more rapid [10, 22]. IV anti-D has recently received a black box warning, given case reports

of severe hemolysis and DIC and it is currently recommended that all patients receiving IV anti-D be observed in the hospital for at least 8 hours after the infusion. Furthermore, IV anti-D is contraindicated in children with a baseline hemoglobin less than 10 g/dL or evidence of hemolytic anemia [26]. Similar to adult guidelines, platelet transfusions are reserved for life-threatening bleeding and ICH.

Chronic and Refractory Immune Thrombocytopenia

Around 70% of patients will respond to first-line therapy with corticosteroids or immunoglobulin; however, in adults, the effect is often transient or requires repeated doses to maintain response. In contrast, only 20% of children will relapse, and late spontaneous remission is well-recognized in this subgroup. Per the IWG, chronic ITP is defined as persistence of thrombocytopenia ($< 100 \times 10^9$/L) for more than 12 months [17]. The definition of refractory ITP is based on splenectomy and is reserved for patients who have severe-persistent thrombocytopenia requiring additional therapy despite splenectomy. Given the emergence of an anti-CD20 antibody (rituximab) and TPO receptor (TPO-R) agonists as second-line therapies, this definition may need to be readdressed.

Splenectomy is the currently accepted second-line approach for adults with chronic ITP, or those who experience unacceptable side-effects from repeated steroid exposure. It is estimated that 60–70% will have a durable response to this procedure. In children, splenectomy is generally deferred for at least 12 months following diagnosis, due to the higher lifelong risk of postsplenectomy sepsis, and the greater chance of remission compared with adults [26]. Numerous therapeutic regimens have been described for those patients who fail to respond or relapse after splenectomy (refractory ITP); however, evidence for efficacy is mostly limited to case series. Examples include high-dose dexamethasone, danazol, dapsone, azathioprine, cyclosporine, mycophenolate, vincristine, and cyclophosphamide.

Rituximab, a monoclonal anti-CD20 chimeric antibody may be used for patients with chronic

ITP as an alternative for splenectomy or where splenectomy has failed. While the optimal dose and frequency of administration for ITP remains debatable, most studies have reported using $375\,mg/m^2$ weekly for 4 weeks. It is estimated that about 60% of patients will have an initial response to rituximab [27], though only 25–30% of patients have a sustained response for longer than 1 year [28,29]. Interestingly, a nonblinded, randomized trial of rituximab in nonsplenectomized adult ITP patients failed to demonstrate a difference in a 6-month composite outcome as defined by any platelet count $<50 \times 10^9/L$, significant bleeding, or the need for rescue treatment [30]. Viral reactivation and progressive multifocal leukoencephalopathy are rare side-effects of rituximab.

Although ITP is predominantly a condition of increased platelet destruction, TPO levels in ITP are not elevated in proportion to the severity of thrombocytopenia, possibly due to faster TPO clearance resulting from rapid platelet turnover. First-generation TPO-R agonists, recombinant forms of human TPO, were withdrawn in 1998 after thrombocytopenia due to anti-TPO antibodies was observed in some healthy volunteers receiving such agents. There are numerous second-generation TPO-R agonists currently in development, and these appear to be nonimmunogenic, well tolerated, and effective at increasing platelet count. Currently, two TPO-R agonists (romiplostim and eltrombopag) are approved for management of adult patients with chronic refractory ITP (Eltrombopag was recently approved for use in children ages 1 year and above with chronic ITP). Romiplostim is administered as a weekly subcutaneous injection and was shown to be superior to both placebo and standard of care in two randomized trials [31,32]. Eltrombopag, an oral TPO-R agonist was also shown to be superior to placebo in a randomized trial with long-term safety data being published as well [33,34]. Recurrent thrombocytopenia on discontinuation, arterial and venous thrombosis, bone marrow reticulin deposition, and hepatotoxicity (with eltrombopag) are known side-effects.

Evan Syndrome

The combination of ITP with autoimmune hemolytic anemia (which may occur simultaneously or sequentially) in the absence of an underlying cause is referred to as Evan syndrome, and has a pathogenesis and clinical course distinct from that of classic ITP [35]. More than half of these patients also have autoimmune neutropenia. Response to standard therapy is poorly sustained, and multiple relapses with significant long-term morbidity is typical. Specific disorders that mimic Evan syndrome must be excluded, as the management of these conditions is different–these include ALPS, CVID, and systemic autoimmune disease (e.g., SLE).

Drug-induced Thrombocytopenia

The incidence of drug-induced thrombocytopenia is estimated to be 1 case per 100 000 annually [36]. This is thought to be an underestimation, either because a platelet count is not measured or thrombocytopenia is attributed to other factors. There are a large number of agents known to cause thrombocytopenia, and most of these can be broadly divided into the following categories:

- drugs that cause predictable dose-dependent marrow suppression;
- drugs that cause idiosyncratic marrow aplasia;
- drugs that specifically inhibit megakaryopoiesis;
- drugs that trigger immune destruction of platelets;
- drugs that cause a TTP-like condition;
- drugs that induce platelet aggregation.

Chemotherapeutic agents used for malignancy or potent immunosuppression often cause dose-dependent thrombocytopenia as a result of generalized bone marrow suppression, although some of these agents can also induce immune-mediated platelet destruction. Although the mechanisms are poorly understood, a number of drugs have been implicated in aplastic anemia, including anticonvulsants, NSAIDs, sulfonamides, and gold salts. Some drugs known to specifically inhibit megakaryopoiesis are listed in Table 10.3. Anagrelide, used in the treatment of thrombocythemia in patients with myeloproliferative diseases, can cause severe thrombocytopenia. Valproic acid, commonly used in seizure disorders, has been associated with dose-dependent thrombocytopenia resulting from direct megakaryocyte suppression. Thiazide diuretics also have a mild inhibitory effect on megakaryocytes.

Many drugs have been implicated in producing a TTP-like condition, with thrombocytopenia, hemolysis, and varying degrees of neurological or renal dysfunction, although for most agents this appears to be an exceedingly rare event [37]. The pathogenesis is poorly understood, although direct or immune-mediated endothelial injury may be an important trigger. Drugs for which a causal association seems likely include mitomycin C (dose-related), calcineurin inhibitors such as cyclosporine and tacrolimus (1–3% incidence), ticlopidine (<0.1% incidence), and clopidogrel (rare). Interestingly, quinine can also cause TTP, although it is better known for inducing antibody-mediated platelet destruction.

Drug-induced, antibody mediated platelet destruction is the most common mechanism of iatrogenic thrombocytopenia [38]. There are several mechanisms of drug-induced immune thrombocytopenia, although the "quinine-type" accounts for the majority:

- Drugs that bind to platelet glycoproteins forming a "compound epitope" include penicillin, quinidine, quinine, and sulfonamide. The antibody binding to such platelets is dependent on the presence of the offending drug.
- Gold salts and procainamide, on the other hand, can induce true autoantibodies which subsequently can bind to platelets in the absence of the original offending drug.
- Antiplatelet agents such as tirofiban, eptifibatide, and abciximab, which specifically target the GPIIb/IIIa (αIIbβ3 integrin) receptor on platelets, cause thrombocytopenia in 1–5% of cardiac patients via antibody-mediated processes.

Diagnosis of drug-induced immune thrombocytopenia requires a high index of suspicion, as systemic illness or other coexistent factors may confuse the clinical picture. Onset of thrombocytopenia within 5–7 days of commencing a new drug is an important clue. Withdrawal of the offending agent leads to resolution of thrombocytopenia in most cases, although rarely IVIG, steroids, or more aggressive management may be indicated. Inadvertent rechallenge with the causative drug may induce rapid and severe thrombocytopenia and should be avoided.

Heparin-induced Thrombocytopenia

In a subset of patients exposure to heparin (unfractionated heparin and low-molecular-weight heparin) may induce a life-threatening immune complication known as heparin-induced thrombocytopenia (HIT) [39]. Though well recognized in adults, HIT is thought to be exceedingly rare in children [40]. HIT differs from other thrombocytopenias in that it is a hypercoagulable state rather than a bleeding condition, manifesting as a sudden decline in platelet count within 5–10 days of heparin exposure with venous and/or arterial thrombosis. This iatrogenic disorder is discussed in more detail in Chapter 28.

Pregnancy-associated Thrombocytopenia

There is a physiological decline in platelet count during the course of a normal pregnancy, most pronounced in the third trimester, although only 6–10% of pregnant women become truly thrombocytopenic (platelet count $< 150 \times 10^9$/L) [41,42]. Mild thrombocytopenia ($100 - 149 \times 10^9$/L) is typical and of little clinical significance, though lower platelet counts warrant closer scrutiny. The most common causes of pregnancy-associated thrombocytopenia include:

- gestational thrombocytopenia (incidental or benign thrombocytopenia of pregnancy), accounts for approximately 75% of cases;
- pre-eclampsia ± HELLP (hemolysis, elevated liver enzymes, low platelets), accounts for approximately 20% of cases;

- ITP ± SLE, accounts for approximately 4% of cases;
- microangiopathic hemolytic anemia (TTP and HUS);
- disseminated intravascular coagulation (DIC).

Gestational thrombocytopenia is a diagnosis of exclusion, but in 95% of cases it manifests as mild thrombocytopenia in an asymptomatic pregnant patient with a previously normal platelet count. This is a benign condition that requires no treatment. Although more severe thrombocytopenia can occasionally be seen, counts below 75×10^9/L should raise strong suspicion of an alternative diagnosis. Similarly, the finding of thrombocytopenia in early pregnancy is more suggestive of ITP or a pre-existing condition. Thrombocytopenia develops in approximately 20% of patients with pre-eclampsia, and there is an inverse relationship between platelet count and severity of disease. The HELLP syndrome can be a serious complication, associated with up to 20% fetal mortality. Thrombocytopenia associated with pre-eclampsia and HELLP syndrome improves following delivery, whereas thrombocytopenia associated with primary microangiopathic hemolytic anemias, TTP, and HUS does not. These conditions may sometimes be difficult to discern from pre-eclampsia or HELLP syndrome in a pregnant woman, and plasma exchange may be required despite an uncertain diagnosis (see below).

DIC complicates a small proportion of cases, and a coagulation screen is an important component of the diagnostic work-up. ITP occurs in 1–2 per 1000 pregnancies and represents approximately 3–5% of the causes of thrombocytopenia during pregnancy. A pregnant patient with ITP can be treated with IVIG (1 g/kg prepregnant weight) and/or prednisone (1 mg/kg prepregnant weight) in the acute setting to raise the platelet count to above 10×10^9/L. Measurement of platelet count in the newborn is important, as 5–10% of infants born to mothers with ITP will have significant thrombocytopenia ($< 50 \times 10^9$/L).

Post-Transfusion Purpura

Post-transfusion purpura (PTP) is a rare disorder, which usually manifests as severe thrombocytopenia occurring 5–10 days following transfusion of a blood product. It is caused by the formation of high-titer alloantibodies against platelet glycoproteins, and represents an anamnestic immune response in a patient previously sensitized through antigen exposure during pregnancy and/or transfusion. The antibodies are most commonly directed against the platelet alloantigen HPA-1a epitope, where the platelet GPIIIa contains a leucine at position 33. Polymorphisms of GPIIIa result in alloantigen HPA-1a and alloantigen HPA-1b (proline at position 33 of GPIIIa), which occur at a frequency of approximately 86% and 14% in Caucasians, respectively. Classically, the affected patient is a homozygous HPA-1b, middle-aged, multiparous woman; however, the condition also occurs in men and nulliparous women. The alloantibodies paradoxically cause destruction of autologous as well as transfused platelets through poorly understood mechanisms.

PTP has been estimated to occur following 1/50–100 000 transfusions; however, this may represent an underestimate as the diagnosis may be overshadowed by coexisting factors such as heparin exposure or sepsis. Interestingly, countries in which universal leukodepletion is practiced have noticed a striking reduction in the incidence of PTP, presumably due to the fact that the process removes platelets from red cell concentrates [43]. Diagnosis of PTP requires a strong index of suspicion, followed by demonstration of high-titer HPA alloantibodies in the transfusion recipient. The observation of a decline in platelet count *below* baseline *following* a platelet transfusion can be an important clue to differentiate this condition from platelet refractoriness which is multifactorial and far more common. Treatment of PTP consists of IVIG, corticosteroids, or plasmapheresis. Platelet transfusions are contraindicated except in rare circumstances, when HPA-1a negative platelets may be used for life-threatening bleeding complications.

HIV-associated Thrombocytopenia

There are multiple factors that contribute to the thrombocytopenia frequently associated with HIV, including immune mechanisms and defective platelet production [44]. The immune-mediated platelet destruction in HIV is indistinguishable from ITP with respect to increased destruction of antibody-coated platelets and the response to prednisone, IVIG, and splenectomy. It does differ from classic ITP with respect to:

- male predominance;
- markedly elevated platelet-associated IgG, IgM, and complement C_3, C_4 ;
- presence of circulating immune complexes; and
- antibody-mediated peroxide lysis of platelets.

Treatment with antiretroviral therapy tends to improve the defective thrombopoiesis in HIV-infected patients. TTP is also found more frequently in HIV-infected patients.

HCV-associated Thrombocytopenia

Thrombocytopenia is a common complication in patients with chronic liver disease, reported in 76% of cirrhotic patients, with moderate thrombocytopenia (platelet count 50×10^9/L to 75×10^9/L) being reported in 13% of cirrhotic patients [3]. Multiple factors contribute to the development of thrombocytopenia in this setting including splenic sequestration secondary to portal hypertension, bone marrow suppression either from the hepatitis C virus or interferon therapy, and thrombopoietin deficiency secondary to hepatic dysfunction [45]. Liver disease is discussed in greater detail in Chapter 23. HCV-associated thrombocytopenia warrants particular mention for several reasons:

- Thrombocytopenia in HCV frequently occurs in the absence of clinical or radiological features to suggest portal hypertension.
- There is an approximately 20-fold increase in the incidence of ITP in patients with HCV, and treatment of ITP with steroids may promote viremia.

- The presence of thrombocytopenia in HCV is an adverse prognostic factor and may limit options for therapy, as antiviral agents such as interferon-α can further reduce platelet count.
- Results from two recently completed phase 3 randomized controlled trials has shown that eltrombopag increases platelet counts in thrombocytopenic patients with HCV and advanced fibrosis and cirrhosis, allowing otherwise ineligible or marginal patients to begin and maintain antiviral therapy [46].

Microangiopathies

Nonimmune, destructive thrombocytopenias include DIC, Kasabach–Merritt syndrome, TTP, HUS, and other conditions listed in Table 10.1. These disorders share the common pathophysiological endpoint of platelet trapping and thrombus formation in the microvasculature, with subsequent fragmentation of red cells due to mechanical damage. They are discussed in greater detail in Chapters 12 and 28.

Disseminated Intravascular Coagulation

DIC is a form of consumptive coagulopathy characterized by the dysregulated systemic activation of coagulation and impairment of fibrinolysis. DIC results in the widespread deposition of microthrombi with occlusion of small to medium-sized blood vessels, and may eventually result in multiorgan failure. Concurrent consumption of platelets and clotting factors from the ongoing coagulation may result in hemorrhage [47]. The diagnosis of DIC is usually made in association with an overt underlying systemic disorder [48]. DIC is discussed in greater detail in Chapter 12.

Kasabach–Merritt Syndrome

Kasabach–Merritt syndrome describes the association of thrombocytopenia with kaposiform hemangioendothelioma or tufted hemangioma. Although poorly understood, the pathogenesis is thought to be caused by platelet trapping and activation within the abnormal endothelium of the hemangioma resulting in thrombocytopenia and laboratory evidence of DIC, including hypofibrinogenemia and increased D-dimers. It is important to highlight that the hemangioma may not be clinically obvious, and investigation of any newborn with microangiopathic hemolysis should include appropriate imaging studies, such as cranial and abdominal ultrasound to exclude the presence of concealed vascular lesions. Kasabach–Merritt hemangiomas tend to grow rapidly for several months followed by spontaneous regression in the first few years of life. However, individualized treatment using vascular ligation, embolization, corticosteroids, α-interferon (IFN-α), or vincristine may be required in some cases of life-threatening thrombocytopenia and coagulopathy.

Thrombotic Thrombocytopenic Purpura and Hemolytic Uremic Syndrome

TTP has been historically characterized by the pentad of microangiopathic hemolytic anemia, thrombocytopenia, fever, neurological deficit, and renal impairment. HUS, another microangiopathic condition, is defined by the simultaneous occurrence of thrombocytopenia, microangiopathic hemolytic anemia, and renal dysfunction. Collectively, TTP and HUS are classified as thrombotic microangiopathies. They are further discussed in Chapter 13.

Hypersplenism

When splenomegaly results in cytopenias and compensatory bone marrow hyperplasia the term "hypersplenism" is appropriate, although bone marrow biopsy in this context is most often performed to exclude hematological malignancy (e.g., leukemia, lymphoma, myeloproliferative disease) rather than to confirm hypersplenism per se. Numerous conditions are associated with splenomegaly and hypersplenism, including portal hypertension secondary to liver disease or portal vein thrombosis, hematological malignancies, chronic hemolytic anemia, storage disorders, leishmaniasis, and malaria. The clinical picture is usually dominated by the underlying disease rather than symptomatic pancytopenia;

however, in the presence of massive splenomegaly thrombocytopenia can be severe and increases following platelet transfusion are poor. Intervention is rarely indicated for management of thrombocytopenia alone; however, improvement in counts usually follows splenectomy or splenic embolization. In the setting of portal hypertension, surgical procedures that redirect or bypass the portal circulation can reduce the risk of bleeding associated with thrombocytopenia and esophageal varices.

Thrombocytopenia in the Newborn Infant

Thrombocytopenia is one of the most common hematological abnormalities observed during the neonatal period, with an estimated incidence of 1–5% in all newborns, though the reported incidence in neonates admitted to the intensive care unit is much higher at 22–35% [49]. Most neonates have mild-to-moderate thrombocytopenia, with only 5–10% presenting with platelet count $< 50 \times 10^9/L$.

The differential diagnosis is broad; however, relatively few conditions account for the majority of cases and many of the rare disorders can be readily identified on the basis of associated clinical and/or laboratory features. A useful approach in determining the etiology of thrombocytopenia in a newborn is to differentiate based on the timing of onset and clinical condition of the infant (Table 10.4). Early-onset thrombocytopenia (<72 hours of age) is most often mild to moderate in severity, and frequently relates to chronic fetal hypoxia (e.g., pre-eclampsia, infant of diabetic mother, IUGR). In the absence of an identifiable precipitant, NAIT should always be considered when early-onset thrombocytopenia is detected in an otherwise well neonate (see below). Severe early-onset thrombocytopenia ($< 50 \times 10^9/L$) in a sick newborn commonly results from perinatal infection (e.g., group B *Streptococcus*, cytomegalovirus) or asphyxia (e.g., meconium aspiration syndrome). Late-onset thrombocytopenia (>72 hours of age) is often due to bacterial or fungal sepsis and/or necrotizing enterocolitis, and is frequently severe in this setting.

Most thrombocytopenia in the neonatal period is self-limited or resolves with treatment of the underlying condition. Treatment of severe nonimmune-mediated thrombocytopenia in neonates consists of platelet transfusion

Table 10.4 Causes of thrombocytopenia in newborns.

Early onset, well infant

Placental insufficiency (e.g., preeclampsia, IUGR)[*]
Alloimmune (NAIT)[*]
Auto-immune (e.g., maternal ITP, SLE)
Artefactual (clumping *ex vivo*)
Renal vein thrombosis
Hereditary thrombocytopenia (see Table 10.2)

Early onset, sick infant

Perinatal asphyxia[*]
Perinatal infection (maternal flora, e.g., GBS, *E. coli*)[*]
DIC (+/− evidence of infection or asphyxia)[*]
Exchange/massive transfusion
Congenital infection (e.g., rubella, CMV, toxoplasmosis)
Severe Rh(D) hemolytic disease
Non-immune hydrops fetalis
Kasabach–Merritt syndrome
Inborn errors of metabolism (e.g., organic acidurias)
Congenital leukemia
Osteopetrosis (severe form)

Early onset, associated congenital anomalies

Aneuploidy (trisomy 21, 13, 18; Turner syndrome)
Hereditary thrombocytopenia (see Table 10.2)
Bone marrow failure syndromes (e.g., Fanconi anemia)
Congenital infection (e.g., rubella)

Late onset, well infant

Late detection of an early onset condition[*]
Drug-induced (antimicrobials, heparin)
Infection (pre-sepsis)

Late onset, sick infant

Infection (skin/gut flora, e.g., *Pseudomonas sp.,
   Candida sp.*)[*]
Necrotizing enterocolitis[*]
Extensive thrombosis
Exchange/massive transfusion
Familial TTP

Early onset < 72 hours of age or present at birth;
late onset > 72 hours of age;
IUGR, intrauterine growth restriction;
GBS, group B *Streptococcus*;
*Most common.

according to transfusion threshold guidelines reviewed by Roberts *et al.* [49].

Neonatal Alloimmune Thrombocytopenia

NAIT is an important cause of thrombocytopenia in an otherwise well-appearing full-term infant. The overall incidence of NAIT in the Caucasian population is estimated to be 1 in 1000–2000 live births, while that of severe NAIT is 1 in 5000 live births. The importance of recognizing and accurately diagnosing NAIT lies not only in the immediate management of the affected infant, but also in the approach to future pregnancies of the affected mother.

In NAIT, the destruction of fetal or neonatal platelets results from transplacental passage of maternal platelet-specific alloantibodies. This is similar to the pathogenesis of Rh(D) hemolytic disease but, in contrast, NAIT frequently affects the first pregnancy (20% of first pregnancies are affected). The most frequent platelet antigen polymorphism in Caucasian populations causing NAIT is the HPA-1a epitope where the platelet GPIIIa contains a leucine at position 33. Alloantibodies (anti-HPA-1a) can form if the mother is homozygous for HPA-1b (proline at position 33 of GPIIIa). HPA-1a incompatibility is estimated to occur in 1 : 350 pregnancies, though thrombocytopenia develops in only 1 : 1000 to 1 : 2000 pregnancies. The ability of a HPA-1b female to form anti-HPA-1a antibodies is significantly increased when she positive for the HLA class II antigen DRB3*0101. HPA-4a alloantibody (arginine at position 143 of GPIIIa) is the most common cause of severe NAIT in Asian populations.

Because ICH may occur antenatally, and because NAIT can present during the first pregnancy, it is often difficult to alter the clinical course of these patients. However, a history of a previously affected infant can be predictive for diagnosing NAIT in a subsequent fetus, with the potential of antenatal intervention. With few exceptions, untreated at-risk fetuses (antigen positive) have more severe disease than their previously affected siblings. Antenatal intervention can effectively ameliorate the disease course, though the ideal approach to management remains unresolved. It is generally accepted that weekly infusions of IVIG (1 g/kg) with or without corticosteroids, given to the mother, can reduce the degree of thrombocytopenia and risk of ICH in the neonate. For high-risk patients (e.g., history of a ICH in a sibling), regular fetal umbilical vein sampling and transfusion of HPA compatible platelets has been suggested, though the risk of fetal blood sampling must be balanced against the risk of exsanguinating hemorrhage after cordocentesis [50,51].

A definitive diagnosis of NAIT requires the serological demonstration of fetomaternal incompatibility for a platelet antigen. Monoclonal antibody-specific immobilization of platelet antigens (MAIPA) is the gold standard for diagnosis, but is labor intensive. Solid-phase ELISA is being increasingly used [52]. However, these serological tests may not be readily available and neonates with suspected NAIT and severe thrombocytopenia should be managed as emergency cases. The treatment of choice is antigen-negative platelets harvested from the mother (washed and irradiated) or a donor known to be compatible through prior HPA-typing. If such a product is not available, random donor (unmatched) platelets may be used. Recent studies have demonstrated efficacy with this approach, and it is not appropriate to delay transfusion in a severely thrombocytopenic neonate whilst waiting for serological confirmation and/or antigen-matched units. For well-appearing neonates with no evidence of hemorrhage, it is recommended to keep the platelet counts greater than $30 \times 10^9/L$. For neonates with clinically significant hemorrhage, a threshold of $50 \times 10^9/L$, and for those with ICH, a threshold of $100 \times 10^9/L$ may be used [52]. If platelet increment following random donor platelet transfusion is suboptimal, concomitant trial of IVIG (1 g/kg for 1–3 days) and/or methylprednisolone (30 mg/kg) may be tried.

Neonatal Autoimmune Thrombocytopenia

Thrombocytopenia may occur in 10–25% neonates born to mothers with a history of ITP though the incidence of ICH in this cohort is rare (<1%) [49]. Similar to NAIT, transplacental transport of maternal antibodies is implicated in the pathogenesis of neonatal autoimmune thrombocytopenia. All infants born to mothers with a history of ITP should have their platelet counts checked at birth and then again at 2–3 days of life when the counts are thought to nadir. Infants with platelet counts less than $30 \times 10^9/L$ in the first week of life and less than $20 \times 10^9/L$ thereafter, should be treated with IVIG (1 g/kg × 1–3 days) with or without added corticosteroids (prednisone 3–4 mg/kg × 3–4 days). Platelet counts usually start rising spontaneously by 7 days, though in some cases thrombocytopenia may persist for 12 weeks [52].

Congenital Thrombocytopenia

Once considered rare, congenital thrombocytopenias are being increasingly recognized as a heterogeneous group of disorders that result in early-onset thrombocytopenia with marked variability in bleeding manifestations ranging from mild to life-threatening hemorrhage [12]. While some of these disorders affect only megakaryocytes and platelets, others involve different cell types and may result in characteristic phenotypic abnormalities. Recent advances in molecular genetics have dramatically improved our understanding of the underlying pathogenesis of several of these conditions [53]. An overview of the molecular basis, mode of inheritance, and associated phenotypic abnormalities of congenital thrombocytopenias is provided in Table 10.2. Summary of MYH9-RD, BSS, congenital amegakaryocytic thrombocytopenia (CAMT), thrombocytopenia with absent radii syndrome (TAR), gray platelet syndrome, and Wiskott–Aldrich Syndrome (WAS) is also elaborated. For a detailed overview of congenital thrombocytopenias the reader is referred to reviews [12,53,54]. Treatment modalities depend on the severity of the bleeding diathesis, and include desmopressin (DDAVP), tranexamic acid, platelet transfusion, and, during life-threatening bleeding episodes, recombinant factor VIIa. Perioperative use of the TPO-R agonist, eltrombopag has been described in a patient with MYH9-RD [55]. Hematopoietic stem cell transplantation is an effective therapeutic modality for diseases with severe long-term sequelae such as progression to aplastic anemia (CAMT) or risk of life-threatening infections (WAS).

MYH9-related Disease (MYH9-RD)

MYH9-RD is an autosomal-dominant condition presenting with macrothrombocytopenia and leukocyte inclusion bodies (Döhle-like bodies) present since birth and a risk of developing nephropathy, sensorineural deafness, and presenile cataracts later in life; it is secondary to heterozygous mutations in the *MYH9* gene encoding for the nonmuscle myosin heavy chain II A (NMMHC-IIA) [56]. Several different eponyms, namely May–Hegglin, Epstein, Sebastian, and Fetchner syndrome were used to describe the association of nephritis, sensorineural deafness, and presenile cataracts with dominantly inherited thrombocytopenia and leukocyte inclusion bodies. It was only in the year 2000, that it was shown by two independent groups that all these syndromes derive from mutations in the *MYH9* gene, and the term MYH9-RD is now preferred [57,58].

Bleeding tendency in patients with MYH9-RD tends to be mild to moderate, with epistaxis, easy bruising, and menorrhagia being the most commonly reported symptoms. Mean platelet counts are typically in the order of $20–130 \times 10^9/L$ with an elevated MPV. Döhle-like inclusion bodies in leukocytes can be appreciated on Wright–Geisma stained blood films in about 40–80% patients. These light blue appearing inclusions are aggregates of NMMHC-IIA observed in the cytoplasm of some neutrophils. However, because these inclusions are not always present, immunofluorescence staining of blood films using anti-NMMHC-IIA antibody is more sensitive, and is able to detect smaller and abnormally localized aggregates (Figure 10.3). The prevalences of nephritis, sensorineural hearing loss, and presenile cataracts in patients with MYH9-RD are estimated to be 28%, 60%, and 16%, respectively [14].

Bernard–Soulier syndrome

BSS is an autosomal recessive macrothrombocytopenia, which occurs secondary to qualitative or quantitative defects in the platelet GPIb-IX-V complex, resulting in decreased adhesion of platelets to the subendothelium. Common bleeding manifestations include petechiae, epistaxis, gingival bleeding, menorrhagia, and hemorrhage with trauma or surgery. Characteristic laboratory findings include moderate thrombocytopenia, giant platelets, and absent ristocetin-induced platelet aggregation. This condition is further discussed in Chapter 11.

Congenital Amegakaryocytic Thrombocytopenia

CAMT is an autosomal recessive disorder due to mutations in the *c-MPL* gene (TPO-R). CAMT typically presents in the newborn period with isolated severe thrombocytopenia, often in association with significant bleeding. Examination of the bone marrow demonstrates marked reduction or complete absence of megakaryocytes, which ultimately progresses to complete bone marrow failure in later life.

Thrombocytopenia with Absent Radii Syndrome

TAR is an autosomal recessive disorder which occurs secondary to compound heterozygous mutations in the *RBM8A* gene. Patients typically have a microdeletion involving a 200-kb region on chromosome 1q21.1 (with loss of one *RBM8A* allele) and hypomorphic mutations on the second *RBM8A* allele [59]. Clinical presentation includes the combination of bilateral radial aplasia with congenital thrombocytopenia, frequently associated with other skeletal or cardiac defects. The platelet count fluctuates over time, with a general trend towards improvement with age.

Gray platelet Syndrome

Gray platelet syndrome is an autosomal recessive bleeding disorder, which occurs secondary to compound heterozygous/homozygous mutations in the *NBEAL2* gene on chromosome 3p21 [60]. There is marked heterogeneity in the clinical presentation, ranging from epistaxis, easy bruising, and postoperative hemorrhage in most patients to severe, fatal hemorrhage in some. Splenomegaly may be appreciated in more than 80% of the patients. The diagnosis is suspected on visualizing large gray-appearing platelets on a May–Giemsa stained blood film and confirmed by thin-section transmission electron microscopy (TEM) showing complete absence of alpha granules, with normal dense granules and other platelet organelles (Figure 10.4). Progressive myelofibrosis on serial bone marrow evaluation may be appreciated.

Wiskott–Aldrich Syndrome and X-linked Thrombocytopenia

WAS is an X-linked disorder characterized by microthrombocytopenia, eczema, and a variable degree of immune deficiency with an increased risk of lymphoid malignancies and autoimmunity, which occurs secondary to mutations in the *WAS* gene located on Xp11. A milder allelic variant of the disease, which occurs secondary to point mutations on the *WAS* gene and presents with isolated microthrombocytopenia and eczema, is known as X-linked thrombocytopenia (XLT).

Thrombocytosis

Thrombocytosis is defined as a platelet count of more than $450 \times 10^9/L$, and may be congenital, reactive, or primary. Congenital thrombocytosis (familial thrombocytosis) is a rare autosomal-dominant disorder that occurs secondary to gain-of-function mutations in either TPO or its receptor (MPL). Reactive thrombocytosis (RT; secondary thrombocytosis), refers to an increase in platelet count associated with conditions other than myeloproliferative or myelodysplastic syndrome, and is much more frequent (90% of cases) as compared to primary thrombocytosis (PT; essential thrombocythemia) in both children and adults [61]. A variety of clinical conditions can lead to RT, including:

- infection;
- malignancy;
- blood loss;
- inflammation;
- tissue damage; and
- splenectomy.

PT is caused by clonal proliferation of megakaryocyte precursors seen in essential thrombocythemia, polycythemia vera, chronic myelogenous leukemia, myelofibrosis, and myelodysplastic syndrome. Myeloproliferative disorders are discussed in detail in Chapter 15. The clinical distinction between primary and reactive thrombocytosis is important given the distinct clinical manifestations and therapeutic strategies, but often difficult and requires proactive identification or exclusion of potential underlying secondary causes. The clinical history and physical examination are of most value in this regard. Thrombosis and/or hemorrhagic symptoms are common in PT but usually absent in RT. Splenomegaly strongly suggests PT. Elevated erythrocyte or leukocyte counts suggest PT in association with a chronic myeloid disorder. In the case of isolated thrombocytosis, persistent or progressive thrombocytosis suggests PT. If RT cannot be confirmed based on the above considerations, a bone marrow examination may be useful, because in RT the bone marrow appears normal whereas it is often abnormal in PT. The identification of a clonal molecular abnormality such as the *JAK2V617F* mutation is diagnostic of PT. However, absence of such a defect does not exclude PT.

Treatment of RT consists of treating the underlying disease, whereas in PT, treatment needs to be stratified based on their risk category. Risk stratification is based on age, past history of thrombosis and severity of thrombocytosis. The management of PT is discussed in detail in Chapter 15.

Acknowledgement

Riten Kumar was a recipient of the Baxter BioScience Pediatric Hemostasis and Thrombosis Fellowship at The Hospital for Sick Children, Toronto (2011–2013).

References

1 Slichter SJ. Relationship between platelet count and bleeding risk in thrombocytopenic patients. *Transfus Med Rev* 2004; 18: 153–167.

2 Deutsch VR, Tomer A. Advances in megakaryocytopoiesis and thrombopoiesis: from bench to bedside. *Br J Haematol* 2013; 161: 778–793.

3 Afdhal N, McHutchison J, Brown R, *et al.* Thrombocytopenia associated with chronic liver disease. *J Hepatol* 2008; 48: 1000–1007.

4 Kuter DJ. New thrombopoietic growth factors. *Blood* 2007; 109: 4607–4616.

5 Diab YA, Wong EC, Luban NL. Massive transfusion in children and neonates. *Br J Haematol* 2013; 161: 15–26.

6 Junt T, Schulze H, Chen Z, *et al.* Dynamic visualization of thrombopoiesis within bone marrow. *Science* 2007; 317: 1767–1770.

7 Chong BH, Ho SJ. Autoimmune thrombocytopenia. *J Thromb Haemost* 2005; 3: 1763–1772.

8 Biss TT, Blanchette VS, Clark DS, *et al.* Use of a quantitative pediatric bleeding questionnaire to assess mucocutaneous bleeding symptoms in children with a platelet function disorder. *J Thromb Haemost* 2010; 8: 1416–1419.

9 Rodeghiero F, Tosetto A, Abshire T, *et al.* ISTH/SSC bleeding assessment tool: a standardized questionnaire and a proposal for a new bleeding score for inherited bleeding disorders. *J Thromb Haemost* 2010; 8: 2063–2065.

10 Neunert C, Lim W, Crowther M, *et al.* The American Society of Hematology 2011 evidence-based practice guideline for immune thrombocytopenia. *Blood* 2011; 117: 4190–4207.

11 Balduini CL, Cattaneo M, Fabris F, *et al.* Inherited thrombocytopenias: a proposed diagnostic algorithm from the Italian Gruppo di Studio delle Piastrine. *Haematologica* 2003; 88: 582–292.

12 Kumar R, Kahr WH. Congenital thrombocytopenia: clinical manifestations, laboratory abnormalities, and molecular defects of a heterogeneous group of conditions. *Hematol Oncol Clin N Am* 2013; 27: 465–494.

13 Noris P, Klersy C, Zecca M, *et al.* Platelet size distinguishes between inherited macrothrombocytopenias and immune thrombocytopenia. *J Thromb Haemost* 2009; 7: 2131–2136.

14 Pecci A, Panza E, Pujol-Moix N, *et al.* Position of nonmuscle myosin heavy chain IIA (NMMHC-IIA) mutations predicts the natural history of MYH9-related disease. *Human mutation* 2008; 29: 409–417.

15 Salvagno GL, Montagnana M, Degan M, *et al.* Evaluation of platelet turnover by flow cytometry. *Platelets* 2006; 17: 170–177.

16 Kistangari G, McCrae KR. Immune thrombocytopenia. *Hematol Oncol Clin N Am* 2013; 27: 495–520.

17 Rodeghiero F, Stasi R, Gernsheimer T, *et al.* Standardization of terminology, definitions and outcome criteria in immune thrombocytopenic purpura of adults and children: report from an international working group. *Blood* 2009; 113: 2386–2393.

18 Barsam SJ, Psaila B, Forestier M, *et al.* Platelet production and platelet destruction: assessing mechanisms of treatment effect in immune thrombocytopenia. *Blood* 2011; 117: 5723–5732.

19 Terrell DR, Beebe LA, Vesely SK, *et al.* The incidence of immune thrombocytopenic purpura in children and adults: A critical review of published reports. *Am J Hematol* 2010; 85: 174–180.

20 Cines DB, Blanchette VS. Immune thrombocytopenic purpura. *N Engl J Med* 2002; 346: 995–1008.

21 Cines DB, Bussel JB, Liebman HA, *et al.* The ITP syndrome: pathogenic and clinical diversity. *Blood* 2009; 113: 6511–6521.

22 Provan D, Stasi R, Newland AC, *et al.* International consensus report on the investigation and management of primary immune thrombocytopenia. *Blood* 2010; 115: 168–186.

23 Glanz J, France E, Xu S, *et al.* A population-based, multisite cohort study of the predictors of chronic idiopathic thrombocytopenic purpura in children. *Pediatrics* 2008; 121: e506–512.

24 Jernas M, Hou Y, Stromberg Celind F, *et al.* Differences in gene expression and cytokine levels between newly diagnosed and chronic pediatric ITP. *Blood* 2013; 122: 1789–1792.

25 Revel-Vilk S, Yacobovich J, Frank S, *et al.* Age and duration of bleeding symptoms at diagnosis best predict resolution of childhood immune thrombocytopenia at 3, 6, and 12 months. *J Pediatr* 2013; 163: 1335–1339.

26 Eimeren VV, Kahr, WHA. Platelet disorders in children. In: Blanchette VS, Breakey VR, Revel-Vilk S, eds. *Sick Kids Handbook of Pediatric Thrombosis and Hemostasis.* Basel: Karger, 2013: 105–123.

27 Garvey B. Rituximab in the treatment of autoimmune haematological disorders. *Br J Haematol* 2008; 141: 149–169.

28 Aleem A, Alaskar AS, Algahtani F, *et al.* Rituximab in immune thrombocytopenia: transient responses, low rate of sustained remissions and poor response to further therapy in refractory patients. *Int J Hematol* 2010; 92: 283–288.

29 Medeot M, Zaja F, Vianelli N, *et al.* Rituximab therapy in adult patients with relapsed or refractory immune thrombocytopenic purpura: long-term follow-up results. *Eur J Haematol* 2008; 81: 165–169.

30 Arnold DM, Heddle NM, Carruthers J, *et al.* A pilot randomized trial of adjuvant rituximab or placebo for nonsplenectomized patients with immune thrombocytopenia. *Blood* 2012; 119: 1356–1362.

31 Kuter DJ, Rummel M, Boccia R, *et al.* Romiplostim or standard of care in patients with immune thrombocytopenia. *N Engl J Med* 2010; 363: 1889–1899.

32 Kuter DJ, Bussel JB, Lyons RM, *et al.* Efficacy of romiplostim in patients with chronic immune thrombocytopenic purpura: a double-blind randomised controlled trial. *Lancet* 2008; 371: 395–403.

33 Cheng G, Saleh MN, Marcher C, *et al.* Eltrombopag for management of chronic immune thrombocytopenia (RAISE): a 6-month, randomised, phase 3 study. *Lancet* 2011; 377: 393–402.

34 Saleh MN, Bussel JB, Cheng G, *et al.* Safety and efficacy of eltrombopag for treatment of chronic immune thrombocytopenia: results of the long-term, open-label EXTEND study. *Blood* 2013; 121: 537–545.

35 Norton A, Roberts I. Management of Evans syndrome. *Br J Haematol* 2006; 132: 125–137.

36 Bussel JB, Thrombocytopenias. In: Goodnight SH, Hathaway WE, eds. *Mechanisms of Hemostasis and Thrombosis*, 2nd edn. Lancester: McGraw Hill Companies, 2001: 76–87.

37 Dlott JS, Danielson CF, Blue-Hnidy DE, *et al.* Drug-induced thrombotic thrombocytopenic purpura/hemolytic uremic syndrome: a concise review. *Ther Apher Dial* 2004; 8: 102–111.

38 Aster RH, Bougie DW. Drug-induced immune thrombocytopenia. *N Engl J Med* 2007; 357: 580–587.

39 Lee GM, Arepally GM. Diagnosis and management of heparin-induced thrombocytopenia. *Hematol Oncol Clin N Am* 2013; 27: 541–563.

40 Avila ML, Shah V, Brandao LR. Systematic review on heparin-induced thrombocytopenia in children: a call to action. *J Thromb Haemost* 2013; 11: 660–669.

41 McCrae KR. Thrombocytopenia in pregnancy. *Hematology Am Soc Hematol Educ Program* 2010; 2010: 397–402.

42 Townsley DM. Hematologic complications of pregnancy. *Semin Hematol* 2013; 50: 222–231.

43 Williamson LM, Stainsby D, Jones H, *et al.* The impact of universal leukodepletion of the blood supply on hemovigilance reports of posttransfusion purpura and transfusion-associated graft-versus-host disease. *Transfusion* 2007; 47: 1455–1467.

44 Liebman HA, Stasi R. Secondary immune thrombocytopenic purpura. *Curr Opin Hematol* 2007; 14: 557–573.

45 Weksler BB. Review article: the pathophysiology of thrombocytopenia in hepatitis C virus infection and chronic liver disease. *Aliment Pharmacol Ther* 2007; 26 Suppl 1: 13–19.

46 Afdhal NH, Dusheiko GM, Giannini EG, *et al.* Eltrombopag increases platelet numbers in thrombocytopenic patients with HCV infection and cirrhosis, allowing for effective antiviral therapy. *Gastroenterology* 2014; 146: 442–452.

47 Kumar R, Steele M. Acquired bleeding disorders in children. In: Blanchette VS, Breakey VR, Revel-Vilk S, eds. *Sick Kids Handbook of Pediatric Thrombosis and Hemostasis*. Basel: Karger, 2013: 105–123.

48 Levi M. Disseminated intravascular coagulation or extended intravascular coagulation in massive pulmonary embolism. *J Thromb Haemost* 2010; 8: 1475–1476.

49 Roberts I, Stanworth S, Murray NA. Thrombocytopenia in the neonate. *Blood Rev* 2008; 22: 173–186.

50 Chakravorty S, Roberts I. How I manage neonatal thrombocytopenia. *Br J Haematol* 2012; 156: 155–162.

51 Peterson JA, McFarland JG, Curtis BR, *et al.* Neonatal alloimmune thrombocytopenia: pathogenesis, diagnosis and management. *Br J Haematol* 2013; 161: 3–14.

52 Avila L, Barnard D. Bleeding in the neonate. In: Blanchette VS, Breakey VR, Revel-Vilk S, eds. *Sick Kids Handbook of Pediatric Thrombosis and Hemostasis*. Basel: Karger, 2013: 105–123.

53 Balduini CL, Pecci A, Noris P. Inherited thrombocytopenias: the evolving spectrum. *Hamostaseologie* 2012; 32: 259–270.

54 Drachman JG. Inherited thrombocytopenia: when a low platelet count does not mean ITP. *Blood* 2004; 103: 390–398.

55 Pecci A, Barozzi S, d'Amico S, Balduini CL. Short-term eltrombopag for surgical preparation of a patient with inherited thrombocytopenia deriving from MYH9 mutation. *Thromb Haemost* 2012; 107: 1188–1189.

56 Balduini CL, Pecci A, Savoia A. Recent advances in the understanding and management of MYH9-related inherited thrombocytopenias. *Br J Haematol* 2011; 154: 161–174.

57 Kelley MJ, Jawien W, Ortel TL, *et al.* Mutation of MYH9, encoding non-muscle myosin heavy chain A, in May-Hegglin anomaly. *Nature Gen* 2000; 26: 106–108.

58 Seri M, Cusano R, Gangarossa S, *et al.* Mutations in MYH9 result in the May-Hegglin anomaly, and Fechtner and Sebastian syndromes. The May-Hegllin/Fechtner Syndrome Consortium. *Nature Gen* 2000; 26: 103–105.

59 Albers CA, Paul DS, Schulze H, *et al.* Compound inheritance of a low-frequency regulatory SNP and a rare null mutation in exon-junction complex subunit RBM8A causes TAR syndrome. *Nature Gen* 2012; 44: 435–439.

60 Kahr WH, Hinckley J, Li L, *et al.* Mutations in NBEAL2, encoding a BEACH protein, cause gray platelet syndrome. *Nature Gen* 2011; 43: 738–740.

61 Sulai NH, Tefferi A. Why does my patient have thrombocytosis? *Hematol Oncol Clin N Am* 2012; 26: 285–301.

11

Qualitative Platelet Disorders

Eti A. Femia Gian Marco Podda and Marco Cattaneo

Key Points

- Qualitative platelet disorders are characterized by impaired platelet-dependent hemostatic function and are associated with mucocutaneous bleeding and excessive early-onset hemorrhage after surgery or trauma.
- Disorders that affect platelet secretion, either due to platelet granule defects or to other abnormalities, are the most common congenital disorders of platelet function.
- Bernard–Soulier syndrome and Glanzmann thrombasthenia are the most severe congenital platelet disorders.
- Acquired defects of platelet function are drug-induced and associated with hematological and nonhematological conditions: in most of these situations, the pathophysiological mechanisms leading to platelet dysfunction are poorly understood.
- Mild bleeding episodes are easily controlled by local measures. Four treatment options are available for moderate/ severe bleeding: platelet transfusions, desmopressin (DDAVP), fibrinolytic inhibitors, and recombinant factor VIIa (rFVIIa).

Introduction

Qualitative platelet disorders are characterized by impaired platelet-dependent hemostatic function, which are associated with bleeding diatheses

of varying severity [1]. Typically, patients with platelet disorders experience mucocutaneous bleeding (e.g., epistaxis, gum bleeding, menorrhagia, and easy bruising) and excessive, early-onset hemorrhage after surgery or trauma [1]. Bleeding into the central nervous system rarely occurs. Qualitative platelet disorders can be either congenital or acquired. In this chapter, the main congenital and acquired qualitative platelet disorders are reviewed. Abnormalities of platelet function resulting from defects of plasma proteins (e.g., von Willebrand disease (VWD), afibrinogenemia) will not be considered here, as they are discussed in Chapters 7 and 8. Acquired von Willebrand syndrome (AVWS) is discussed in Chapter 9.

Congenital Qualitative Platelet Defects

The prevalence of congenital platelet disorders among the general population is unknown, but it might be much higher than generally assumed, probably as high as VWD. They are more commonly diagnosed in women, likely because the added hemostatic challenges of menstruation and childbirth affect the burden of living with a bleeding disorder and the likelihood of referral for evaluation [2].

Congenital disorders of platelet function have been generally classified according to the functions or responses that are abnormal. However,

Practical Hemostasis and Thrombosis, Third Edition. Edited by Nigel S. Key,Michael Makris and David Lillicrap.
© 2017 John Wiley & Sons, Ltd. Published 2017 by John Wiley & Sons, Ltd.

because platelet functions are intimately related, a clear distinction between disorders of platelet adhesion, aggregation, activation, secretion, and procoagulant activity is, in many instances, problematic. For this reason, a classification of the congenital disorders of platelet function was proposed based on abnormalities of platelet components that share common characteristics [1] (Table 11.1):

- platelet receptors for adhesive proteins;
- platelet receptors for soluble agonists;
- platelet granules;
- signal-transduction pathways;
- procoagulant phospholipids;
- miscellaneous disorders (less well characterized).

Abnormalities of the Platelet Receptors for Adhesive Proteins

Abnormalities of GPIb-V-IX Complex (VWF Binding Site)

Bernard–Soulier syndrome (BSS) is a relatively severe bleeding disorder, caused by qualitative and quantitative defects in the glycoprotein (GP) Ib-V-IX complex [3]. It is a rare disease (prevalence 1 : 1 million), which is characterized by:

- autosomal recessive inheritance (with few exceptions of autosomal dominant inheritance);
- prolonged bleeding time;
- variable degree of thrombocytopenia;
- giant platelets (often not detected by automatic counters);
- decreased platelet survival;
- lack of platelet agglutination induced by ristocetin.

The lack of ristocetin-induced agglutination is not corrected by the addition of normal plasma. The platelet responses to physiological agonists are normal, with the exception of low concentrations of thrombin, because GPIbα (one of the two components of GPIb) has a critical role in the platelet aggregatory, secretory, and procoagulant responses to thrombin.

Table 11.1 Congenital platelet defects.

Abnormalities of the platelet receptors for adhesive proteins:

GPIb-V-IX complex (Bernard–Soulier syndrome, platelet-type VWD, Bolin–Jamieson syndrome)

GPIIb/IIIa (α_{IIb}/β_3) (Glanzmann thrombasthenia)

GPIa/IIa (α_2/β_1)

GPVI

Abnormalities of the platelet receptors for soluble agonists:

Thromboxane A_2 receptor

α_2-Adrenergic receptor

$P2Y_{12}$ receptor

Abnormalities of the platelet granules:

δ-Granules (δ-SPD, HPS, CHS, TAR syndrome, Wiskott–Aldrich syndrome)

α-Granules (gray platelet syndrome, Quebec platelet disorder, Paris–Trousseau syndrome, Jacobsen syndrome)

α- and δ-Granules (α,δ-SPD)

Abnormalities of the signal-transduction pathways:

Abnormalities of cytosolic phospholipase A2α, defects of cyclooxygenase, Gqα deficiency, partial selective PLC-β2 isoenzyme deficiency, defects in pleckstrin phosphorylation, defective Ca^{2+} mobilization, hyperresponsiveness of platelet Gsα, defects of CalDAG-GEFI

Abnormalities of membrane phospholipids:

Scott syndrome

Stormorken syndrome

Miscellaneous abnormalities of platelet function:

Primary secretion defects

Other platelet abnormalities (osteogenesis imperfecta, Ehlers–Danlos syndrome, Marfan syndrome, hexokinase deficiency, glucose-6-phosphate deficiency)

CHS, Chédiak–Higashi syndrome; HPS , Hermansky–Pudlak syndrome; PLC, phospholipase C; SPD, storage pool deficiency; TAR, thrombocytopenia with absent radii; VWD, von Willebrand disease.

BSS is due to molecular defects (frameshifts, deletions and point mutations) in the genes *GP1BA* on chromosome 17, *GP1BB* on chromosome 22, or *GP9* on chromosome 3. No cases of mutations in *GP5* have been described so far. Some variants with autosomal dominant inheritance have been described: the most common is the A156V mutation on *GP1AB*, known as Bolzano variant, which is the most frequent cause of macrothrombocytopenia in Italy [4]. Diagnosis of BSS is based on the demonstration of GPIb-V-IX deficiency by flow cytometry or immunoblotting.

Bleeding events, which may be very severe in homozygous BSS, can be controlled by platelet transfusions. Most heterozygotes, with few exceptions, do not have a bleeding diathesis, but have macrothrombocytopenia [5].

Platelet-type von Willebrand disease (VWD) or pseudo VWD is not caused by defects of VWF, but by a gain-of-function phenotype of the platelet GPIbα [6]. This abnormal receptor has an increased avidity for VWF, leading to the binding of the largest VWF multimers to the resting platelets and their clearance from the circulation. Because the high-molecular-weight VWF multimers are the most hemostatically active, their loss is associated with an increased bleeding risk, like in type 2B VWD (which is caused by a gain-of-function abnormality of the VWF molecule; see Chapter 7). Platelet-type VWD is an autosomal dominant disease caused by gain-of-function missense mutations of *GPIBA* and associated with amino acid substitutions (G233V, G233S, and M239V) occurring within the disulfide-bonded double loop region of GPIbα [6]. A family with a 27-base pair in-frame deletion in the *GP1BA* has also been described [7]. The defect should be suspected when increased sensitivity to ristocetin is present. The diagnosis is confirmed by genetic studies.

Bolin–Jamieson syndrome is a rare, autosomal dominant, mild bleeding disorder associated with a larger form of GPIbα in one allele [8]. It has been proposed that it is associated with a large multimer form of the size polymorphism occurring in the mucin-like domain.

Abnormalities of GPIIb/IIIa (α_{IIb}/β_3)

Glanzmann thrombasthenia (GT) is an autosomal recessive disease caused by lack of expression or qualitative defects of one of the two glycoproteins forming the integrin α_{IIb}/β_3, which

binds, in activated platelets, adhesive glycoproteins (e.g., fibrinogen, VWF) that bridge adjacent platelets, securing platelet aggregation. Severe forms are associated to the lack of platelet fibrinogen stored in the α-granules, as its uptake from the plasma is mediated by α_{IIb}/β_3.

The diagnostic hallmark is the lack, or severe impairment, of platelet aggregation induced by all agonists. Platelet clot retraction is defective and although GT platelets bind to the subendothelium, they fail to spread and to build up a thrombus.

The GT defect is caused by mutations or deletions in the genes encoding one of the two glycoproteins forming the α_{IIb}/β_3 integrin: *ITGA2B* and *ITGB3*. In GT caused by mutations in the α_3 integrin, the levels of the platelet vitronectin receptor (α_v/β_3) are also decreased, but the platelet phenotype of these patients is no different from that of the other GT patients.

The disease is associated with bleeding manifestations similar to those of patients with BSS, although of lower severity [9], characterized by mucocutaneous bleeding and bleeding after trauma or surgery. Heterozygotes do not have a bleeding diathesis. Although platelet count and platelet volume (and morphology) are normal in classic GT, some novel but rare point mutations in either *ITGA2B* or *ITGB3* have been associated with mild thrombocytopenia [10].

Diagnosis of GT is confirmed by evaluating GPIIb/IIIa expression by flow cytometry or immunoblotting, and sequencing the genes *ITGA2B* and *ITGB3*.

Abnormalities of GPIa/IIa (α_2/β_1)

Two patients with mild bleeding disorders associated with deficient expression of the platelet receptor for collagen, GPIa/IIa (α_2/β_1), and selective impairment of platelet responses to collagen have been described [11]. Their platelet defect spontaneously recovered after the menopause, suggesting that α_2/β_1 expression is under hormonal control.

Abnormalities of GPVI

A selective defect of collagen-induced platelet aggregation was described in a patient with a mild bleeding disorder [1], characterized by deficiency of the platelet GPVI, a member of the immunoglobulin superfamily of receptors, which mediates platelet activation by collagen [12].

Both acquired defects due to the inhibition or antibody-mediated depletion of GPVI in circulating platelets, and congenital defects linked to mutations in the *GP6* gene have been described [13]. The gene encoding for the Fcα receptor, which is the signaling subunit of GPVI, may also be implicated.

Abnormalities of the Platelet Receptors for Soluble Agonists

Thromboxane A$_2$ Receptor

Thromboxane (Tx) A$_2$, synthesized from arachidonic acid released by membrane phospholipids, mediates vasoconstriction and induces platelet aggregation and secretion. TxA$_2$ binds the T-prostanoid receptor (TP), a G-protein coupled receptor (GPCR), which activates a phosphatidylinositol–calcium second messenger system. Two isoforms (α and β) have been identified in different cells of vascular tissues: both are expressed on platelets.

Genetic variations affecting the TP receptor are associated with a mild bleeding phenotype. To date, two quantitative defects causing reduced TP receptor expression (c167dupG) [14] and (W29C) [15] and a qualitative defect caused by point mutation (R60L) [16] in the first cytoplasmic loop of TP have been identified; another mutation (D304N) [17] associated with reduced ligand binding to TP has been described.

The defects may be suspected in patients with defective aggregation response to the TxA$_2$ analog U46619, arachidonic acid, and collagen.

α$_2$-Adrenergic Receptors

Subjects with a selective impairment of platelet response to epinephrine, a decreased number of the platelet α$_2$-adrenergic receptors, and mildly prolonged bleeding times have been described [18]. However, the relationship between this

defect and bleeding manifestations still needs to be defined.

P2Y$_{12}$ Receptor for ADP

Human platelets express three distinct P2 receptors stimulated by adenosine nucleotides:

- P2X$_1$ receptor for ATP
- P2Y$_1$ receptor for ADP with a role in the initiation of platelet activation;
- P2Y$_{12}$ receptor for ADP essential for a sustained, full aggregation response to ADP.

The concurrent activation of both P2Y receptors is necessary for full platelet aggregation induced by ADP. P2Y$_{12}$ also mediates the potentiation of platelet secretion by ADP and the stabilization of thrombin-induced platelet aggregates.

Only patients with congenital defects of the platelet P2Y$_{12}$ receptor have been described. The first patient [19] had a life-long history of excessive bleeding, prolonged bleeding time, and abnormalities of platelet aggregation similar to those observed in patients with defects of platelet secretion (reversible aggregation in response to weak agonists and impaired aggregation in response to low concentrations of collagen or thrombin), except that the aggregation response to ADP was severely impaired.

Five additional patients belonging to four kindreds with severe P2Y$_{12}$ deficiency were later described: all of them displayed base pair deletions in the P2Y$_{12}$ gene, shifting the reading frame for several residues before introducing a premature stop codon, causing an early truncation of the protein [20].

The study of molecular abnormalities associated with inherited qualitative defects of the P2Y$_{12}$ receptor protein is useful to unravel structure–function relationships of the receptor. Mutations in the region that spans the transition between transmembrane helix (TM) 6 and extracellular loop (EL) 3 are associated with receptor dysfunction despite normal ligand binding, suggesting that this region of the molecule plays a role in signal transduction [20]. A heterozygous mutation, predicting a lysine to glutamate (Lys174Glu) substitution in P2Y$_{12}$, was identified in one patient with reduced and reversible aggregation in response to ADP and an approximate 50% reduction in binding of agonist radioligand [^{3}H] 2-MeSADP. Considering that Lys174 is situated in the EL2 of P2Y$_{12}$, adjacent to Cys175, which may be important for the integrity of the ADP binding site on the receptor, and that a hemagglutinin-tagged Lys174Glu P2Y$_{12}$ variant showed surface expression in Chinese hamster ovary cells, the Lys174Glu mutation is likely responsible for disruption of the ADP binding site. In one patient, with no personal history of abnormal bleeding, reduced expression of P2Y$_{12}$ was associated with the heterozygous mutation Pro341Ala, in a putative postsynaptic density 95/ disc large/ zonula occludens-1 (PDZ)-binding motif, most likely as a consequence of significantly compromised P2Y$_{12}$ recycling [20].

The diagnosis of P2Y$_{12}$ defects should be suspected when ADP, even at high concentrations ($\geq 10\,\mu M$), fails to induce full and irreversible platelet aggregation, but induces normal platelet shape change. Confirmation of the diagnosis is based on tests that evaluate the degree of inhibition of adenyl cyclase by ADP, through the Gi-coupled P2Y$_{12}$ receptor. Measurement of the phosphorylation of vasodilator-stimulated phosphoprotein (VASP) after the exposure of platelets to prostaglandin E$_1$ (PGE$_1$) and ADP [21] is probably preferable to measurement of cAMP levels under the same experimental conditions, because it is cheaper and easier to perform. Combining measurement of radioligand binding to P2Y$_{12}$ allows the distinction between quantitative and qualitative abnormalities of the receptor.

Abnormalities of the Platelet Granules

Abnormalities of the δ-Granules (δ-Storage Pool Deficiency)

The term δ-storage pool deficiency (δ-SPD) defines a congenital abnormality characterized by deficiency of dense granules in megakaryo-cytes and platelets [22]. It may present as an isolated platelet function defect or be associated with congenital disorders. Between 10% and 18% of patients with congenital abnormalities of platelet function have nonsyndromic SPD. The inheritance is autosomal recessive in some families and autosomal dominant in others. δ-SPD is characterized by:

- variable degree of bleeding diathesis;
- mildly to moderately prolonged skin bleeding time, inversely related to the amount of ADP or serotonin contained in the granules;
- abnormal platelet secretion induced by several platelet agonists;
- impaired platelet aggregation in 75% of cases (only 33% have aggregation tracings typical for a platelet secretion defect);
- decreased levels of δ-granule constituents: ATP and ADP, serotonin, calcium, and pyrophosphate.

Lumiaggregometry, which measures platelet aggregation and secretion simultaneously, may prove a more accurate technique than platelet aggregometry for diagnosing patients with δ-SPD and, more generally, with platelet secretion defects [23].

Molecular defects responsible for δ-SPD have not been identified yet [24]. The diagnosis is essentially based on the finding of defective platelet secretion induced by several agonists and decreased platelet δ-granules content.

Hermansky–Pudlak syndrome (HPS) and Chédiak–Higashi syndrome (CHS) are rare syndromic forms of δ-SPD [25].

HPS is a disease of subcellular organelles involving abnormalities of many tissues: melanosomes, platelet δ-granules, and lysosomes, characterized by:

- autosomal recessive inheritance;
- tyrosinase-positive oculocutaneous albinism;
- bleeding diathesis;
- ceroid–lipofuscin lysosomal storage disease.

HPS can arise from mutations in different genetic loci [22] that characterize nine HPS subtypes (HSP-1 through HSP-9). All known HPS proteins are components of one of four protein complexes: biogenesis of lysosome-related organelles complex (BLOC) and adaptor protein complex (AP)-3.

CHS is a lethal disorder (death usually in the first decade of life) with:

- autosomal recessive inheritance;
- variable degrees of oculocutaneous albinism;
- very large peroxidase-positive cytoplasmic granules in a variety of hematopoietic (neutrophils) and nonhematopoietic cells;
- easy bruisability;
- recurrent infections, associated with neutropenia, impaired chemotaxis, and bactericidal activity;
- abnormal natural killer (NK) cell function.

Molecular defects of CHS involve mutations in the lysosomal traffic regulator (*LYST*) gene, which encodes a large cytoplasmic protein with distinct structural domains including BEACH and HEAT, involved in trafficking among lysosomes and δ-granules [26].

Two types of hereditary thrombocytopenia may be associated with δ-SPD: thrombocytopenia with absent radii syndrome (TAR) and Wiskott–Aldrich syndrome (WAS) [27].

Abnormalities of the α-Granules

Gray platelet syndrome (GPS) derives its name from the gray appearance of the patient's platelets in peripheral blood smears as a consequence of the absent or ghostly platelet α-granules. The inheritance pattern seems to be autosomal recessive, although in a single family it seemed to be autosomal dominant. Since its first description in 1971, more than 100 cases have been reported. Affected patients have a lifelong history of mucocutaneous bleeding, which may vary from mild to moderate in severity, and prolonged bleeding time [28]. They have mild thrombocytopenia with abnormally large platelets and isolated reduction of the platelet α-granule content. Mild to moderate myelofibrosis has been described in some patients (hypothetically ascribed to the action of cytokines released by the hypogranular platelets and megakaryocytes in the bone marrow). Recently, three independent

groups identified missense, nonsense, and frameshift mutations in the *NBEAL2* gene, which is likely involved in vesicular trafficking. Diagnosis is confirmed by electron microscopy and quantification of α-granules content.

The Quebec platelet disorder is an autosomal dominant qualitative platelet abnormality, characterized by [29]:

- severe post-traumatic bleeding complications unresponsive to platelet transfusion;
- abnormal proteolysis of α-granule proteins;
- severe deficiency of platelet factor V;
- deficiency of multimerin;
- reduced to normal platelet counts (macrothrombocytopenia);
- decreased platelet aggregation induced by epinephrine.

Multimerin, one of the largest proteins found in the human body, is present in platelet α-granules and in endothelial cell Weibel–Palade bodies [30]. It binds factor V and its activated form, factor Va. Its deficiency in patients with the Quebec platelet disorder is probably responsible for the defect in platelet factor V, which is likely to be degraded by abnormally regulated platelet proteases, notably urokinase plasminogen activator [31].

Jacobsen and Paris–Trousseau syndrome are rare syndromes [32] associated with:

- a mild hemorrhagic diathesis;
- congenital thrombocytopenia with normal platelet life span;
- increased number of marrow megakaryocytes (many presenting with signs of abnormal maturation and intramedullary lysis);
- a deletion of the distal part of one chromosome 11 [del(11)q23.3→qter] has been found in affected patients.

Abnormalities of the α- and δ-Granules

α,δ-SPD is characterized by deficiencies of both α- and δ-granules [33,34]. The clinical picture and the platelet aggregation abnormalities are similar to those of patients with GPS or δ-SPD.

Abnormalities of the Platelet Signal-Transduction Pathways

Congenital abnormalities of the arachidonate–thromboxane A_2 pathway, involving the liberation of arachidonic acid from membrane phospholipids (defects of cytosolic phospholipase A_2), defects of cyclooxygenase ("aspirin-like defects") or thromboxane synthase, are associated with platelet function defects and mild bleeding [1].

Other congenital abnormalities of the platelet signal-transduction pathways have been described involving [1]:

- G-proteins ($G\alpha q$ deficiency)
- phosphatidylinositol metabolism (partial selective phospholipase $C-\beta_2$ isozyme deficiency)
- defects in pleckstrin phosphorylation and hyper-responsiveness of platelet $Gs\alpha$
- defects of CalDAG-GEFI

Abnormalities of Membrane Phospholipids

Scott Syndrome

This is a very rare autosomal recessive bleeding disorder associated with lack of calcium-induced rearrangement of the platelet membrane phospholipids, necessary to govern the bidirectional exchange of phospholipids between the two leaflets of the bilayer. This defect causes the failure to expose negatively charged phosphatidylserine (PS) at the outer surface of membranes of blood cells, including platelets [35] leading to reduced production of microparticles and impaired activation of factor X and prothrombin; hence, thrombin generation and fibrin formation are reduced and platelets lose their procoagulant activity. To date, only a few patients have been identified. Suzuki *et al.* showed that TMEM16F [36] is an essential component for the Ca^{2+} dependent exposure of PS on the cell surface and showed that a patient with Scott syndrome carries a mutation at a splice-acceptor site of the gene encoding TMEM16F, causing the premature termination of the protein [37]. Prothrombin consumption during clotting of whole blood is defective in Scott syndrome, and clotting time after recalcification of kaolin-activated platelet-rich plasma in the presence of Russell's viper venom is prolonged. In contrast, platelet count and structure are normal, and no abnormalities of platelet secretion, aggregation, metabolism, granule content, or platelet adhesion to subendothelium have been described [38].

Stormorken Syndrome

In Stormorken syndrome, resting, unstimulated platelets from patients with this syndrome display a full procoagulant activity. Therefore, this condition represents the exact opposite in terms of platelet membrane function to the Scott syndrome; yet, surprisingly, it is also associated with a bleeding tendency. Platelets from patients with this condition respond normally to all agonists, with the exception of collagen [39].

Miscellaneous Abnormalities of Platelet Function

Primary Secretion Defects

The term primary secretion defect was probably used for the first time by Weiss, to indicate all those ill-defined abnormalities of platelet secretion not associated with platelet granule deficiencies. The term was later used to indicate the platelet secretion defects not associated with platelet granule deficiencies and abnormalities of the arachidonate pathway, or all the abnormalities of platelet function associated with defects of signal transduction [40]. With the progression of our knowledge of platelet pathophysiology, this heterogeneous group, which brings together the majority of patients with congenital disorders of platelet function, will become progressively smaller, losing those patients with better defined biochemical abnormalities responsible for their platelet secretion defect. An example is the heterozygous $P2Y_{12}$ deficiency state, which was included in this group of disorders until its biochemical abnormality was identified.

Other Platelet Abnormalities

Platelet function abnormalities have also been reported in osteogenesis imperfecta, Ehlers–Danlos syndrome, Marfan syndrome, hexokinase deficiency, and glucose-6-phosphate deficiency [1].

Acquired Platelet Defects

Platelet function can be impaired in several hematological and nonhematological conditions and by medications [41] (Table 11.2). In most of these situations, the pathophysiological mechanisms leading to platelet dysfunction are poorly understood.

Uremia

The bleeding time (BT) may be severely prolonged in patients with uremia, but it can be corrected by increasing the hematocrit with red blood cell (RBC) transfusions [42] or with erythropoietin [43], suggesting that, in many instances, the defective primary hemostasis in uremia is a consequence of anemia. It is generally accepted that RBCs normally facilitate the platelet interaction with the vessel wall.

Table 11.2 Acquired platelet defects.

Medications affecting platelet function
Uremia
Dysproteinemias
Acute leukemias and myelodysplastic syndromes
Cardiopulmonary bypass
Liver disease
Antiplatelet antibodies
Myeloproliferative disorders
Essential thrombocythemia
Polycythemia vera
Chronic myelogenous leukemia
Agnogenic myeloid metaplasia

However, correction of the hematocrit fails to correct the BT in some patients, suggesting that other factors impair platelet–vessel wall interaction in this condition. The following platelet abnormalities have been described in uremia [44]:

- abnormalities of interaction of adhesive glycoproteins with their platelet receptors;
- defective platelet activation;
- defective platelet procoagulant activity.

Both dialyzable and nondialyzable substances (i.e., antibiotics, antiplatelet agents, heparin) may be responsible.

Acute Leukemia and Myelodysplastic Syndromes

Bleeding complications are very common in acute leukemia and in myelodysplastic syndromes (MDS). The mechanisms responsible for bleeding events in patients with leukemia are complex, involving leukemic cell infiltration of the vessel wall, reduction in platelet number, coagulation dysfunction, and platelet function defects. The following abnormalities of platelet function have been reported in patients with acute leukemia or MDS [45,46]:

- decreased platelet aggregation in response to most platelet agonists;
- reduced surface expression of GPIb;
- impaired platelet secretion;
- deficiency of platelet granules;
- reduced TXA_2 production.

Myeloproliferative Disorders

The *BCR-ABL*-negative classical myeloproliferative neoplasms (MPNs), which include myelofibrosis, essential thrombocythemia, and polycythemia vera, share a tendency toward thrombotic and hemorrhagic complications. In a study of 494 MPD patients, 5.5% suffered from major bleeding. The bleeding tendency is multifactorial: thrombocytopenia, acquired von Willebrand disease, antiplatelet medications, and acquired platelet defects are involved [47].

Functional and biochemical abnormalities of platelets that have been described in patients with myeloproliferative disorders include:

- decreased release of arachidonic acid from membrane phospholipids;
- reduced conversion of arachidonic acid to its active metabolites;
- reduced responsiveness to TxA_2;
- deficiency of platelet granules;
- deficiency of the α_2/β_1 integrin and impaired fibrinogen binding;
- decreased number of α_2-adrenergic receptors.

The hemostatic and thrombotic complications of MPNs are discussed further in Chapter 15.

Cardiopulmonary Bypass

Cardiopulmonary bypass causes transient thrombocytopenia and platelet function defects, which contribute to the increased bleeding risk of these patients. Platelet function defects associated with extracorporeal circulation include [48]:

- defective *in vitro* aggregation;
- platelet granule deficiencies;
- abnormal interaction with VWF;
- generation of platelet-derived microparticles.

These abnormalities result from platelet activation and fragmentation, hypothermia, contact with the blood–air interface, and exposure to traces of platelet agonists such as thrombin, ADP, and plasmin.

Medications

Many drugs affect platelet function (Table 11.3), sometimes causing a prolongation of the BT and are associated with a potential increased risk of bleeding. In some instances, the inhibition of platelet function is the intended target of the drug, as in the case of antiplatelet agents that are given to reduce the risk of cardiovascular or cerebrovascular accidents. In other cases, the induced abnormalities of platelet function are considered side-effects of the drug, which are in most instances without obvious clinical consequences.

Table 11.3 Drugs affecting platelet function.

NSAIDs:

Aspirin, indomethacin, ibuprofen, sulindac, naproxen, phenylbutazone

Thienopyridines:

Ticlopidine, clopidogrel, prasugrel

Reversible $P2Y_{12}$ antagonists:

Ticagrelor, Cangrelor

GPIIb/IIIa antagonists:

Abciximab, eptifibatide, tirofiban

Drugs that increase the platelet cAMP or cGMP levels:

Prostacyclin, iloprost, dipyridamole, theophylline, nitric oxide, nitric oxide donors

Cardiovascular drugs:

Nitroglycerin, isosorbide dinitrate, propranolol, furosemide, calcium-channel blockers, quinidine, ACE inhibitors, verapamil, diltiazem

Antimicrobials:

Penicillins, cephalosporins, nitrofurantoin, hydroxychloroquine, miconazole

Volume expanders:

Dextran, hydroxyethyl starch

Psychotropic drugs, anesthetics:

Imipramine, amitriptyline, nortriptyline, chlorpromazine, promethazine, fluphenazine, trifluoperazine, selective serotonin reuptake inhibitors, haloperidol, halothane, dibucaine, tetracaine, butacaine, nupercaine, procaine, plaquenil

Chemotherapeutic agents:

Mitomycin, daunorubicin, BCNU, dasatinib

Miscellaneous drugs:

Antihistamines, radiographic contrast agents, clofibrate

ACE, angiotensin-converting enzyme; cGMP cyclic guanosine 3',5'-monophosphate; cAMP, cyclic adenosine 3',5'-monophosphate; BCNU, 1,3-bis(2-chloroethyl)-1-nitrosurea.

Liver Disease

Chronic liver disease is associated with a prolongation of the BT disproportionate to the degree of thrombocytopenia that usually complicates this condition [49]. Whether the described defects are caused by intrinsic or extrinsic abnormalities of the platelets is unclear.

Therapy

Treatment of patients with qualitative platelet disorders is needed to prevent bleeding complications in situations at risk, and to control severe/moderate spontaneous bleeding manifestations such as menorrhagia, epistaxis, and gastrointestinal bleeding, especially in GT and BBS patients. Therapy is not warranted for bruising.

General principles of treatment of patients with qualitative platelet disorders are:

- avoid drugs that interfere with platelet function or other components of the hemostatic system;
- avoid intramuscular injections;
- good dental care to prevent or minimize gum bleeding;
- use of oral contraceptives for the control of menorrhagia.

Four treatment options are available for moderate/ severe bleeding: platelet transfusions, desmopressin (DDAVP), fibrinolytic inhibitors, and recombinant factor VIIa (rFVIIa).

Platelet transfusions should be reserved for patients with serious bleeding unresponsive to medical therapies or the most severe platelet function defects, such as BSS, GT, and Scott syndrome and patients with platelet-type VWD. In individuals with deficient platelet membrane glycoproteins, there is an increased risk of allo-immunization against HLA antigens and/or platelet a $\alpha_{IIb}\beta_3$ from platelet transfusion therapy, which limits future responses to platelet transfusion. This risk appears to be higher for GT than for BSS [2].

Recombinant FVIIa can be used for management of serious bleeding in patients with BSS or GT who no longer respond to platelet transfusions because of alloimmunization [2,50].

Desmopressin, which increases the plasma concentrations of von Willebrand factor (VWF) and factor VIII, can be used in the management of less severe platelet disorders and for milder bleeding manifestations. However, the evidence for its clinical effectiveness in the prophylaxis and treatment of bleeding in these patients is based on case reports and clinical experience only [13,49].

Fibrinolytic inhibitors (epsilon–aminocaproic acid and tranexamic acid) are useful as adjunctive therapy for prevention of bleeding following minor surgery. A short course (5–7 days) may be helpful for recurrent epistaxis. Fibrinolytic inhibitors should not be used to treat hematuria and they should be avoided for operative procedures associated with thrombotic high risks (e.g., orthopedic surgery). Fibrinolytic inhibitors are very useful to prevent and control bleeding in the Quebec platelet disorder [2].

When severe bleeding cannot be adequately controlled, bone marrow transplantation can be taken into consideration for patients with severe disorders, such as CHS, WAS, and GT.

References

1 Cattaneo M. Inherited platelet-based bleeding disorders. *J Thromb Haemost* 2003; 1: 1628–1636.
2 Hayward CP, Rao AK, Cattaneo M. Congenital platelet disorders: overview of their mechanisms, diagnostic evaluation and treatment. *Haemophilia* 2006; 12 (Suppl. 3): 128–136.
3 Lopez JA, Andrews RK, Afshar-Kharghan V, *et al.* Bernard-Soulier syndrome. *Blood* 1998; 91: 4397–4418.
4 Savoia A, Balduini CL, Savino M, *et al.* Autosomal dominant macrothrombocytopenia in Italy is most frequently a type of heterozygous Bernard-Soulier syndrome. *Blood* 2001; 97: 1330–1335.
5 Berndt MC, Andrews RK. Bernard-Soulier syndrome. *Haematologica* 2011; 96: 355–359.
6 Budde U. Diagnosis of von Willebrand disease subtypes: implications for treatment. *Haemophilia* 2008; 14 (Suppl. 5): 27–38.
7 Othman M, Notley C, Lavender FL, *et al.* Identification and functional characterization of a novel 27-bp deletion in the macroglycopeptide-coding region of the GPIBA gene resulting in platelet-type von Willebrand disease. *Blood* 2005; 105: 4330–4336.
8 Bolin RB, Okumra T, Jamieson GA. New polymorphism of platelet membrane glycoproteins. *Nature* 1977; 269: 69–70.

9 Nair S, Ghosh K, Kulkarni B, *et al.* Glanzmann's thrombasthenia: updated. *Platelets* 2002; 13: 387–393.

10 Nurden AT, Pillois X, Fiore M, *et al.* Glanzmann thrombasthenia-like syndromes associated with Macrothrombocytopenias and mutations in the genes encoding the alphaIIbbeta3 integrin. *Semin Thromb Hemost* 2011; 37: 698–706.

11 Moroi M, Jung SM. Platelet receptors for collagen. *Thromb Haemost* 1997; 78: 439–444.

12 Clemetson JM, Polgar J, Magnenat E, *et al.* The platelet collagen receptor glycoprotein VI is a member of the immunoglobulin superfamily closely related to FcalphaR and the natural killer receptors. *J Biol Chem* 1999; 274: 29019–29024.

13 Podda G, Femia EA, Pugliano M, *et al.* Congenital defects of platelet function. *Platelets* 2012; 23: 552–563.

14 Kamae T, Kiyomizu K, Nakazawa T, *et al.* Bleeding tendency and impaired platelet function in a patient carrying a heterozygous mutation in the thromboxane A2 receptor. *J Thromb Haemost* 2011; 9: 1040–1048.

15 Mumford AD, Nisar S, Darnige L, *et al.* Platelet dysfunction associated with the novel Trp29Cys thromboxane A2 receptor variant. *J Thromb Haemost* 2013; 11: 547–554.

16 Hirata T, Kakizuka A, Ushikubi F, *et al.* Arg60 to Leu mutation of the human thromboxane A2 receptor in a dominantly inherited bleeding disorder. *J Clin Invest* 1994; 94: 1662–1667.

17 Mumford A, Dawood B, Daly M, *et al.* A novel thromboxane A2 receptor D304N variant that abrogates ligand binding in a patient with a bleeding diathesis. *Blood* 2010; 115: 363–369.

18 Tamponi G, Pannocchia A, Arduino C, *et al.* Congenital deficiency of alpha-2-adrenoceptors on human-platelets - description of 2 cases. *Thromb Haemost* 1987; 58: 1012–1016.

19 Cattaneo M, Lecchi A, Randi AM, *et al.* Identification of a new congenital defect of platelet-function characterized by severe impairment of platelet responses to adenosine-diphosphate. *Blood* 1992; 80: 2787–2796.

20 Cattaneo M. The platelet P2Y(12) receptor for adenosine diphosphate: congenital and drug-induced defects. *Blood* 2011; 117: 2102–2112.

21 Zighetti ML, Carpani G, Sinigaglia E, *et al.* Usefulness of a flow cytometric analysis of intraplatelet vasodilator-stimulated phosphoprotein phosphorylation for the detection of patients with genetic defects of the platelet P2Y(12) receptor for ADP. *J Thromb Haemost* 2010; 8: 2332–2334.

22 Nurden P, Nurden AT. Congenital disorders associated with platelet dysfunctions. *Thromb Haemost* 2008; 99: 253–263.

23 Cattaneo M. Light transmission aggregometry and ATP release for the diagnostic assessment of platelet function. *Semin Thromb Hemost* 2009; 35: 158–167.

24 Bunimov N, Fuller N, Hayward CPM. Genetic loci associated with platelet traits and platelet disorders. *Semin Thromb Hemost* 2013; 39: 291–305.

25 Huizing M, Helip-Wooley A, Westbroek W, *et al.* Disorders of lysosome-related organelle biogenesis: clinical and molecular genetics. *Annu Rev Genomics Hum Genet* 2008; 9: 359–386.

26 Introne W, Boissy RE, Gahl WA. Clinical, molecular, and cell biological aspects of Chediak-Higashi syndrome. *Mol Genet Metab* 1999; 68: 283–303.

27 Gunay-Aygun M, Huizing M, Gahl WA. Molecular defects that affect platelet dense granules. *Semin Thromb Hemost* 2004; 30: 537–547.

28 Nurden AT, Nurden P. The gray platelet syndrome: clinical spectrum of the disease. *Blood Rev* 2007; 21: 21–36.

29 Diamandis M, Veljkovic DK, Maurer-Spurej E, *et al.* Quebec platelet disorder: features, pathogenesis and treatment. *Blood Coagul Fibrinolysis* 2008; 19: 109–119.

30 Hayward CP, Bainton DF, Smith JW, *et al.* Multimerin is found in the alpha-granules of resting platelets and is synthesized by a megakaryocytic cell line. *J Clin Invest* 1993; 91: 2630–2639.

31 Diamandis M, Paterson AD, Rommens JM, *et al.* Quebec platelet disorder is linked to the

urokinase plasminogen activator gene (PLAU) and increases expression of the linked allele in megakaryocytes. *Blood* 2009; 113: 1543–1546.

32 Breton-Gorius J, Favier R, Guichard J, *et al.* A new congenital dysmegakaryopoietic thrombocytopenia (Paris-Trousseau) associated with giant platelet alpha-granules and chromosome 11 deletion at 11q23. *Blood* 1995; 85: 1805–1814.

33 Weiss HJ, Lages B, Vicic W, *et al.* Heterogeneous abnormalities of platelet dense granule ultrastructure in 20 patients with congenital storage pool deficiency. *Br J Haematol* 1993; 83: 282–295.

34 Weiss HJ, Witte LD, Kaplan KL, *et al.* Heterogeneity in storage pool deficiency: studies on granule-bound substances in 18 patients including variants deficient in alpha-granules, platelet factor 4, beta-thromboglobulin, and platelet-derived growth factor. *Blood* 1979; 54: 1296–1319.

35 Weiss HJ. Scott syndrome: a disorder of platelet coagulant activity. *Semin Hematol* 1994; 31: 312–319.

36 Lhermusier T, Chap H, Payrastre B. Platelet membrane phospholipid asymmetry: from the characterization of a scramblase activity to the identification of an essential protein mutated in Scott syndrome. *J Thromb Haemost* 2011; 9: 1883–1891.

37 Suzuki J, Umeda M, Sims PJ, *et al.* Calcium-dependent phospholipid scrambling by TMEM16F. *Nature* 2010; 468: 834–838.

38 Toti F, Satta N, Fressinaud E, *et al.* Scott syndrome, characterized by impaired transmembrane migration of procoagulant phosphatidylserine and hemorrhagic complications, is an inherited disorder. *Blood* 1996; 87: 1409–1415.

39 Stormorken H, Holmsen H, Sund R, *et al.* Studies on the hemostatic defect in a complicated syndrome - an inverse Scott syndrome platelet membrane abnormality. *Thromb Haemost* 1995; 74: 1244–1251.

40 Rao AK. Inherited defects in platelet signaling mechanisms. *J Thromb Haemost* 2003; 1: 671–681.

41 Rao AK. Acquired disorders of platelet function. In: Michelson AD, ed. *Platelets*, 3rd edn. London: Academic Press, 2013, pp. 1049–1074.

42 Livio M, Gotti E, Marchesi D, *et al.* Uraemic bleeding: role of anaemia and beneficial effect of red cell transfusions. *Lancet* 1982; 2: 1013–1015.

43 Moia M, Mannucci PM, Vizzotto L, *et al.* Improvement in the haemostatic defect of uraemia after treatment with recombinant human erythropoietin. *Lancet* 1987; 2: 1227–1229.

44 Bennett J. Acquired platelet function defects. In: Gresele P, Page C, Fuster V, Vermylen J, eds. *Platelets in Thrombotic and Non-Thrombotic Disorders.* Cambridge, UK: Cambridge University Press, 2002, pp. 674–688.

45 Psaila B, Bussel JB, Frelinger AL, *et al.* Differences in platelet function in patients with acute myeloid leukemia and myelodysplasia compared to equally thrombocytopenic patients with immune thrombocytopenia. *J Thromb Haemost* 2011; 9: 2302–2310.

46 Gerrard JM, McNicol A. Platelet storage pool deficiency, leukemia, and myelodysplastic syndromes. *Leuk Lymphoma* 1992; 8: 277–281.

47 Elliott MA, Tefferi A. Thrombosis and haemorrhage in polycythaemia vera and essential thrombocythaemia. *Br J Haematol* 2005; 128: 275–290.

48 Smith BR, Rinder HM. Cardiopulmonary bypass. In: Michelson AD, ed. *Platelets*, 3rd edn. London: Academic Press, 2013, pp. 1075–1096.

49 Mannucci PM, Vicente V, Vianello L, *et al.* Controlled trial of desmopressin in liver cirrhosis and other conditions associated with a prolonged bleeding time. *Blood* 1986; 67: 1148–1153.

50 Poon M-C. Factor VIIa. In: Michelson AD, editor. *Platelets*, 3rd edn. London: Academic Press, 2013, pp. 1257–1274.

12

Disseminated Intravascular Coagulation

Raj S. Kasthuri and Nigel S. Key

Key Points

- DIC is a clinicopathological syndrome that is not in itself a disease but a manifestation of another underlying disorder.
- Patients with DIC can develop thrombotic and/or hemorrhagic manifestations depending to some extent on the underlying cause.
- There is no diagnostic test for DIC. It is recommended that one of the DIC scoring systems be used to establish the diagnosis.
- Management of DIC is centered on treating the underlying cause and providing supportive care including transfusion of blood products.

Introduction

Disseminated intravascular coagulation (DIC) is an acquired clinicopathological syndrome characterized by chaotic activation of the coagulation system, resulting in widespread intravascular deposition of fibrin-rich thrombi. DIC is not itself a disease state, but rather is a secondary manifestation of some other underlying disorder. Depending on the underlying cause and rapidity of the process, the clinical spectrum may range from subclinical laboratory abnormalities (compensated DIC or nonovert DIC) to multiorgan failure, metabolic derangement, hemodynamic instability, widespread bleeding, and death.

The following definition of DIC has been proposed by the DIC Scientific and Standardization Committee (SSC) of the International Society on Thrombosis and Hemostasis (ISTH): "DIC is an acquired syndrome characterized by the intravascular activation of coagulation with loss of localization arising from different causes. It can originate from and cause damage to the microvasculature, which if sufficiently severe, can produce organ dysfunction" [1].

Synonyms for DIC in the medical literature include the defibrination syndrome, consumption coagulopathy, generalized intravascular coagulation, thrombohemorrhagic phenomenon, and disseminated intravascular fibrin formation.

Etiology

A broad range of pathological conditions may trigger DIC. Sepsis syndromes are among the most frequently encountered causes. Although the highest risk is seen with Gram-negative bacterial infections, Gram-positive infections as well as nonbacterial infections can also be associated with DIC. Complications of pregnancy and malignancy are other common causes of DIC in clinical practice. Pathological conditions associated with the development of DIC are listed in Table 12.1.

Practical Hemostasis and Thrombosis, Third Edition. Edited by Nigel S. Key, Michael Makris and David Lillicrap.
© 2017 John Wiley & Sons, Ltd. Published 2017 by John Wiley & Sons, Ltd.

Table 12.1 Conditions associated with disseminated intravascular coagulation (DIC).

Infection

    Sepsis syndromes (Gram-positive and Gram-negative bacteria)
    Viral infections (e.g., dengue, Ebola)
    Other (e.g., ricketsial, malarial infections)

Trauma/ tissue damage

    Head injury
    Pancreatitis
    Fat embolism
    Any other serious tissue damage (crush or penetrating injury)

Malignancy

    Solid tumors
    Acute leukemias (especially AML-M3)
    Chronic leukemias (CMML)

Obstetric complications

    Abruptio placentae
    Amniotic fluid embolism
    Eclampsia and pre-eclampsia
    Retained dead fetus

Vascular disorders

    Giant hemangiomas (Kasabach–Merritt syndrome)
    Other vascular malformations
    Large aortic aneurysm

Severe allergic/toxic reactions

    Toxic shock syndrome
    Snake, spider venoms

Severe immunological reactions

    Acute hemolytic transfusion reactions
    Heparin-induced thrombocytopenia, type II

AML-M3, acute myelogenous leukemia, M3 subtype; CMML, chronic myelomonocytic leukemia.

Pathogenesis

The pathogenesis of DIC is complex and involves simultaneous dysregulation of several homeostatic mechanisms (Figure 12.1). These can be broadly divided into:

- excessive activation of coagulation;
- downregulation of physiological anticoagulant pathways; and
- dysregulation of fibrinolysis.

Dysfunction of the vascular endothelium, a vast and pervasive organ, is prominent as both a cause and a consequence of these processes. The net result is widespread generation of thrombin and conversion of circulating fibrinogen to insoluble fibrin thrombi, aggravated by the relative inability of the fibrinolytic mechanism to remove intravascular fibrin.

Obstruction of small and medium-sized vessels caused by intravascular fibrin deposition may lead to (multiple) organ dysfunction, especially affecting the kidneys, brain, lung, liver, and heart. The widespread activation of coagulation leads to consumption of clotting factors, natural anticoagulants, and platelets, a process that is aggravated by simultaneous impaired hepatic production of these factors. Thus, abnormal prolongation of coagulation screening tests, thrombocytopenia, and a seemingly paradoxical bleeding tendency may occur in some patients with more advanced forms of DIC.

The passage of erythrocytes through the fibrin meshwork in the microvascular circulation may lead to red cell fragmentation. This microangiopathic hemolytic anemia is much less common in DIC than in the group of disorders known as the "thrombotic microangiopathies," where it is, in fact, a *sine qua non*.

Excessive Activation of Coagulation

Although coagulation may be initiated *in vitro* by both the intrinsic (contact) and extrinsic (tissue factor) pathways, the tissue factor pathway is the primary initiator of coagulation *in vivo* [2]. Unlike most other soluble clotting factors circulating in plasma, tissue factor (TF) is a cell-bound transmembrane protein. By virtue of its predominant extravascular location, TF is normally present on cells that are relatively inaccessible to blood clotting factors in the absence of vessel injury, such as smooth muscle cells and fibroblasts. However, the systemic response to infection and injury results in the synthesis and release of proinflammatory cytokines, such as tumor necrosis factor (TNF-α), interleukin 1 (IL-1), and IL-6, which trigger TF synthesis by monocytes and endothelial cells (Figure 12.1) [2]. In the case of DIC from other causes, it is likely that additional stimuli capable of activating

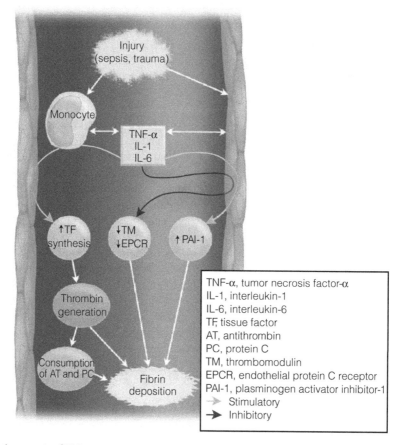

Figure 12.1 Pathogenesis of DIC.

and/or propagating coagulation (such as fat, brain lipids, cancer procoagulant protein, or amniotic fluid) are released into the circulation.

Downregulation of Physiological Anticoagulation Pathways

DIC is associated with an acquired deficiency of naturally occurring anticoagulants, particularly antithrombin and protein C. Plasma levels are decreased secondary to consumption and increased enzymatic degradation by activated neutrophils [3]. Endothelial dysfunction also adversely affects the protein C/ protein S/ thrombomodulin (TM) pathway. The same proinflammatory cytokines that upregulate TF synthesis simultaneously downregulate endothelial synthesis of the cofactors TM and endothelial

cell protein C receptor [4]. The end result is decreased conversion of protein C to activated protein C on the endothelial cell surface.

Dysregulation of Fibrinolysis

The role of the fibrinolytic system is to generate plasmin on fibrin surfaces, in an effort to restore vascular patency via enzymatic digestion of fibrin strands. The excessive thrombin generation in DIC also leads to activation of the fibrinolytic system, resulting in an increase in circulating fibrin degradation products. However, in many forms of DIC, fibrinolysis is insufficient to clear intravascular fibrin thrombi because of elevated levels of plasminogen activator inhibitor type 1 (PAI-1) [5]. PAI-1 inhibits the plasminogen activators tissue plasminogen activator and urokinase, preventing the generation of plasmin from plasminogen. Thus, the inhibition of fibrinolysis by PAI-1 contributes to the net procoagulant state and end-organ hypoperfusion in DIC.

DIC Versus Trauma-Induced Coagulopathy

In recent years, it has been suggested that the acute hemostatic dysfunction that occurs following major trauma is distinct from the changes seen in other forms of DIC. This rapid-onset condition is referred to as trauma-induced coagulopathy (also called coagulopathy of trauma) [6]. While there are similarities between DIC and trauma-induced coagulopathy [7], the proposed pathophysiological mechanism underlying trauma-induced coagulopathy involves excessive thrombin-TM driven activation of the protein C pathway with subsequent inactivation of coagulation factors Va and VIIIa. It is postulated that the resulting systemic endogenous anticoagulation and hyperfibrinolysis leads to an increased risk for bleeding and death [6]. However, differentiating DIC from trauma-induced coagulopathy can be challenging, and is a controversial topic [7].

Clinical Manifestations

As predicted from the complex underlying pathophysiological derangements, patients with DIC may suffer thrombotic and/or hemorrhagic manifestations. Clinical features are determined to some extent by the underlying etiology. Thus, whereas vaso-occlusive manifestations are significantly more prevalent overall, certain subtypes of DIC may be more commonly associated with bleeding, usually in the form of microvascular oozing from mucocutaneous surfaces. In obstetric disorders, bleeding may be explained by the hyperacuity of the process leading to rapid consumption of clotting factors and platelets, whereas in acute promyelocytic leukemia (AML-M3), production of plasminogen activators by leukemic cells may lead to hyperfibrinolytic bleeding [8].

The most common result of microvascular occlusion is end-organ dysfunction, as is typical of sepsis syndromes. This process may lead to renal, cardiac, and/or pulmonary failure. Vaso-occlusion may occasionally lead to more clinically overt thrombotic manifestations, such as purpura fulminans in meningococcal or pneumococcal sepsis, which is a clinical syndrome presenting as skin necrosis and digital gangrene (Figure 12.2). The systemic prothrombotic state

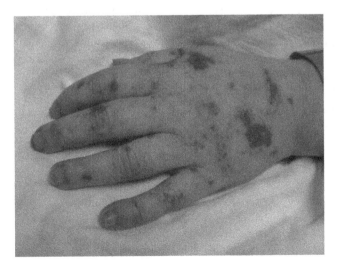

Figure 12.2 Purpura fulminans in a patient with meningococcemia. Purpura fulminans is associated with underlying DIC and is characterized by widespread ecchymosis and ischemic infarction of the skin. *Source:* courtesy of Dr Stephan Moll. *See Plate section for color representation of this figure.*

may also lead to the development of a localized large-vessel arterial or venous thromboembolic event.

It is important to realize that a substantial subset of patients with DIC may suffer only subclinical laboratory abnormalities, with insidious or even absent clinical features. This condition has been referred to as compensated DIC or nonovert DIC (discussed below).

Diagnosis

The diagnosis of DIC should take into account both the clinical presentation as well as laboratory findings. It is important to appreciate that DIC is a syndrome that is *always secondary* to another underlying pathological condition and that there is no single diagnostic laboratory test for DIC.

A number of laboratory tests can be abnormal in patients with DIC. However, none of them are specific for the diagnosis of DIC. The prothrombin time (PT) has been shown to be prolonged in over 50% of patients with DIC at some point during their illness [9] but this can also be due to other reasons such as liver dysfunction and vitamin K deficiency, both of which are not uncommon in situations associated with development of DIC (critical illness, massive trauma, etc.). Similarly, the increase in fibrin degradation products is also a nonspecific finding in acutely ill, hospitalized patients. And although perceived as a classic finding, a low plasma fibrinogen level is not a sensitive marker of DIC [10]. In fact, high plasma fibrinogen levels are much more frequently encountered. Fibrinogen levels are probably influenced more by the degree of activation of secondary fibrino(geno) lysis than the degree of consumption during thrombus formation.

Scoring Systems for the Diagnosis of DIC

Two diagnostic algorithms using widely available coagulation tests have been proposed and validated for the diagnosis of DIC, as follows.

International Society on Thrombosis and Hemostasis DIC Score

The design of this scoring system has a pathophysiological basis, incorporating the concept of "overt" (Table 12.2) and "nonovert" (Table 12.3) DIC as distinct entities [1]. To some extent, these subsets reflect different points in the continuum, although nonovert DIC may be associated with adverse outcomes in critically ill patients independently of progression to overt DIC. It should be noted that the term "fibrin-related products" in the scoring system includes:

- direct assays for the presence of fibrin (e.g., soluble fibrin monomers); and
- indirect assays of fibrin generation (e.g., D-dimer, fibrin degradation products (FDPs)).

Importantly, the ISTH scoring algorithm should be applied only if an underlying disorder known to be associated with DIC (e.g., sepsis, cancer) exists. This scoring system has been validated prospectively in the diagnosis of DIC, and it has been shown that DIC is an independent predictor of mortality in sepsis patients. Additionally, the severity of DIC based on the DIC score also correlates with poor outcomes in these patients [11]. This scoring system is useful for the diagnosis of DIC regardless of the underlying etiology (i.e., both infective and noninfective causes).

Overt DIC: This is defined as a state in which the vascular endothelium, and blood and its components, have lost the ability to compensate and restore homeostasis in response to injury. The result is a progressively decompensating state that is manifest as thrombotic multiorgan dysfunction and/or bleeding. Under the scoring system, a score of 5 or more meets the definition of "overt" DIC.

Nonovert DIC: This is defined as a clinical vascular injury state that results in great stress to the hemostatic system, the response to which, for the moment, is sufficient to forestall further rampant inflammatory and hemostatic activation.

Table 12.2 Diagnostic scoring system for overt disseminated intravascular coagulation (DIC). Do not use this algorithm unless the patient has an underlying disorder that is associated with DIC.

Global coagulation test	Results	Score (0, 1, or 2 points)
Platelet count	$>100 \times 10^9$/L	= 0
	$50-100 \times 10^9$/L	= 1
	$<50 \times 10^9$/L	= 2
Elevated fibrin-related markers(soluble fibrin monomers, D-dimers, fibrin degradation products)	No increase	= 0
	Moderate increase	= 1
	Strong increase	= 2
Prolonged prothrombin time (in seconds above upper limit of normal)	<3 s	= 0
	3–6 s	= 1
	>6 s	= 2
Fibrinogen level	>1.0 g/L	= 0
	<1.0 g/L	= 1
Total score		=

If score ≥ 5, compatible with overt DIC, recommend repeating score daily.

If score < 5, suggestive (not affirmative) for nonovert DIC, repeat scoring in 1–2 days.

Source: Adapted from Taylor *et al.* 2001 [1].

The scoring system for the diagnosis of nonovert DIC includes, in addition to global studies of coagulation (PT, FDPs), more specific (but less widely available) tests that are surrogate markers of intravascular thrombin generation (thrombin–antithrombin (TAT) complexes) and ongoing consumption of coagulation inhibitors (such as antithrombin (AT) and protein C (PC) levels). However, the value of including AT and PC levels in the "nonovert DIC" scoring system is unclear and modifications to the nonovert DIC score to improve its ability to diagnose early overt DIC have been proposed [12, 13].

Japanese Association for Acute Medicine DIC Score

The Japanese Association for Acute Medicine (JAAM) DIC score was developed based on the Japanese Ministry for Health and Welfare's original scoring system specifically for critically ill patients and, as such, incorporates systemic inflammatory response criteria in the DIC score (Table 12.4) [14]. This score has been validated in critically ill patients. The two DIC scores have also been compared in patients with sepsis-associated DIC with a high level of agreement demonstrated between the two [15, 16].

In summary, in the absence of a gold standard for the diagnosis of DIC, current recommendations are to use one of the scoring systems that correlate with "key clinical observations and outcomes" [17]. Furthermore, it is recommended that the dynamic nature of DIC be assessed by calculation of the score on a daily basis in affected patients.

Table 12.3 Diagnostic scoring system for nonovert DIC. Score of 0, 1, or 2 is assigned for criteria plus a score for rising, stable, or falling.

Criteria	Score	
1. *Risk assessment*		
Is there an underlying disorder that is associated with DIC?	Yes = 2 No – 0	
2. *Major criteria*		
Platelet count	$> 100 \times 10^9 / L = 0$	Rising = –1
	$< 100 \times 10^9 / L = 1$	Stable = 0 Falling = 1
Prothrombin time (in seconds above upper limit of normal)	<3 s = 0 >3 s = 1	Falling = –1 Stable = 0 Rising = 1
Soluble fibrin or FDPs	Normal = 0 Raised = 1	Falling = –1 Stable = 0 Rising = 1
3. *Specific criteria*		
Antithrombin	Normal = –1 Low = 1	
Protein C	Normal = –1 Low = 1	
TAT complexes	Normal = –1 High = 1	
	Total score =	

Source: Adapted from Taylor *et al.* 2001 [1].
FDP, fibrin degradation product; TAT, thrombin–antithrombin complex.
At the present time, although this scoring system has been proposed, interpretations with regards to cut-off scores for diagnosis of nonovert DIC are unclear. In general, trends over time will be more useful than individual single point scores.

Treatment

The development of DIC in patients with sepsis or trauma has been shown to be independently associated with increased morbidity and mortality. Thus, prompt and at times pre-emptive therapy becomes important in these patients.

DIC treatment guidelines have been developed by the British Committee for Standards in Haematology (BCSH) [18, 19], the Italian Society for Haemostasis and Thrombosis (SISET) [20], and the Japanense Society of Thrombosis and Hemostasis (JSTH) [21]. Recently, the DIC Scientific Subcommittee of the ISTH reviewed these guidelines and published harmonized recommendations on the diagnosis and management of DIC [17]. All the guidelines recommend the use of a DIC scoring system to make the diagnosis. While there is considerable agreement between the different guidelines in regards to treatment, some differences exist. These differences are discussed under the specific sections below.

Management of the Underlying Disease

The mainstay of treatment in patients with DIC is management of the underlying disease. The reversibility of DIC depends to a large degree on the underlying cause. Delivery of the fetus and placenta may promptly restore homeostasis in patients with obstetric DIC. Although essential, eradication of infection with antibiotics and/or surgery may not necessarily have the same rapid effect in sepsis syndromes,

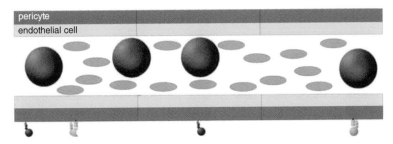

Figure 1.1 *Vessel.* An intact blood vessels is pictured with the endothelial cells (tan) and surrounding pericytes (dark brown). Within the vessel are red blood cells and platelets (blue). Associated with the pericytes, tissue factor complexed with factor VII(a) is shown in green. Factor IX, shown in blue, is associated with collagen IV in the extravascular space.

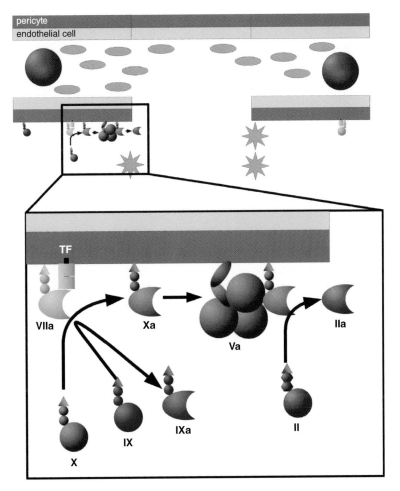

Figure 1.2 *Initiation.* A break in the vasculature brings plasma coagulation factors and platelets into contact with the extravascular space. Unactivated platelets within the vessel are shown as blue disks. Platelets adhering to collagen in the extravascular space are activated and are represented as blue star shapes to indicate cytoskeletal-induced shape change. The expanded view shows the protein reactions in the initiation phase. Factor VIIa–tissue factor activates both factor IX and factor X. Factor Xa, in complex with factor Va released from platelets, can activate a small amount of thrombin (IIa).

Practical Hemostasis and Thrombosis, Third Edition. Edited by Nigel S. Key, Michael Makris and David Lillicrap.
© 2017 John Wiley & Sons, Ltd. Published 2017 by John Wiley & Sons, Ltd.

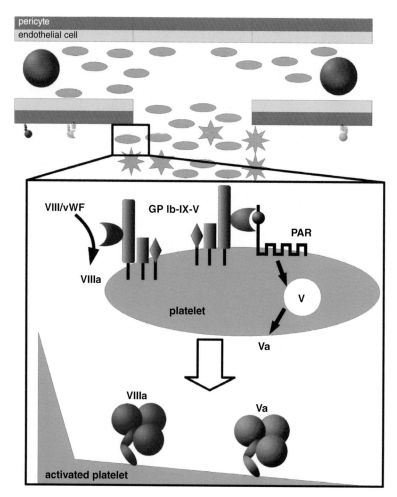

Figure 1.3 *Amplification.* Platelets, shown as blue discs, aggregate to stop blood loss from the break in the vasculature. Activated platelets are shown as star shapes. The expanded view shows thrombin (red) generated during the initiation phase binding to the glycoprotein Ib–IX–V complex (GP Ib–IX–V) on platelets. When bound, thrombin is somewhat protected from inhibition and can cleave protease activated receptor (PAR) 1 at the recognition site (black sphere). When the new amino terminal folds back on the seven transmembrane domain, a signaling cascade is initiated leading to surface exposure of phosphatidylserine as well as degranulation of alpha (white circle) or dense (not shown) granules. Factor Va is released from alpha granules and further activated by thrombin. Also, factor VIII is activated by cleavage and release from von Willebrand factor (vWF).

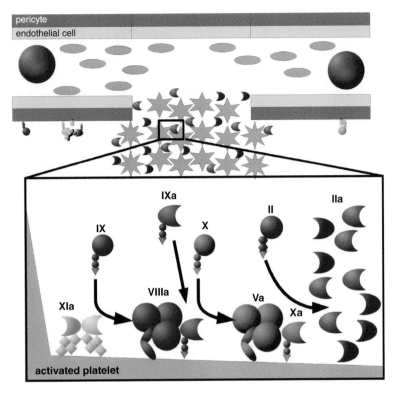

Figure 1.4 *Propagation.* The expanded view shows platelet surface thrombin generation. Factor IXa, formed during the initiation phase, can move into a complex with factor VIIIa formed during the amplification phase. This IXa–VIIIa complex cleaves factor X. Factor Xa, in complex with platelet surface factor Va, generates a burst of thrombin (IIa). This thrombin can feed back and activate platelet surface bound factor XI; the resulting factor XIa can feed more factor IXa into the reaction. This additional factor IXa enhances factor Xa and thrombin generation. As shown in the overview, the burst of thrombin stabilizes the initial platelet plug as all of the platelets are now activated (represented as blue star shapes as opposed to the disc shaped platelets in circulation). The factor VIIa–tissue factor complex with associated factor Xa is inhibited by TFPI.

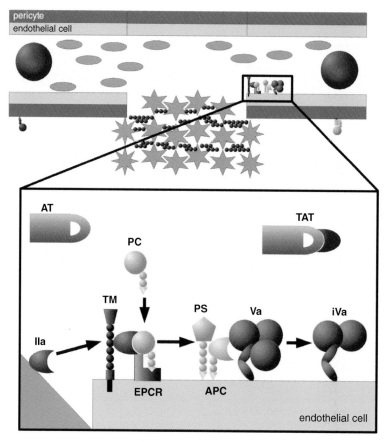

Figure 1.5 *Localization.* Thrombin generated during the propagation phase cleaves fibrinopeptides A and B leading to fibrin assembly (shown as brown distributed among and associated with the blue star shapes that represent activated platelets). The result is a stable platelet plug with fibrin and bound thrombin distributed throughout the plug. The expanded view shows the interface between the platelet plug (blue) and healthy endothelium. Thrombin released into the circulation is inhibited by antithrombin (AT) to form a thrombin–antithrombin complex (TAT). Also, thrombin (IIa) that reaches the endothelial cell surface binds tightly to thrombomodulin (TM). The thrombin–thrombomodulin complex activates protein C (PC) in a reaction enhanced by the endothelial cell protein C receptor (EPCR). Activated protein C (APC) in a reaction enhanced by protein S (PS) can cleave factor Va to inactivated factor Va (iVa). So thrombin on healthy endothelium participates in a negative feedback process that prevents thrombin generation away from the platelet plug that seals an injury.

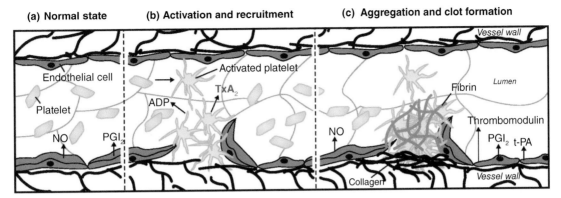

(a) Normal state   **(b) Activation and recruitment**   **(c) Aggregation and clot formation**

Figure 4.2 Platelet adhesion, activation, and aggregation. (a) Normal endothelium releases antiaggregant molecules promoting hemostasis and nonthrombogenic state. (b) Injured endothelium exposes platelets to thrombogenic subendothelium. Activated platelets release proaggregant molecules. (c) Clot formation at site of injury. Endothelium releases factors that stabilize the clot and limit the haemostatic process to the site of injury. ADP, adenosine diphosphate; NO, nitric oxide; PGI_2, prostacyclin; t-PA, tissue plasminogen activator; TxA_2, thromboxane A_2. Source: Lordkipanidzé, 2006 [11]. Reproduced with permission of Elsevier.

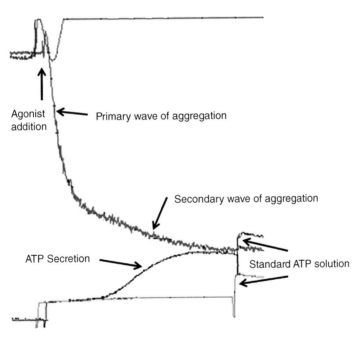

Figure 4.3 Example lumiaggregometry traces from a patient with an ADP $P2Y_{12}$ receptor mutation and from a healthy volunteer (control). The agonist used in this trace was a very high concentration of adenosine diphosphate (ADP) (100 μM). Control aggregation is shown in blue, patient aggregation is shown in red. Control adenosine triphosphate (ATP) secretion is shown in black, patient ATP secretion is shown in green. Secondary wave of aggregation is seen in the healthy volunteer and is labeled, whereas the patient shows no ATP secretion and no secondary wave of aggregation, with deaggregation noted after initial primary wave formation. Addition of the ATP standard to allow calculation of secretion to normalized platelet count is also labeled.

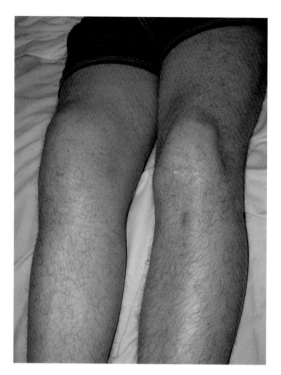

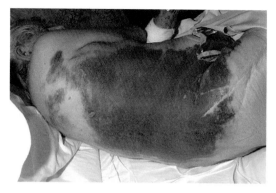

Figure 6.3 Extensive spontaneous subcutaneous hematoma in a patient with acquired hemophilia A. In contrast to congenital hemophilia, these patients often present with extensive subcutaneous bleeds and rarely have hemarthroses.

Figure 6.1 Right knee hemarthrosis in a severe hemophilia A patient. Bleeds such as this are unusual in countries where patients have home treatment with clotting factor concentrates. Usually the there are no physical signs and the only symptoms are pain and limitation of joint movement.

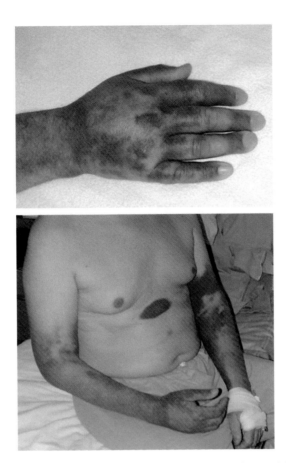

Figure 9.2 Patient presenting with acquired hemophilia having typical large soft tissue bleeds, after sleeping on his left side and exerting his left arm. The photograph is from the time of diagnosis, which was delayed for several days. Source: With permission from Duodecim Medical Journal, Finland, 2003.

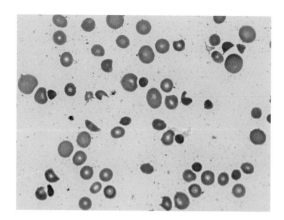

Figure 10.2 Peripheral blood smear in a patient with microangiopathic hemolytic anemia showing helmet cells, schistocytes, and microspherocytes. Source: Kumar *et al.* 2013 [47]. Reproduced with permission of Karger Medical and Scientific Publishers.

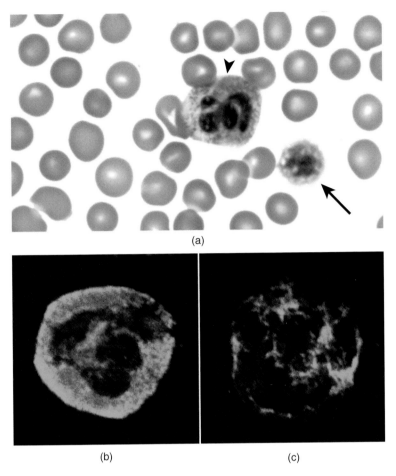

(a)

(b)   (c)

Figure 10.3 (a) Peripheral blood smear from a patient with MYH9-RD demonstrating giant platelet (arrow) and neutrophil inclusion (arrowhead). Immunofluorescent visualization of nonmuscle myosin heavy chain IIA aggregates: (b) normal homogenous cytoplasmic staining (lower left) and (c) abnormal variable speckled cytoplasmic staining.

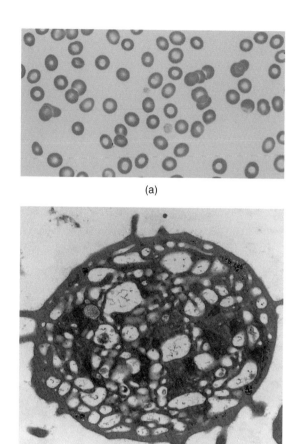

(a)

(b)

Figure 10.4 (a) Peripheral blood smear from a patient with gray platelet syndrome demonstrating large gray-appearing platelets. (b) Platelet transmission electron micrograph from a patient with gray platelet syndrome showing complete absence of alpha granules with increased vacuoles. Scale bar represents 5 nanometers. Source: Kumar and Kahr 2013 [12]. Reproduced with permission of Elsevier.

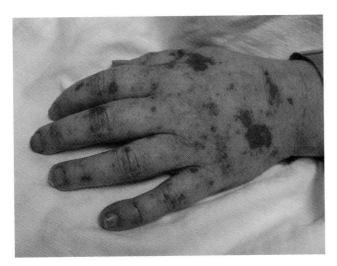

Figure 12.2 Purpura fulminans in a patient with meningococcemia. Purpura fulminans is associated with underlying DIC and is characterized by widespread ecchymosis and ischemic infarction of the skin. Source: courtesy of Dr Stephan Moll.

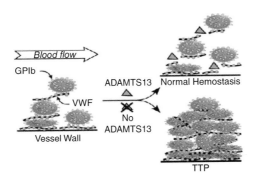

Figure 13.1 The role of ADAMTS13 in the pathophysiology of thrombotic thrombocytopenic purpura (TTP). VWF, von Willebrand factor. Source: adapted from Sadler 2008 [44].

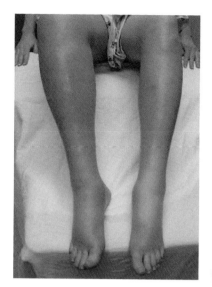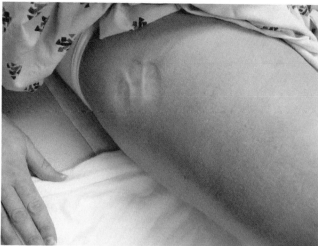

Figure 14.1 Acute right lower extremity deep vein thrombosis. Note the swelling, erythema, and pitting edema. Source: reproduced with permission of Dr. Stephan Moll.

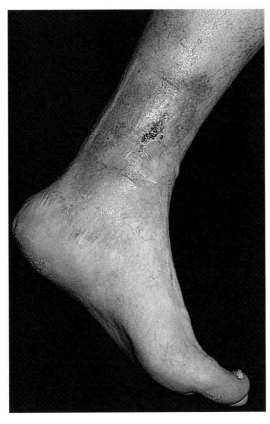

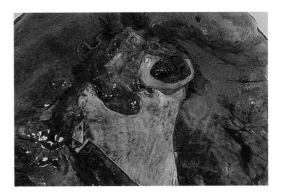

Figure 14.3 Pulmonary embolus in the pulmonary artery causing sudden death in a young woman who was using the combined pill. Source: Makris and Greaves, 1997 [4]. Reproduced with permission of Elsevier.

Figure 14.2 Post-thrombotic syndrome. Although usually the symptoms are confined to itching, mild swelling and pain, when severe there is pigmentation and ulceration over the medial malleolus. Source: Makris and Greaves, 1997 [4]. Reproduced with permission of Elsevier.

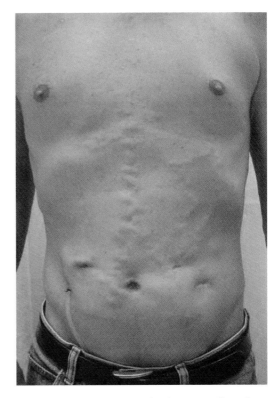

Figure 14.6 Prominent superficial venous collaterals in a patient with inferior vena caval (IVC) thrombotic occlusion, occurring as a late complication of an IVC filter. Source: reproduced with permission of Dr. Stephan Moll.

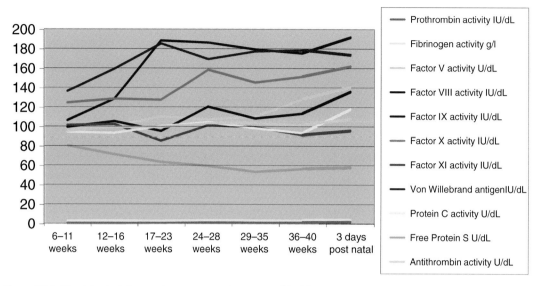

Figure 26.1 Physiological changes in pregnancy. Source: modified from Pavord and Hunt, 2010 [1].

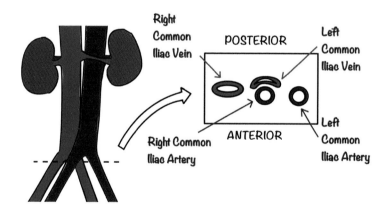

Figure 26.2 Diagram of iliac vessels.

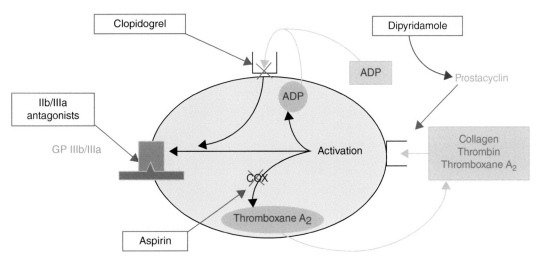

Figure 27.1 Receptor sites for antiplatelet agents.

Immediate management of suspected heparin-induced thrombocytopenia (hit)

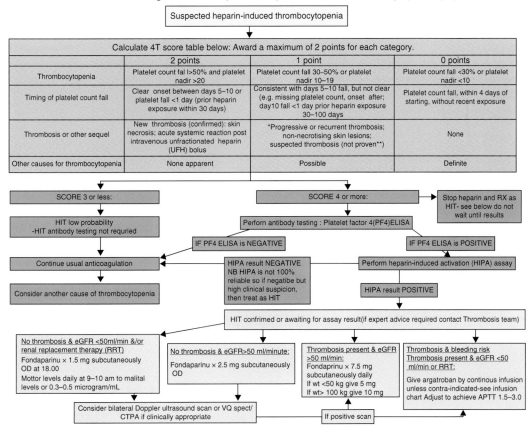

Figure 28.1 A local management protocol for heparin-induced thrombocytopenia (HIT). APTT, activated partial thromboplastin time; CTPA, computed tomographic pulmonary angiography; eGFR, estimated glomerular filtration rate; ELISA, enzyme-linked immunosorbent assay.

Management of Acute Massive Pulmonary Embolism

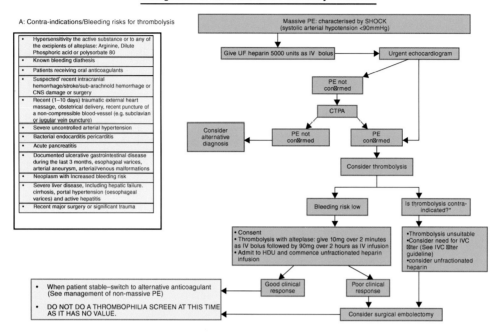

A: Contra-indications/Bleeding risks for thrombolysis

- Hypersensitivity the active substance or to any of the excipients of alteplase: Arginine, Dilute Phosphoric acid or polysorbate 80
- Known bleeding diathesis
- Patients receiving oral anticoagulants
- Suspected' recent intracranial hemorrhage/stroke/sub-arachnold hemorrhage or CNS damage or surgery
- Recent (1–10 days) traumatic external heart massage, obstetrical delivery, recent puncture of a non-compressible blood-vessel (e.g. subclavian or jugular vein puncture)
- Severe uncontrolled arterial hypertension
- Bacterial endocarditis pericarditis
- Acute pancreatitis
- Documented ulcerative gastrointestinal disease during the last 3 months, esophageal varices, arterial aneurysm, arterial/venous malformations
- Neoplasm with Increased bleeding risk
- Severe liver disease, Including hepatic failure. cirrhosis, portal hypertension (oesophageal varices) and active hepatitis
- Recent major surgery or significant trauma

Massive PE: characterised by SHOCK (systolic arterial hypotension <90mmHg)

Give UF heparin 5000 units as IV bolus → Urgent echocardiogram

PE not confirmed

CTPA

Consider alternative diagnosis ← PE not confirmed | PE confirmed

Consider thrombolysis

Bleeding risk low | Is thrombolysis contra-indicated?*

- Consent
- Thrombolysis with alteplase: give 10mg over 2 minutes as IV bolus followed by 90mg over 2 hours as IV infusion
- Admit to HDU and commence unfractionated heparin infusion

- Thrombolysis unsuitable
- Consider need for IVC filter (See IVC filter guideline)
- consider unfractionated heparin

- When patient stable–switch to alternative anticoagulant (See management of non-massive PE)
- DO NOT DO A THROMBOPHILIA SCREEN AT THIS TIME AS IT HAS NO VALUE.

Good clinical response | Poor clinical response

Consider surgical embolectomy

Figure 28.2 A local management algorithm for managing massive pulmonary embolism (PE). CTPA, computed tomographic pulmonary angiography; IVC, inferior vena cava.

Table 12.4 The Japanese Association for Acute Medicine disseminated intravascular coagulation (DIC) score.

Criteria	Score
SIRS criteria	
≥3	1
0–2	0
Platelet count (10^9/L)	
<80 or >50% decrease in last 24 hours	3
≥80 and <120 or >30% decrease in last 24 hours	1
>120	0
Prothrombin time (patients value/ normal value)	
≥1.2	1
<1.2	0
Fibrinogen (g/L)	
<3.5	1
≥3.5	0
Fibrin(ogen) degradation products (mg/L)	
≥25	3
≥10 and <25	1
<10	0
	Total score =

A total score of ≥ 5 is suggestive of DIC

Source: Adapted from Gando *et al.* 2006 [14].

possibly because of established widespread endothelial injury.

Supportive Care and Blood Products

Good supportive care in the management of patients with DIC includes adequate hemodynamic support to maintain perfusion and appropriate transfusion of blood products. Given the mechanisms involved in the development of DIC, there is always the theoretical fear of "fueling the fire" with transfused blood cells and plasma products, although the evidence that this occurs in practice is underwhelming. The approach to these patients should be individualized based on their clinical and laboratory manifestations.

Treatment of patients with DIC who are actively bleeding or at high risk for bleeding should include platelet transfusions (with goal platelet count of 50×10^9 /L), fresh frozen plasma (FFP, 15–30 mL/kg), cryoprecipitate (for fibrinogen ≤1.0 g/L), and packed red cells as needed. Patients requiring invasive procedures should be covered periprocedurally with plasma and platelet transfusions as needed. Reasonable transfusion triggers in these circumstances are platelet counts ≤ 50×10^9 /L , fibrinogen ≤1.0 g/L, and maintenance of PT and activated partial thromboplastin time (APTT) as close to the normal range as possible. The role for the prophylactic administration of blood products in patients with DIC who are not bleeding is more controversial [22], but generally there is no evidence to support their routine use.

FFP is the preferred product for replacement of coagulation factors. There are insufficient data on the use of prothrombin complex concentrates in DIC, and FFP is deemed superior as it contains a fuller complement of clotting factors and natural anticoagulants. The efficacy of recombinant factor VIIa in the DIC patient with life-threatening bleeding is unknown and it should be used with caution and preferably under the auspices of a clinical trial.

There is generally good consensus between the different treatment guidelines for the above recommendations.

Systemic Anticoagulation

On the basis of the pathophysiology of DIC, an argument may be made for the use of systemic heparin anticoagulation. Although the literature remains divided about this approach, the few available controlled trials have failed to demonstrate a clear benefit [17]. The routine use of therapeutic heparin in DIC not associated with a clinical thrombotic event is generally discouraged, given the risk of bleeding complications in these patients. However, there is some consensus that treatment is indicated for those with a documented thromboembolic event or extensive deposition of fibrin leading to acral ischemia or purpura fulminans. In the case of large-vessel thromboembolic events, therapeutic doses of heparin are indicated, whereas in microvascular occlusive syndromes, lower doses may be preferable. Low-molecular-weight heparins have been successfully used as an alternative to unfractionated heparin and have become the preferred agent in most of the treatment guidelines. Thromboprophylactic doses of either unfractionated or low–molecular-weight heparin is recommended in acutely ill patients to prevent thrombosis. The role of direct thrombin inhibitors (such as hirudin or argatroban) in DIC also remains to be established in controlled trials. Although these agents might theoretically be more effective than heparins, they also carry a higher risk of bleeding.

Antifibrinolytic Therapy

Because fibrinolysis is generally relatively down-regulated concomitant with excessive fibrin formation in DIC, treatment with antifibrinolytic agents (such as ε-aminocaproic acid or tranexamic acid) is generally contraindicated. There may be exceptions to the rule, such as patients with acute promyelocytic leukemia who may develop a form of DIC characterized by hyperfibrinolytic bleeding. In this instance, use of antifibrinolytics may be effective [23]. Similarly, in patients with trauma, the early administration of tranexamic acid has been demonstrated to reduce bleeding and death [24].

Specific Inhibitors of Coagulation

In view of the depletion of natural anticoagulants during DIC, it is logical to suppose that replacement therapy using one or more of the missing natural anticoagulants may be of clinical benefit.

Antithrombin: Several preliminary trials with antithrombin, mainly in patients with sepsis, demonstrated some improvement in the duration of DIC and resolution of laboratory abnormalities. However, a significant benefit in mortality could not be demonstrated in a large, randomized controlled study of sepsis (the KyberSept Trial) [25]. Although a *post hoc* subgroup analysis in this trial suggested a benefit of AT without concomitant heparin in a subset of patients with DIC [26], the role of AT therapy in

patients with DIC remains unclear. Specifically, the BCSH and SISET guidelines do not recommend the use of AT in DIC. However, the JSTH guidelines recommend its use in DIC patients with sepsis and evidence of organ dysfunction, and the ISTH harmonized guidelines suggest there may be a role, although additional data are needed [17].

Recombinant Human Activated Protein C: A large, randomized, controlled trial (the PROWESS Study) using recombinant activated PC (rhAPC, Drotrecogin alfa, activated) to treat patients with sepsis demonstrated improved survival compared with placebo [27]. This benefit was probably mediated not only by an antithrombotic effect, but also by anti-inflammatory and profibrinolytic effects of this agent. However, excess bleeding was seen in patients treated with rhAPC, which inactivates factors Va and VIIIa. Therefore, it is not recommended in patients with severe thrombocytopenia (platelets $\leq 30 \times 10^9$/L) or otherwise at high risk of bleeding. A subsequent clinical trial evaluating the role of rhAPC in less severe sepsis (APACHE II score <25, the ADDRESS study) showed no benefit to the use of rhAPC. Further, the concomitant use of heparin and rhAPC in patients with severe sepsis was also evaluated (the XPRESS study) and this study failed to demonstrate significant differences with use of heparin [28–30]. Finally, the benefit of rhAPC in patients with septic shock was evaluated in the PROWESS-SHOCK study [31]. This study failed to show a benefit of rhAPC in patients with septic shock, including those with decreased levels of protein C. Based on these findings, the drug was withdrawn from the market worldwide and its use is no longer recommended in patients with DIC.

Recombinant Soluble Thrombomodulin (TM): Recombinant human TM (rhTM, ART-123 or Recomodulin) was evaluated against unfractionated heparin in a phase III randomized controlled trial in patients with DIC (related to hematological malignancies or sepsis) [32]. RhTM resulted in faster resolution of DIC in this trial. However, a recent large multicenter, randomized, placebo controlled trial in septic patients with DIC failed to show a significant benefit with the use of rhTM [33]. At present, the role of rhTM in the treatment of DIC is unresolved, and the drug is only approved for use in Japan.

In conclusion, the mainstay of treatment in patients with DIC remains treatment of the underlying cause and supportive care, including administration of blood products on a case-by-case basis as dictated by the clinical situation. There is a role for prophylactic anticoagulation with heparins and for therapeutic anticoagulation in a selected subpopulation. The role of AT and rhTM in the treatment of DIC remains unclear.

References

1 Taylor FB, Jr., Toh CH, Hoots WK, Scientific Subcommittee on Disseminated Intravascular Coagulation of the International Society on Thrombosis and Hemostasis, *et al*. Towards definition, clinical and laboratory criteria, and a scoring system for disseminated intravascular coagulation. *Thromb Haemost* 2001; 86: 1327–1330.

2 Mackman N, Tilley RE, Key NS. Role of the extrinsic pathway of blood coagulation in hemostasis and thrombosis. *Arterioscler Thromb Vasc Biol* 2007; 27: 1687–1693.

3 Levi M, de Jonge E, van der Poll T. Rationale for restoration of physiological anticoagulant pathways in patients with sepsis and disseminated intravascular coagulation. *Crit Care Med* 2001; 29 (Suppl.): S90–94.

4 Levi M. Disseminated intravascular coagulation. *Crit Care Med* 2007; 35: 2191–2195.

5 Biemond BJ, Levi M, Ten Cate H, *et al*. Plasminogen activator and plasminogen activator inhibitor I release during experimental endotoxaemia in chimpanzees: effect of interventions in the cytokine and coagulation cascades. *Clin Sci* 1995; 88: 587–594.

6 Frith D, Brohi K. The pathophysiology of trauma-induced coagulopathy. *Curr Opin Crit Care* 2012; 18: 631–636.

7 Gando S, Wada H, Thachil J, Scientific, Standardization Committee on DICotISoT, Haemostasis. Differentiating disseminated intravascular coagulation (DIC) with the fibrinolytic phenotype from coagulopathy of trauma and acute coagulopathy of trauma-shock (COT/ACOTS). *J Thromb Haemost* 2013; 11: 826–835.

8 Menell JS, Cesarman GM, Jacovina AT, *et al*. Annexin II and bleeding in acute promyelocytic leukemia. *N Engl J Med* 1999; 340: 994–1004.

9 Bick RL. Disseminated intravascular coagulation: objective clinical and laboratory diagnosis, treatment, and assessment of therapeutic response. *Semin Thromb Haemost* 1996; 22: 69–88.

10 Levi M, de Jonge E, van der Poll T, *et al*. Disseminated intravascular coagulation. *Thromb Haemost* 1999; 82: 695–705.

11 Angstwurm MW, Dempfle CE, Spannagl M. New disseminated intravascular coagulation score: A useful tool to predict mortality in comparison with Acute Physiology and Chronic Health Evaluation II and Logistic Organ Dysfunction scores. *Crit Care Med* 2006; 34: 314–320; quiz 28.

12 Toh CH, Hoots WK, ISTH SSCoDICot. The scoring system of the Scientific and Standardisation Committee on Disseminated Intravascular Coagulation of the International Society on Thrombosis and Haemostasis: a 5-year overview. *J Thromb Haemost* 2007; 5: 604–606.

13 Wada H, Hatada T, Okamoto K, *et al*. Modified non-overt DIC diagnostic criteria predict the early phase of overt-DIC. *Am J Hematol* 2010; 85: 691–694.

14 Gando S, Iba T, Eguchi Y, *et al*. A multicenter, prospective validation of disseminated intravascular coagulation diagnostic criteria for critically ill patients: comparing current criteria. *Crit Care Med* 2006; 34: 625–631.

15 Singh RK, Baronia AK, Sahoo JN, *et al*. Prospective comparison of new Japanese Association for Acute Medicine (JAAM) DIC and International Society of Thrombosis and Hemostasis (ISTH) DIC score in critically ill

septic patients. *Thromb Res* 2012; 129: e119–125.

16 Takemitsu T, Wada H, Hatada T, *et al.* Prospective evaluation of three different diagnostic criteria for disseminated intravascular coagulation. *Thromb Haemost* 2011; 105: 40–44.

17 Wada H, Thachil J, Di Nisio M, *et al.* Harmonized guidance for disseminated intravascular coagulation from the International Society on Thrombosis and Haemostasis and the current status of anticoagulant therapy in Japan: a rebuttal. *J Thromb Haemost* 2013; 11: 2078–2079.

18 Levi M, Toh CH, Thachil J, *et al.* Guidelines for the diagnosis and management of disseminated intravascular coagulation. British Committee for Standards in Haematology. *Br J Haematol* 2009; 145: 24–33.

19 Thachil J, Toh CH, Levi M, *et al.* The withdrawal of activated protein C from the use in patients with severe sepsis and DIC (Amendment to the BCSH guideline on disseminated intravascular coagulation). *Br J Haematol* 2012; 157: 493–494.

20 Di Nisio M, Baudo F, Cosmi B, *et al.* Diagnosis and treatment of disseminated intravascular coagulation: guidelines of the Italian Society for Haemostasis and Thrombosis (SISET). *Thromb Res* 2012; 129: e177–184.

21 Wada H, Asakura H, Okamoto K, *et al.* Expert consensus for the treatment of disseminated intravascular coagulation in Japan. *Thromb Res* 2010; 125: 6–11.

22 Squizzato A, Hunt BJ, Kinasewitz GT, *et al.* Supportive management strategies for disseminated intravascular coagulation. An international consensus. *Thromb Haemost* 2016: 115; 896–904.

23 Schwartz BS, Williams EC, Conlan MG, *et al.* Epsilon-aminocaproic acid in the treatment of patients with acute promyelocytic leukemia and acquired alpha-2-plasmin inhibitor deficiency. *Ann Intern Med* 1986; 105: 873–877.

24 Collaborators C-T, Shakur H, Roberts I, *et al.* Effects of tranexamic acid on death, vascular occlusive events, and blood transfusion in trauma patients with significant haemorrhage (CRASH-2): a randomised, placebo-controlled trial. *Lancet* 2010; 376: 23–32.

25 Warren BL, Eid A, Singer P, *et al.* Caring for the critically ill patient. High-dose antithrombin III in severe sepsis: a randomized controlled trial. *JAMA* 2001; 286: 1869–1878.

26 Kienast J, Juers M, Wiedermann CJ, *et al.* Treatment effects of high-dose antithrombin without concomitant heparin in patients with severe sepsis with or without disseminated intravascular coagulation. *J Thromb Haemost* 2006; 4: 90–97.

27 Bernard GR, Vincent JL, Laterre PF, *et al.* Efficacy and safety of recombinant human activated protein C for severe sepsis. *N Engl J Med* 2001; 344: 699–709.

28 Abraham E, Laterre PF, Garg R, *et al.* Drotrecogin alfa (activated) for adults with severe sepsis and a low risk of death. *N Engl J Med* 2005; 353: 1332–1341.

29 Ely EW, Laterre PF, Angus DC, *et al.* Drotrecogin alfa (activated) administration across clinically important subgroups of patients with severe sepsis. *Crit Care Med* 2003; 31: 12–19.

30 Levi M, Levy M, Williams MD, *et al.* Prophylactic heparin in patients with severe sepsis treated with drotrecogin alfa (activated). *Am J Respir Crit Care Med* 2007; 176: 483–490.

31 Ranieri VM, Thompson BT, Barie PS, *et al.* Drotrecogin alfa (activated) in adults with septic shock. *N Engl J Med* 2012; 366: 2055–2064.

32 Saito H, Maruyama I, Shimazaki S, *et al.* Efficacy and safety of recombinant human soluble thrombomodulin (ART-123) in disseminated intravascular coagulation: results of a phase III, randomized, double-blind clinical trial. *J Thromb Haemost* 2007; 5: 31–41.

33 Vincent JL, Ramesh MK, Ernest D, *et al.* A randomized, double-blind, placebo-controlled, Phase 2b study to evaluate the safety and efficacy of recombinant human soluble thrombomodulin, ART-123, in patients with sepsis and suspected disseminated intravascular coagulation. *Crit Care Med* 2013; 41: 2069–2079.

13

Thrombotic Microangiopathies

Marie Scully and David Kavanagh

Key Points

- Thrombotic thrombocytopenic purpura (TTP) and atypical hemolytic uremic syndrome (aHUS) are acute life-threatening illnesses that require treatment with plasma exchange, without delay, at first presentation.
- Differentiation between these conditions can be made by ADAMTS13 analysis. Creatinine levels do not always correctly categorize these disorders.
- Immunosuppression for most cases of TTP and complement inhibitors for aHUS, respectively, are the mainstay of therapy, once diagnosis is confirmed.
- Specific therapy for subgroups of TTP or HUS may be required.
- Molecular diagnostics are required to confirm the underlying pathogenesis, and to guide prognosis and treatment in aHUS.

Introduction

The thrombotic microangiopathies (TMAs) are a group of disorders that present clinically with thrombocytopenia and microangiopathic hemolytic anemia (MAHA) with distinctive blood film features (polychromasia and fragmented red blood cells) and clinical features of microvascular thrombosis. There are a number of disorders that need to be considered in the differential diagnosis (Table 13.1). The most common is disseminated intravascular coagulation (DIC), which typically is associated with an abnormal coagulation screen, not seen in thrombotic thrombocytopenic purpura (TTP) or atypical hemolytic uremic syndrome (aHUS). DIC is discussed in greater detail in Chapter 12. An autoimmune profile (e.g., antinuclear autoantibodies, antineutrophil cytoplasmic antibodies, and extractable nuclear antibodies screens) may be helpful in excluding scleroderma, systemic lupus erythematosus, or less common conditions such as Wegener granulomatosis or Goodpasture syndrome. A number of drugs have been associated with MAHA, and their effect may be idiosyncratic. Pregnancy needs to be excluded in all women of child bearing age to help differentiate TTP or aHUS from pre-eclampsia or HELLP syndrome (hemolysis, elevated liver enzymes, low platelets). Certain infections can cause an MAHA picture, particularly in immunosuppressed patients, such as in association with bone marrow or solid organ transplant. Such infections are often viral or fungal. Acute bacterial infections such as *Streptococcus* can present with a picture similar to HUS. TTP and aHUS need to be excluded, as these are life-threatening conditions, with high mortality rates, requiring urgent treatment. They are acute medical emergencies and are the primary focus of this chapter.

Confirmation of Diagnosis

Confirmation of TMAs may include histological confirmation, but this is not always practical or

Practical Hemostasis and Thrombosis, Third Edition. Edited by Nigel S. Key, Michael Makris and David Lillicrap.
© 2017 John Wiley & Sons, Ltd. Published 2017 by John Wiley & Sons, Ltd.

Table 13.1 Differential diagnosis of thrombotic microangiopathies.

Disseminated Intravascular coagulation

Infections, typically viral (influenza, cytomegalovirus, adenovirus, herpes simplex virus) or severe bacterial (*Meningococcus, Pneumococcus*), fungal

Autoimmune disease (lupus nephritis, acute scleroderma)

Vasculitis

Malignancy (usually adenocarcinomas)

Malignant hypertension

Drugs, e.g., ciclosporin, chemotherapy, antibiotics, e.g., trimethoprim

Autoimmune hemolysis/ Evans syndrome

Pregnancy-associated thrombotic microangiopathies, e.g., HELLP (hemolysis, elevated liver enzymes and low platelets) pre-eclampsia, hemolytic uremic syndrome

Thrombotic thrombocytopenic purpura

Hemolytic uremic syndrome

---

conclusive. ADAMTS13 activity <10% and, most commonly, the presence of anti-ADAMTS13 IgG antibodies are specific for TTP. However, in congenital TTP no antibodies will be detected. In HUS, the ADAMTS13 activity will not be reduced to this level, although may be reduced below the normal range for a number of reasons, similar to all the other TMAs.

In Shiga-like toxin-associated hemolytic uremic syndrome (STEC-HUS), stool culture or rectal swab may detect STEC although false-negative results may be encountered due to the bacteria's limited duration in the stools. Serological tests for Shiga toxin and antilipopolysaccharide (LPS) antibodies and polymerase chain reaction (PCR) for Shiga toxin genes should also undertaken.

In aHUS, the initial laboratory analysis should include serum levels of C3, C4, complement factor H (CFH), and complement factor I (CFI) as well as analysis for factor H autoantibodies prior to plasma exchange. Flow cytometry to assess CD46 levels on peripheral blood mononuclear cells should also be performed, if available. Although low antigenic levels of complement proteins may point to a mutation in the complement system, genetic screening, including copy number variation, is required to definitively exclude a mutation. However, only about 50% of aHUS cases have a confirmed mutation in complement.

Pathophysiology

Thrombotic Thrombocytopenic Purpura

Thrombotic thrombocytopenic purpura is a rare disease, occurring in 6–10/million of the population and resulting from a deficiency of the enzyme ADAMTS13, a metalloprotease required to cleave von Willebrand factor (VWF) [1–3]. VWF is a large glycoprotein that binds to platelets during hemostasis. On initial release from endothelial cells, ultralarge VWF is cleaved to multimeric forms of various sizes by ADAMTS13. Deficiency of ADAMTS13 occurs in patients with congenital deficiency states, or plasma levels may be low due to the formation of IgG autoantibodies, which is a more frequent cause (Figure 13.1). The precise trigger for antibody formation is unknown and a number of hypotheses have been proposed. There appears to be a genetic predisposition, with HLA-DQ7, DRB1*11, and HLA-DRB3 all significantly increased in Caucasians. However, there is also a suggestion that certain HLA types (HLA-DRB1*04 and HLA-DR53) are protective factor against the development of TTP [4]. Viral and infective disease trigger(s) have been hypothesized; however, this possibility has not been well defined in cohort studies. Secondary causes of TTP are frequently described but account for a smaller proportion of cases (10–15%). Nevertheless, HIV, pregnancy, and certain drugs are known precipitants.

Shiga-like Toxin-associated Hemolytic Uremic Syndrome

STEC-HUS is the most common cause of HUS in children, accounting for ~90% of cases. The incidence of STEC-HUS is approximately 1 to 3 cases/100 000 of the general population per annum [5].

Shiga toxins consist of a single A subunit and 5 B subunits. Uncertainty exists as to the mechanism

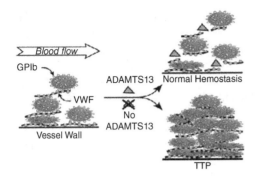

Figure 13.1 The role of ADAMTS13 in the pathophysiology of thrombotic thrombocytopenic purpura (TTP). VWF, von Willebrand factor. Source: adapted from Sadler 2008 [44]. *See Plate section for color representation of this figure.*

by which the Shiga toxin reaches the kidney; however, current theories favor transport from the intestine bound to polymorphonuclear leukocytes. In the glomerular endothelium, mesangium, and podocytes, the B subunits bind to globotriaosyl ceramide (Gb3) resulting in internalization of the A subunit that inhibits protein synthesis. This results in a change in the phenotype of the endothelial cell to a procoagulant state and predisposes to the development of thrombotic microangiopathy.

Bacteria Causing HUS

In North America and Western Europe, ~70% of cases of STEC-HUS is secondary to infection with the *E. coli* O157: H7 [6]. A recent large epidemic in Germany was due to a newly described strain, *E. coli* O104: H4 [7]. However, many other *E. coli* serotypes (O111: H8, O103: H2, O121, O145, O26, and O113) have also been shown to cause STEC-HUS.

Infection by Shiga toxin-producing *Shigella dysenteriae* serotype 1 has been commonly linked to HUS in developing countries of Asia and Africa but rarely in industrialized countries.

Shiga toxin-producing *E. coli* colonize healthy cattle intestine, and meat contamination at slaughter is the most common method of human infection. Other vehicles for transmission include contaminated vegetables and fruit and unpasteurized dairy products.

Atypical Hemolytic Uremic Syndrome

Atypical HUS is a term that has been used to describe any non-STEC-related HUS. Mutations in genes encoding proteins in the complement system have been shown to predispose to disease in the majority of cases of aHUS [8] (Figure 13.2). As such, aHUS has become synonymous for complement-mediated HUS, although the term

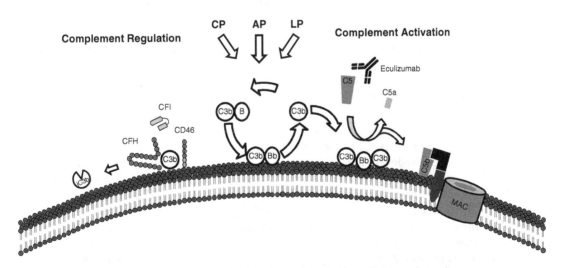

Figure 13.2 The role of complement in the pathophysiology of atypical hemolytic uremic syndrome.

aHUS also includes other noncomplement genetic defects (e.g., cblC and DGKε) and *Streptococcus* pneumonia-mediated disease. The best estimate of aHUS incidence is $2/10^6$ in a North American population [9].

Complement System

Complement activation can be mediated through the classical, alternative, and lectin pathways. The classical pathway is initiated via IgM, IgG, and C1q. In the lectin pathway, mannose binding lectin and ficolins bind carbohydrates, triggering complement activation. The alternative pathway continually "ticks over," depositing C3b on surfaces. C3b is subsequently inactivated on host cells and amplified on foreign cells. The alternative pathway is also recruited by C3 convertases formed by the classical and lectin pathways and, as such, it serves as an amplification step accounting for ~80% of all complement activation regardless of the initial trigger [10].

These pathways converge to produce the common terminal pathway effector molecules. This positive feedback loop of the alternative pathway has evolved to rapidly attack invading pathogens. Host cell-associated complement regulatory molecules prevent bystander damage. It is the disparity between complement activation and regulation on the glomerular vasculature that leads to aHUS.

Loss-of-function Mutations in Complement Regulatory Proteins

The most frequently occurring genetic abnormality seen in aHUS is in the gene encoding complement factor H (*CFH*) (up to 30%). CFH is the principal fluid phase regulator of the alternative pathway pathway. It acts as a cofactor for factor I (CFI) mediated proteolytic inactivation of C3b, competes with factor B (CFB) for C3b binding, and accelerates the decay of the C3 convertase into its components. It can also bind to and protect host cells surfaces via glycosaminoglycans and C3b through its C-terminal domain (CCP19-20). In aHUS, mutations in *CFH* are usually heterozygous and cluster in CCP19-20. These mutations do not usually result in a quantitative deficiency of CFH but instead result in a protein that can control complement in the fluid phase but cannot bind to and regulate complement on host endothelium and platelets.

Membrane cofactor protein (MCP:CD46) is a ubiquitously expressed membrane bound complement regulator that acts as a cofactor for the CFI-mediated inactivation of both alternative and classical pathways on host cells. Mutations in *CD46* account for approximately 15% of aHUS. Most mutations described to date result in a quantitative deficiency of CD46 with only a few resulting in a secreted nonfunctional protein.

CFI is a serum serine protease that cleaves C3b and C4b in the presence of its cofactors. Mutations in *CFI* account for up to 12% of aHUS cases [11].

Gain-of-function Mutations in Complement Regulatory Proteins

Gain of function mutations in factors C3 and CFB have been reported. C3 is the core component of the complement cascade. C3 is cleaved to form the anaphylatoxin C3a and the highly reactive C3b that binds to cell surfaces via its reactive thioester. CFB can bind to C3b, which in the presence of factor D forms the alternative pathway C3 convertase (C3bBb) that cleaves further C3, introducing a positive-feedback loop.

Mutations in C3 have been reported in around 10% of aHUS cases [12]. Many of these mutants either have increased resistance to regulation or bind to CFB with higher affinity, resulting in increased C3 convertase formation. Mutations in *CFB* are much rarer, but again either increase convertase formation or result in a C3 convertase that is more resistant to regulation.

Ultimately, CFB and C3 mutations in aHUS result in increased complement activation on platelets and glomerular endothelium.

Inhibitory Autoantibodies in aHUS

As in TTP, inhibitory autoantibodies are also found in aHUS, although at a lower frequency. Autoantibodies to CFH are found in 4–14% of aHUS patients. CFH autoantibodies in aHUS are associated with genomic deletion of *CFHR*1 and *CFHR*3. The autoantibodies predominantly bind to the C-terminal of CFH thereby impairing protection at the cell surface. Autoantibodies to CFI have also been described in aHUS but are much rarer (~2%) than anti-CFH Abs [13].

Penetrance of aHUS

The penetrance of mutations in aHUS is ~50%, suggesting that other genetic and environmental modifiers play a role. It is increasingly recognized that patients may carry more than one mutation and that penetrance increases as the number of mutations in the DNA of a patient increases. Additionally, a number of single nucleotide polymorphisms (SNPs) and haplotypes in *CFH* and *CD46* have been associated with aHUS in several studies. Even when a patient has several genetic risk factors, disease may not present until middle age, suggesting that a trigger is required for aHUS to manifest. Recent analyses of cohorts of aHUS patients with complement mutations have identified upper respiratory tract infections, fevers, pregnancy, and drugs as potential triggers. In individuals with genetic risk factors, these triggers likely initiate the alternative pathway, setting off the positive amplification loop that cannot be adequately controlled, resulting in aHUS.

Genotype–phenotype Correlations

Historically, the prognosis for patients with aHUS was poor, with ~66% of adults dying or reaching end-stage renal disease (ESRD) within 5 years. The outlook can now be predicted based on the specific mutation; individuals with mutations in *CFH, CFI, C3*, and *CFB* generally have a poor outcome while those with *CD46* mutations have a better prognosis. No patient with an *MCP* mutation from either the French or Italian cohorts died at first episode, and none of the children and only 25% of adults with an *MCP* mutation developed ESRD at first episode. At 3 years, only 6% of all patients with *MCP* mutations had developed ESRD and by 5 years, only 35% [14].

Noncomplement-mediated Genetic Causes of aHUS

Combined Methylmalonic Aciduria and Homocystinuria

Combined methylmalonic aciduria and homocystinuria (cblC) is a rare hereditary cause of aHUS [15]. It is a disorder of cobalamin (vitamin B_{12}) metabolism characterized by neurological, metabolic, and developmental symptoms. The pathophysiological mechanism of HUS is obscure, with striking endothelial abnormalities on kidney biopsies. However, only a proportion of patients develop aHUS. Long-term management is with intramuscular hydroxycobalamin, oral folic acid, and betaine

Diacylglycerol Kinase ε and HUS

Complete deficiency of diacylglycerol kinase ε (DGKε) has been shown to cause aHUS [16]. All affected individuals present in the first year of life. In those recovering from the acute episode of aHUS, microscopic hematuria and proteinuria persist and progression to chronic kidney disease (CKD) is common. As would be expected from a noncomplement-mediated disease, eculizumab did not prevent disease in individuals with DGKε mutations. Recurrence was not seen following renal transplantation.

Streptococcus Pneumonia-associated HUS

Pneumococcal HUS is a common cause of non-STEC-HUS [17]. The incidence of HUS following invasive pneumococcal infections is estimated at 0.5%.

S. pneumoniae produces the enzyme neuraminidase, which has been postulated to play a role in the development of disease. Neuraminidase cleaves *N*-acetyl neuraminic acid residues from glycoproteins on the cell membrane of erythrocytes, platelets, and glomeruli, exposing the normally hidden Thomsen–Freidenreich antigen (T-antigen). This then reacts with anti-T IgM antibodies, normally present in plasma. It has been hypothesized that binding of anti-T IgM to platelets and endothelial cells causes aHUS by platelet aggregation and direct endothelial cell damage.

Pneumococcal HUS usually occurs 7–9 days after the onset of pneumococcal symptoms. In one series, 10% developed ESRD and 12% died in the acute phase of the illness.

Diagnosis

Diagnosis of TTP

TTP typically presents with a low platelet count, with a median of approximately $20 \times 10^9 / L$, anemia, fragmented red cells, and polychromasia, and often signs of microvascular thrombi.

Differentiation can be very difficult and exclusion of other TMAs needs to be undertaken (Table 13.1). Furthermore, in a clinical presentation suggestive of aHUS, congenital TTP needs to be excluded by ADAMTS13 analysis, and conversely, in a clinical presentation of TTP, aHUS or another TMA need to be considered if the ADAMTS13 levels are not reduced to <10%. Congenital TTP can present with end-organ damage, which typically affects the brain, kidneys, and heart, especially in cases with recurrent MAHA from childhood [18,19]. Furthermore, the increasing observation of late-onset TTP in adulthood, especially in relation to pregnancy, requires differentiation from other pregnancy-associated TMAs by an ADAMTS13 assay. Lastly, aHUS can present with mild renal impairment, which can be reversed with plasma exchange (PEX). Differentiation from TTP is only possible by ADAMTS13 analysis. Furthermore, diagnostic confirmation by defining complement mutations helps to understand the pathogenesis of these cases and ensure correct treatment protocols.

There is often no obvious difference in the presenting parameters between primary autoimmune TTP and those with an underlying precipitant such as infection or drugs. Presenting features can be vague and nonspecific, and typically have a short prodrome. Ten percent of cases present in a coma, with neurological features accounting for approximately 70% of presentations, with renal impairment and abdominal symptoms in 30–40%, and features of thrombocytopenia in more than half of cases [20].

The median creatinine at presentation in TTP is not above the normal range. However, TTP cases can present with renal impairment that responds to therapy and results in normalization of kidney function. These patients will have low ADAMTS13 activity (<10%) at presentation. However, severe acute presentations can be associated with acute temporary renal failure requiring dialysis; while this situation is not common, the ADAMTS13 level will be the guide to diagnosis. A third scenario is renal impairment at presentation that may deteriorate despite PEX. The ADAMTS13 is not reduced (i.e., to <10%). These patients may have an underlying complement mutation.

The primary cause of death in acute TTP is arrhythmia, resulting from microvascular thrombi affecting the cardiac conduction system. Clinically, patients may be asymptomatic and cardiac investigations may be normal. However, troponin levels in those with severe disease are raised. They mirror patients with high anti-ADAMTS13 antibody levels and can be used as a prognostic marker. Indeed, patients with raised troponin and anti-ADAMTS13 antibody levels are more likely to die or be admitted to an intensive care unit [21].

Diagnosis of STEC-HUS

The interval between ingestion of a contaminated vehicle and the onset of diarrhea ranges from 2 to 12 days. Typically, *E. coli* O157: H7 infections cause 1–3 days of nonbloody diarrhea, after which the diarrhea becomes bloody in about 90% of cases [22]. The colon can be quite severely affected. However, mild infections can occur, and *E. coli* O157: H7 has been recovered from the stools of patients with HUS without diarrhea.

The risk that a child younger than 10 years with *E. coli* O157: H7 infection will develop HUS is between 1 and 15%. In a recent German outbreak, this was much higher (22%), probably due to the novel properties of the O104: H4 strain [23].

Diagnosis of aHUS

As a general rule, patients with aHUS will have a higher platelet count and higher serum creatinine than patients with TTP. It has been suggested that a creatinine >150–200 μmol/L and a platelet count >30 000/mm^3 almost always eliminates ADAMTS13 deficiency [24].

Although correct on a population basis, such criteria will lead to incorrect diagnosis of individual patients, and ADAMTS13 activity assays are required prior to initiation of eculizumab treatment.

Extrarenal manifestations in aHUS are not common, occurring in ~10–20% of patients. Of these, neurological sequelae are most frequently reported (~10%) with symptoms ranging from irritability to coma. It is unclear how many of these symptoms are the direct result of a cerebral TMA, with severe hypertension and posterior reversible encephalopathy syndrome (PRES) a possible differential diagnoses. Rarely, other organ involvement may occur (e.g., digital gangrene, cerebral artery thrombosis/ stenosis, ocular involvement) but in the majority of reported cases definitive biopsy evidence of TMA in the organ is lacking.

Diagnosis of Pneumococcal HUS

In contrast to other forms of HUS, the direct Coombs' test is positive due to the exposed T-antigen. T-antigen exposure can be confirmed by a peanut lectin- agglutination test. Pneumococcal HUS usually occurs 7–9 days after the onset of pneumococcal symptoms. In one series, 10% developed ESRD and 12% died in the acute phase of the illness.

Treatment

Treatment of TTP

The mainstay of treatment for acute TTP is PEX. Plasma infusion as the only therapeutic modality is not appropriate, although it can be used as a holding strategy while transferring to an apheresis unit. The Canadian Aphereis Group demonstrated, over 20 years ago, the benefit of PEX over plasma infusion in terms of morality [25]. At presentation, 1.5 × plasma volume exchange should be initiated, at least for the first three procedures. Patients are then assessed to determine if this should be continued, reduced to single plasma volume, or increased to twice-daily PEX, depending on the clinical response.

As the majority of patients have antibody-mediated disease, concomitant use of steroid therapy is often appropriate. These agents have a prompt onset of action, but long-term use should be avoided. The precise formulation of steroids will depend on the clinical presentation, and either pulsed methylprednisolone or oral therapy (e.g., 1 mg/kg of prednisolone) can be instigated. Despite the frequent use of steroids in TTP, there is limited published evidence for their efficacy, and no comparison of PEX to PEX and steroid therapy have been completed.

Given the risk of relapse or exacerbation, further immunosuppressive therapy may need to be considered. In the past, there have been a number of anecdotal reports or small case series, but no formal trials of immunosuppression. For example, vincristine, cyclophosphamide, or splenectomy have all been reported to be beneficial. Vincristine used in refractory TTP was associated with a rapid increase in platelet counts and ADAMTS13 activity by reducing VWF-platelet interaction and inhibiting autoantibodies [26]. A schedule of 1 mg intravenously, repeated every 3–4 days for a total of four doses is popular. Peripheral neuropathy remains an unacceptable side-effect. Splenectomy previously had a high mortality, which has been reduced with laparoscopic techniques. Ten-year relapse-free survival was 70%. However, there are very limited numbers of published cases in the literature [27].

In recent years, rituximab, a monoclonal anti-CD 20 antibody, and cyclosporine have been preferred immunosuppressive options. Rituximab has been used in cases with refractory/relapsed TTP, but has been shown to be beneficial at acute presentation and prophylactically to prevent relapse [28–31]. A potential side-effect is recurrent infections. However, in TTP, it does not appear to have a significant effect on serum immunoglobulin levels. Indeed, side-effects appear minimal, although rigors are more common with the first infusion. Patients who have serological evidence of previous hepatitis B infection are at potential risk of virus reactivation, such that coadministration of lamivudine is required. Very rarely, serum sickness and neutropenia occur. A particular potential risk is progressive multifocal leukoencephalopathy. However, TTP patients do not usually need prolonged intensive immunosuppressive therapy and rarely need immunosuppressive agents that act on T lymphocytes.

Rituximab has been shown to reduce anti-ADAMTS13 IgG antibodies and increase enzyme activity levels. Furthermore, with monitoring of levels, any reduction from the normal range of activity can be treated with prophylactic rituximab therapy to prevent relapse. There is evidence that sustained, low ADAMTS13 activity despite clinical remission is associated with an increased risk of relapse [32].

As rituximab is an IgG antibody, it is expected to be removed by PEX. Indeed, approximately 65% is removed. Based on the pharmacokinetics of rituximab during PEX, therapy can be given every 3 to 4 days [33].

A review of the benefit of rituximab in relapsed/ refractory TTP or during the acute presentation (within 3 days of admission) has shown that the number of PEX to remission ($P = 0.046$), the median length of admission ($P = 0.008$), and time to complete remission from admission ($P = 0.001$) were all significantly reduced. However, the median time to complete response after the first infusion (9–10 days for both groups) was no different [34]. Furthermore, the risk of relapse appears to be reduced.

At higher doses, cyclosporine is associated with an MAHA picture, but its use has also been beneficial in refractory and relapsing TTP, with effects seen within 7–14 days. The optimal target therapeutic range is also unknown, although trough serum levels between 200 and 300 µg/L have been used. The potential medium and long-term side-effect profile must be considered. In a randomized comparison with steroids during PEX, remission occurred in 89% of patients receiving cyclosporine, but there was a 14% relapse during therapy and a 33% relapse rate in patients who stopped therapy after 6 months. In the steroid group, 83% achieved remission but 60% had an exacerbation (within 30 days) [35]. Tacrolimus is an alternative therapy, but side-effects may again preclude medium and

long-term use. There is one case report of the use of mycophenolate in refractory disease.

Folic acid should be given to compensate for that lost due to hemolysis. Low-dose aspirin (75 mg daily) and thromboprophylaxis are started once the platelet count is greater than 50×10^9 / L to prevent thrombotic sequelae during platelet recovery. Fever is a feature of TTP, which appears to be cytokine/ inflammatory mediated rather than due to an underlying infection. However, vigilance is required to ensure any acquired infections are treated promptly.

Given the significant volumes of plasma used during an acute admission, it is important to use the safest product available with respect to acute and longer-term pathogen transmission and also anaphylactic reactions during the procedure, which can be life-threatening. Methylene blue-treated fresh frozen plasma (MB-FFP) from a single donor, developed for its viral inactivation and pathogen protection properties, possesses comparable hemostatic variables. However, in a retrospective analysis of TTP cases treated with MB-FFP, patients required significantly more PEX to remission, were more likely to relapse, and, although not significant, more deaths occurred in the MB-FFP group. A prospective trial of standard FFP to MB-FFP showed an increased number of PEX to remission in the MB-FFP group, more plasma to remission, and increased recurrences on treatment [36]. Currently, Octaplas™, which has a double viral inactivation step and preservation of hemostatic parameters, is the preferred therapy.

Treatment of STEC-HUS

Supportive therapy, including control of hypertension and correction of fluid and electrolyte abnormalities, remains the mainstay in STEC–HUS. Mechanical ventilation and renal replacement therapy may also be required. Early volume replacement is associated with improved renal outcome.

Plasma Exchange

In complement-mediated aHUS or TTP, PEX provides a logical treatment to replace complement regulatory or ADAMTS13 activity, respectively. In STEC-HUS, the rationale for the use of PEX is less clear and there are no randomized controlled studies demonstrating its efficacy. In an uncomplicated episode of STEC-HUS, PEX is not used, although some have advocated its use if there is severe neurological involvement.

Eculizumab

Following the successful use of the complement inhibitor, eculizumab in aHUS, its use in STEC-HUS was reported in three children. Contemporaneously, the German O104:H4 outbreak prompted the National Society of Nephrology to recommend its use in the sickest STEC-HUS patients. The nonrandomized nature of the trial in a self-limiting condition makes analysis of its use in STEC-HUS difficult; however, initial reports do not support a role for eculizumab [23].

Antibiotics

Antibiotic eradication of STEC in the pre-HUS phase of disease is not recommended. In a recent investigation in a pediatric cohort with *E. coli* O157:H7, children given antibiotics developed STEC-HUS more frequently than those that did not [37]. It has been suggested that this was due to increased toxin release during treatment. The role of antibiotics in individuals who have already developed STEC-HUS has yet to be investigated. In the German O104:H4 outbreak, patients with STEC-HUS who received antibiotics exhibited fewer seizures and a lower morbidity.

Treatment of Atypical HUS

Plasma Exchange

Despite the introduction of eculizumab, initial presentation with aHUS continues to require immediate treatment with PEX. The removal of inhibitory autoantibodies and hyperfunctional complement components, and replacement of nonfunctional complement regulators will control disease until ADAMTS13 deficiency can be excluded (reviewed in European [38] and UK [39] guidelines on aHUS treatment).

Eculizumab

Eculizumab is an anti-C5 monoclonal antibody that prevents the cleavage of C5 into its effector components, C5a and C5b. Initially introduced for the treatment of aHUS in 2009, the publication of a prospective trial in aHUS has recently confirmed its efficacy [40]. In patients treated with eculizumab, ~85% become disease free in both plasma-resistant and plasma-dependent aHUS. It is effective in patients with and without identified complement mutations. As with PEX, the earlier eculizumab is commenced, the better the long-term renal outcome.

Treatment with eculizumab should only be instituted once ADAMTS13 deficiency can be eliminated and current treatment protocols suggest lifelong therapy. Pre-emptive eculizumab strategies are now also employed to prevent aHUS recurrence following renal transplantation. As eculizumab prevents the terminal pathway of complement functioning, patients are at risk from infections with encapsulated organisms. Vaccination against *Neisseria meningitides* is therefore required, with most groups also suggesting long-term prophylactic antibiotic cover.

Management of pneumococcal HUS is supportive with antibiotic treatment of the infection and fluid and electrolyte management, possibly including dialysis. There is no evidence that PEX is effective. Indeed there is a theoretical disadvantage of giving plasma products as they contain anti-T IgM that may exacerbate the disease.

Outcomes

STEC-HUS Outcomes

STEC-HUS is not a benign disease. Seventy percent of patients who develop HUS require red blood cell transfusions, 50% need dialysis, and 25% have neurological involvement, including stroke, seizure, and coma [41]. Although mortality for infants and young children in industrialized countries decreased when improvements in intensive care and availability of dialysis, still

~3% of patients die during the acute phase. A case–control study of children with *E. coli* O157:H7 HUS has shown a significant increase in microalbuminuria 3 years after recovery. A recent meta-analysis of 49 published studies described death or permanent ESRD in 12% of patients and glomerular filtration rate $< 80\,\text{mL}/\text{min}\ per\ 1.3\text{m}^2$ in 25%. The severity of acute illness, particularly central nervous system symptoms, and the need for initial dialysis were strongly associated with a worse long-term prognosis [42].

Renal Transplantation in aHUS

In the pre-eculizumab era, the outcome of renal transplantation in patients with aHUS was poor, with the death-censored 5-year graft survival ~51% and a 7% mortality at 5 years. This was predominantly due to aHUS recurrence in the first year following transplant.

In addition to predetermining the outcome of aHUS in the native kidneys, the genetic defect also affects the outcome following transplantation. The complement regulators CFH and CFI and the components CFB and C3 are produced in the liver and therefore a renal transplant does not correct the defect, thus the recurrence rate is high. In contrast, the complement regulatory defect in those with mutations in the membrane-bound CD46 is corrected by an allograft bearing wild-type CD46, giving a low recurrence rate [42,43].

TTP Outcomes

The acute mortality remains unchanged and is still between 10 and 20%. Newer therapies in development include novel anti-VWF treatments targeting platelet VWF binding and the consequences of microthrombi formation. They cause an acquired VWD state, with low VWF activity levels. To date, these agents have not associated with an increase in bleeding. Overall, time to remission and relapse rates have continued to improve with the use of immunosuppressive therapies.

Further developments include the possible future availability of recombinant ADAMTS13,

which will be a major improvement and reduce the need for PEX. However, this can only be given in cases where TTP has been clearly defined.

References

1 Scully M, Hunt BJ, Benjamin S, *et al.* Guidelines on the diagnosis and management of thrombotic thrombocytopenic purpura and other thrombotic microangiopathies. *Br J Haematol* 2012; 158: 323–335.

2 Furlan M, Robles R, Lamie B. Partial purification and characterization of a protease from human plasma cleaving von Willebrand factor to fragments produced by in vivo proteolysis. *Blood* 1996; 87: 4223–4234.

3 Tsai HM. Deficiency of ADAMTS13 and thrombotic thrombocytopenic purpura. *Transfusion* 2002; 42: 1523–1524.

4 Scully M, Brown J, Patel R, *et al.* Human leukocyte antigen association in idiopathic thrombotic thrombocytopenic purpura: evidence for an immunogenetic link. *J Thromb Haemost* 2010; 8: 257–262.

5 Corrigan JJ Jr, Boineau FG. Hemolytic-uremic syndrome. *Pediatr Rev* 2001; 22: 365–369.

6 Karmali MA, Steele BT, Petric M, *et al.* Sporadic cases of haemolytic-uraemic syndrome associated with faecal cytotoxin and cytotoxin-producing Escherichia coli in stools. *Lancet* 1983; 1(8325): 619–620.

7 Rasko DA, Webster DR, Sahl JW, *et al.* Origins of the E. coli strain causing an outbreak of hemolytic-uremic syndrome in Germany. *N Engl J Med* 2011; 3658: 709–717.

8 Kavanagh D, Goodship T. Genetics and complement in atypical HUS. *Pediatr Nephrol* 2010; 25: 2431–2442.

9 Constantinescu AR, Bitzan M, Weiss LS, *et al.* Non-enteropathic hemolytic uremic syndrome: causes and short-term course. *Am J Kidney Dis* 2004; 43: 976–982.

10 Richards A, Kavanagh D, Atkinson JP. Inherited complement regulatory protein deficiency predisposes to human disease in acute injury and chronic inflammatory statesthe examples of vascular damage in

atypical hemolytic uremic syndrome and debris accumulation in age-related macular degeneration. *Adv Immunol* 2007; 96: 141–177.

11 Richards A, Kathryn LM, Kavanagh D, *et al*. Implications of the initial mutations in membrane cofactor protein (MCP; CD46) leading to atypical hemolytic uremic syndrome. *Mol Immunol* 2007; 44: 111–122.

12 Fremeaux-Bacchi V, Miller EC, Liszewski MK, *et al*. Mutations in complement C3 predispose to development of atypical hemolytic uremic syndrome. *Blood* 2008; 112: 4948–4952.

13 Kavanagh D, Richards A, Fremeaux-Bacchi V, *et al*. Screening for complement system abnormalities in patients with atypical hemolytic uremic syndrome. *Clin J Am Soc Nephrol* 2007; 2: 591–596.

14 Noris M, Caprioli J, Bresin E, *et al*. Relative role of genetic complement abnormalities in sporadic and familial aHUS and their impact on clinical phenotype. *Clin J Am Soc Nephrol* 2010; 5: 1844–1859.

15 Kind T, Levy J, Lee M, *et al*. Cobalamin C disease presenting as hemolytic-uremic syndrome in the neonatal period. *J Pediatr Hematol Oncol* 2002; 24: 327–329.

16 Lemaire M, Fremeaux-Bacchi V, Schaefer F, *et al*. Recessive mutations in DGKE cause atypical hemolytic-uremic syndrome. *Nat Genet* 2013; 45: 531–536.

17 Copelovitch L, Kaplan BS. Streptococcus pneumoniae-associated hemolytic uremic syndrome. *Pediatr Nephrol* 2008; 23: 1951–1956.

18 Loirat C, Veyradier A, Girma JP, *et al*. Thrombotic thrombocytopenic purpura associated with von Willebrand factor-cleaving protease (ADAMTS13) deficiency in children. *Semin Thromb Hemost* 2006; 32: 90–97.

19 Veyradier A, Obert B, Haddad E, *et al*. Severe deficiency of the specific von Willebrand factor-cleaving protease (ADAMTS 13) activity in a subgroup of children with atypical hemolytic uremic syndrome. *J Pediatr* 2003; 142: 310–317.

20 Scully M, Yarranton H, Liesner R, *et al*. Regional UK TTP registry: correlation with laboratory ADAMTS 13 analysis and clinical features. *Br J Haematol* 2008; 142: 819–826.

21 Hughes C, McEwan JR, Longair I, *et al*. Cardiac involvement in acute thrombotic thrombocytopenic purpura: association with troponin T and IgG antibodies to ADAMTS 13. *J Thromb Haemost* 2009; 7: 529–536.

22 Tarr PI, Gordon CA, Chandler WL. Shiga-toxin-producing Escherichia coli and haemolytic uraemic syndrome. *Lancet* 2005; 365: 1073–1086.

23 Menne J, Nitschke M, Stingele R, *et al*. Validation of treatment strategies for enterohaemorrhagic Escherichia coli O104: H4 induced haemolytic uraemic syndrome: case-control study. *BMJ* 2012; 345: e4565.

24 Zuber J, Fakhouri F, Roumenina LT, *et al*. Use of eculizumab for atypical haemolytic uraemic syndrome and C3 glomerulopathies. *Nat Rev Nephrol* 2012; 8: 643–657.

25 Rock GA, Shumak KH, Buskard NA, *et al*. Comparison of plasma exchange with plasma infusion in the treatment of thrombotic thrombocytopenic purpura. Canadian Apheresis Study Group. *N Engl J Med* 1991; 325: 393–397.

26 Bohm M, Betz C, Miesbach W, *et al*. The course of ADAMTS-13 activity and inhibitor titre in the treatment of thrombotic thrombocytopenic purpura with plasma exchange and vincristine. *Br J Haematol* 2005; 129: 644–652.

27 Kappers-Klunne MC, Wijermans P, Fijnheer R, *et al*. Splenectomy for the treatment of thrombotic thrombocytopenic purpura. *Br J Haematol* 2005; 130: 768–776.

28 Bresin E, Gastoldi S, Daina E, *et al*. Rituximab as pre-emptive treatment in patients with thrombotic thrombocytopenic purpura and evidence of anti-ADAMTS13 autoantibodies. *Thromb Haemost* 2009; 101: 233–238.

29 Fakhouri F, Vernant JP, Veyradier A, *et al*. Efficiency of curative and prophylactic treatment with rituximab in ADAMTS13-deficient thrombotic thrombocytopenic purpura: a study of 11 cases. *Blood* 2005; 106: 1932–1937.

30 Froissart A, Buffet M, Veyradier A, *et al*. Efficacy and safety of first-line rituximab in

severe, acquired thrombotic thrombocytopenic purpura with a suboptimal response to plasma exchange. Experience of the French Thrombotic Microangiopathies Reference Center. *Crit Care Med* 2012; 40: 104–111.

31 Scully M, Cohen H, Cavenagh J, *et al.* Remission in acute refractory and relapsing thrombotic thrombocytopenic purpura following rituximab is associated with a reduction in IgG antibodies to ADAMTS-13. *Br J Haematol* 2007; 136: 451–461.

32 Peyvandi F, Lavoretano S, Palla R, *et al.* ADAMTS13 and anti-ADAMTS13 antibodies as markers for recurrence of acquired thrombotic thrombocytopenic purpura during remission. *Haematologica* 2008; 93: 232–239.

33 McDonald V, Manns K, MacKie IJ, *et al.* Rituximab pharmacokinetics during the management of acute idiopathic thrombotic thrombocytopenic purpura. *J Thromb Haemost* 2010; 8: 1201–1208.

34 Westwood JP, Webster H, McGuckin S, *et al.* Rituximab for thrombotic thrombocytopenic purpura: benefit of early administration during acute episodes and use of prophylaxis to prevent relapse. *J Thromb Haemost* 2013; 11: 481–490.

35 Cataland SR, Peyvandi F, Mannucci PM, *et al.* Initial experience from a double-blind, placebo-controlled, clinical outcome study of ARC1779 in patients with thrombotic thrombocytopenic purpura. *Am J Hematol* 2012; 87: 430–432.

36 Alvarez-Larran A, Rio-Garma J, Pujol M, *et al.* Newly diagnosed versus relapsed idiopathic thrombotic thrombocytopenic purpura: a comparison of presenting clinical characteristics and response to treatment. *Ann Hematol* 2009; 88: 973–978.

37 Wong CS, Jelacic S, Habeeb RL, *et al.* The risk of the hemolytic-uremic syndrome after antibiotic treatment of Escherichia coli O157: H7 infections. *N Engl J Med* 2000; 342: 1930–1936.

38 Ariceta G, Besbas N, Johnson S, *et al.* Guideline for the investigation and initial therapy of diarrhea-negative hemolytic uremic syndrome. *Pediatr Nephrol* 2009; 24: 687–696.

39 Taylor CM, Machin S, Wigmore SJ, *et al.* Clinical practice guidelines for the management of atypical haemolytic uraemic syndrome in the United Kingdom. *Br J Haematol* 2010; 148: 37–47.

40 Legendre CM, Licht C, Muus P, *et al.* Terminal complement inhibitor eculizumab in atypical hemolytic-uremic syndrome. *N Engl J Med* 2013; 368: 2169–2181.

41 Mead PS, Griffin PM. Escherichia coli O157: H7. *Lancet* 1998; 352: 1207–1212.

42 Garg AX, Suri RS, Barrowman N, *et al.* Long-term renal prognosis of diarrhea-associated hemolytic uremic syndrome: a systematic review, meta-analysis, and meta-regression. *JAMA* 2003; 290: 1360–1370.

43 Kavanagh D, Richards A, Goodship T, *et al.* Transplantation in atypical hemolytic uremic syndrome. *Semin Thromb Hemost* 2010; 36: 653–659.

44 Sadler JE. Von Willebrand factor, ADAMTS13, and thrombotic thrombocytopenic purpura. *Blood* 2008; 112: 11–18.

14

Venous Thromboembolism

Sarah Takach Lapner, Lori-Ann Linkins and Clive Kearon

Key Points

- Assessment of clinical probability of venous thromboembolism (VTE) is the first step in the diagnosis of deep vein thrombosis or pulmonary embolism.
- Clinical probability is combined with other results, such as D-dimer testing or imaging, to exclude or diagnose VTE.
- VTE can be treated with either a combination of parenteral anticoagulation, such as heparin, and a vitamin K antagonist or with a novel oral anticoagulant (sometimes preceeded by parenteral anticoagulation).
- Three months of anticoagulant therapy is considered sufficient for VTE associated with a transient risk factor, such as surgery.
- Indefinite anticoagulation is indicated in patients with malignancy or unprovoked VTE who are at a low risk of bleeding.

Pathogenesis of Venous Thromboembolism

Virchow was the first to identify stasis, vessel wall injury, and hypercoagulability as the pathogenic triad responsible for thrombosis. This classification of risk factors for venous thromboembolism (VTE) remains valuable. A summary of risk factors for VTE is given in Table 14.1.

Inherited Predisposition to VTE

The most important inherited biochemical disorders that are associated with VTE result from:

- defects in the naturally occurring inhibitors of coagulation: deficiencies of antithrombin, protein C, or protein S; and
- resistance to activated protein C, caused by the factor V Leiden mutation in the majority of cases, and the G20210A prothrombin gene mutation.

The first three of these disorders are rare in the general population (combined prevalence of <1%), have a combined prevalence of approximately 5% in patients with a first episode of VTE, and are associated with a 10- to 40-fold increase in the risk of VTE [1]. The factor V Leiden mutation is common, occurring in approximately 5% of Caucasions and approximately 20% of patients with a first episode of VTE (i.e., an approximate fourfold increase in VTE risk). A mutation in the 3′ untranslated region of the prothrombin gene (G20210A), which is associated with an approximately 25% increase in prothrombin levels, is also common, occuring in about 2% of Caucasians and approximately 5% of those with a first episode of VTE (i.e., an approximate 2.5-fold increase in risk).

Elevated levels of a number of coagulation factors (II, VIII, IX, XI, and fibrinogen) are associated with thrombosis in a "dose-dependent" manner. It is probable that such elevations are often inherited, with strong evidence for this in the case of factor VIII.

Practical Hemostasis and Thrombosis, Third Edition. Edited by Nigel S. Key, Michael Makris and David Lillicrap.
© 2017 John Wiley & Sons, Ltd. Published 2017 by John Wiley & Sons, Ltd.

Table 14.1 Risk factors for venous thromboembolism (VTE).

Patient factors:

Previous VTE[a]

Age over 40

Pregnancy, purpureum

Obesity

Inherited hypercoagulable state

Underlying condition and acquired factors:

Malignancy[a]

Estrogen therapy

Chronic inflammatory conditions

Cancer chemotherapy

Paralysis[a]

Prolonged immobility

Major trauma[a]

Lower limb injuries[a]

Heparin-induced thrombocytopenia

Antiphospholipid antibodies

Lower limb orthopedic surgery[a]

Surgery requiring general anesthesia >30 minutes

Combinations of factors have at least an additive effect on the risk of VTE.
a) Common major risk factors for VTE.

Acquired Predisposition to VTE

Acquired hypercoagulable states include estrogen therapy, antiphospholipid antibodies (anticardi-olipin antibodies and/or lupus anticoagulants), systemic lupus erythematosus, inflammatory bowel disease, malignancy, combination chemotherapy, and surgery [2]. Patients who develop heparin-induced thrombocytopenia (HIT) also have a very high risk of developing arterial and venous thromboembolism [3].

Prevalence and Natural History of VTE

VTE is rare before the age of 16 years, likely because the immature coagulation system is resistant to thrombosis. However, the risk of VTE increases exponentially with advancing age (i.e., 1.9-fold per decade), rising from an annual incidence of approximately 30 in 100 000 at 40 years, to 90 in 100 000 at 60 years, and 260 in 100 000 at 80 years. Clinically important components of the natural history of VTE are summarized in Table 14.2.

Management of VTE

Diagnosis of VTE

Objective testing for deep vein thrombosis (DVT) and pulmonary embolism (PE) is essential because clinical assessment alone is unreliable. Failure to diagnose VTE is associated with a high mortality, whereas inappropriate anticoagulation can lead to serious complications, including fatal hemorrhage.

Diagnosis of DVT

The clinical features of DVT include localized swelling, erythema, tenderness, and distal edema

Table 14.2 Natural history of venous thromboembolism (VTE).

VTE usually starts in the calf veins

About 75% of symptomatic DVTs are proximal

Two-thirds of asymptomatic DVT detected postoperatively by screening venography are confined to the distal (calf) veins

About 20% of symptomatic isolated calf DVTs subsequently extend to the proximal veins, usually within a week of presentation

PE usually arises from proximal DVT

70% of patients with symptomatic proximal DVT have asymptomatic PE (high probability lung scans in 40%), and at least 75% of patients with symptomatic PE have asymptomatic (~50%) or symptomatic (~25%) DVT

50% of untreated symptomatic proximal DVTs are expected to cause symptomatic PE

10% of symptomatic PE are rapidly fatal

30% of untreated symptomatic nonfatal PE will have a fatal recurrence

PE, pulmonary embolism; DVT, deep vein thrombosis.

(Figure 14.1). However, these features are non-specific, and approximately 85% of ambulatory patients with suspected DVT will have another cause for their symptoms. The differential diagnosis for DVT includes:

- cellulitis;
- ruptured Baker cyst;
- muscle tear, muscle cramps, muscle hematoma;
- external venous compression;
- superficial thrombophlebitis; and
- post-thrombotic syndrome (Figure 14.2).

Venography

Venography is the reference standard test for the diagnosis of DVT, but it is now rarely performed. It has advantages over other tests in that it is capable of detecting both proximal vein thrombosis and isolated calf vein thrombosis. However, the disadvantages are that it:

- is invasive, expensive, and requires technical expertise; and
- exposes patients to the risks associated with contrast media, including the potential for an allergic reaction or renal impairment.

For these reasons, noninvasive tests such as venous ultrasonography and D-dimer testing, alone or in combination with clinical assessment, have largely replaced venography [5]. A summary of the test results that effectively confirm or exclude DVT is given in Table 14.3.

Clinical Assessment

Although clinical assessment cannot unequivocally confirm or exclude DVT, clinical evaluation using empiric assessment or a structured clinical model (Table 14.4) can stratify patients as having:

- low probability of DVT (prevalence of DVT approximately 5%);
- moderate probability of DVT (prevalence of DVT approximately 25%); or
- high probability of DVT (prevalence of DVT approximately 60%) [6].

Such categorization is useful in guiding the performance and interpretation of objective testing [7].

Compression Venous Ultrasonography

This is the noninvasive method of choice for diagnosing DVT. The common femoral vein, superfi-

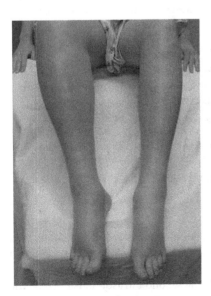
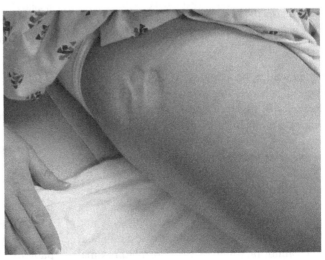

Figure 14.1 Acute right lower extremity deep vein thrombosis. Note the swelling, erythema, and pitting edema. *Source:* reproduced with permission of Dr. Stephan Moll. *See Plate section for color representation of this figure.*

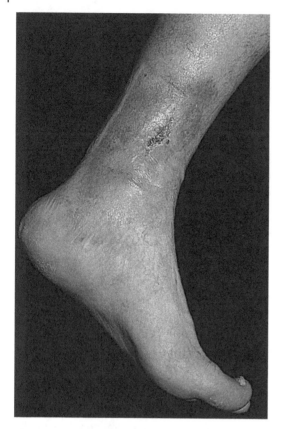

Figure 14.2 Post-thrombotic syndrome. Although usually the symptoms are confined to itching, mild swelling and pain, when severe there is pigmentation and ulceration over the medial malleolus. *Source: Makris and Greaves, 1997 [4]. Reproduced with permission of Elsevier. See Plate section for color representation of this figure.*

Table 14.3 Test results that confirm or exclude deep vein thrombosis (DVT).

Diagnostic for first DVT

Venography: intraluminal filling defect

Venous ultrasound: noncompressible proximal veins at two or more of the common femoral, popliteal, and calf trifurcation sites

Excludes first DVT

Venography: all deep veins seen, and no intraluminal filling defects

D-dimer: normal test which has a very high sensitivity (i.e., ≥98%)

Venous ultrasound: fully compressible proximal veins *and* (a) fully compressible distal veins; *or* (b) low clinical suspicion for DVT at presentation; *or* (c) normal D-dimer test which has a moderate sensitivity (i.e., ≥85%) *or* (d) normal repeat proximal vein ultrasound at 7 days (i.e., normal serial testing)

Low clinical suspicion for DVT at presentation *and* (a) normal D-dimer test which has moderate sensitivity (i.e., ≥85%) at presentation; *or* (b) D-dimer <1000 µg/L using a quantitative D-dimer assay

Moderate clinical suspicion for DVT at presentation *and* a D-dimer <500 µg/L using a quantitative D-dimer assay

Diagnostic for recurrent DVT

Venography: intraluminal filling defect

Venous ultrasound: (a) a new noncompressible common femoral or popliteal vein segment or (b) >4.0 mm increase in diameter of the common femoral or popliteal vein during compression compared to a previous test

Excludes recurrent DVT

Venogram: all deep veins seen and no intraluminal filling defects

Venous ultrasound: normal or ≤4.0 mm increase in diameter of the common femoral or popliteal veins on venous ultrasound compared to a previous test, *and* remains normal (or no progression) at 2 and 7 days

D-dimer: normal test which has a very high sensitivity (i.e., ≥98%)

cial femoral vein, popliteal vein, and proximal deep calf veins are imaged in real time and compressed with the transducer probe. Inability to compress the vein fully is diagnostic of venous thrombosis. Ultrasound may also identify an alternative reason for the patient's symptoms.

Venous ultrasonography is highly accurate for the detection of proximal vein thrombosis with a sensitivity of approximately 97%, specificity of approximately 94%, and negative predictive value of approximately 98% in symptomatic patients. If DVT cannot be excluded by a normal proximal venous ultrasound in combination with other results (e.g., low clinical probability or normal D-dimer), a follow-up ultrasound is performed after 1 week to check for extending calf vein thrombosis (present in approximately 2% of patients). If the second ultrasound is normal, the risk of symptomatic VTE during the next 6 months is less than 2%.

Table 14.4 Wells' model for determining clinical suspicion of deep vein thrombosis (DVT).

Variables	Points
Active cancer (treatment ongoing or within previous 6 months or palliative)	1
Paralysis, paresis, or recent plaster immobilization of the lower extremities	1
Bedridden >3 days or major surgery within 4 weeks	1
Localized tenderness along the distribution of the deep venous system	1
Entire leg swollen	1
Calf swelling 3 cm > asymptomatic side (measured 10 cm below tibial tuberosity)	1
Pitting edema confined to the symptomatic leg	1
Collateral dilated superficial veins (nonvaricose)	1
Previously documented DVT	1
Alternative diagnosis as likely or more likely than DVT	−2

Pretest probability calculated using two scoring methods

	Total points		**Total points**
High	≥3	DVT likely	≥2
Moderate	1 or 2	DVT unlikely	0 or 1
Low	≤0		

Source: modified from Wells *et al.*, 2003 [6].
Note: in patients with symptoms in both legs, the more symptomatic leg is used.

The accuracy of venous ultrasonography is substantially lower if its findings are discordant with the clinical assessment [5] and/or if abnormalities are confined to short segments of the deep veins. Ideally, these patients should have a venogram because the result of the venogram will differ from the venous ultrasound in approximately 25% of these cases. If venography is not available, additional testing (e.g., D-dimer, serial venous ultrasonography) may help to clarify the diagnosis and avoid inappropriate anticoagulant therapy.

Venous ultrasonography of the calf veins is more difficult to perform and less accurate than examination of the proximal veins. A negative "whole-leg" (proximal and distal veins) ultrasound by an experienced examiner excludes DVT without the need for a follow-up examination [5]. However, whole-leg ultrasound leads to diagnosis of calf DVT that would have spontaneously lysed without treatment and to false-positive results, thereby exposing patients to the risk

of bleeding due to anticoagulant therapy without clear benefit. For this reason, we prefer not to perform whole-leg ultrasound examinations.

D-dimer Blood Testing

D-dimer is formed when crosslinked fibrin is broken down by plasmin, and levels are usually elevated with DVT and/or PE. Normal levels can help to exclude VTE, but elevated D-dimer levels are nonspecific and have low positive predictive value (PPV) [5].

D-dimer assays differ markedly in their diagnostic properties for VTE. A normal result with a highly sensitive D-dimer assay (i.e., sensitivity approximately 98%) excludes VTE on its own (i.e., it has a high negative predictive value (NPV)). However, highly sensitive D-dimer tests have low specificity (approximately 40%), which limits their use because of high false-positive rates. In order to exclude DVT and/or PE, a normal result with a less sensitive D-dimer assay (i.e., approximately 85%) needs to be *combined* with either a low clinical probability or another objective test that has a high NPV (e.g., negative venous ultrasound of the proximal veins) [5]. As less sensitive D-dimer assays are more specific (approximately 70%), they yield fewer false-positive results.

Traditionally, irrespective of which quantitative D-dimer assay is selected, a single D-dimer cut-off level is used to exclude DVT in all patients. More recently, it has been shown that varying D-dimer cut-off levels according to clinical probability of DVT is more efficient. The prevalence of DVT in patients with low clinical probability is less than in patients with moderate or high clinical probability. For this reason, a more liberal D-dimer threshold of <1000 µg/L can be used to exclude DVT in patients with low clinical probability. In patients with a moderate clinical probability who have a higher prevalence of disease, a D-dimer of <500 µg/L is required to exclude DVT [8].

Specificity of D-dimer decreases with aging and with comorbid illness, such as cancer. Consequently, D-dimer testing has limited value as a diagnostic test for VTE in hospitalized patients (more false-positive results) and is unhelpful in the early postoperative period.

Computed Tomography and Magnetic Resonance Venography

Computed tomography (CT) and magnetic resonance (MR) venography have the potential to diagnose DVT in settings where the accuracy of compression ultrasonography is limited (e.g., isolated pelvic DVT). However, given the cost, exposure to radiation, and limited availability of these modalities, neither currently play a significant role in the diagnosis of DVT.

Diagnosis of Recurrent DVT

Persistent abnormalities of the deep veins on ultrasound examination are common following DVT. Therefore, diagnosis of recurrent DVT requires evidence of new clot formation. Tests that can diagnose or exclude recurrent DVT are noted in Table 14.3.

Diagnosis of DVT in Pregnancy

Pregnant patients with suspected DVT can generally be managed in the same way as nonpregnant patients, although diagnostic approaches have not been well evaluated in this population. Normal serial compression ultrasound with visualization of the iliac veins appears to have a high NPV and can be used to exclude DVT [9]. Pregnant patients with normal noninvasive tests who still have a high clinical suspicion of isolated iliac DVT should be considered for venography or an MRI.

Diagnosis of PE

The clinical features of PE (Figure 14.3) may include:

- pleuritic chest pain;
- shortness of breath;
- syncope;
- hemoptysis; and
- palpitations.

As with DVT, these features are nonspecific and objective testing must be performed to confirm or exclude the diagnosis of PE.

Pulmonary Angiography

Pulmonary angiography, with injection of contrast directly into the pulmonary arteries, is the reference standard test for the diagnosis of PE (Figure 14.4). However, it has many of the same limita-

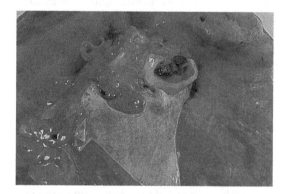

Figure 14.3 Pulmonary embolus in the pulmonary artery causing sudden death in a young woman who was using the combined pill. *Source:* Makris and Greaves, 1997 [4]. Reproduced with permission of Elsevier. *See Plate section for color representation of this figure.*

tions as venography. A diagnostic algorithm for PE is given in Figure 14.5 and a summary of tests that confirm or exclude PE is given in Table 14.5.

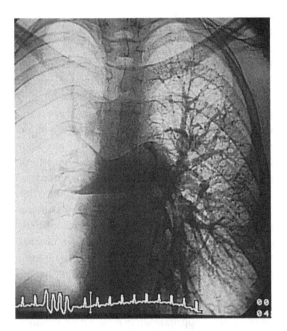

Figure 14.4 Pulmonary angiogram showing massive pulmonary embolism in the right pulmonary artery. *Source:* Makris and Greaves, 1997 [4]. Reproduced with permission of Elsevier.

Computed Tomographic Pulmonary Angiography

Multislice spiral CT (also know as helical CT) with peripheral injection of radiographic contrast is the current standard diagnostic test for PE [10,11]. In comparison with traditional ventilation–perfusion lung scanning, computed tomographic pulmonary angiography (CTPA) is less likely to be "nondiagnostic" (i.e., approximately 10% vs. 60%) and has the potential to identify an alternative etiology for the patient's symptoms. This technique has a sensitivity of 83%, specificity of 96%, NPV of 95%, and PPV of 86% for PE.

Accuracy of CTPA varies according to the size of the largest pulmonary artery involved and according to clinical pretest probability.

In management studies that used CTPA to diagnose PE, less than 2% of patients who had anticoagulant therapy withheld based on a negative CTPA went on to have symptomatic VTE during follow-up. Taken together, these observations suggest the following:

- A good-quality, normal CTPA excludes PE.
- Lobar or larger pulmonary artery intraluminal defects are generally diagnostic for PE (PPV 97%).

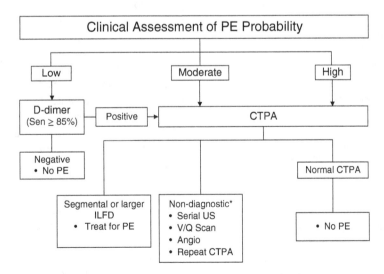

Figure 14.5 Diagnostic algorithm for PE. *Choice of additional diagnostic testing depends on clinical presentation and local expertise. CTPA, computerized tomographic pulmonary angiography (multidetector); US, ultrasound; V/Q, ventilation–perfusion; angio, angiography; ILFD, intraluminal filling defect.

Table 14.5 Test results that confirm or exclude pulmonary embolism (PE).

Diagnostic for PE

Pulmonary angiography: intraluminal filling defect

CTPA: lobar or main pulmonary artery intraluminal filling defect. Segmental intraluminal filling defect and moderate or high clinical suspicion

Ventilation-perfusion scan: high probability scan and moderate/ high clinical suspicion

Diagnostic test positive for DVT: with non-diagnostic ventilation-perfusion scan or CTPA

Excludes PE

Pulmonary angiography: normal

Ventilation-perfusion scan: normal

D-*dimer*: normal test which has a very high sensitivity (i.e., ≥98%)

Low clinical suspicion for PE at presentation *and* (a) normal D-dimer test which has moderate sensitivity (i.e., ≥85%) at presentation

CTPA: negative good-quality study

Non-diagnostic CTPA *and* normal proximal venous ultrasound *and*

a) low clinical suspicion, *or*

b) normal D-dimer with sensitivity ≥85%, *or*

c) negative bilateral leg ultrasounds at day 7 and day 14 *or*

d) nonhigh probability ventilation-perfusion scan

(Could consider repeating CTPA 24 hours later, if inadequate due to technical reasons)

Nondiagnostic ventilation-perfusion scan *and* normal proximal venous ultrasound *and*

a) low clinical suspicion for PE, *or*

b) normal D-dimer test which has at least a moderately high sensitivity (i.e., ≥85%), *or*

c) negative bilateral leg ultrasounds at day 7 and day 14, *or*

d) negative CTPA

CTPA, computed tomographic pulmonary angiography; DVT, deep vein thrombosis.

- Segmental pulmonary artery intraluminal defects are generally diagnostic for PE if clinical suspicion is moderate or high, but should be considered nondiagnostic if clinical suspicion is low, if there are discordant findings (e.g., negative D-dimer), or if the intraluminal defects are small or are atypical in appearance (PPV 68%).

- Subsegmental pulmonary artery intraluminal defects are nondiagnostic, and patients with such findings require further testing (PPV 25%).

Ventilation–Perfusion Lung Scanning

In the past, planar (two dimensional) ventilation–perfusion lung scanning was the initial investigation in patients with suspected PE, and it is still useful in patients with contraindications to X-ray contrast dye (e.g., renal failure) and patients at higher risk for developing breast cancer from CT radiation exposure (e.g., women under 40 years old). A normal perfusion scan excludes PE, but is only found in a minority of patients (10–40%). Perfusion defects are nonspecific; approximately one-third of patients with perfusion defects have PE. The probability that a perfusion defect is caused by PE increases with size and number and the presence of a normal ventilation scan ("mismatched" defect). A lung scan with mismatched segmental or larger perfusion defects is termed "high probability." A single mismatched defect is associated with a prevalence of PE of approximately 80%. Three or more mismatched defects are associated with a prevalence of PE of approximately 90%. Lung scan findings are highly age dependent, with a relatively high proportion of normal scans and a low proportion of nondiagnostic scans in younger patients. A high frequency of normal lung scans are also seen in pregnant patients who are investigated for PE.

Many centers now perform SPECT (single-photon emision CT; three dimensional imaging) rather than planar ventilation–perfusion scanning. SPECT appears to be more accurate for PE diagnosis than planar imaging and to yield fewer nondiagnostic interpretations. However, criteria for interpretation of SPECT scans are poorly standardized, and the accuracy of SPECT or the safety of using it to manage patients with suspected PE has not been evaluated in large, prospective multicenter studies.

Clinical Assessment

As with suspected DVT, clinical assessment is useful for categorizing probability of PE (Table 14.6) [12].

Table 14.6 Wells' model for determining clinical suspicion of pulmonary embolism (PE).

Variables		Points		
Clinical signs and symptoms of deep vein thrombosis (minimum leg swelling and pain with palpation of the deep veins)		3.0		
Pulmonary embolism is the most likely diagnosis.		3.0		
Heart rate >100 bpm		1.5		
Immobilization or surgery in the previous 4 weeks		1.5		
Previous DVT/PE		1.5		
Hemoptysis		1.0		
Malignancy (treatment ongoing or within previous 6 months or palliative)		1.0		
Pretest probability calculated using two scoring methods				
	Total points		**Total points**	
High	>6			
Moderate	4.5–6	PE likely	≥4.5	
Low*	≤4.0	PE unlikely	≤4.0	

Source: modified from Wells *et al.*, 2000 [13].

*In the original derivation of the Wells PE model, patients were required to have a score less than 1.5 to be categorized as low CPTP, but a score of <4 has subsequently been used for low CPTP DVT, deep vein thrombosis.

D-dimer Testing

As previously discussed when considering the diagnosis of DVT, a normal D-dimer result, alone or in combination with another negative test, can be used to exclude PE (Table 14.5).

Patients with Nondiagnostic Combinations of Noninvasive Tests for PE

Patients with nondiagnostic test results for PE at presentation have a prevalence of PE of approximately 20%; therefore, further investigations to exclude PE are required. The first step is to perform venous ultrasonography to look for DVT. If DVT is confirmed, it can be concluded that the patient's symptoms are due to PE. Negative tests for DVT do not rule out PE, but they do reduce the probability of PE and suggest that the short-term risk of recurrent PE is low.

If imaging studies are negative for DVT, we recommend one of the management strategies outlined in Table 14.5.

Magnetic Resonance Angiography (MRA)

Current evidence suggests that MRA has about an 80% sensitivity and a high specificity for PE,

and that this translates into a high PPV (establishing a diagnosis of PE) but an inadequate NPV (for exclusion of PE).

Diagnosis of PE in Pregnancy

Pregnant patients with suspected PE can be managed similarly to nonpregnant patients, with the following modifications [14]:

- Venous ultrasound of the legs should be performed first followed by ventilation–perfusion lung scanning if there is no DVT.
- Ventilation perfusion scanning is preferred over CTPA because it exposes the breast tissue to less radiation. Even though ventilation perfusion scanning delivers slightly more radiation to the fetus than CTPA, neither technique delivers a sufficient dose to increase the risk of birth defects or childhood cancers.
- The amount of radioisotope used for the perfusion scan should be reduced and the duration of scanning extended.
- CTPA is suggested in pregnant patients who are acutely unwell or unstable to allow prompt diagnosis.

Advice to Patients After Negative Testing for Supected DVT or PE

Recognizing that even after optimal diagnostic testing there is a small possibilty of a missed diagnosis, patients who have had PE and/or DVT excluded should routinely be asked to return for re-evaluation if symptoms of PE and/or DVT persist or recur.

Treatment of VTE

Initiation of Anticoagulant Therapy

Heparin, low-molecular-weight heparin (LMWH), and fondaparinux are commonly used for the initial treatment of VTE. Advantages of LMWH and fondaparinux over heparin include administration as a once-daily subcutaneous injection, lack of need for laboratory monitoring, and a lower risk of HIT. The advantages of heparin include a short half-life when given intravenously, reversibility, and lack of dependence on renal clearance. Current clinical practice is to treat patients with acute VTE for a minimum of 5 days with: (i) intravenous heparin in a regimen of at least 30 000 IU/day or 18 IU/kg/hour adjusted to achieve an activated partial thromboplastin time (APTT) ratio of 1.5 to 2.5; (ii) LMWH at a weight-adjusted dose of either approximately 100 IU/kg every 12 hours or approximately 150–200 IU/kg once daily; (iii) subcutaneous heparin administered twice daily, either monitored (initial dose of 17 500 IU twice daily or a weight-adjusted dose of 250 IU/kg twice daily, with dose adjustment to achieve an APTT ratio of 1.5 to 2.5 6 hours after injection) or unmonitored (initial dose of 333 IU/kg followed by a twice daily dose of 250 IU/kg); or (iv) fondaparinux 7.5 mg (5 mg if <50 kg; 10 mg if >100 kg) once daily by subcutaneous injection [15]. This initial treatment is usually overlapped with a course of oral anticoagulants.

Long-term Therapy with Vitamin K Antagonists

Vitamin K antagonists (e.g., warfarin) produce their anticoagulant effect through the production of hemostatically defective vitamin K-dependent coagulant proteins (prothrombin, factor VII, factor IX, and factor X). The dose of warfarin must be monitored closely using the international normalized ratio (INR) because the anticoagulant response is influenced by interactions with other medications and changes in diet [16]. The target INR for treatment of acute VTE is 2.0–3.0.

Vitamin K antagonists are typically started on day 1 or 2 of treatment of acute VTE and continued for a length of time determined on an individual basis (discussed below).

Novel Oral Anticoagulants

Novel oral anticoagulants include factor Xa inhibitors (rivaroxaban, apixaban) and direct thrombin inhibitors (dabigatran). These agents inhibit factor Xa or thrombin directly without binding to antithrombin. The advantages of the novel oral anticoagulants over vitamin K antagonists include lack of need for laboratory monitoring of anticoagulant effect, absence of dietary restrictions and far fewer drug interactions.

The novel oral anticoagulants have been shown to be as effective as heparin and warfarin in the treatment of acute VTE [17]. Factor Xa inhibitors are given at a higher dose during the initial treatment period (rivaroxaban 15 mg twice daily for three weeks, apixaban 10 mg twice daily for 7 days), followed by a lower maintenance dose (rivaroxaban 20 mg once daily, apixaban 5 mg twice daily). An initial 5-day course of heparin, LMWH, or fondaparinux is required before dabigatran, which is given as 150 mg twice daily throughout treatment. These three novel anticoagulants are contraindicated with marked renal impairment (i.e., estimated creatinine clearance <30 mL per minute). The risk of intracranial bleeding is about half with each of the novel agents compared to warfarin. Use of the novel anticoagulants for acute and long-term treatment of VTE is influenced by cost and local licensing.

Duration of Anticoagulant Therapy

Conceptually, treatment of VTE can be divided into two phases. The first phase, which is common to all episodes of VTE, is treatment of the acute thrombosis and lasts 3 months. Treatment for less than 3 month is associated with an increased risk of recurrence in the first 6 months after stopping therapy [18]. The second phase, which is optional, is to continue anticoagulation beyond 3 months to prevent new unrelated epsiodes of VTE. Extending anticoagulation beyond 3 months is very effective at preventing recurrence but, if treatment is subsequently stopped, there will be a risk of recurrence similar to if treatment was stopped at 3 months. Consequently, for most patients, the question is whether to stop treatment at 3 months or to continue treatment indefinetely (i.e., no scheduled stop date, but ongoing review of risks and benefits of extended therapy). The decision to continue anticoagulation indefinitely is determined by balancing the increased risk of recurrent VTE if anticoagulants are stopped, against the increased risk of bleeding if they are continued, while also considering cost and individual patient preference.

Major Transient Risk Factors

These include surgery with general anesthesia within 3 months, major trauma, and plaster cast immobilization of a leg. The risk of recurrence after stopping anticoagulant therapy is very low, approximately 2% in the first year and 5% in the first 5 years. Three months of anticoagulant therapy is adequate for these patients.

Minor Transient Risk Factors

These include estrogen therapy, prolonged travel (i.e., >10 hours), pregnancy, less marked leg injuries, and medical illness with immobilization (including in hospital). The risk of recurrence after stopping anticoagulant therapy is expected to be higher than in those patients with a major transient risk factor, but lower than those patients with an unprovoked VTE (e.g., approximately 5% in the first year and 15% in the first 5 years). Three months of anticoagulant therapy is also considered adequate for most of these patients.

Unprovoked VTE

The risk of recurrent VTE after stopping anticoagulant therapy in patients with a first unprovoked proximal DVT or PE is approximately 10% in the first year and 30% after 5 years. Given this high risk of recurrence, and the greater than 90% risk reduction with anticoagulant therapy, indefinite therapy is the preferred option for patients who have a low risk of bleeding, provided this is consistent with patient preference. The rationale for indefinite anticoagulation is stronger for patients with unprovoked PE compared to DVT, and after a second compared to a first episode of thrombosis. As patients with isolated calf DVT have half the risk of recurrence of those with proximal DVT, 3 months of anticoagulant therapy is considered adequate. There is evolving evidence that the risk of recurrence among patients with a first unprovoked proximal DVT or PE can be further stratified according to patient sex and whether D-dimer level becomes abnormal a month after stopping anticoagulant therapy: the risk of recurrence is low enough in females with a persistently negative D-dimer level that anticoagulants can be stopped after 3 months [19].

Active Malignancy

Patients with cancer who have VTE are threefold more likely to have recurrent VTE than patients who do not have cancer. Those at highest risk of recurrence (e.g., metastatic disease, poor mobility, or ongoing chemotherapy) should generally be treated indefinitely. Extended LMWH is preferred over treatment with a vitamin K antagonist because of a lower risk of recurrence, and greater compatibility with chemotherapy and the need for invasive interventions [20]. There is inadequate experience to recommend treatment of cancer-associated VTE with the novel anticoagulants.

Hypercoagulable States

Patients who are persistently positive for antiphospholipid antibody (e.g., anticardiolipin antibodies and/or lupus anticoagulant) appear to have a higher risk of recurrence. Patients heterozygous for factor V Leiden or the G20210A prothrombin gene mutation do not appear to have a clinically important increased risk for recurrence. The implications for duration of treatment of other abnormalities, such as homozygous factor V Leiden, double heterozygosity for factor V Leiden, and the G20210A prothrombin gene mutation, as well as elevated levels of clotting factors VIII, IX, XI, and deficiencies of protein C, protein S, and antithrombin, are uncertain. We rarely test for hypercoagulable states in order to guide duration of anticoagulant therapy [21].

Risk of Bleeding on Anticoagulant Therapy

The risk of bleeding on anticoagulants differs markedly among patients, depending on the prevalence of risk factors (e.g., age >75 years, previous bleeding or stroke, renal failure, anemia, antiplatelet therapy that cannot be stopped, malignancy, poor anticoagulant control) [22]. A meta-analysis in patients who received oral anticoagulant therapy for VTE for at least 3 months (at a target INR range of 2.0–3.0) demonstrated a case-fatality of major bleeding of 11% [23]. Consequently, the case-fatality with an episode of major bleeding appears to be at least twice the case-fatality of recurrent VTE after a DVT, and probably similar to the case-fatality after a PE.

Treatment of VTE During Pregnancy

Heparin and LMWH do not cross the placenta and are safe for the fetus, whereas oral anticoagulants cross the placenta and can cause fetal bleeding and malformations. Compared to heparin, prolonged therapeutic-dose LMWH is associated with a lower risk of osteoporosis, requires less or no laboratory monitoring, and can be given once rather than twice daily. Therefore, pregnant women with acute VTE should be treated with LMWH throughout pregnancy. Care should be taken to avoid delivery while the mother is therapeutically anticoagulated; one management approach involves stopping subcutaneous LMWH 24 hours prior to induction of labor and switching to intravenous heparin, if there is a high risk of embolism. After delivery, warfarin, which is safe for infants of nursing mothers, should be given (with initial heparin overlap) for 6 weeks and until a minimum of 3 months of treatment has been completed.

Thrombolytic Therapy

Systemic thrombolytic therapy accelerates the rate of resolution of PE, which can be life-saving for patients with hemodynamic compromise (i.e., severe hypotension and/or hypoxia). However, this benefit comes at the cost of about a twofold increase in the frequency of major bleeding, and a five- to tenfold increase in intracranial bleeding [24]. Catheter-based techiques, with or without thrombolytic therapy (i.e., if there is a high risk of bleeding), can be used to disrupt acute PE and improve outflow from the right ventricle. Similarly, catheter-directed thrombolysis, with or without mechanical disruption of thrombus, has the potential to reduce the risk of the post-thrombotic syndrome following DVT and may be indicated in patients with extensive thrombosis, severe symptoms, and without risk factors for bleeding.

When thrombolysis is indicated for treatment of PE, regimens that are given within 2 hours or less, such as 100 mg rt-PA over 2 hours, appear preferable to more prolonged infusions (bolus regimens should be used with impending cardiac arrest). Catheter-directed thrombolysis for DVT generally uses much lower dose of drug and requires operator expertese.

Major contraindications to thrombolytic therapy include:

- active internal bleeding;
- stroke within the past 3 months; and
- intracranial disease.

Relative contraindications include:

- major surgery within the past 10 days;
- recent organ biopsy;
- recent puncture of a noncompressible vessel;

- recent gastrointestinal bleeding;
- liver or renal disease;
- severe arterial hypertension; and
- severe diabetic retinopathy.

Surgical Treatment

Pulmonary endarterectomy is highly beneficial in selected patients with chronic thromboembolic pulmonary hypertension. Urgent pulmonary embolectomy in patients with acute PE is reserved for patients with shock whose blood pressure cannot be maintained despite administration of systemic or catheter-directed thrombolytic therapy or use of catheter-based therapy alone (e.g., if there is an absolute contraindication to thrombolytic therapy).

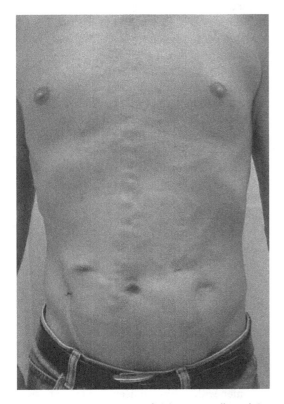

Figure 14.6 Prominent superficial venous collaterals in a patient with inferior vena caval (IVC) thrombotic occlusion, occurring as a late complication of an IVC filter. *Source:* reproduced with permission of Dr. Stephan Moll. *See Plate section for color representation of this figure.*

Inferior Vena Caval Filters

A randomized trial demonstrated that a filter, as an adjunct to anticoagulation in patients with proximal DVT, reduced the rate of PE (asymptomatic and symptomatic) from 4.5% to 1.0% during the 12 days following insertion, with a suggestion of fewer fatal episodes (0% vs. 2%). However, after 8 years of follow up, despite a reduction in PE (6% vs. 15%) there was an increase in DVT (36% vs. 28%), no difference in DVT and PE combined, and no reduction in mortality [25]. This study supports the use of vena caval filters to prevent PE in patients with acute DVT and/or PE who cannot be anticoagulated (i.e., bleeding) but does not support more liberal use of filters. Patients should receive a course of anticoagulation if this subsequently becomes safe, which should be continued for the same duration as if the patient did not have a vena caval filter in situ. A rare late complication of inferior vena cava filters is extensive inferior vena cava thrombosis (Figure 14.6).

Prevention of VTE

VTE Prophylaxis Following Surgery

Low Risk

This category includes patients under 40 years of age who undergo uncomplicated surgery and have no additional risk factors. The rate of asymptomatic proximal DVT detected by surveillance bilateral venography is estimated to be 0.4%, and the rate of symptomatic PE and fatal PE is 0.2% and <0.01%, respectively. Recommended VTE prophylaxis in this group is limited to early mobilization.

Moderate Risk

This category includes patients over 40 years of age who undergo prolonged and/or complicated surgery or have additional minor risk factors. The rate of asymptomatic proximal DVT is estimated to be 5%, and the rate of symptomatic PE and fatal PE is 2% and 0.5%, respectively. Recommended VTE prophylaxis in this group includes unfractionated heparin (5000 IU/day preoperatively, and two to three times daily postoperatively), LMWH (approximately 3000 IU/day), or graduated compression stockings alone or in combination with pharmacological methods.

High Risk

This category includes patients who undergo major surgery for malignancy, hip or knee surgery, or those who have a history of previous VTE. The rate of asymptomatic proximal DVT is estimated to be 15%, and the rate of symptomatic PE and fatal PE is 5% and 1%, respectively. Recommended VTE prophylaxis in this group includes: unfractionated heparin (5000 IU two to three times daily postoperatively); LMWH (4000 to 6000 IU/day, as a single or divided dose); warfarin (usually started postoperatively and adjusted to achieve an INR of 2.0–3.0) or fondaparinux (2.5 mg once daily, usually started postoperatively); or intermittent pneumatic compression devices alone or in combination with other methods of prophylaxis. Mechanical methods of prophylaxis should be used in patients who have a moderate or high risk of VTE if anticoagulants are contraindicated (e.g., neurosurgical patients). Novel oral anticoagulants, such as rivaroxaban (10 mg once daily), dabigatran (150–220 mg once daily), or apixaban (2.5 mg twice daily), are increasingly being used for prevention of VTE in patients who undergo hip or knee replacement.

VTE prophylaxis in Medical Patients

Primary prophylaxis with anticoagulants should be used in hospitalized patients who are confined to bed, have a history of VTE, or who have other major risk factors for VTE. Meta-analyses have shown that heparin, LMWH, and fondaparinux reduce the rate of symptomatic VTE by about 50% compared with placebo in acutely ill medical patients. While rivaroxaban is as effective as LMWH, it appears to increase the risk of bleeding. Mechanical methods of prophylaxis, particularly intermittent pneumatic compression devices, should be considered in patients who cannot receive anticoagulants because of

bleeding, but they increase the risk of skin ulceration.

References

1 Kearon C, Crowther M, Hirsh J. Management of patients with hereditary hypercoagulable disorders. *Ann Rev Med* 2000; 51: 169–185.
2 Anderson FA, Jr., Spencer FA. Risk factors for venous thromboembolism. *Circulation 2003*; 107 (23 Suppl. 1): 19–16.
3 Linkins LA, Dans AL, Moores LK, *et al.* Treatment and prevention of heparin-induced thrombocytopenia: Antithrombotic therapy and prevention of thrombosis, 9th ed: American College of Chest Physicians evidence-based clinical practice guidelines. *Chest* 2012; 141 (2 Suppl.): e495S–530S.
4 Makris M, Greaves M. *Blood in Systemic Disease.* Saint Louis, MO: Mosby, 1997.
5 Bates SM, Jaeschke R, Stevens SM, *et al.* Diagnosis of DVT: Antithrombotic therapy and prevention of thrombosis, 9th ed: American College of Chest Physicians evidence-based clinical practice guidelines. *Chest* 2012; 141 (2 Suppl.): e351S–418S.
6 Wells PS, Anderson DR, Rodger M, *et al.* Evaluation of D-dimer in the diagnosis of suspected deep-vein thrombosis. *N Engl J Med* 2003; 349: 1227–1235.
7 Wells PS, Owen C, Doucette S, *et al.* Does this patient have deep vein thrombosis? *JAMA* 2006; 295: 199–207.
8 Linkins LA, Bates SM, Lang E, *et al.* Selective D-dimer testing for diagnosis of a first suspected episode of deep venous thrombosis: a randomized trial. *Ann Intern Med* 2013; 158: 93–100.
9 Chan WS, Spencer FA, Lee AY, *et al.* Safety of withholding anticoagulation in pregnant women with suspected deep vein thrombosis following negative serial compression ultrasound and iliac vein imaging. *CMAJ* 2013; 185: E194–200.
10 Stein PD, Fowler SE, Goodman LR, *et al.* Multidetector computed tomography for

acute pulmonary embolism. *N Engl J Med* 2006; 354: 2317–2327.

11 van Belle A, Buller HR, Huisman MV, *et al.* Effectiveness of managing suspected pulmonary embolism using an algorithm combining clinical probability, D-dimer testing, and computed tomography. *JAMA* 2006; 295: 172–179.

12 Lucassen W, Geersing GJ, Erkens PM, *et al.* Clinical decision rules for excluding pulmonary embolism: a meta-analysis. *Ann Intern Med* 2011; 155: 448–460.

13 Wells PS, Anderson DR, Rodger M, *et al.* Derivation of a simple clinical model to categorize patients probability of pulmonary embolism: increasing the models utility with the SimpliRED D-dimer. *Thromb Haemost* 2000; 83: 416–420.

14 Bourjeily G, Paidas M, Khalil H, *et al.* Pulmonary embolism in pregnancy. *Lancet* 2010; 375: 500–512.

15 Kearon C, Akl EA, Comerota AJ, *et al.* Antithrombotic therapy for VTE disease: Antithrombotic therapy and prevention of thrombosis, 9th ed: American College of Chest Physicians evidence-based clinical practice guidelines. *Chest* 2012; 141 (2 Suppl.): e419S–494S.

16 Ageno W, Gallus AS, Wittkowsky A, *et al.* Oral anticoagulant therapy: Antithrombotic therapy and prevention of thrombosis, 9th ed: American College of Chest Physicians evidence-based clinical practice guidelines. *Chest* 2012; 141 (2 Suppl.): e44S–88S.

17 Fox BD, Kahn SR, Langleben D, *et al.* Efficacy and safety of novel oral anticoagulants for treatment of acute venous thromboembolism: direct and adjusted indirect meta-analysis of randomised controlled trials. *BMJ* 2012; 345: e7498.

18 Boutitie F, Pinede L, Schulman S, *et al.* Influence of preceding length of anticoagulant treatment and initial presentation of venous thromboembolism on risk of recurrence after stopping treatment: analysis of individual participants' data from seven trials. *BMJ* 2011; 342: d3036.

19 Douketis J, Tosetto A, Marcucci M, *et al.* Risk of recurrence after venous thromboembolism in men and women: patient level meta-analysis. *BMJ* 2011; 342: d813.

20 Lyman GH, Khorana AA, Kuderer NM, *et al.* Venous thromboembolism prophylaxis and treatment in patients with cancer: American Society of Clinical Oncology clinical practice guideline update. *J Clin Oncol* 2013; 31: 2189–2204.

21 Kearon C. Influence of hereditary or acquired thrombophilias on the treatment of venous thromboembolism. *Curr Opin Hematol* 2012; 19: 363–370.

22 Schulman S, Beyth RJ, Kearon C, *et al.* Hemorrhagic complications of anticoagulant and thrombolytic treatment: American College of Chest Physicians evidence-based clinical practice guidelines (8th edition). *Chest* 2008; 133 (6 Suppl.): 257S–298S.

23 Carrier M, Le Gal G, Wells PS, *et al.* Systematic review: case-fatality rates of recurrent venous thromboembolism and major bleeding events among patients treated for venous thromboembolism. *Ann Intern Med* 2010; 152: 578–589.

24 Dong BR, Hao Q, Yue J, *et al.* Thrombolytic therapy for pulmonary embolism. *Cochrane Database Syst Rev* 2009; (3): CD004437.

25 PREPIC Study Group. Eight-year follow-up of patients with permanent vena cava filters in the prevention of pulmonary embolism: the PREPIC (Prevention du Risque d'Embolie Pulmonaire par Interruption Cave) randomized study. *Circulation* 2005; 112: 416–422.

15

Myeloproliferative Neoplasms: Thrombosis and Hemorrhage

Brandi Reeves and Stephan Moll

Key Points

- Polycythemia vera (PV) and essential thrombocythemia (ET) are generally associated with a normal life expectancy, while that of primary myelofibrosis (PMF) is significantly reduced.
- Thrombosis is the major cause of mortality in PV and ET, and the majority are arterial events.
- Splanchnic vein thrombosis/Budd–Chiari syndrome is a hallmark of *BCR-ABL*-negative myeloproliferative neoplasms.
- Treatment of PV and ET is primarily based on the thrombotic risk, while that of PMF is based on general symptom management.
- Clinically focused summarizing tables are provided in this chapter on diagnostic criteria, diagnostic work-up and risk stratification to decide which patients to treat with antiplatelet agents with or without cytoreductive therapy.

Introduction

Myeloproliferative neoplasms (MPNs) are chronic disorders characterized by autonomous myeloproliferation and complicated by thrombosis, hemorrhage, constitutional symptoms, and fibrotic and leukemic transformation. The "classic" *BCR-ABL*-negative MPNs (polycythemia vera (PV), essential thrombocythemia (ET) and primary myelofibrosis (PMF)) are a phenotypically diverse group of disorders with acquired Janus kinase–signal transducer and activator of transcription (JAK-STAT) protein activation central to their pathogenesis resulting in cellular proliferation and resistance to apoptosis. This chapter will focus on the practical aspects of diagnosis and management of the thrombohemorrhagic complications of each.

Clinical Manifestations

Polycythemia Vera

Polycythemia vera (PV) is generally first suspected on the basis of erythrocytosis with or without leukocytosis and thrombocytosis on complete blood count (CBC). The abnormality is often discovered coincidentally on CBC testing, with no symptoms present.

Symptoms of PV range from nonspecific fatigue to the more specific aquagenic (also known as postbath) pruritus, and to potentially life-threatening thrombosis. Aquagenic pruritus is characterized by a sometimes intense itching/burning/tickling sensation, especially of the trunk and extremities, and generally noted within 10 minutes of hot water contact. It is seen in up to 70% of PV patients and can be an early sign of the disease. Another hallmark of MPN/PV is splanchnic vein thrombosis in the absence of a provoking risk factor such as cirrhosis or abdominal surgery. Less specific symptoms include fatigue, bone pain, left upper quadrant pain, early satiety, weight loss, and

Practical Hemostasis and Thrombosis, Third Edition. Edited by Nigel S. Key, Michael Makris and David Lillicrap.
© 2017 John Wiley & Sons, Ltd. Published 2017 by John Wiley & Sons, Ltd.

gout. Microvascular symptoms are present in approximately 30% and include migrainous headaches, tinnitus, dizziness, visual disturbances, and painful burning of the hands and feet accompanied by a reddish or bluish skin discoloration known as erythromelalgia. Twenty percent of patients will have had a thrombotic event by the time of diagnosis, with the majority being arterial events: transient ischemic attacks (TIA), strokes, and myocardial infarctions (MI) (Table 15.1). The incidence of thrombosis by the time of MPN diagnosis is the same for younger patients as for those over age 65 years, though Budd–Chiari syndrome is more common among patients less than 45 years and arterial clots are more common in those over age 65 years [1].

Essential Thrombocythemia

Essential thrombocythemia (ET) is often first suspected due to incidental discovery of thrombocytosis on CBC. The symptoms and signs of ET overlap significantly with those of PV, though ET has a lower incidence of pruritus and

Table 15.1 Comparison of classic (*BCR-ABL*-negative) myeloproliferative neoplasms.

	Polycythemia vera	Essential thrombocythemia	Primary myelofibrosis
Incidence	1.9 per 100 000	2.5 per 100 000	1.5 per 100 000
Age at initial presentation	60 years	60 years	60 years
Men : women	2 : 1	1 : 1.5	2 : 1
Mutation status			
JAK2 V617F	97%	50–60%	50–60%
JAK2 exon12	3%	Rare	Rare
CALR exon 9	0%	25%	25%
MPL mutation	–	5%	5%
Major cause of mortality	Thrombosis (40%)	Thrombosis (40%)	Leukemic transformation, infection
Median overall survival[a]	Slightly reduced	Normal	Very reduced (5 year)
10-year risk of fibrotic/leukemic transformation (overall) [29,36]	10% / 3%	1% / 1%	Not applicable/12–31%
Prevalence of thrombosis [23,37]			
At diagnosis	19–34%	7–26%	7–22%
Type (% of total events)	Arterial 66–80%	Arterial 59–85%	Arterial 46–78%
	Venous 25–35%	Venous 15–41%	Venous 22–54%
during follow-up	9–19%	8–22%	7–21%
Type (% of total events)	Arterial 55–67%	Arterial 56–94%	Arterial 48–75%
	Venous 33–42%	Venous 6–44%	Venous 25–53%
Prevalence of major hemorrhage [6,7,8]			
at diagnosis	5%	2–5%	7%[b]
during follow-up period	1–2%	1–10%	9–12%[b]

a) Median overall survival may be overestimated due to reporting of immature data. Survival in PMF variable depending upon disease characteristics.
b) Prefibrotic primary myelofibrosis only included in these studies.
   JAK, Janus kinase; PV, polycythemia vera; PMF, primary myelofibrosis; *CALR*, calreticulin.

splenomegaly. Rates of thrombosis and hemorrhage are similar to PV (Table 15.1).

Primary Myelofibrosis

Patients with primary myelofibrosis (PMF) tend to be the most symptomatic of patients with *BCR-ABL*-negative MPNs. Patients with PMF often come to the attention of a hematologist when cytopenias are noted, especially when associated with teardrop cells and nucleated red blood cells on the peripheral blood smear. Nearly all patients are affected by fatigue, with half also experiencing night sweats or weight loss, and 20% with fever. Splenomegaly is common, causing early satiety, abdominal pain, and portal hypertension. Thrombotic complications are slightly less prevalent at diagnosis than in PV or ET at 10–15%, while major hemorrhagic events tend to be higher (Table 15.1).

Diagnosis

Diagnostic Criteria

The *BCR-ABL*-negative MPNs are diagnosed by a combination of laboratory and clinical findings, most recently detailed in the WHO 2016 criteria (Table 15.2) [2]. In patients with suspected ET, PV, or PMF, the evaluation begins with peripheral blood genetic testing for the Janus kinase-2 (*JAK2*) V617F mutation. Calreticulin exon 9 (*CALR*) mutation analysis from peripheral blood is next considered for suspected ET or PMF. Figure 15.1 summarizes the diagnostic steps.

Molecular Testing

Two mutations are present in the majority of MPN: *JAK2* V617F and *CALR* exon 9. They are mutually exclusive, with *JAK2* V617F being most prevalent (Table 15.1).

The *JAK2*V617F mutation is an acquired mutation in exon 14 of the Janus kinase-2 gene. JAK2 is a nonreceptor tyrosine kinase that is activated by several growth factors including erythropoietin, thrombopoietin, and granulocyte colony stimulating factor as well as numerous cytokines.

Activated JAK2 activates STAT protein, which ultimately results in cellular proliferation. In the normal state, JAK2 must be activated by the growth factor or cytokine; however, presence of the *JAK2*V617F mutation leads to the constitutive activation of JAK2, resulting in unchecked cellular proliferation.

While the *JAK2*V617F mutation has been shown to be quite specific for an underlying MPN, it does appear at a low prevalence in the general population without apparent MPN. The allele burden in these individuals is very low at <0.05% (allele burden is defined as the percentage of V617F alleles among the sum of V617F plus wild type *JAK2* alleles) suggesting that the typically accepted laboratory cut-off of ≥ 1% for a "positive" test result is reasonable to distinguish a "true positive" from a "false positive", especially when combined with clinical presentation.

There are several methods in widespread clinical use to detect the *JAK2*V617F mutation, each with varying sensitivity, though most are generally able to detect the mutation at a level of at least 5% allele burden. Quantification should be interpreted with caution, as the assays are often not standardized across different laboratories. Currently, there is little value in obtaining a quantitative allele burden analysis due to a lack of test standardization and current uncertainty as to its prognostic value. Allele quantification may be helpful in cases of monitoring for treatment response/residual disease after bone marrow transplant, perhaps interferon treatment, or in the research setting.

*JAK2*V617F mutation testing is generally carried out on the peripheral blood as it has essentially 100% concordance with testing from bone marrow aspirate. Granulocyte enrichment can be used to increase the test sensitivity (whole blood may be diluted by nonclonal lymphocytes and monocytes), but given the excellent sensitivity of the detection methods, is usually unnecessary. Note that samples collected into lithium heparin tubes may produce false-negative results as this anticoagulant may interfere with the assay.

Mutations in exon 9 of the calreticulin (*CALR*) gene were described in 2013 in approximately half of *JAK2* V617F-negative ET or PMF cases [3,4].

Table 15.2 World Health Organization (WHO) 2016 Diagnostic Criteria for the *BCR-ABL* negative myeloproliferative neoplasms [2].

	Polycythemia vera	Essential thrombocythemia	Primary myelofibrosis
Major criteria	1) Men: Hgb >16.5 g/dL or Hct > 49% Women: Hgb >16.0 g/dL or Hct >48%; or red cell mass >25% above predicted 2) BM biopsy[a] showing hypercellularity for age with trilineage growth including prominent erythroid, granulocytic, and megakaryocytic proliferation with pleomorphic, mature megakaryocytes 3) Presence of *JAK2V617F* or *JAK2* exon 12 mutation	1) Platelet count ≥450 × 10⁹/L 2) BM biopsy showing proliferation mainly of the megakaryocyte lineage with increased numbers of enlarged, mature megakaryocytes with hyperlobulated nuclei. No significant increase or left shift in neutrophil granulopoiesis or erythropoiesis and very rarely minor (grade 1) increase in reticulin fibers 3) Not meeting WHO criteria for CML, PV, PMF, MDS or other myeloid neoplasm 4) Presence of *JAK2, CALR,* or *MPL* mutation	1) BM biopsy with megakaryocyte proliferation and atypia, usually accompanied by reticulin and/or collagen fibrosis grade 2 or 3 2) Not meeting WHO criteria for ET PV, CML, MDS, or other myeloid neoplasm 3) Presence of *JAK2, CALR,* or *MPL* mutation or in the absence of these mutations, presence of another clonal marker,[b] or absence of reactive myelofibrosis[c]
Minor criteria	1) Low serum erythropoietin level	1) Presence of a clonal marker or absence of evidence for reactive thrombocytosis	1) Leukoerythroblastosis 2) Increased serum LDH 3) Anemia not attributable to another cause 4) Palpable splenomegaly 5) Leukocytosis (WBC ≥11.0 × 10⁹/L)
Diagnosis	1) All three major criteria *or* 2) First two major criterion + minor criterion	1) All four major criteria *or* 2) Three major criteria and minor criterion	1) All three major criteria + at least one minor criterion

a) BM biopsy may not be required in cases with sustained absolute erythrocytosis: Hgb levels >18.5 g/dL in men (Hct 55.5%) or >16.5 g/dL in women (Hct 49.5%) if major criterion 3 and the minor criterion are present. However, initial myelofibrosis (present in up to 20% of patients) can only be detected by performing a BM biopsy; this finding may predict progression to PMF.
b) In the absence of any of the 3 major clonal mutations, the search for the most frequent accompanying mutations (e.g., *ASXL1, EZH2, TET2, IDH1/IDH2, SRSF2, SF3B1*) are of help in determining the clonal nature of the disease.
c) BM fibrosis secondary to infection, autoimmune disorder, or other chronic inflammatory conditions, hairy cell leukemia or other lymphoid neoplasm, metastatic malignancy, or toxic (chronic) myelopathies.
BM, bone marrow; CML, chronic myelogenous leukemia; Hct, hematocrit; Hgb, hemoglobin; LDH, lactate dehydrogenase; MDS, myelodysplastic syndrome; PMF, primary myelofibrosis; PV, polycythemia vera; WHO, World Health Organization.

Though multiple mutations have been found in *CALR* exon 9, all have caused the same frameshift mutation and resultant mutant protein. The mechanism of mutated *CALR* on cellular proliferation has not yet been elucidated, though it appears to act on the JAK-STAT pathway. Patients with *CALR* mutations tend to have a phenotype of isolated thrombocytosis, with decreased risk of thrombosis and perhaps a better prognosis in PMF. As with *JAK2* testing, *CALR* testing is performed on the peripheral blood and is not expected to be found in healthy volunteers.

Several other mutations have been identified in MPN, with the most important being *JAK2* exon 12 mutations and *MPL* mutations. *JAK2* exon 12 mutations are present in 3% of *JAK2*V617F

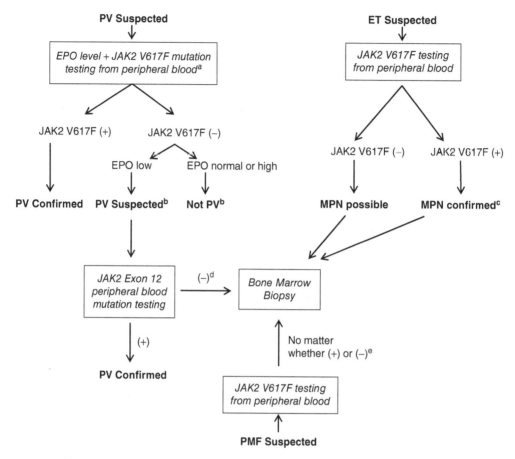

Figure 15.1 The diagnostic algorithm for the classic *BCR-ABL*-negative myeloproliferative neoplasms (MPNs) begins with peripheral blood *JAK2* V617F mutation testing, as the test has a good sensitivity and specificity for these diseases. A bone marrow biopsy should be considered in all patients both for diagnosis and prognosis. [a] The *JAK2* V617F mutation test is augmented by serum erythropoietin (EPO) testing in polycythemia vera (PV), as approximately 5% of PV patients will lack the mutation. [b] A further 3% of PV patients will have a mutation in the *JAK2* exon 12 and essentially all of these will have a low serum EPO level [35]. [c] Though an MPN is confirmed, a bone marrow biopsy is needed to distinguish between ET and prefibrotic primary myelofibrosis (PMF). [d] If clinical suspicion for PV remains high despite negative *JAK2* mutation testing, *CALR* mutation testing should be done. If mutation testing is negative, a bone marrow biopsy to evaluate for erythroid hyperplasia and bizarre megakaryocyte clusters is indicated. [e] Bone marrow biopsy needed for diagnostic and prognostic purposes.

(exon 14)-negative PV and generally impart a phenotype of isolated erythrocytosis without increase in platelets or white cells. The prevalence of thrombotic complications appears to be similar to the patient population with *JAK2* V617F mutation. Testing for *JAK2* exon 12 mutations should be performed for the evaluation of *JAK2* V617F-negative erythrocytosis in the presence of a low serum erythropoietin level. *JAK2* exon 12 mutations are very rare in ET and PMF

and should not be tested when evaluating for these disorders. The myeloproliferative leukemia (*MPL*) gene encodes the thrombopoietin receptor, and various *MPL* mutations have been found in ET and PMF, but not PV. *MPL* mutations are present in approximately 5% of ET and PMF and testing can be considered for *JAK2* V617F and *CALR* nonmutated cases if one is hesitant to proceed to a bone marrow biopsy or if bone marrow biopsy is equivocal. *MPL* gene mutations can be found in approximately 3% of *JAK*2V617F-negative ET and 10% of PMF cases (Table 15.1).

Which Patients Presenting with Thrombosis should be Tested for an MPN?

Up to 20% of patients with an MPN will have a thrombotic event at or prior to the diagnosis of their MPN disease. Nearly 15% of these patients will have no hematological manifestations of an underlying MPN [5]. In the absence of increased cell counts on CBC, certain thrombotic presentations should raise one's awareness for an underlying MPN (Table 15.3): splanchnic vein thrombosis in the absence of cirrhosis, trauma, or surgery, and to a lesser degree cerebral and sinus vein thrombosis (CSVT) in the absence of provoking factors. In such patients, *JAK*2V617F testing is indicated given the sensitivity, specificity, and noninvasiveness of the test and that a positive result changes management. To date, there has not been an investigation on the prevalence of *CALR* exon 9 mutations in unexplained thrombotic events. Neither the *JAK*2 exon 12 nor *MPL*515 mutation have been prevalent in thrombosis at unusual sites, though the literature is scant [6].

Pathophysiology of Thrombotic and Hemorrhagic Complications

The pathogenesis of thrombosis in the *BCR-ABL*-negative MPNs is complex. In the simplest terms, it is thought to result from overly active clonal cells and the host's inflammatory reaction to them. Especially in PV, the increased red cell mass may marginalize the already active platelets, allowing them to interact with the noninjured endothelium. As a result of the hyperactive cellular components, the level of procoagulant microparticles in the circulation is elevated, leading to increased thrombin generation, which is further sustained by an acquired activated protein C resistance[7]. It has been speculated that the *JAK*2V617F mutation plays a role in the pathogenesis of thrombotic events, especially arterial

events, though this is yet to be prospectively demonstrated and the mechanism explained. Though it is well recognized that splanchnic vein thrombosis is a hallmark of *BCR-ABL*-negative MPNs, the pathogenesis is poorly understood. Changes in endothelial cells, endothelial progenitor cells, and the splanchnic microenvironment may contribute to the underlying predisposition to clots in the splanchnic district.

Contrary to past beliefs, thrombocytosis does not result in a prothrombotic phenotype, but rather has been implicated in microvascular symptoms (i.e., erythromelalgia) and an increased bleeding tendency, especially in patients who are "platelet millionaires" (i.e., platelets >1000 × 10^9/L). Platelets in the *BCR-ABL*-negative MPNs appear to be hyper-responsive to arterial shear stress as found in the microvasculature where they can become activated, trapped, and release their contents, causing vasomotor disturbance and a local inflammatory response [8]. These platelets may then be released into the circulation in a "spent" form with reduced granular content and, thus, appear hypofunctioning on platelet aggregation assays.

The pathogenesis of hemorrhage also appears to be complex. Bleeding is often multifactorial, secondary to qualitative platelet abnormalities, thrombocytopenia (as the consequences of portal hypertension from splenomegaly or from bone marrow fibrosis), and use of antiplatelet agents. Additionally, acquired von Willebrand syndrome (AVWS) occurs in up to 11% of patients. Diminished von Willebrand factor (VWF) activity becomes more prevalent at higher platelet concentrations, presumably because the larger VWF multimers are adsorbed by the increased numbers of platelets and proteolyzed by myeloid enzymes.

Treatment – General Approach

The only currently known cure for the *BCR-ABL*-negative MPNs is bone marrow transplantation. MPN treatment is targeted at preventing or treating disease complications without promoting

Table 15.3 Patients with unexplained thrombosis – whom to test for an occult myeloproliferative neoplasm (MPN)?

Patient group	JAK2 V617F Prevalence of mutation	Test for mutation?	Perform a bone marrow biopsy?	Comments
PE or DVT of the extremity, initial event	0.2–0.9% [5,38]	No	No	
PE or DVT of the extremity, recurrent event	2% [39,40]	No	No	JAK2 positivity associated with age >70 years. It may therefore be reasonable to test selected older patients, though there may be no change in management as cytoreduction may not be indicated, beneficial or tolerated in the setting of a normal CBC
Splanchnic vein thrombosis	30–50% [5,6]	Yes	Yes	15% of JAK2V617F positive patients will present without overt features of an MPN, sometimes due to a relative normalization of the CBC from splenomegaly or variceal bleeding. Half of these patients will develop an overt MPN. JAK2 V617F prevalence is highest in BCS and young women. 7% of patients will have a JAK2V617F-negative MPN, so bone marrow biopsy is indicated in the evaluation
Cerebral and sinus vein thrombosis	0–7% [41]	Yes	No	Prevalence of JAK2V617F mutation in 2 largest series: ~6% Incidence of CSVT in general population: 3 : 1 000 000 Incidence of CVST in ET 1 : 100, suggesting an increased risk in this population [42,43] Despite overall low prevalence of the JAK2 mutation, testing positive will likely change management
Nonarteriosclerotic arterial thrombosis	<1% [44,45]	No	No	Very low prevalence of JAK2V617F mutation, even in patients less than 50 years old with ACS or with recurrent unexplained arterial thrombosis
Unexplained miscarriage	<1% [46,47]	No	No	Slight increase in JAK2V617F mutation prevalence over control (1% vs. 0.2%), but when population was enriched to include only ≥ 3 miscarriages before 10 weeks or ≥1 loss after 10 weeks, the mutation was found in 0/385 cases

In the absence of myeloproliferation on CBC, certain thrombotic presentations should raise one's awareness for an underlying overt MPN: splanchnic vein thrombosis/BCS in the absence of cirrhosis, trauma, or surgery; and to a lesser degree CSVT in the absence of provoking factors. Given the sensitivity, specificity, and noninvasiveness of the JAK2V617F mutation test, it serves as a useful screen for MPN in these otherwise occult situations. Neither the JAK2 exon 12 nor MPL515 mutations have thus far been prevalent in these conditions, though the literature is scant [6]. Testing for CALR exon 9 mutations is reasonable in JAK2 V617F-negative cases given the prevalence of the mutation ET; however, there is no literature to support this and CALR is associated with a lower rate of venous thrombosis overall.
ACS, acute coronary syndrome; BCS, Budd–Chiari syndrome; CSVT, cerebral sinus vein thrombosis; ET, essential thrombocytosis; CALR, calreticulin.

fibrotic or leukemic transformation or hemorrhage. As thrombosis is the major cause of mortality for patients with PV and ET, treatment decisions are primarily based on thrombotic risk in addition to disease symptoms, such as pruritus and erythromelalgia. The major cause of mortality in PMF is leukemic transformation followed by infections and thrombosis. As there is currently no way to halt leukemic transformation, therapy is intended for symptom management and prevention of thrombosis. Treatment decisions are further influenced by the individual's estimated life expectancy, which aids in the decision for bone marrow transplant, and tolerability of drugs. Enrollment into a clinical trial should always be considered.

Polycythemia Vera

Thrombosis Risk Stratification

Current laboratory tests are unfortunately unable to discern which patients will develop a thrombotic event. Instead, stratification relies on the nondisease-specific patient characteristics of advancing age and history of thrombosis (Table 15.4). This simple two-characteristic system stratifies patients into a "low" or "high" risk thrombosis category. To date, neither the presence of cardiovascular risk factors nor inherited thrombophilias are included in the risk stratification schema, as variable results have been obtained.

General Treatment

Patients at Low Risk for Thrombosis: In PV patients classified as "low risk", therapy consists of low-dose aspirin (assuming no increased bleeding tendency – refer to Table 15.4), phlebotomy to maintain hematocrit <45%, and optimization of cardiovascular health [9,10]. Cytoreductive therapy is not indicated in low-risk PV, unless the patient is intolerant of phlebotomy, the hematocrit cannot be effectively controlled with phlebotomy alone, there is symptomatic or progressive splenomegaly, progressive leukocytosis, bleeding diathesis due to AVWS, or there are severe disease-related symptoms not controlled with aspirin or other measures [9]. Phlebotomy will ultimately result in iron deficiency, which is the main mechanism by which it is effective in reducing the hematocrit. The resultant iron deficiency should,

Table 15.4 Management of polycythemia vera (PV) and essential thrombocythemia (ET).

Thrombotic risk category	Polycythemia vera	Essential thrombocythemia
Low No history of thrombosis Age <60 *(thrombotic risk: 1–2% per patient year)* [48,49]	Aspirin 81 to 100 mg + Phlebotomy to goal Hct <45%[a]	Aspirin 81 to 100 mg[b]
Low but with extreme thrombocytosis No history of thrombosis Age <60 Platelets >1000 × 10^9/L	Aspirin 81 to 100 mg[c] + Phlebotomy to goal Hct <45%	Aspirin 81 to 100 mg[c]
High History of thrombosis *or* Age ≥ 60 *(thrombotic risk: >5% per patient year)* [48,50]	Aspirin 81 to 100 mg + Phlebotomy to goal Hct <45% + Pharmacological cytoreduction	Aspirin 81 to 100 mg[d] + Pharmacological cytoreduction

Because there is currently no cure for ET or PV, the aim of management is to minimize thrombotic risk while not increasing bleeding risk or accelerating the transformation to acute leukemia. For ET, IPSET-thrombosis is undergoing validation to further refine the thrombotic risk classification with the addition of cardiovascular risk factors and *JAK2* V617F mutation status (Figure 15.2) [51].

a) In women, a hematocrit target of <42% should be considered [52]. Pharmacological cytoreduction should be initiated if the hematocrit goal is not reached with phlebotomy alone.

b) Recent expert opinion suggests that no aspirin therapy is advised in low-risk ET patients who are *JAK2* V617F negative and without cardiovascular risk factors [17].

c) If no history of unusual mucocutaneous bleeding and von Willebrand factor activity >30%.

d) Twice-daily aspirin is considered in high-risk *JAK2* V617F mutation positive patients, as once-daily dosing may be inadequate given the increase in platelet turnover [17]. In those patients already anticoagulated for prior VTE, the addition of aspirin is considered for patients with cardiovascular risk factors or *JAK2* V617F mutation.

Hct, hematocrit.

therefore, not be treated unless the patient becomes symptomatic. Iron deficiency may lead to thrombocytosis but should not alter therapy unless a bleeding tendency develops, at which point cytoreductive therapy is indicated.

Patients at high risk for thrombosis: In high-risk patients treatments/interventions are as for low-risk patients, plus the addition of a cytoreductive agent. The cytoreductive agent of choice is hydroxyurea or IFN-α at all ages, with busulfan, ^{32}P, and pipobroman reserved for the second line. Busulfan is the least leukemogenic of the second-line agents, with data showing no overall increased risk of leukemic transformation [11]. Patients whose symptoms are resistant to once-daily aspirin may benefit from twice daily low-dose aspirin because of increased platelet turnover [8].

Summary of Clinical Trials in Polycythemia Vera

Phlebotomy: As an elevated hematocrit leads to increased blood viscosity, reducing the hematocrit is a rational treatment approach in PV. Illustrative is that reducing the hematocrit from 53% to 45% results in a 73% increase in mean cerebral blood flow and a 30% reduction in blood viscosity. There has been one randomized trial evaluating the target hematocrit in PV, called "CYTO-PV". In this study, patients who maintained a hematocrit of <45% had significantly fewer major thrombotic events or death than those maintained at 45–50% [10]. It is, therefore, recommended that all PV patients maintain a hematocrit of <45%. Though CYTO-PV established that achieving a target hematocrit of <45% was beneficial, it was less clear if the methods to reach this goal (phlebotomy versus pharmacological cytoreduction) were equivalent. Additionally, there is speculation that a hematocrit of <42% is more appropriate for women, given that they, in general, have lower hematocrits than men, though this was not addressed in CYTO-PV [12].

Aspirin: Aspirin is indicated in all PV patients, as it reduces the risk of both arterial and venous

thrombosis and treats microvascular symptoms. This recommendation stems from the European Collaboration on Low-Dose Aspirin in Polycythemia Vera (ECLAP) trial, which randomized 518 low-risk PV patients to low-dose (100 mg) aspirin or placebo. Patients who received aspirin daily had a 60% reduction of significant thrombotic events and death without a significant increase in bleeding as compared to placebo [13]. Very-high-dose aspirin is not more effective than low-dose aspirin in PV: in a trial combining phlebotomy with high-dose aspirin (300 mg three times daily) plus dipyridamole versus ^{32}P, there was no increased efficacy in preventing thrombotic events with high-dose aspirin but there was a significant increase in bleeding events [14].

Hydroxyurea: Initial treatment trials in PV compared phlebotomy to ^{32}P, or chlorambucil, and demonstrated better thrombotic risk reduction with the cytoreductive agents over phlebotomy, but an increased incidence of acute leukemia and decreased survival with ^{32}P or chlorambucil. In an attempt to improve upon the efficacy of phlebotomy, which had a 23% risk of thrombotic events at 2 years (when hematocrit maintained <52%), a Phase II trial of hydroxyurea to maintain a hematocrit below 50% was conducted, which showed a 9% 2-year incidence of thrombosis in hydroxyurea-treated patients, a seeming improvement over treatment with phlebotomy alone. Additionally, leukemic transformation was not statistically different between hydroxyurea-treated patients and those receiving phlebotomy alone, suggesting an improvement in safety profile over the alkylating agents that had previously been investigated [14]. Further support to use hydroxyurea stems from the laboratory as it has been shown that hydroxyurea reduces some prothrombotic laboratory parameters in MPN patients (Table 15.5) [7,14].

Interferon-α: IFN-α is also used as a first-line cytoreductive agent in PV, especially in younger or pregnant patients, as it is not thought to be teratogenic or leukemogenic [9]. IFN-α has been

Table 15.5 Drugs used in the treatment of *BCR-ABL*-negative myeloproliferative neoplasms (MPNs).

	Hydroxyurea	Interferon-α	Anagrelide	Busulfan
Mechanism of action	Antimetabolite affecting all lines	Antiproliferative, affecting all lines	Phosphodiesterase-3 inhibitor, targets megakaryocytes	DNA alkylating agent, affects all lines
Usual dose	15 mg/kg/day PO	3 million units SC three times per week	0.5 mg–1.0 mg twice daily PO	2–4 mg/day PO
Toxicities	Pregnancy category D[a] Neutropenia, anemia, oral ulcers, rash, nail changes, hyperpigmentation	Pregnancy category C Dose-dependent flu-like and depressive symptoms	Pregnancy category C Fluid retention, diarrhea, nausea, palpitations, tachycardia, congestive heart failure, headache	Pregnancy category D Skin hyperpigmentation, xerostomia, ovarian suppression, myelosuppression
Tolerability	Good	Fair–poor 10–20% will discontinue due to side-effects	Fair	Fair
Leukemogenecity	Most recent data suggest no increased risk when used as a single agent [53]	Not implicated	Not implicated, though perhaps increased fibrotic transformation	Most recent data suggest no increase [11]
Comments	First-line treatment in high-risk PV and ET	Can induce molecular remissions Pegylated form may result in better tolerability Presently in trial vs. hydroxyurea[b]	Used in ET, generally as a second-line agent due to tolerability issues	Second-line agent, generally reserved for those >65 years

a) Despite this classification, there have been no reports of teratogenicity in MPN patients receiving hydroxyurea [32].
b) Clinical Trial NCT01259856, registered at *clinicaltrials.gov*
 PO, per os, orally; SC, subcutaneously.

shown in several small cohort studies to be very effective in achieving a complete hematological response, reducing splenomegaly and pruritus, and in some cases inducing a durable molecular remission. Additionally, in a long-term follow-up study of 55 PV patients treated with IFN-α (median follow-up of 13 years), none had thrombotic complications [15]. Given the potential disease-modifying capability of IFN-α as compared to hydroxyurea, clinical trials comparing the two are ongoing. A Phase III study comparing hydroxyurea with pegylated IFN-α 2a in newly diagnosed high-risk ET and PV patients is ongoing (NCT01259856), as is a Phase III study comparing low-dose IFN-α with HU in *BCR-ABL*-negative MPN (NCT01387763).

JAK-STAT Inhibitors: Inhibitors of the JAK/STAT pathway are under active study. As is the case with IFN-α, this class of drugs may alter the disease course in addition to providing symptomatic relief. Ruxolitinib has been compared to best available therapy (BAT) in hydroxyurea-resistant or intolerant patients with PV. Ruxolitinib resulted in phlebotomy independence in 60% of patients versus 20% treated with BAT, with durable responses [16]. Although not a primary endpoint, thromboembolic events were reduced in patients receiving ruxolitinib, with 1.8 thromboembolic events per 100 patient-years versus 8.2 per 100 patient-years in those receiving BAT. Ruxolitinib is now FDA-approved for PV patients intolerant of, or refractory to, hydroxyurea.

Essential Thrombocythemia

Thrombosis Risk Stratification

The cornerstones of thrombosis risk stratification in ET, as in PV, are also advancing age and prior history of thrombosis (Table 15.4). In 2012, the International Prognostic Score of Thrombosis in ET (IPSET-Thrombosis) further defined a three-tiered system that also considers the *JAK*2V617F mutation status and the presence of generic cardiovascular risk factors, though this has yet to be validated in prospective trials. In this system, 1 point each is given for age >60 years and cardiovascular risk factors and 2 points each for prior thrombosis and *JAK*2V617F mutation positivity. Low-risk (0–1 points), intermediate risk (2 points), or high risk (≥3 points) patients had a thrombosis risk of 1.0%, 2.4%, and 3.6% per year, respectively.

General Treatment

Patients at Low Risk for Thrombosis: ET patients at low risk for thrombosis are in general treated only with aspirin therapy (Table 15.4). In a recently proposed, tailored approach to ET that incorporates IPSET-thrombosis risk factors, stratification begins with the presence or absence of thrombosis (including whether arterial or venous), followed by further refinement with age ≥ 60 years, presence of cardiovascular risk factors and presence of the *JAK*2V617F mutation (Figure 15.2) [17]. For low-risk ET patients (age <60 years and no history of thrombosis), aspirin is indicated if the *JAK*2V617F mutation or cardiovascular risk factors are present.

Patients at High Risk for Thrombosis: Treatment is as for low-risk patients, with the addition of a cytoreductive agent. The cytoreductive treatment of choice is hydroxyurea. Anagrelide may also be considered in the first-line setting as it has been shown to be noninferior to hydroxyurea; however, it is ideally reserved for the second-line setting given its side-effect profile and limitation of targeting only the megakaryocytic lineage (Table 15.5). IFN-α may also be used, though its

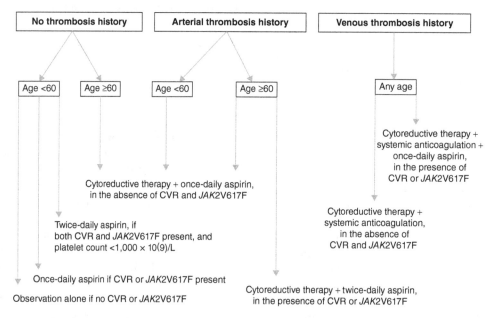

Figure 15.2 Tailored treatment for essential thrombocythemia (ET). A proposed algorithm for the treatment of ET incorporates *JAK*2V617F mutation status and the presence of cardiovascular risk factors to tailor therapy. Twice-daily aspirin may be considered in some cases, as there may be incomplete platelet inhibition by aspirin due to increased platelet turnover. CVR, cardiovascular risk factors. *Source:* Tefferi 2013, Figure 1 [31]. Reproduced with permission of Macmillan Publisher.

side-effect profile in general limits its front-line use. In the more tailored approach to ET, even patients younger than 60 years without prior thrombosis are considered "high risk" and cytoreduction is considered (Figure 15.2).

Summary of Clinical Trials in Essential Thrombocythemia

Aspirin: In a retrospective study of 300 patients with low-risk ET (as defined by age <60 and no history of prior thrombosis) who were either given low-dose aspirin therapy or no aspirin therapy, there was no difference in the incidence of thrombotic or bleeding complications among the groups; however, patients with the *JAK*2V617F mutation or cardiovascular risk factors had a higher incidence of thrombosis if they did not receive aspirin [18]. This study forms the recommendation to treat ET patients who have the *JAK*2V617F mutation or cardiovascular risk factors with low-dose aspirin therapy. Twice-daily dosing of aspirin may prove beneficial in aspirin-refractory or otherwise high-risk ET patients, because they have increased platelet turnover.

Hydroxyurea and Anagrelide: As in PV, hydroxyurea is generally the first-line cytoreductive agent. Recommendations are derived from the results of three clinical trials. In the first, 114 patients with high-risk ET were randomized to receive hydroxyurea or no cytoreductive therapy. The addition of hydroxyurea resulted in a 20% absolute risk reduction of thrombotic events, thus establishing its use in ET [19]. Hydroxyurea has also been compared to anagrelide in two randomized controlled trials: PT-1 and ANAHYDRET. In the first, 815 ET patients were randomized to receive aspirin plus either hydroxyurea or anagrelide. Hydroxyurea was better tolerated and was superior to anagrelide in reducing arterial (but not venous) thrombosis [20]. Additionally, there was a tendency for more fibrotic transformation in those treated with anagrelide. The classification of ET was updated in the WHO 2008 schema, and the ANAHYDRET study revisited the question of hydroxyurea versus anagrelide in this new classification system (which

excluded prefibrotic PMF), finding that anagrelide was noninferior to hydroxyurea [21].

Interferon-α: As in PV, IFN-α has been shown to induce molecular remissions in ET. It is not yet known how IFN-α treatment outcomes compare to the standard first-line agent hydroxyurea; as noted in the PV section above, a clinical trial to address this issue is ongoing.

JAK-STAT Inhibitors: Although *JAK1/2* inhibition is expected to result in control of platelet counts and symptomatic relief in patients with ET, no *JAK* inhibitor is presently approved for this indication. The RUXO-BEAT trial is underway comparing ruxolitinib to BAT in patients with high-risk ET or PV (NCT02577926).

Primary Myelofibrosis

Thrombosis Risk Stratification
Unlike PV and ET, there is not a dedicated thrombosis risk-stratification schema for PMF. Though thrombotic events seem to occur at a similar rate to ET and PV, the major causes of death are leukemic transformation and infection; thus, the disease risk stratification for PMF is based on survival prognosis rather than thrombotic risk. In a study of 700 PMF patients, advancing age, *JAK*2V617F mutation, and leukocytosis were associated with increased thrombotic risk [22]. However, in a separate study of 200 PMF patients, only history of thrombosis was associated with increased thrombotic risk [23]. Thus, it is unclear what characteristics confer the highest thrombotic risk in PMF.

General Treatment
There are no guidelines for thromboprophylaxis in patients with PMF. In this population, aspirin should be used with caution, given the bleeding tendency not only from thrombocytopenia but also from esophageal varices due to portal hypertension. In addition, it is not known whether prefibrotic PMF may have a different bleeding phenotype than PMF: aspirin was found to exacerbate the rate of hemorrhage in prefibrotic PMF patients [24]. Whether the risk of thrombosis can be altered with cytoreductive strategies, including

ruxolitinib, is unknown. Cytoreductive therapy should, however, be strongly considered in PMF patients over age 60 years or with prior thrombosis as tolerated by the peripheral blood counts. Thrombotic events in PMF are often in "provoked" settings such as surgery, and adequate prophylaxis in these high-risk situations is warranted.

Treatment – Specifics

Treatment of Established Thrombosis

As previously described, the risk of recurrent thrombotic events is increased in ET and PV patients older than 60 years and approaches >5 per 100 patient-years. Recurrent events tend to occur in the same vascular district as the initial clot [25].

Arterial

As noted in Table 15.1, the majority of thromboses among MPN patients occur in the arterial system, primarily in the cerebral and coronary vasculature. Primary prevention of thrombotic events consists of aspirin with or without cytoreductive therapy, depending on thrombosis risk, as discussed above. Secondary prevention, that is prevention of recurrent events, consists of the combination of low-dose aspirin and cytoreductive therapy (in addition to phlebotomy for PV). Interestingly, cytoreduction has retrospectively been shown to decrease the risk of recurrent acute coronary syndrome (ACS) by 70% but did not significantly reduce the risk of recurrent cerebrovascular accidents (CVA). The opposite was true for aspirin: an approximate 70% risk reduction was seen with aspirin in cerebrovascular accidents while a nonsignificant 25% risk reduction was seen in acute coronary syndrome [25].

Venous

The acute management of deep venous thrombosis (DVT) or pulmonary embolism (PE) is the same in the MPN population as in the general population. Though low-molecular-weight heparins (LMWH) are generally the preferred anticoagulant in cancer-associated VTE, there have been no studies comparing LMWH to warfarin in MPN patients. Presently, no data exist on the efficacy of the new oral anticoagulants for the treatment of DVT in MPNs.

Deep Venous Thrombosis of the Extremities or Pulmonary Embolism: The optimal length of anticoagulation for a first event of VTE in patients with MPN is somewhat controversial. It is generally agreed that all patients with either a provoked or unprovoked event should receive at least 3 months of anticoagulant therapy. Long-term anticoagulation can be considered in all MPN patients with venous thrombosis, given that they have a clonal disorder with a continued underlying thrombotic tendency. However, the circumstances of the VTE event (triggered by transient risk factors or unprovoked), bleeding risk factors, and patient preference are also factors to consider when deciding on length of anticoagulation.

Though thrombophilia testing is not universally recommended for patients with MPN, it may be reasonable to further risk-stratify patients with a provoked event because an additive effect seems to exist. Similarly, D-dimer testing may also be helpful to guide decision making; however, this has not been specifically studied in MPNs.

For many patients with VTE, cytoreduction in addition to anticoagulation will be instituted to normalize platelet count, hematocrit, and perhaps leukocyte count. Anticoagulation and cytoreduction appear to have similar efficacy in preventing recurrent thrombosis, approximately halving the risk; however, data behind this conclusion are sparse and come from retrospective analyses only. The combination of cytoreduction and long-term anticoagulation is better at preventing VTE recurrence than either alone, resulting in a 75% risk reduction at a median of 5 years [25]. Antiplatelet agents also reduced the risk of recurrence by over half; however, there was little additional protection afforded when combined with cytoreduction [25]. Though prospective studies are needed, the combination of cytoreductive therapy plus anticoagulation seems most prudent to reduce the thrombotic risk. In the patient who cannot tolerate anticoagulation, aspirin should be chosen.

Venous Thrombosis at Unusual Sites

MPN patients who have VTE at unusual sites are generally treated with long-term anticoagulation coupled with cytoreductive therapy, given the presumed associated high recurrence rate and morbidity in this population [26,27].

Splanchnic Vein Thrombosis: Thrombosis of hepatic, portal, splenic, or mesenteric veins is referred to as splanchnic vein thrombosis. When splanchnic vein thrombosis affects the liver outflow tract, Budd–Chiari syndrome (BCS) may occur. BCS may present with right upper quadrant pain, hepatomegaly, liver failure, and variceal bleeding and has a high mortality rate if untreated. Reports in all-comers of noncirrhotic patients with splanchnic vein thrombosis have shown a rate of up to 5 per 100 patient-years, and MPN was a risk factor for recurrence [26–28]. The risk of VTE recurrence in MPN patients with prior splanchnic vein thrombosis was 25% in one series, with 70% of events recurring in the splanchnic veins; anticoagulation was protective [27]. Though the recurrence rate is not well defined, because MPN is a risk factor for recurrence, it is reasonable to consider long-term anticoagulant therapy in addition to cytoreduction and aspirin in this group.

Cerebral and Sinus Vein Thrombosis: Among all-comers with cerebral and sinus vein thrombosis (CVST), the overall incidence of recurrent VTE at any site is approximately 2 per 100 patient-years. There are no specific studies examining the recurrence rate in MPN patients [28]. The role of long-term anticoagulation in the MPN patient with CVST therefore remains unclear, though cytoreduction plus aspirin should be continued long term.

Hemorrhage: Prevention and Management

Controversy exists as to whether or not cytoreductive therapy should be initiated for otherwise low-thrombotic-risk patients with extreme thrombocytosis [9,29,30]. Platelet counts in this range have not been shown to increase thrombotic risk, but, instead, seem to put patients at higher risk for hemorrhagic events secondary to platelet hypofunction, in part due to AVWS, especially when coupled with aspirin therapy. As such, the decision to begin cytoreductive therapy in patients who are asymptomatic, low thrombotic risk, and with extreme thrombocytosis is made on a case-by-case basis. If there are bleeding symptoms, cytoreduction should be initiated. Anagrelide should be used with caution in this setting until the platelet count is reduced and/or the AVWS resolves as it can further exacerbate bleeding risk. Prior to surgical procedures or before the initiation of aspirin in patients with extreme thrombocytosis, a VWF activity assay should be performed to ensure adequate hemostatic levels.

Treatment of hemorrhage associated with AVWS is aimed at (i) immediate correction of hemostasis and (ii) reduction of platelet count, as extreme thrombocytosis is associated with a reduction of high-molecular-weight VWF multimers. The best management of acute bleeding beyond routine supportive care is not known. Noteworthy is that (i) in a registry of AVWS patients with MPNs, desmopressin was effective in only 21% of cases (3/14 cases); (ii) factor VIII/VWF concentrates was effective in only 14% (2/14 cases); (iii) it is not known whether higher doses of factor VIII/VWF concentrate would be more effective; and (iv) while recombinant factor VIIa has been reported effective in >90% of AVWS of any cause, it is not known how often it is effective in the MPN subpopulation. Thus, in emergent bleeding settings, any of these treatment options, including antfibrinolytic therapy and platelet pheresis, can and should be considered [31].

Special Situations

Pregnancy

Pregnancy in patients with MPNs combines two thrombophilic states, leading to an increased risk of complications to both mother and fetus. The data on pregnancy outcomes in MPNs are sparse. These pregnancies have an increased rate of both hemorrhage and thrombosis over non-MPN pregnancies, with a 5% risk of postpartum

VTE as well as pre- or postpartum hemorrhage [32]. In ET approximately 25–40% of pregnancies end in first trimester loss, 10% late trimester loss, and approximately 5% are complicated by placental abruption or intrauterine growth restriction, all of which are higher than in non-MPN pregnancies [32]. Pregnancy outcomes appear similar to ET in PV and PMF.

Management guidelines in pregnancy are based on expert opinion and few retrospective studies and case reports, but no prospective studies. Management should begin in the pre-conception stage, with collaboration between hematology and high-risk obstetrics, because cytoreductive treatments may be teratogenic and because most pregnancy losses occur in the first trimester. Pregnancies are categorized as low risk or high risk based on maternal risk factors and prior pregnancy outcomes (Table 15.6). In the absence of a clear contraindication, low-dose daily aspirin is recommended for all patients. Prophylactic LMWH is generally commenced after delivery until 6 weeks postpartum for all patients and antepartum for those with a history of thrombotic events or recurrent miscarriage [9]. Cytoreduction is controversial given the inherent risks to the fetus and the uncertain

improvement to outcomes. If cytoreduction is chosen, IFN-α is the drug of choice (after the first trimester) bearing in mind that it is pregnancy category C. The hematocrit should be kept below 45%, and phlebotomy can be employed if needed.

In breast feeding, aspirin and LMWH are generally safe; however, the safety of cytoreductive therapies is less clear. Hydroxyurea is excreted in breast milk but the degree of excretion of anagrelide and IFN-α in breast milk is uncertain.

Contraception and Hormone Replacement Therapy

Estrogen-based oral contraceptives are associated with an increased risk of VTE and should be avoided if possible in women with MPN [33]. Though not specifically studied in MPNs, alternative forms of contraception, such as a progestin-releasing intrauterine device, would be a reasonable alternative because they have not been associated with an increased risk for VTE in the general population.

Estrogen hormone replacement therapy in a small study of women with ET was not associated with an increased risk of thrombotic events in MPN patients [33]. However, as in the general population, if hormone replacement therapy is

Table 15.6 Pregnancy management in myeloproliferative disorders – considerations.[a]

Risk category	Antepartum	Postpartum
Low risk	Aspirin (81–100 mg per day)[c] *plus* Phlebotomy to maintain Hct <45%	Aspirin (81–100 mg)
High risk[b]	Aspirin (81–100 mg per day)[c] *plus* Phlebotomy to maintain Hct <45% *plus* LMWH[c] (best dose unclear) *plus* IFN-α[d]	*plus* LMWH (best dose unclear) × 6 weeks

a) The best ante- and postpartum management is not known. Existing recommendations are based on expert opinion [9,32], rather than extensive data. Individualized decisions need to be made, weighing risk factors for thrombosis and bleeding, as well as patient preference. The strategy of LMWH combined with aspirin appears safe based on studies in antiphospholipid syndrome, but the use of cytoreductive agents is more controversial, with only anecdotal case reports.
b) High risk is defined as at least one of the following: (i) platelet count >1500 × 10^9/L, (ii) previous major thrombotic or bleeding complication in pregnancy or otherwise, (iii) previous severe pregnancy complications (>3 first trimester or >1 second or third trimester losses, birth weight less than 5th percentile for gestation, severe pre-eclampsia, placental abruption), (iv) diabetes or hypertension requiring treatment.
c) Consider no aspirin and no LMWH if previous major bleeding or platelet count >1500 × 10^9/L during pregnancy and in spite of IFN-α.
d) IFN-α is also considered if cytoreductive therapy was indicated prior to pregnancy.
   Hct, hematocrit; LMWH, low molecular weight heparin; IFN, interferon.

necessary, use of the lowest dose for the least amount of time is prudent.

Perioperative Management
Surgery poses a potential risk to MPN patients, with increased perioperative thrombotic and bleeding risk. Few data have been published on which to base risk assessments and treatment recommendations: one retrospective study of 255 ET or PV patients undergoing surgery and one case–control study of 13 MPN patients are reported [34]. In these studies, there was an overall fivefold increased risk of VTE in patients with MPNs undergoing surgery and a 30% rate of stroke in MPN patients undergoing cardiovascular surgery. Paradoxically, there was also an increased risk of perioperative bleeding at nearly 8%. Cytoreductive therapy is continued in high-risk patients and is initiated to control the blood counts to normal levels preoperatively in those who are not high risk. Antiplatelet therapy may need to be discontinued (anagrelide should not cause bleeding at the doses used to treat ET), and LMWH prophylaxis should be considered in the pre- and postoperative setting. However, decisions on best VTE prophylaxis (pharmacological versus mechanical method, anticoagulation intensity and length) need to be individualized.

Patient Resources

An excellent repository of information regarding MPNs can be found at www. MPNResearchFoundation.org and www. MPDinfo.org. A comprehensive patient brochure on *Thrombosis in Myeloproliferative Neoplasms* is in development by *Clot Connect* (www.clotconnect.org).

References

1 Stein BL, Saraf S, Sobol U, Halpern A, Shammo J, Rondelli D, *et al.* Age-related differences in disease characteristics and clinical outcomes in polycythemia vera. *Leukemia & lymphoma.* 2013;54(9):1989-95.

2 Arber DA, Orazi A, Hasserjian R, Thiele J, Borowitz MJ, Le Beau MM, *et al.* The 2016 revision to the World Health Organization classification of myeloid neoplasms and acute leukemia. *Blood.* 2016;127(20):2391-405.

3 Klampfl T, Gisslinger H, Harutyunyan AS, Nivarthi H, Rumi E, Milosevic JD, *et al.* Somatic mutations of calreticulin in myeloproliferative neoplasms. *The New England journal of medicine.* 2013;369(25):2379-90.

4 Nangalia J, Massie CE, Baxter EJ, Nice FL, Gundem G, Wedge DC, *et al.* Somatic CALR mutations in myeloproliferative neoplasms with nonmutated JAK2. *The New England journal of medicine.* 2013;369(25):2391-405.

5 Dentali F, Squizzato A, Brivio L, Appio L, Campiotti L, Crowther M, *et al.* JAK2V617F mutation for the early diagnosis of Ph– myeloproliferative neoplasms in patients with venous thromboembolism: a meta-analysis. *Blood.* 2009;113(22):5617-23.

6 Smalberg JH, Arends LR, Valla DC, Kiladjian J-J, Janssen HLA, Leebeek FWG. Myeloproliferative neoplasms in Budd-Chiari syndrome and portal vein thrombosis: a meta-analysis. *Blood.* 2012;120(25):4921-8.

7 Falanga A, Marchetti M. Thrombotic disease in the myeloproliferative neoplasms. *ASH Education Program Book.* 2012;2012(1): 571-81.

8 Michiels JJ, Berneman Z, Schroyens W, Koudstaal PJ, Lindemans J, Neumann HA, *et al.* Platelet-mediated erythromelalgic, cerebral, ocular and coronary microvascular ischemic and thrombotic manifestations in patients with essential thrombocythemia and polycythemia vera: a distinct aspirin-responsive and coumadin-resistant arterial thrombophilia. *Platelets.* 2006;17(8):528-44.

9 Barbui T, Barosi G, Birgegard G, Cervantes F, Finazzi G, Griesshammer M, *et al.* Philadelphia-negative classical myeloproliferative neoplasms: critical concepts and management recommendations from European LeukemiaNet. *Journal of clinical oncology : official journal of the American Society of Clinical Oncology.* 2011;29(6):761-70.

10 Marchioli R, Finazzi G, Specchia G, Cacciola R, Cavazzina R, Cilloni D, *et al.* Cardiovascular Events and Intensity of Treatment in Polycythemia Vera. *New England Journal of Medicine.* 2013;368(1):22-33.

11 Tefferi A, Rumi E, Finazzi G, Gisslinger H, Vannucchi AM, Rodeghiero F, *et al.* Survival and prognosis among 1545 patients with contemporary polycythemia vera: an international study. *Leukemia.* 2013.

12 Spivak JL. Polycythemia vera: myths, mechanisms, and management. *Blood.* 2002;100(13):4272-90.

13 Landolfi R, Marchioli R, Kutti J, Gisslinger H, Tognoni G, Patrono C, *et al.* Efficacy and Safety of Low-Dose Aspirin in Polycythemia Vera. *New England Journal of Medicine.* 2004;350(2):114-24.

14 Fruchtman SM, Mack K, Kaplan ME, Peterson P, Berk PD, Wasserman LR. From efficacy to safety: a Polycythemia Vera Study group report on hydroxyurea in patients with polycythemia vera. *Seminars in hematology.* 1997;34(1):17-23.

15 Silver RT. Long-term effects of the treatment of polycythemia vera with recombinant interferon-α. *Cancer.* 2006;107(3):451-8.

16 Verstovsek S, Vannucchi AM, Griesshammer M, Masszi T, Durrant S, Passamonti F, *et al.* Ruxolitinib versus best available therapy in patients with polycythemia vera: 80-week follow-up from the RESPONSE trial. *Haematologica.* 2016;101(7):821-9.

17 Tefferi A, Barbui T. Personalized management of essential thrombocythemia-application of recent evidence to clinical practice. *Leukemia.* 2013;27(8):1617-20.

18 Alvarez-Larran A, Cervantes F, Pereira A, Arellano-Rodrigo E, Perez-Andreu V, Hernandez-Boluda JC, *et al.* Observation versus antiplatelet therapy as primary prophylaxis for thrombosis in low-risk essential thrombocythemia. *Blood.* 2010;116(8):1205-10; quiz 387.

19 Cortelazzo S, Finazzi G, Ruggeri M, Vestri O, Galli M, Rodeghiero F, *et al.* Hydroxyurea for Patients with Essential Thrombocythemia and a High Risk of Thrombosis. *New England Journal of Medicine.* 1995;332(17):1132-7.

20 Harrison CN, Campbell PJ, Buck G, Wheatley K, East CL, Bareford D, *et al.* Hydroxyurea Compared with Anagrelide in High-Risk Essential Thrombocythemia. *New England Journal of Medicine.* 2005;353(1):33-45.

21 Gisslinger H, Gotic M, Holowiecki J, Penka M, Thiele J, Kvasnicka H-M, *et al.* Anagrelide compared with hydroxyurea in WHO-classified essential thrombocythemia: the ANAHYDRET Study, a randomized controlled trial. *Blood.* 2013;121(10):1720-8.

22 Barbui T, Carobbio A, Cervantes F, Vannucchi AM, Guglielmelli P, Antonioli E, *et al.* Thrombosis in primary myelofibrosis: incidence and risk factors. *Blood.* 2010;115(4):778-82.

23 Elliott MA, Pardanani A, Lasho TL, Schwager SM, Tefferi A. Thrombosis in myelofibrosis: prior thrombosis is the only predictive factor and most venous events are provoked. *Haematologica.* 2010;95(10):1788-91.

24 Finazzi G, Carobbio A, Thiele J, Passamonti F, Rumi E, Ruggeri M, *et al.* Incidence and risk factors for bleeding in 1104 patients with essential thrombocythemia or prefibrotic myelofibrosis diagnosed according to the 2008 WHO criteria. *Leukemia.* 2012;26(4):716-9.

25 De Stefano V, Za T, Rossi E, Vannucchi AM, Ruggeri M, Elli E, *et al.* Recurrent thrombosis in patients with polycythemia vera and essential thrombocythemia: incidence, risk factors, and effect of treatments. *Haematologica.* 2008;93(3):372-80.

26 Miranda B, Ferro JM, Canhao P, Stam J, Bousser MG, Barinagarrementeria F, *et al.* Venous thromboembolic events after cerebral vein thrombosis. *Stroke; a journal of cerebral circulation.* 2010;41(9):1901-6.

27 Amitrano L, Guardascione MA, Scaglione M, Pezzullo L, Sangiuliano N, Armellino MF, *et al.* Prognostic Factors in Noncirrhotic Patients With Splanchnic Vein Thromboses. *Am J Gastroenterol.* 2007;102(11):2464-70.

28 Riva N, Dentali F, Donadini MP, Squizzato A, Ageno W. Risk of recurrence of unusual site venous thromboembolism. *Hämostaseologie.* 2013;33(3):225-31.

29 Tefferi A. Polycythemia vera and essential thrombocythemia: 2013 update on diagnosis, risk-stratification, and management. *American journal of hematology*. 2013;88(6):507-16.

30 Tefferi A, Gangat N, Wolanskyj AP. Management of extreme thrombocytosis in otherwise low-risk essential thrombocythemia; does number matter? *Blood*. 2006;108(7):2493-4.

31 Tiede A, Rand JH, Budde U, Ganser A, Federici AB. How I treat the acquired von Willebrand syndrome. *Blood*. 2011;117(25):6777-85.

32 Harrison CN, Robinson SE. Myeloproliferative Disorders in Pregnancy. *Hematology/Oncology Clinics of North America*. 2011;25(2):261-75.

33 Gangat N, Wolanskyj AP, Schwager SM, Mesa RA, Tefferi A. Estrogen-based hormone therapy and thrombosis risk in women with essential thrombocythemia. *Cancer*. 2006;106(11):2406-11.

34 Ruggeri M, Rodeghiero F, Tosetto A, Castaman G, Scognamiglio F, Finazzi G, *et al.* Postsurgery outcomes in patients with polycythemia vera and essential thrombocythemia: a retrospective survey. *Blood*. 2008;111(2):666-71.

35 Scott LM. The JAK2 exon 12 mutations: A comprehensive review. *American journal of hematology*. 2011;86(8):668-76.

36 Gangat N, Caramazza D, Vaidya R, George G, Begna K, Schwager S, *et al.* DIPSS plus: a refined Dynamic International Prognostic Scoring System for primary myelofibrosis that incorporates prognostic information from karyotype, platelet count, and transfusion status. *Journal of clinical oncology : official journal of the American Society of Clinical Oncology*. 2011;29(4):392-7.

37 Casini A, Fontana P, Lecompte TP. Thrombotic complications of myeloproliferative neoplasms: risk assessment and risk-guided management. *Journal of Thrombosis and Haemostasis*. 2013;11(7):1215-27.

38 Rodger MA, Kekre N, Le Gal G, Kahn SR, Wells PS, Anderson DA, *et al.* Low prevalence of JAK2 V617F mutation in patients with first unprovoked venous thromboembolism. *British Journal of Haematology*. 2011;155(4):511-3.

39 Pardanani A, Lasho TL, Schwager S, Finke C, Hussein K, Pruthi RK, *et al.* JAK2V617F prevalence and allele burden in non-splanchnic venous thrombosis in the absence of overt myeloproliferative disorder. *Leukemia*. 2007;21(8):1828-9.

40 Remacha AF, Estivill C, Sarda MP, Mateo J, Souto JC, Canals C, *et al.* The V617F mutation of JAK2 is very uncommon in patients with thrombosis. *Haematologica*. 2007;92(2):285-6.

41 Casini A, Fontana P, Lecompte TP. Thrombotic complications of myeloproliferative neoplasms: risk assessment and risk-guided management. *Journal of thrombosis and haemostasis : JTH*. 2013;11(7):1215-27.

42 Bazzan M, Tamponi G, Schinco P, Vaccarino A, Foli C, Gallone G, *et al.* Thrombosis-free survival and life expectancy in 187 consecutive patients with essential thrombocythemia. *Annals of hematology*. 1999;78(12):539-43.

43 De Stefano V, Rossi E, Za T, Ciminello A, Betti S, Luzzi C, *et al.* JAK2 V617F mutational frequency in essential thrombocythemia associated with splanchnic or cerebral vein thrombosis. *American journal of hematology*. 2011;86(6):526-8.

44 Sène D, Elalamy I, Ancri A, Cacoub P. JAK2V617F mutation is not associated with unexplained recurrent arterial and venous thrombosis. *Thrombosis Research*. 2008;122(3):427-8.

45 Dentali F, Squizzato A, Appio L, Brivio L, Ageno W. JAK2V617F mutation in patients with arterial thrombosis in the absence of overt myeloproliferative disease. *Journal of Thrombosis and Haemostasis*. 2009;7(4):722-5.

46 Dahabreh IJ, Jones AV, Voulgarelis M, Giannouli S, Zoi C, Alafakis-Tzannatos C, *et al.* No evidence for increased prevalence of JAK2 V617F in women with a history of recurrent miscarriage. *Br J Haematol*. 2009;144(5):802-3.

47 Mercier E, Lissalde-Lavigne G, Gris JC. JAK2 V617F mutation in unexplained loss of first pregnancy. *The New England journal of medicine*. 2007;357(19):1984-5.

48 Marchioli R, Finazzi G, Landolfi R, Kutti J, Gisslinger H, Patrono C, *et al.* Vascular and Neoplastic Risk in a Large Cohort of Patients

With Polycythemia Vera. *Journal of Clinical Oncology*. 2005;23(10):2224-32.

49 Ruggeri, Finazzi, Tosetto, Riva, Rodeghiero, Barbui. No treatment for low-risk thrombocythaemia:results from a prospective study. *British Journal of Haematology*. 1998;103(3):772-7.

50 Cortelazzo S, Viero P, Finazzi G, D'Emilio A, Rodeghiero F, Barbui T. Incidence and risk factors for thrombotic complications in a historical cohort of 100 patients with essential thrombocythemia. *Journal of Clinical Oncology*. 1990;8(3):556-62.

51 Barbui T, Finazzi G, Carobbio A, Thiele J, Passamonti F, Rumi E, *et al*. Development and validation of an International Prognostic Score of thrombosis in World Health Organization–essential thrombocythemia (IPSET-thrombosis). *Blood*. 2012;120(26):5128-33.

52 Spivak JL. Polycythemia vera, the hematocrit, and blood-volume physiology. *The New England journal of medicine*. 2013;368(1):76-8.

53 Bjorkholm M, Derolf AR, Hultcrantz M, Kristinsson SY, Ekstrand C, Goldin LR, *et al*. Treatment-related risk factors for transformation to acute myeloid leukemia and myelodysplastic syndromes in myeloproliferative neoplasms. *Journal of clinical oncology : official journal of the American Society of Clinical Oncology*. 2011;29(17):2410-5.

16

Arterial Thrombosis

R. Campbell Tait and Catherine N. Bagot

Key Points

- All manifestations of cardiovascular disease share the traditional risk factors of smoking, hypertension, diabetes, abdominal obesity, and dyslipidemia.
- Primary prevention of cardiovascular disease should focus on lifestyle advice and pharmacological treatments to correct remedial risk factors.
- Antiplatelet therapy is no longer recommended for primary prevention of cardiovascular disease.
- Antiplatelet agents remain the primary treatment for secondary prevention of cardiovascular disease.
- Most atrial fibrillation patients, even those with relatively low stroke risk (CHA_2DS_2-VASc score >1), will likely receive overall net benefit from anticoagulant therapy.

Introduction

Arterial thrombosis is a common cause of hospital admission, death, and disability in developed countries and increasingly in developing nations. It usually follows spontaneous rupture of an atherosclerotic plaque or embolization of preformed thrombus, and may:

- be clinically silent;

- contribute to atherosclerotic progression resulting in coronary artery stenosis and stable angina, or lower limb artery stenosis and claudication;
- present as acute ischemia in the heart (acute coronary syndromes: unstable angina, myocardial infarction), brain (transient cerebral ischemic attack or stroke), or limb (acute limb ischemia).

There is now good evidence that patients with acute ischemic syndromes have lower morbidity and mortality if they are promptly diagnosed, admitted as soon as possible to specialist acute units, undergo risk stratification, and receive appropriate treatment. This includes antithrombotic drugs and consideration of thrombolysis, thrombectomy, angioplasty, or vascular reconstruction in the acute phase and subsequent early, multidisciplinary rehabilitation.

Hematologists are commonly asked to develop local guidelines on investigation and management of patients with arterial thrombosis. In addition, they are often referred patients with arterial thrombosis that is premature, recurrent, or which occurs at multiple or unusual sites. This review therefore focuses on the recognized modifiable risk factors and appropriate hematological investigations in patients with arterial thrombosis, and appropriate antithrombotic therapy in various patient groups.

Practical Hemostasis and Thrombosis, Third Edition. Edited by Nigel S. Key, Michael Makris and David Lillicrap.
© 2017 John Wiley & Sons, Ltd. Published 2017 by John Wiley & Sons, Ltd.

Risk Factors

Cardiovascular Disease

Traditional risk factors (Table 16.1) remain the most important markers for arterial disease and together account for up to 90% of population attributable risk [1,2]. Every opportunity should be taken to encourage patients to adjust their lifestyles and consider pharmacological secondary prevention in those with clinical evidence of arterial disease (Table 16.2).

There are a number of existing systematic reviews and evidence-based national guidelines, such as those produced by the American Heart Association / American College of Chest Physicians, the British Committee for Standards in Haematology (BCSH), the European Society of Cardiology, the National Institute for Health and Clinical Excellence (NICE), and the Scottish Intercollegiate Guidelines Network (SIGN).

Atrial Fibrillation

Atrial fibrillation (AF) is the most common cardiac arrhythmia, with a prevalence of around 1.5% in the adult population. Recognized precipitants include thyrotoxicosis, cardiomyopathy, and rheumatic heart disease, especially that causing mitral stenosis; however, the majority of cases are nonvalvular showing a strong association with increasing age. AF confers a fivefold increased risk of stroke and is estimated to be responsible for 20% of all stroke events. Furthermore, stroke occurring in the presence of AF carries a higher morbidity and mortality rate. Anticoagulant therapy with a vitamin K antagonist (VKA) provides a 68% relative risk reduction of stroke events in patients with AF [3], but at a cost of increased major bleeding. Therefore, careful assessment of a patient's risk of stroke without anticoagulation and of bleeding with anticoagulation is required.

Key factors influencing stroke risk have been identified from epidemiological and randomized controlled trials, and a variety of scoring systems have been developed and compared [4]. Over the last decade the most widely used has been the $CHADS_2$ scheme which recognizes congestive cardiac failure, hypertension, age >75 years, diabetes, and prior stroke or systemic embolism as key risk factors [5]. However, this has been updated as the CHA_2DS_2VASc score, which adds more weight to increasing age and also recognizes the relevance of existing vascular disease (e.g., prior myocardial infarction or peripheral vascular disease) and female sex [6].

Table 16.1 Risk factors for cardiovascular disease [2,47,48].

Risk factor	Adjusted odds ratio[a]	95% confidence interval
Dyslipidemia	3.25	2.81–3.76
Current smoker	2.87	2.58–3.19
Diabetes	2.37	2.07–2.71
Hypertension	1.91	1.74–2.10
Abdominal obesity	1.62	1.45–1.80
Psychosocial factors	2.67	2.21–3.22
Previous venous thrombosis	1.60	1.35–1.91
Hormone replacement therapy (estrogen and progestogen)	1.81	1.09–3.01
Daily fruit and vegetables	0.70	0.62–0.79
Regular exercise	0.86	0.76–0.97
Alcohol intake	0.91	0.82–1.02

a) Odds ratios quoted are for coronary heart disease, however these risk factors are also significant for ischaemic stroke [49].

Table 16.2 Summary of lifestyle advice and pharmacological prevention of cardiovascular disease [50,51].

Lifestyle advice (primary and secondary prevention)

Stop or reduce smoking (cigarette, cigar, or pipe)

Take regular exercise (e.g., walk 30 minutes most days per week)

Lose weight if overweight (BMI >25 kg/m^2) or obese (BMI >30 kg/m^2)

Diet: reduce salt and saturated fat; increase fruit, vegetables, and fish

Moderate alcohol consumption (<2–3 units/day for women, <3–4 units/day for men); avoid binge drinking

Pharmacological

Antiplatelet agents are not recommended for primary prevention of cardiovascular disease

Antiplatelet agents are indicated for secondary prevention in all patients with clinical cardiovascular disease (unless vitamin K antagonist or new oral anticoagulant also indicated)

Blood pressure reduction (if not achieved by lifestyle advice) to a target of <140/90 mmHg

Beta-blocker following acute coronary syndrome (unless contraindicated)

ACE inhibitor following acute coronary syndrome with or without LV dysfunction

Cholesterol reduction (usually with a statin at dose of proven efficacy in cardiovascular reduction)

Aspirin + P2Y12 inhibitor (e.g., clopidogrel, ticagrelor, or prasugrel) for 3–12 months following acute coronary syndrome with/without addition of PCI + stent, with continuation of aspirin 75 mg/day indefinitely

Clopidogrel 75 mg/day alone or dipyridamole slow-release (200 mg bd) + aspirin 75 mg/day in patients with ischemic stroke or TIA

Oral anticoagulation, e.g., with warfarin (at target INR 2.0–3.0), dabigatran, rivaroxaban or apixaban in patients with atrial fibrillation with previous history of ischemic stroke or other thromboembolic event; or at high risk of thromboembolism (CHA$_2$DS$_2$-VASc score ≥ 2)

ACE, angiotensin-converting enzyme; BMI, body mass index; INR, international normalized ratio; LV, left ventricle; PCI, percutaneous intervention; TIA, transient ischemic attack.

The CHA$_2$DS$_2$VASc risk scoring system, summarized in Table 16.3, has been validated in large cohorts (Table 16.4) and is now the preferred

Table 16.3 CHA$_2$DS$_2$-VASc risk stratification index for patients with nonvalvular atrial fibrillation [6,52].

Risk factor	Allocated score
Congestive heart failure/ left ventricle dysfunction	1
Hypertension	1
Age ≥75 years	2
Diabetes mellitus	1
Stroke / transient ischemic attack / arterial embolism	2
Vascular disease (prior myocardial infarction, peripheral artery disease, or aortic plaque)	1
Age 65–74	1
Sex **c**ategory (female)	1

risk assessment scheme for patients with AF as recommended by the European Society of Cardiology [7]. It is particularly helpful in identifying very low risk patients (men scoring 0 or women scoring 1) who are unlikely to benefit

Table 16.4 Stroke risk according to CHA$_2$DS$_2$-VASc score – Danish data from 73 538 hospitalized patients with atrial fibrillation who were not treated with vitamin K antagonists.

CHA$_2$DS$_2$-VASc score	Thromboembolism rate[a] per 100 person years (95% confidence interval)
0	0.78 (0.58–1.04)
1	2.01 (1.70–2.36)
2	3.71 (3.36–4.09)
3	5.92 (5.53–6.34)
4	9.27 (8.71–9.86)
5	15.26 (14.35–16.24)
6	19.74 (18.21–21.41)
7	21.50 (18.75–24.64)
8	22.38 (16.29–30.76)
9	23.64 (10.62–52.61)

Source: Olesen *et al.* 2011 [53]. Reproduced with permission of BMJ.
a) Includes peripheral artery embolism, ischemic stroke, and pulmonary embolism.

from anticoagulation [8]. AF is also discussed in Chapter 20.

Laboratory Investigations

Table 16.5 outlines routine and specialist investigations that are applicable to patients with arterial thrombosis or ischemia.

Routine Laboratory Investigations

Routine hematology investigations include:

- full blood count as a screen for anemia, polycythemia, hyperleukocytic leukemias, and thrombocytosis [9];
- erythrocyte sedimentation rate (ESR) or plasma viscosity as a screen for hyperviscosity syndromes and connective tissue disorders and/ or vasculitis, e.g., temporal arteritis, systemic lupus erythematosus, polyarteritis nodosa. Hyperviscosity syndromes may require urgent plasma exchange, plasmapheresis, or cytapheresis; vasculitis may require urgent steroid or cytotoxic therapy and biopsy [9].

Acute elevations in white cell count and platelet counts, ESR, or plasma viscosity, and other acute phase reactants, such as C-reactive protein and fibrinogen, are common in acute ischemic syndromes; but persistent elevations (e.g., more than 1 month that are unexplained by complications, such as infections, limb necrosis, or venous thromboembolism) should raise the suspicion of underlying connective tissue disorder or malignancy.

Routine biochemical investigations include:

- lipid profile, specifically low-density lipoprotein and high-density lipoprotein cholesterol;
- glucose, or another measure of insulin resistance; and
- thyroid screen for evidence of underlying thyrotoxicosis in patients with atrial fibrillation.

Careful control of diabetes and reduction of cholesterol have proven value in reduction of both primary and secondary vascular disease in affected individuals.

Table 16.5 Summary of laboratory tests in persons with arterial thromboembolism.

Routine
Full blood count
anemia (promotes ischemia)
polycythemia
hyperleukocytic leukemias
thrombocytosis
ESR/ plasma viscosity
hyperviscosity syndromes
vasculitis/ connective tissue disorders
Cholesterol
total cholesterol or LDL : HDL ratio predicts arterial disease
Glucose
diabetes mellitus
Thyroid function tests
thyrotoxicosis is a cause of atrial fibrillation
Specialized
Homocysteine
if arterial thrombosis at age <30 years
Sickle cell screening
in persons at ethnic risk
Lupus anticoagulant and anticardiolipin antibodies
if arterial events at age under 50 years, without prominent clinical risk factors
Congenital thrombophilias
utility unproven
Coagulation factors
utility unproven
Fibrin D-dimer
utility unproven
Fibrinolytic factors
utility unproven
Platelet function studies
utility unproven (e.g., for aspirin resistance)

ESR, erythrocyte sedimentation rate; HDL, high-density lipoprotein; LDL, low-density lipoprotein.

Specialized Laboratory Investigations

These should be reserved for patients in whom clinical assessment suggests a reasonable expectation of finding a "thrombophilia" that may alter clinical management. Overinvestigation will result in identification of laboratory "abnormalities" that are irrelevant to clinical management. Table 16.5 summarizes indications for particular tests in adults.

Thrombosis in childhood (apart from that associated with central venous catheters) is uncommon and requires specialist assessment by a pediatric hematologist. The reader is referred to Chapter 27 for more information.

Homocysteine Measurement

This is indicated in all patients with premature (age under 30) arterial thrombosis, to exclude homocystinuria, a rare autosomal recessive disorder. If this diagnosis is confirmed, the patient should be managed by a specialist in metabolic medicine. In contrast, the value of screening for mild–moderate hyperhomocysteinemia in the secondary prevention of arterial thrombosis in patients aged over 30 years is unproven.

Sickle Cell Screening

This may be appropriate in persons at ethnic risk, although, in practice, a diagnosis of sickle cell disease will usually have been made long before adulthood. Large- and small-vessel vaso-occlusive events are responsible for the protean manifestations of sickle cell disease.

Screening for Lupus Anticoagulant and Anticardiolipin Antibodies

This is appropriate in all patients with premature (<50 years) cerebral or limb thrombosis or ischemia, provided there are no other identifiable risk factors [10]. Management of the antiphospholipid syndrome is considered in Chapter 19.

Screening for Congenital Thrombophilia

Conflicting results have been obtained when investigating the link between arterial disease and the factor V Leiden and prothrombin G20210A mutations: some studies have shown modest but statistically significant associations with coronary heart disease (CHD), stroke, and peripheral arterial events, especially in younger persons (<55 years) and in women, whereas others have

demonstrated no link using multivariate analysis [11]. However, these findings may have relevance to the increase in risk of coronary and stroke events during pregnancy or with use of combined oral contraceptives or oral hormone replacement therapy, because both are associated with an acquired resistance to activated protein C.

There is little evidence that other congenital thrombophilias are associated with increased risk of arterial disease, and the clinical value of screening for such abnormalities in patients with arterial thrombosis is at present unproven [12]. Furthermore, there is no evidence that secondary prevention with oral anticoagulants in such patients is more effective than routine antithrombotic prevention with aspirin (Table 16.2).

Ischemic stroke may be associated with a right-to-left intracardiac shunt, for example patent foramen ovale or atrial septal defect in younger patients, suggesting the possibility of "paradoxical" cerebral arterial embolism from venous thrombosis. Whether such events are commonly associated with thrombophilia is unknown, as are the relative benefits and risks of prophylaxis with aspirin, oral anticoagulants, or shunt closure [13].

Coagulation Factors

Plasma fibrinogen levels are associated with CHD, stroke, and peripheral arterial events; the risks increase by 30–40% per 1 g/L increase [14]. Although there are several plausible biological mechanisms through which increased circulating fibrinogen levels might promote such risk (atherogenic, thrombogenic, and rheological via increased blood viscosity), the lack of association of functional genetic polymorphisms with risk of CHD argues against causality. The association of fibrinogen with arterial risk may therefore be coincidental (because of mutual associations with multiple risk factors) or consequential (reverse causality, resulting from effects of atherosclerosis on plasma fibrinogen) [15]. The clinical utility of plasma fibrinogen assessment in the assessment of arterial thrombosis is therefore unproven.

Von Willebrand factor (VWF) is weakly associated with risk of CHD, and reduced VWF levels have been demonstrated to have a protective effect against both coronary artery disease (odds ratio (OR) 0.28; 95% confidence interval (CI) 0.14–0.54, P <0.0001) and cerebrovascular disease (OR 0.28; 95% CI 0.10–0.77, P = 0.01) [16,17]. Female carriers of hemophilia who have plasma levels of factor VIII or IX that are 50% lower than noncarriers have an estimated 35% lower risk of CHD [18]. Similarly, males with hemophilia have approximately 80% lower risk of fatal CHD compared with unaffected men.

However, it remains unproven that assessment of plasma levels of VWF, factor VIII, or factor IX in patients with arterial disease will affect outcome or alter management.

Coagulation Activation Markers
Plasma fibrin D-dimer levels are associated with increased risks of incident CHD and stroke, including in patients with atrial fibrillation [19–21]. Although D-dimer levels might therefore be useful in predicting stroke in atrial fibrillation, further management studies are required.

Fibrinolytic Tests
Circulating levels of tissue plasminogen activator (tPA) antigen, but not of plasminogen activator inhibitor type 1 (PAI-1), are associated with increased risk of CHD in population studies. However, this association is markedly reduced after adjustment for associated CHD risk factors such as obesity and other markers of insulin resistance [22]. Elevated alpha 2-antiplasmin levels have been shown to be independently associated with an increased risk of myocardial infarction, and thrombin activatable fibrinolysis inhibitor (TAFI) appears to be a risk factor for ischaemic stroke, although less consistent results have been obtained with the latter for coronary artery disease [23,24]. Overall, the clinical utility of measuring plasma components of the fibrinolytic system in the management of arterial thrombosis remains unproven.

Platelet Function Tests
Platelet aggregation studies and measures of platelet activation are not useful in the prediction of arterial thrombosis. Although there is

increasing evidence that aspirin resistance, defined as a laboratory measure of the failure of aspirin to inhibit platelet synthesis of thromboxane A_2, platelet aggregation, or the skin bleeding time, is associated with increased risk of recurrent cardiovascular events, further work is required to define the place of such laboratory measures in clinical practice [25].

Thrombin Generation
Thrombin generation as measured by calibrated automated thrombography (CAT) is a promising marker of thrombotic phenotype compared to measurement of individual factor levels. Most work to date has evaluated its role in the prediction of first and recurrent venous thrombosis, but there is also evidence that patients with arterial disease demonstrate increased thrombin generation [26–29]. However, it is unknown how thrombin generation assays correlate with clinical outcomes. Furthermore, significant work is still required to standardize thrombin generation before it can be used in routine clinical care.

Treatment

Primary Prevention of Arterial Thrombosis

Until 2009, most guidelines recommended aspirin for primary prevention of cardiovascular disease in asymptomatic individuals if their estimated 10-year risk of cardiovascular disease exceeded 30%, or of coronary heart disease exceeded 20%. However, recent re-evaluation of aspirin in high-risk patients, including diabetics, showed no or minimal cardiovascular benefit and a trend to increased bleeding risk [30–32]. A subsequent meta-analysis by the Antithrombotic Trialists' Collaboration demonstrated that primary prevention with aspirin reduced the vascular event rate by 6/10 000 patient years but increased the rate of major bleeding events by 3/10 000 patient years [33]. Currently, therefore, primary prevention with antiplatelet agents cannot be recommended.

Secondary Prevention of Arterial Thrombosis

Acute treatment and secondary prevention strategies of cardiovascular disease primarily involve antiplatelet agents. Treatment of acute coronary syndromes is discussed in more detail in Chapter 20, with secondary prevention also summarized in Table 16.2. There have been recent advances in acute management of myocardial infarction and other acute coronary syndromes using other anticoagulant (low-molecular-weight heparins or fondaparinux) or antiplatelet agents (glycoprotein IIb/IIIa and P2Y12 inhibitors) [34]. Clopidogrel is now favored over the combination of aspirin and dipyridamole in the treatment and secondary prevention of ischemic stroke [35], while the evidence for the use of aspirin (although common practice) in secondary prevention in patients with peripheral arterial disease remains weak [36]. In patients with recurrent events despite aspirin, possible empirical approaches are to add a second antiplatelet agent, to increase the dose of aspirin, or to change to oral anticoagulant therapy.

Atrial Fibrillation

Randomized controlled trials and subsequent meta-analyses in the 1990s demonstrated the superiority of VKAs over aspirin in the primary and secondary prevention of stroke and systemic thromboembolism in patients with AF. Recently, the threshold at which VKAs are thought to have overall net benefit has fallen from a CHADS$_2$ score of ≥ 2 to a CHA$_2$DS$_2$-VASc score >1 (Figure 16.1). Furthermore, the role of aspirin in patients with very low stroke risk is now debated, with recommendations for no antithrombotic therapy in patients with a CHA$_2$DS$_2$-VASc score of zero [7].

In addition to estimating the thromboembolism risk, it is also recommended that each patient has a bleeding risk assessment so that patients with a relatively low stroke risk but high bleeding risk can be advised against anticoagulant therapy. A variety of bleeding risk scores have been developed with the HAS-BLED score being the simplest [37].

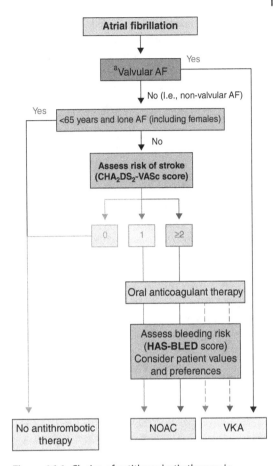

Figure 16.1 Choice of antithrombotic therapy in patients with atrial fibrillation. Antiplatelet therapy with aspirin plus clopidogrel, or less effectively aspirin only, should be considered in patients who refuse any oral anticoagulant, or cannot tolerate anticoagulants for reasons unrelated to bleeding. If there are contraindications to VKA, NOAC or antiplatelet therapy, left atrial appendage occlusion, closure or excision may be considered. [a] Includes rheumatic valvular disease and prosthetic valves. AF, atrial fibrillation; NOAC, novel oral anticoagulant; VKA, vitamin K antagonist. Solid line, best option; dashed line, alternative option. *Source:* Camm *et al.* 2012 [7]. Reproduced with permission of Oxford University Press.

The role of VKAs as first-choice anticoagulants for AF is now being challenged by the novel oral anticoagulant agents dabigatran (a direct thrombin inhibitor) and direct factor Xa inhibitors (rivaroxaban, apixaban, and edoxaban), which are discussed in detail in Chapter 18.

These new agents, which have a wide therapeutic window, few drug and food interactions, and require no anticoagulant monitoring, have been shown in large randomized trials to be at least as efficacious and possibly safer than warfarin [38–40]. Indeed, the latest recommendations from the European Society of Cardiology [7] favor these new agents over warfarin (Figure 16.1).

Combination Therapy with Vitamin K Antagonists and Antiplatelet Agents

An increasingly problematic issue in clinical practice has been to determine the risk–benefit ratios for combination treatment, either in patients already receiving a VKA who develop an indication for aspirin (e.g., a patient being treated for recent DVT who then suffers an acute coronary syndrome) or a patient on aspirin who develops an indication for a VKA (e.g., a patient with previous myocardial infarction developing atrial fibrillation). Management of such patients has to be individualized, considering the patient's thrombotic and bleeding risks. However, there is evidence in the literature that can inform decision making:

- In patients with AF, the combination of aspirin + clopidogrel is inferior to VKA (INR 2-3) in terms of stroke prevention, and is associated with similar bleeding rates [41].
- In patients with AF, the addition of aspirin to VKA is associated with a higher risk of major bleeding [42].
- In patients with peripheral arterial disease treated with aspirin, the addition of VKA does not reduce the cardiovascular event rate, but does increase the rate of life-threatening bleeding [43].
- In patients with stable coronary artery disease, VKAs are as effective as aspirin at reducing the risk of further ischemic events, albeit with an increased risk of major bleeding. Aspirin plus VKA is not significantly better than VKA alone [44].
- In high thrombotic risk patients with prosthetic heart valves (e.g., metal prosthetic valves, tissue prosthesis plus AF, or previous stroke), the benefit of adding aspirin to VKA outweighs the increased risk of major bleeding [45].

Therefore, it would seem reasonable to treat with VKA alone in stable coronary artery disease patients who have an indication for VKA (e.g., AF or venous thrombosis). The problem arises in acute coronary syndromes and in the presence of coronary artery stents where there is insufficient evidence comparing the relative efficacies and safeties of aspirin plus clopidogrel against VKA alone. A pragmatic approach is required where possible, such as using bare metal stents (that require shorter exposure to combination antiplatelet therapy); using VKA plus single-agent antiplatelet therapy in lower thrombotic risk patients; and short-term triple therapy with VKA plus aspirin plus clopidogrel in patients at highest thrombotic risk [46].

Conclusions

At present, risk stratification for arterial disease continues to rely on assessment of traditional clinical and routine laboratory risk factors. The role of thrombophilia screening in patients with arterial disease is unproven, although selective testing for homocystinuria and antiphospholipid syndrome is indicated in patients with premature arterial thrombosis, especially in the absence of traditional risk factors.

The mainstay of treatment is control or eradication of risk factors, coupled with antithrombotic therapy – primarily antiplatelet agents, but also anticoagulation with either a VKA or direct oral anticoagulant for patients with AF and additional risk factors (Figure 16.1).

References

1 Lowe GD, Danesh J. The need for risk factor assessment in atherothrombotic vascular disease. *Semin Vasc Med* 2002; 2: 231–232.
2 Yusuf S, Hawken S, Ounpuu S, *et al*. Effect of potentially modifiable risk factors associated with myocardial infarction in 52 countries (the INTERHEART study): case-control study. *Lancet* 2004; 364: 937–952.

3 Anon. Risk factors for stroke and efficacy of antithrombotic therapy in atrial fibrillation. Analysis of pooled data from five randomized controlled trials. *Arch Intern Med* 1994; 154: 1449–1457.

4 Gage BF, van Walraven C, Pearce L, *et al*. Selecting patients with atrial fibrillation for anticoagulation: stroke risk stratification in patients taking aspirin. *Circulation* 2004; 110: 2287–2292.

5 Gage BF, Waterman AD, Shannon W, *et al*. Validation of clinical classification schemes for predicting stroke: results from the National Registry of Atrial Fibrillation. *JAMA* 2001; 285: 2864–2870.

6 Lip GY, Nieuwlaat R, Pisters R, *et al*. Refining clinical risk stratification for predicting stroke and thromboembolism in atrial fibrillation using a novel risk factor-based approach: the euro heart survey on atrial fibrillation. *Chest* 2010; 137: 263–272.

7 Camm AJ, Lip GY, De Caterina R, *et al*. 2012 focused update of the ESC Guidelines for the management of atrial fibrillation: an update of the 2010 ESC Guidelines for the management of atrial fibrillation. Developed with the special contribution of the European Heart Rhythm Association. *Eur Heart J* 2012; 33: 2719–2747.

8 Coppens M, Eikelboom JW, Hart RG, *et al*. The CHA2DS2-VASc score identifies those patients with atrial fibrillation and a CHADS2 score of 1 who are unlikely to benefit from oral anticoagulant therapy. *Eur Heart J* 2013; 34: 170–176.

9 Lowe GD. Blood rheology in vitro and in vivo. *Baillieres Clin Haematol* 1987; 1: 597–636.

10 Keeling D, Mackie I, Moore GW, *et al*. Guidelines on the investigation and management of antiphospholipid syndrome. *Br J Haematol* 2012; 157: 47–58.

11 Sode BF, Allin KH, Dahl M, *et al*. Risk of venous thromboembolism and myocardial infarction associated with factor V Leiden and prothrombin mutations and blood type. *CMAJ* 2013; 185: E229–237.

12 Baglin T, Gray E, Greaves M, *et al*. Clinical guidelines for testing for heritable thrombophilia. *Br J Haematol* 2010; 149: 209–220.

13 Wu LA, Malouf JF, Dearani JA, *et al*. Patent foramen ovale in cryptogenic stroke: current understanding and management options. *Arch Intern Med* 2004; 164: 950–956.

14 Danesh J, Lewington S, Thompson SG, *et al*. Plasma fibrinogen level and the risk of major cardiovascular diseases and nonvascular mortality: an individual participant meta-analysis. *JAMA* 2005; 294: 1799–1809.

15 Previtali E, Bucciarelli P, Passamonti SM, *et al*. Risk factors for venous and arterial thrombosis. *Blood Transfus* 2011; 9: 120–138.

16 Danesh J, Wheeler JG, Hirschfield GM, *et al*. C-reactive protein and other circulating markers of inflammation in the prediction of coronary heart disease. *N Engl J Med* 2004; 350: 1387–1397.

17 Qureshi W, Hassan S, Dabak V, *et al*. Thrombosis in VonWillebrand disease. *Thromb Res* 2012; 130: e255–258.

18 Sramek A, Kriek M, Rosendaal FR. Decreased mortality of ischaemic heart disease among carriers of haemophilia. *Lancet* 2003; 362: 351–354.

19 Danesh J, Whincup P, Walker M, *et al*. Fibrin D-dimer and coronary heart disease: prospective study and meta-analysis. *Circulation* 2001; 103: 2323–2327.

20 Vene N, Mavri A, Kosmelj K, *et al*. High D-dimer levels predict cardiovascular events in patients with chronic atrial fibrillation during oral anticoagulant therapy. *Thromb Haemost* 2003; 90: 1163–1172.

21 Lowe GD. Fibrin D-dimer and cardiovascular risk. *Semin Vasc Med* 2005; 5: 387–398.

22 Lowe GD, Danesh J, Lewington S, *et al*. Tissue plasminogen activator antigen and coronary heart disease. Prospective study and meta-analysis. *Eur Heart J* 2004; 25: 252–259.

23 Meltzer ME, Doggen CJ, de Groot PG, *et al*. Plasma levels of fibrinolytic proteins and the risk of myocardial infarction in men. *Blood* 2010; 116: 529–536.

24 Heylen E, Willemse J, Hendriks D. An update on the role of carboxypeptidase U (TAFIa) in

fibrinolysis. *Front Biosci (Landmark Ed)* 2011;
16: 2427–2450.

25 Hankey GJ, Eikelboom JW. Aspirin resistance.
BMJ 2004; 328: 477–479.

26 Haidl H, Cimenti C, Leschnik B, *et al.*
Age-dependency of thrombin generation
measured by means of calibrated automated
thrombography (CAT). *Thromb Haemost*
2006; 95: 772–775.

27 Tripodi A, Legnani C, Chantarangkul V,
et al. High thrombin generation measured in
the presence of thrombomodulin is associated
with an increased risk of recurrent venous
thromboembolism. *J Thromb Haemost* 2008;
6: 1327–1333.

28 Orbe J, Zudaire M, Serrano R, *et al.* Increased
thrombin generation after acute versus
chronic coronary disease as assessed by the
thrombin generation test. *Thromb Haemost*
2008; 99: 382–387.

29 Carcaillon L, Alhenc-Gelas M, Bejot Y, *et al.*
Increased thrombin generation is associated
with acute ischemic stroke but not with
coronary heart disease in the elderly: the
Three-City cohort study. *Arterioscler Thromb
Vasc Biol* 2011; 31: 1445–1451.

30 Fowkes FG, Price JF, Stewart MC, *et al.*
Aspirin for prevention of cardiovascular
events in a general population screened for a
low ankle brachial index: a randomized
controlled trial. *JAMA* 2010; 303: 841–848.

31 Belch J, MacCuish A, Campbell I, *et al.* The
prevention of progression of arterial disease
and diabetes (POPADAD) trial: factorial
randomised placebo controlled trial of aspirin
and antioxidants in patients with diabetes and
asymptomatic peripheral arterial disease. *BMJ*
2008; 337: a1840.

32 De Berardis G, Sacco M, Strippoli GF, *et al.*
Aspirin for primary prevention of
cardiovascular events in people with diabetes:
meta-analysis of randomised controlled trials.
BMJ 2009; 339: b4531.

33 Baigent C, Blackwell L, Collins R, *et al.* Aspirin
in the primary and secondary prevention of
vascular disease: collaborative meta-analysis of
individual participant data from randomised
trials. *Lancet* 2009; 373: 1849–1860.

34 SIGN. *Acute Coronary Syndromes. A National
Clinical Guideline.* SIGN, 2007, pp. 93.

35 NICE. *Clopidogrel and Modified-Release
Dipyridamole for the Prevention of Occlusive
Vascular Events.* NICE technology appraisal
guidance, TA210, 2010.

36 Berger JS, Krantz MJ, Kittelson JM, *et al.*
Aspirin for the prevention of cardiovascular
events in patients with peripheral artery
disease: a meta-analysis of randomized trials.
JAMA 2009; 301: 1909–1919.

37 Olesen JB, Lip GY, Hansen PR, *et al.* Bleeding
risk in 'real world' patients with atrial
fibrillation: comparison of two established
bleeding prediction schemes in a nationwide
cohort. *J Thromb Haemost* 2011; 9: 1460–1467.

38 Connolly SJ, Ezekowitz MD, Yusuf S, *et al.*
Dabigatran versus warfarin in patients with
atrial fibrillation. *N Engl J Med* 2009; 361:
1139–1151.

39 Patel MR, Mahaffey KW, Garg J, *et al.*
Rivaroxaban versus warfarin in nonvalvular
atrial fibrillation. *N Engl J Med* 2011; 365:
883–891.

40 Granger CB, Alexander JH, McMurray JJ,
et al. Apixaban versus warfarin in patients
with atrial fibrillation. *N Engl J Med* 2011; 365:
981–992.

41 Connolly S, Pogue J, Hart R, *et al.* Clopidogrel
plus aspirin versus oral anticoagulation for atrial
fibrillation in the Atrial fibrillation Clopidogrel
Trial with Irbesartan for prevention of Vascular
Events (ACTIVE W): a randomised controlled
trial. *Lancet* 2006; 367: 1903–1912.

42 Douketis JD, Arneklev K, Goldhaber SZ, *et al.*
Comparison of bleeding in patients with
nonvalvular atrial fibrillation treated with
ximelagatran or warfarin: assessment of
incidence, case-fatality rate, time course and
sites of bleeding, and risk factors for bleeding.
Arch Intern Med 2006; 166: 853–859.

43 Anand S, Yusuf S, Xie C, *et al.* Oral
anticoagulant and antiplatelet therapy and
peripheral arterial disease. *N Engl J Med* 2007;
357: 217–227.

44 Hurlen M, Abdelnoor M, Smith P, *et al.*
Warfarin, aspirin, or both after myocardial
infarction. *N Engl J Med* 2002; 347: 969–974.

45 Little SH, Massel DR. Antiplatelet and anticoagulation for patients with prosthetic heart valves. *Cochrane Database Syst Rev* 2003; (4): CD003464.

46 Eikelboom JW, Hirsh J. Combined antiplatelet and anticoagulant therapy: clinical benefits and risks. *J Thromb Haemost* 2007; 5 Suppl 1: 255–263.

47 Sorensen HT, Horvath-Puho E, Pedersen L, *et al.* Venous thromboembolism and subsequent hospitalisation due to acute arterial cardiovascular events: a 20-year cohort study. *Lancet* 2007; 370: 1773–1779.

48 Manson JE, Hsia J, Johnson KC, *et al.* Estrogen plus progestin and the risk of coronary heart disease. *N Engl J Med* 2003; 349: 523–534.

49 O'Donnell MJ, Xavier D, Liu L, *et al.* Risk factors for ischaemic and intracerebral haemorrhagic stroke in 22 countries (the INTERSTROKE study): a case-control study. *Lancet* 2010; 376: 112–123.

50 Perk J, De Backer G, Gohlke H, *et al.* European Guidelines on cardiovascular disease prevention in clinical practice (version 2012). The Fifth Joint Task Force of the European Society of Cardiology and Other Societies on Cardiovascular Disease Prevention in Clinical Practice (constituted by representatives of nine societies and by invited experts). *Eur Heart J* 2012; 33: 1635–1701.

51 Smith SC, Jr., Benjamin EJ, Bonow RO, *et al.* AHA/ACCF Secondary Prevention and Risk Reduction Therapy for Patients with Coronary and other Atherosclerotic Vascular Disease: 2011 update: a guideline from the American Heart Association and American College of Cardiology Foundation. *Circulation* 2011; 124: 2458–2473.

52 Camm AJ, Kirchhof P, Lip GY, *et al.* Guidelines for the management of atrial fibrillation: the Task Force for the Management of Atrial Fibrillation of the European Society of Cardiology (ESC). *Europace* 2010; 12: 1360–1420.

53 Olesen JB, Lip GY, Hansen ML, *et al.* Validation of risk stratification schemes for predicting stroke and thromboembolism in patients with atrial fibrillation: nationwide cohort study. *BMJ* 2011; 342: d124.

17

Anticoagulation: Heparins and Vitamin K Antagonists

Gualtiero Palareti and Benilde Cosmi

Key Points

- Heparin, low-molecular-weight heparins, and fondaparinux are parenteral anticoagulants that are usually employed for prophylaxis and treatment of the acute phase of venous thromboembolism.
- Heparin requires strict laboratory monitoring for dose adjustment, while low-molecular-weight heparins and fondaparinux can be administered in weight-adjusted fixed doses without laboratory monitoring in the majority of patients for treatment of venous thromboembolism and also in acute coronary syndromes.
- Vitamin K antagonists have been available for 60 years and are the most widely employed oral anticoagulants for long-term treatment of thromboembolic diseases.
- Vitamin K antagonist have a wide inter- and intraindividual variability and require periodic laboratory testing with the prothrombin time (International Normalized Ratio) for dose adjustment.
- Optimal vitamin K antagonists monitoring requires skilled physicians, adequate laboratory facilities, and patient education on the benefits and risks of oral anticoagulation to ensure optimal compliance.

Heparins

Heparin is one of the naturally occurring glycosaminoglycans (GAGs), which are polysaccharides composed of alternating and variously sulfated residues of uronic acid and aminosugar or hexosamine [1]. Connective tissue mast cells of several mammals synthesize heparin, which is still extracted from tissues such as intestine, lung, and liver. Nowadays, porcine intestinal mucosa is the usual source for commercial (unfractionated) heparin, which is a mixture of highly sulfated chains of disaccharide repeating units consisting of 1→4 linked residues of uronic acid and D-glucosamine [1]. Heparin chains vary in length and structure with a range of 15 to 100 monosaccharide residues per chain and molecular weight ranging from 5000 to 30 000 Da.

The anticoagulant and antithrombotic properties of heparin depend on its ability to enhance the activity of the natural occurring serine protease inhibitor, antithrombin (AT). As a result, heparin catalyzes the inhibition of all the serine proteases of the intrinsic coagulation pathway such as factor IXa, factor XIa, factor XIIa and also of the common pathway such as thrombin and factor Xa [2]. A specific pentasaccharide sequence present in only about a third of commercial heparin chains is required for AT binding [1]. Heparin is not absorbed orally and must be administered parenterally by either continuous intravenous infusion, which allows an immediate anticoagulant effect, or by subcutaneous injection, which is associated with a reduced bioavailability. Heparin chains are negatively charged and bind to a number of plasma proteins other than AT, as well as to endothelial cells and macrophages. This nonspecific binding of heparin reduces its anticoagulant activity and explains the variability of its anticoagulant response, which therefore requires strict laboratory monitoring [1]. Endothelial cells and macrophages bind and depolymerize heparin through a rapid saturable mechanism of clearance, while the kidney clears heparin via a much slower nonsaturable mechanism. As a result, heparin's anticoagulant effect is nonlinear and dose dependent at therapeutic doses, with both the intensity and duration of effect rising with increasing doses [1].

Heparin is an effective, relatively safe, inexpensive, parenteral antithrombotic agent, but it has several limitations. These arise from: (i) its marked intra- and interpatient variability in anticoagulant response; (ii) its poor bioavailability at low doses; (iii) its relatively narrow risk to benefit ratio, which is partly related to the interference of heparin with platelet aggregation and with vessel wall permeability that both serve to increase the risk of bleeding; (iv) the risk of heparin-induced thrombocytopenia; and (v) the risk of osteoporosis during long-term treatment.

Low-molecular-weight heparins (LMWHs) have been developed to overcome some of unfractionated heparin's limitations, and are obtained by chemical or enzymatic depolymerization or size fractionation of heparin. LMWHs have a shorter polysaccharide chain, a lower molecular weight (4000–6500 Da) and a lower proportion of pentasaccharide-containing chains (between 10% and 20%). Only 25–50% of the molecules of commercial LMWHs contain at least 18 saccharide units, which is the minimum length required to promote thrombin inhibition by providing a template to which both AT and thrombin bind [1]. This accelerates the rate of the reaction by about 1000-fold. Shorter chains are unable to catalyze thrombin inhibition, but still bind AT, thus producing an AT conformational change which accelerates factor Xa inhibition [1]. LMWHs differ from heparin in their biochemical and pharmacological properties. In particular, LMWHs' dose response is more predictable than that of heparin, and this allows their administration in weight-adjusted fixed doses without laboratory monitoring. They also have a better bioavailability at low doses when administered subcutaneously, a reduced hemorrhagic to antithrombotic ratio, and a lower risk of developing thrombocytopenia. The half-life of LMWHs, which is 3 to 6 hours after subcutaneous injection, is dose independent, as they are cleared only by the kidneys, so that their biological half-life is prolonged in patients with renal failure.

LMWHs share similar antithrombotic properties but are produced by different processes with distinct biochemical and pharmacological properties, and therefore they may not be completely interchangeable for their heterogeneity [1]. Few studies have compared LMWHs for clinical equivalence. Some trials have reported comparable efficacy between LMWHs in the prophylaxis and treatment of venous thromboembolism (VTE), while others have reported significant differences in efficacy or pharmacological properties [1]. Clinical guidelines on VTE prevention and treatment provide recommendations on the use of LMWHs as a class [1] and recommend that clinicians follow the manufacturer-suggested dosing guidelines for each of the antithrombotic agents. Clinical guidelines from the American College of Cardiology Foundation/ American Heart Association for the treatment of acute coronary syndromes (ACS) specifically recommend enoxaparin [2].

Fondaparinux is a synthetic analogue of the AT-binding pentasaccharide found in heparin with a modified structure that increases its affinity for AT [1], a molecular weight of 1728, and a longer half-life after subcutaneous injection than LMWHs (17 hours and 4 hours, respectively). Fondaparinux is rapidly and completely absorbed after subcutaneous injection. It has minimal nonspecific binding and it can be given in weight-adjusted fixed doses without laboratory monitoring. It is cleared only through the renal route and is contraindicated in renal failure. No antidote is available for fondaparinux in the event of serious bleeding, while protamine sulfate can neutralize heparin completely and LMWHs partially.

LMWHs and fondaparinux have been approved for use in VTE (i.e., deep vein thrombosis (DVT) and pulmonary embolism (PE)) prophylaxis and treatment and ACS treatment.

Prophylaxis of Venous Thromboembolism

Major General Surgery

Both heparin and LMWHs reduce the risk of asymptomatic DVT and symptomatic VTE by at least 60% compared with no thromboprophylaxis [3]. Most trials employed low-`dose unfractionated heparin (LDUH) 5000 IU SC 1–2 hours before surgery, followed by 5000 U b.i.d. or t.i.d. for approximately 1 week. LDUH and LMWHs have been shown to have similar efficacy and safety, but LMWHs can be administered only once daily and have a significant lower risk of heparin-induced thrombocytopenia [3].

Fondaparinux at 2.5 mg SC once daily started postoperatively was compared with dalteparin at 5000 U SC once daily started before surgery in a randomized, blinded clinical trial [3] among almost 3000 patients undergoing major abdominal surgery, with similar efficacy and safety.

Major Orthopedic Surgery

Although LDUH thromboprophylaxis is superior to no thromboprophylaxis, LDUH is less effective than other thromboprophylaxis regimens in this high-risk group. Vitamin K antagonists (VKAs) were shown to be less effective than LMWHs in elective total hip and total knee replacement and hip fracture surgery in preventing total and proximal DVT [4]. In a meta-analysis, fondaparinux at a dose of 2.5 mg once daily was associated with a lower incidence of

symptomatic or asymptomatic VTE, compared with enoxaparin, albeit with higher incidence of major bleeding [4].

Medical Patients

A meta-analysis [5] of randomized trials including almost 20 000 medical patients found that thromboprophylaxis (with either heparin, LMWH, or fondaparinux) reduced fatal PE by 64%, symptomatic PE by 58%, and symptomatic DVT by 53%, without an increase in major bleeding compared with no thromboprophylaxis.

Therapy of Venous Thromboembolism

Acute Phase

Treatment should start with an initial parenteral anticoagulation to overlap with a long-term oral anticoagulation with VKAs. The introduction of new oral anticoagulants such as rivaroxaban or apixaban with a single drug approach from the start is another recent option (see Chapter 18). VKAs are usually started on the same day of diagnosis. Parenteral anticoagulation should continue for no less than 5 days and be stopped when the patient's International Normalized Ratio (INR) is >2.0 for two consecutive days [6,7]. Parenteral anticoagulation has been performed for many years with IV heparin, then substituted with SC heparin and with LMWHs or recently with fondaparinux. Intravenous unfractionated heparin therapy should start with a bolus (5000 IU or 70–80 IU/kg to overcome nonspecific binding) followed by a continuous infusion (with a pump) of 18 IU/kg/h, with dose adjustment according to the activated partial thromboplastin time (APTT) test, to be performed at least once daily and repeated at 4 hours after any dose adjustment, in order to achieve and maintain an APTT ratio of 1.5–2.0 times of normal. Such a treatment requires hospitalization, strict laboratory monitoring, and skilful dose adjustment, and has a higher burden of bleeding complications. It is currently reserved for particular conditions, such as severe renal insufficiency, where monitoring is necessary to avoid heparin accumulation and excessive anticoagulation. Other conditions are when surgery, or delivery, or other invasive maneuvers are planned or highly probable in a short interval time, and in patients with a very high risk of bleeding. In all these conditions, heparin has the advantage of a short half-life after stopping the infusion and the possibility of complete reversal of its anticoagulant effect with protamine sulfate (1 mg of protamine neutralizes 80–100 U of heparin when administered within 15 minutes of the heparin dose) [1]. These advantages are clinically important because they allow the provider to treat for a short interval without therapeutic cover, or to start soon and safely a different antithrombotic treatment, or to immediately reverse anticoagulation if necessary.

Fixed-dose unfractionated heparin for VTE treatment has also been proposed (5000 IU bolus IV or 333 IU/kg SC followed by 250 IU/kg/12 h) and has been evaluated in only a single study [6].

Anticoagulant treatment is currently initiated with LMWH or fondaparinux in most cases. The subcutaneous administration twice or once daily at weight-adjusted fixed doses, without laboratory monitoring, allows an immediate or early home treatment for many patients. Several trials addressing LMWHs instead of heparin for initial treatment of patients with acute VTE (either DVT or PE) have shown lower mortality, VTE recurrence, major bleeding, and a lower potential for heparin-induced thrombocytopenia (10 times less than heparin). Fondaparinux can also be safely and effectively used for the initial treatment of DVT or PE with a once-daily SC dose (7.5 mg if 50–100 kg; 5.0 mg if <50 kg; 10 mg if >100 kg) for at least 5 days [6].

Both LMWHs and fondaparinux are cleared by the kidney and are contraindicated in the presence of severe renal insufficiency, due to the difficulties in monitoring treatment. LMWHs' effect on APTT is nonspecific and the test cannot be used for dosage monitoring, while the anti-Xa activity assay is more informative, although not completely standardized and not widely available. Samples for the anti-Xa activity assay should be taken at peak levels, that is at 4 hours after an injection. A target range of 0.6–1.0 IU/mL is suggested for twice-daily and 1.0–2.0 IU/mL for once-daily administration. LMWHs can be administered without laboratory monitoring in the majority of patients. However, in certain clinical situations, anti-Xa activity measurement could be indicated, such as in renal insufficiency, pregnancy, obesity, neonates and infants for LMWH dose adjustment, or in case of unexpected bleeding or before emergency surgery in subjects receiving LMWHs. Fondaparinux can also be measured with fondaparinux-specific anti-Xa assays.

Long-term Treatment

Adjusted-dose SC heparin or LMWHs can be an alternative to VKAs for long-term treatment of DVT. LMWHs are preferable for their once-daily administration without monitoring and their lower potential for osteoporosis. A meta-analysis of studies comparing LMWHs or VKAs, each administered for 3 months after initial heparin therapy, has shown a trend toward less recurrent VTE and major bleeding with LMWHs [7]. In cancer-associated VTE, therapeutic dose LMWHs for the first 3 or 6 months were associated with lower recurrence, bleeding, and mortality than with VKAs. As a result, LMWHs instead of VKAs are recommended for the first 3 to 6 months in cancer-related VTE, with indefinite subsequent anticoagulation with VKAs or LMWHs or until the underlying cancer is resolved [7].

Treatment of Arterial Diseases

Intravenous heparin in ACS reduces the risk of recurrent ischemic events. The dose is lower than that used in VTE (60–70 IU/kg maximum 5000 IU, followed by 12–15 IU/kg/h maximum 1000 IU/h). Enoxaparin was compared to heparin (both agents being used at therapeutic dose and in conjunction with aspirin) with a reduced incidence of the composite endpoint (death, myocardial infarction, or recurrent angina) with LMWH in ACS [2].

Fondaparinux (2.5 mg OD) has been compared with enoxaparin (1 mg/kg SC b.i.d.) or intravenous heparin in patients with ACS with efficacy in reducing the risk of ischemic events but substantially reduced major bleeding, including fatal bleeding, and improved long-term mortality and morbidity [2].

Oral Anticoagulants: Vitamin K Antagonists

VKAs are 4-hydroxycoumarin compounds, which have been the only orally available anticoagulants since their introduction for the treatment of thrombotic disorders in the 1950s and until the recent development of new oral anticoagulants (see Chapter 18). Warfarin, acenocoumarol, and phenprocoumon are the compounds currently in clinical use, with warfarin being the most prescribed world-wide.

VKAs interfere with the vitamin K-dependent hepatic synthesis of coagulation factors II, VII, IX, and X as well as the coagulation inhibitors protein C and S. Vitamin K-dependent post-translational carboxylation is critical for coagulation factors to acquire the calcium-mediated ability to bind to negatively charged phospholipid surfaces [8].

Carboxylation of vitamin K-dependent coagulation factors depends on a carboxylase requiring a reduced form of vitamin K (vitamin KH2), oxygen, and carbon dioxide. During this reaction, vitamin KH2 is oxidized to vitamin K epoxide, which is reduced to vitamin K by epoxide reductase and then to vitamin KH2 by vitamin K reductase. VKAs inhibit vitamin K epoxide reductase and possibly vitamin K reductase. As a result, intracellular depletion of vitamin KH2 takes place and only partially carboxylated and decarboxylated proteins are secreted. The antagonizing effect on vitamin K with the production of biologically inactive coagulation factors is the basis for VKAs therapeutic use [8].

The metabolism of warfarin is almost exclusively mediated by the activity of the enzyme CYP2C9, which accounts for ~85% of its catabolism. Several genetic polymorphisms of CYP2C9 have been identified and two of

them, the CYP2C9*2 and CYP2C9*3, relatively frequent among Caucasians, are clinically relevant because carriers of these variants metabolize warfarin more slowly than carriers of the wild type allele (CYP2C9*1) and require lower warfarin doses [8].

Numerous polymorphisms of the gene encoding for vitamin K epoxide reductase subunit 1 were also found to induce a different sensitivity, highly increased or reduced, of the enzyme to VKAs action [8]. Prewarfarin initiation genetic testing has been proposed but it is not recommended over traditional INR monitoring [9].

The therapeutic effect of VKAs is delayed because time is required for the normal coagulation factors to be cleared from plasma and replaced by partially carboxylated or decarboxylated factors. This delay in the onset of VKAs' effect varies according to the coagulation factor's half-life, which is only 6–7 hours for factor VII and 60–72 hours for prothrombin.

Animal studies have shown that the reduction of prothrombin and possibly of factor X is more important than the reduction of factor VII and IX for the *in vivo* antithrombotic effect of VKAs. As a result, the initial effect of VKAs as measured by the prolongation of the prothrombin time primarily reflects factor VII reduction, while the antithrombotic effect is only observed after the reduction of prothrombin, which requires 60–72 hours. In addition, in the first days of treatment with VKAs, a reduction of the levels of protein C and protein S is also observed, as the synthesis of these natural anticoagulants is also vitamin K dependent. Protein C's half-life is similar to that of factor VII; as a result, in the initial phase of treatment with VKAs, protein C levels can be reduced significantly before achieving an efficient antithrombotic effect. This can result in warfarin induced skin necrosis (Figure 17.1).

The delayed onset of the antithrombotic effect of VKAs, and the potentially prothrombotic effect in the first 24–48 hours provide the rationale for overlapping heparin with VKAs for 4–5 days until their full antithrombotic effect is obtained.

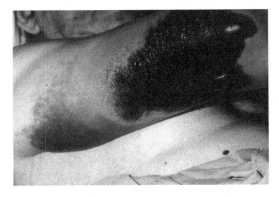

Figure 17.1 Skin necrosis of the elbow in a patient who just started warfarin.

Initiation and Dosing of Warfarin Anticoagulation

The anticoagulant effect of VKAs shows high inter- and intraindividual variability. Even though the average daily dose of warfarin is approximately 5 mg, individual patient's daily dosage may range between 0.5 and 60 mg. Furthermore, VKAs have a narrow therapeutic window, and over- or underdosage can result in overanticoagulation, with increased risk of hemorrhage, or under anticoagulation, with increased risk of thrombosis, respectively. The INR range is 2.0–3.0 for the majority of indications for VKAs (Table 17.1).

The quality of VKA monitoring is certainly an important factor influencing the risk of bleeding or thrombotic complications. Guiding VKA therapy requires skill and practice [9]. Techniques to reduce the risk of inappropriate warfarin dosing include:

- warfarin regimen nomograms;
- computer-generated warfarin regimens;
- dedicated anticoagulation clinics.

Several nomograms have been proposed to help warfarin regimens either during the induction phase or during the stabilized phase of

Table 17.1 Indications and contraindications (absolute or relative) for anticoagulant treatment with vitamin K antagonists.

Proven indications	Primary and secondary prevention of venous thromboembolism Prevention of systemic embolism in atrial fibrillation or in patients with tissue or mechanical heart valves Prevention of stroke or death in patients with acute myocardial infarction Prevention of acute myocardial reinfarction in men at high risk
Other accepted indications	Prevention of thrombotic complications in high-risk patients with: prosthetic heart valves mitral stenosis systemic embolism of unknown etiology intraventricular thrombosis dilated cardiomyopathy
Absolute contraindications	Pregnancy between the 6th and 12th week Major bleeding (within 30 days)
Relative contraindications	All the conditions that increase the risk of bleeding or of insufficient quality of treatment severe hepatic or renal insufficiency severe uncontrolled hypertension severe heart failure bleeding diathesis recent central venous system surgery or trauma active peptic ulcer or bowel inflammatory disease bacterial endocarditis or pericarditis tendency to fall chronic alcoholism poor compliance psychiatric disorders or dementia (if not supported by family or social services)

anticoagulation. Nomograms require that baseline INR is normal or near normal (not more than 1.4). Nomograms with either a 10 mg or 5 mg loading dose were proposed, in the latter case with subsequent doses determined by the INR response, which can be checked on the third or fourth day [9]. The rate of lowering of prothrombin levels was similar when warfarin was started with either loading dose. However, the larger dose produced a more rapid reduction in protein C levels and a higher frequency of overanticoagulation (INR > 3.0). A smaller loading dose of warfarin might therefore be less likely to produce a potentially prothrombotic effect in the first 24–48 hours of treatment. However, patients who receive a 10 mg initial dose of warfarin achieve an INR in the target range earlier than patients initially treated with 5 mg. Also, fewer INR assessments are performed in the 10 mg group with no significant differences in recurrent events or major bleeding [9].

Some authors have demonstrated that a reduced dose is required in the elderly, while patients starting VKAs after heart valve replacement are more sensitive to warfarin than nonsurgical patients, and initial warfarin doses lower than 5 mg may be appropriate.

Computer-guided dosing has been shown to be effective, both during long-term maintenance and in the early, highly unstable phase of treatment. Computer-guided dosing increases the amount of time spent in the therapeutic range compared with exclusive management by doctors [9].

It is a general experience, confirmed by some studies, that the quality of anticoagulation control is higher and the rate of bleeding lower when patients are monitored by dedicated anticoagulation clinics [9], where the specialized training and experience of medical and paramedical staff, proper patient education, and the use of computer programs can ensure optimization of anticoagulation.

Patients with Highly Unstable Response to VKAs

Some patients may have a highly unstable response to VKAs, although universally accepted criteria for instability of response to VKAs are lacking. Some criteria have been proposed [10]: (i) less than 50% of INR results within the intended therapeutic range, with the other INR results both above or below the range; and/or (ii) weekly dose changes (at least 15% of the previously prescribed coumarin weekly dose) in at least 40% of visits during the previous 4 months.

Instability is more frequently associated with working status people versus retirees, use of acenocoumarol, and distribution of CYP2C9. Instability is more frequent in patients with lower scores in the Abbreviated Mental Test administered to assess the degree of attention, with lack of awareness of reasons for VKAs, and of the mechanisms and possible side-effects of VKAs [10].

Patient education and knowledge of VKAs and its management is a primary determinant of the quality of anticoagulation, and appropriate education and information of patients is one of the most important tasks of anticoagulation clinics. The distribution of patient education brochures at the beginning of anticoagulant treatment may not be sufficient and further education by personal interview should be considered for unstable patients [10].

Fluctuations in dietary vitamin K intake can also lead to changes in the INR. Additionally, patients with fluctuating INRs generally have a lower oral vitamin K intake than patients with stable INRs. Some patients on oral anticoagulants have fluctuating INRs that cannot be explained by changes in concomitant medications, intercurrent illness, or obvious dietary changes. Supplementation with low-dose oral vitamin K in such patients is sometimes used in clinical practice, and some studies have shown that vitamin K supplementation (500 µg) daily decreases INR variability.

Complications of Anticoagulation with VKAs: Bleeding

The risk of bleeding on VKAs in prospective studies has been reported to be:

- 0.1–1.0% patient years of treatment for fatal episodes;
- 0.5–6.5% for major episodes;

- 6.2–21.8% for minor bleeding.

Differences in the adopted classification of bleeding events (Table 17.2) and populations may explain the wide range of bleeding rates reported in clinical studies. Although the criteria for major bleeding were different in different studies, in all studies the most consistent risk factors for major bleeding were:

- intensity of anticoagulation;
- age;
- the first 90 days of treatment.

An INR >4.5 increases the risk of hemorrhage sixfold and the risk of major hemorrhage increases by 42% for each one point increase in INR.

The intended intensity, and especially the actually achieved intensity of anticoagulation, is the major determinant of anticoagulation-induced bleeding with VKAs [12], with the lowest rate of bleeding associated in the 2.0–2.9 INR range. Although many bleeding events occur at a very low anticoagulation intensity (<2.0 INR), the increase in bleeding increases exponentially for INR values >4.5.

Intracranial hemorrhage is the most feared bleeding complication (Figure 17.2) with high mortality and morbidity. The rate of intracranial hemorrhage in randomized trials of atrial fibrillation and post myocardial infarction was 0.3%, while it was 0.5–0.6% in observational studies of patients on VKAs for arterial and venous thromboembolic indications. The rate of intracranial bleeding was 1.15 per 100 patient years in a meta-analysis evaluating studies in patients taking oral anticoagulant therapy for venous thromboembolism [13].

Risk factors for intracranial bleeding are:

- older age;
- intensity of anticoagulation; the risk increases fourfold for each unit increase in the prothrombin time ratio, and is particularly high for INR >4.0;
- ischemic cerebrovascular disease;
- hypertension;
- neurological pathologies such as leukoaraiosis (a diffuse white matter abnormality seen on computed tomography or magnetic resonance)

Table 17.2 Classification of bleeding complications.

Major bleeding (according to the Control of Anticoagulation Subcommittee of the ISTH [11])	Fatal bleeding Symptomatic bleeding in a critical area or organ, such as intracranial, intraspinal, intraocular, retroperitoneal, intraarticular or pericardial, or intramuscular with compartment syndrome Bleeding causing a fall in hemoglobin level of 20 g/L or more, or leading to transfusion of two or more units of whole blood or red cells.
Minor bleeding	Any overt hemorrhage not included among the major bleeds

Bruising, small ecchymoses, nosebleed (not requiring tamponade), occasional hemorrhoidal bleeding and microscopic hematuria should not be considered as clinically relevant bleeds.

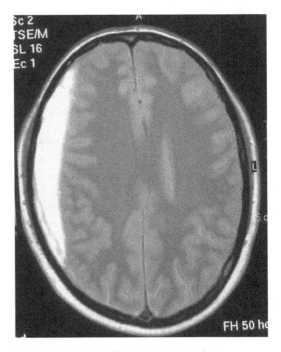

Figure 17.2 Subdural hematoma in a patient on warfarin.

and amyloid angiopathy (increases with age and is associated with asymptomatic microhemorrhages and with spontaneous lobar intracerebral hemorrhage in the elderly).

Management of Overanticoagulation and Bleeding

Anticoagulation Reversal

The coumarin drugs have very different half-lives: acenocoumarol has the shortest, phenprocoumon the longest, and warfarin in between.

Discontinuing coumarin intake will result in a slow reversal of anticoagulation, proportional to the half-life of the particular agent. The majority of overanticoagulated patients (INR >4.5) will take 3 days to return to the therapeutic range. For subjects already within the therapeutic range, it will take 3–5 days for the anticoagulation to be completely reversed.

Temporary withdrawal of coumarin administration alone is useful in overanticoagulated patients, especially if they are treated with acenocoumarol, are at low risk of bleeding, and are due to undergo elective surgery. This option cannot be used alone in actively bleeding patients because of the long period necessary for anticoagulation reversal.

Vitamin K (phytonadione) is the antidote of choice for coumarin drugs reversal. However, response to vitamin K varies, depending on the pretreatment INR value, the route of administration, and the dose used. Vitamin K can be administered intravenously, orally, or subcutaneously [14].

The intramuscular route is not recommended because of unpredictable absorption and the risk of intramuscular hematoma while higher doses and longer reversion times are needed with subcutaneous administration when compared with intravenous and oral administration. Vitamin K can be administered intravenously as a slow injection or infused in 5% glucose solution. Intravenous administration can cause anaphylaxis; however, this risk is much lower with the new vitamin K preparation that is stabilized with a mixed micelle vehicle (Konakion® MM) instead of castor oil (Konakion®).

Vitamin K administration in anticoagulated patients is indicated in:

- cases of excessive overanticoagulation, especially in patients at a higher bleeding risk [8];
- patients who need to undergo invasive procedures that require an INR value <1.5;
- cases with active major bleeding.

In overanticoagulated patients, oral vitamin K was demonstrated to be much more effective than placebo in correcting excessive INRs. Small amounts of oral vitamin K can produce a major correction in the INR at 24 hours, but the correction is insufficient at 4 hours or for cases of major bleeding.

In patients on acenocoumarol, administration of low-dose oral vitamin K offers no advantage to simple omission of a single dose of the drug and may result in an excessive risk of underanticoagulation.

Intravenous vitamin K administration leads to an effective reversal of anticoagulation within 6–8 hours, and is therefore the treatment of choice in life-threatening bleeding.

Prothrombin Complex Concentrates

Concentrates of factors II, VII, IX, and X, known as prothrombin complex concentrates (PCCs), are available and should be the first choice for their high effectiveness in replacing deficient clotting factors in anticoagulated patients with major bleeding, especially in those with intracranial hemorrhage in whom an immediate correction of the coagulopathy is mandatory [14]. The optimal dose of PCC is uncertain but a range of 25–50 U/kg has been suggested on the basis of INR values.

Despite all the precautions taken (selection of donors as well as specific viral inactivation procedures), an extremely small risk of viral infection can still persist. Thrombotic events have been reported after PCC transfusion in anticoagulated patients; however, this risk is also small, especially in preparations with added antithrombin and heparin.

Fresh frozen Plasma

Administration of fresh frozen plasma (FFP) is intended to correct the deficiency of factors II,

VII, IX, and X resulting from the effect of VKAs. The recommended FFP dose for warfarin reversal is 15 mL/kg body weight. However, FFP should only be employed in cases where PCCs are unavailable because of the risk of volume overload for the large quantities (e.g., approximately 1000 mL for an adult weighing 70 kg) needed, and failure to significantly correct the coagulopathy, especially for persistently low factor IX levels even with administration of the recommended dose, delays in transfusion, and the lack of viral inactivation of FFP.

Clinical Management of Overanticoagulation and Bleeding

The risk of bleeding increases sharply in association with very high INR values and it is desirable for a patient to spend as little time as possible in a state of overanticoagulation. In these cases, the clinical management should be as follows in nonbleeding patients:

- In case of very high INR values (>8.0), or with more moderately high INR values but at high risk of bleeding, the patient should receive 1–5 mg vitamin K orally; the INR should be measured the following day and oral vitamin K given again if necessary [14].
- In case of INR of 4.5–7.9, and in those treated with acenocoumarol regardless of the INR, withholding the coumarin drug for 1–2 days followed by a reduction of the weekly dose is usually sufficient.
- In cases of major although not life-threatening bleeding, a complete reversal of anticoagulation with intravenous vitamin K is advisable.
- Emergency anticoagulation reversal is recommended in patients with life-threatening bleeding. PCC infusion will completely correct the coagulopathy within 5–10 minutes with 5–10 mg vitamin K also administered intravenously.

Notably, FFP is nor recommended in this situation. Similarly, recombinant factor VIIa is also not recommended for emergency reversal.

Management of Patients Treated with VKAs Who Require Surgery or Invasive Procedures

No universally accepted guidelines for the management of anticoagulated patients requiring surgery or invasive procedures are available. Clear indications are lacking for the different patient groups, procedures, anticoagulant regimens, event definition, and duration of follow-up, as well as the absence of randomized clinical trials in this setting.

The general strategy for VKA management in patients undergoing invasive procedures requires the careful evaluation of three elements:

- the individual thromboembolic risk in case of VKA interruption in relation to its initial indication and the risk of postoperative thromboembolism;
- the bleeding risk of the procedure itself, as well as the added risk if/ when anticoagulation is continued;
- the necessity of alternative anticoagulation (bridging therapy) and its relative efficacy and safety.

The substantial difference between the consequences of major bleeding events and thromboembolic complications should also be taken into account. Permanent disability and death are common after arterial thromboembolism, especially in cases of cerebrovascular events (70–75%), while they are less frequent in cases of venous thromboembolic complications (4–10%), or major postoperative hemorrhage (1–6%).

The attitude of the specialist performing the procedure is also crucial, for his/her concern about bleeding if oral anticoagulation is continued rather than the risk of thromboembolism if oral anticoagulation is stopped. In the absence of certain indications, a careful evaluation by several specialists is warranted (hematologist, internist, cardiologist, surgeon, and anesthesiologist).

Three options are possible [15] (Table 17.3).

Continuation of VKA Treatment: In procedures at low risk of bleeding, such as interventions

Table 17.3 Strategies to manage patients treated with VKAs who require surgery or invasive procedures.

Continuation of VKA treatment	*In conditions at low risk of bleeding complications* Punctures and catheterization of superficial veins and arteries (e.g., femoral artery and Seldinger catheter) Sternal punctures and bone marrow aspirates Skin biopsies, minor dermatological surgery, biopsy of mucosa that is easily accessible and explorable (oral cavity, vagina), minor eye surgery Endoscopic examinations without surgery Simple tooth extraction in the absence of infection or surgical incisions In the latter cases, it is recommended to use local hemostatic agents, suturing of alveolar edges and mouth rinses with a 5% tranexamic acid solution, 4–5 minutes every 6 hours for 5–6 days, combined with antibiotic therapy
Temporary discontinuation of VKA treatment	*In patients with low risk of thrombotic complications in conditions at risk of bleeding* Major elective surgery, general or specialist Explorative cavity punctures (thoracocentesis, paracentesis) Biopsies of deep tissues (liver, kidney, bone) or mucosa (gastroenteric, respiratory, genital) not accessible Epidural anesthesia
Perioperative anticoagulant bridging therapy	*In patients with high risk of thrombotic complications* Prosthetic heart valves Atrial fibrillation with high/ moderate CHADS2 score (especially if with previous systemic embolism) Recent (within 30 days) or at high risk of recurrence venous thromboembolism Multiple risk factors

on superficial tissues, as indicated in Table 17.3, local hemostatic measures (e.g., pressure, antifibrinolytics, fibrin glue) can be applied and VKAs can be continued; it is often advisable to lower the INR to approximately 2 to decrease the hemorrhagic risk without an increase in the thromboembolic risk.

If the expected risk of bleeding is higher (e.g., multiple teeth extractions in the presence of infection, closed biopsy, endo-ocular surgery, or cataract with retrobulbar anesthesia) and the risk of thromboembolism is not high (in most cases, excluding patients with prosthetic heart valves or cardiac endocavitary thrombosis), VKAs can be temporarily reduced, aiming at INR values between 1.5 and 2.

Patients being treated with VKAs should be told to avoid, whenever possible, intramuscular injections so to avoid the risk of hematomas (especially if the patient needs many injections). Cataract surgery can be performed for its practically null risk of bleeding with topical or general anesthesia, avoiding if possible retro- and peribulbar anesthesia for the risk of hematomas.

Temporary Discontinuation of VKA Treatment: This is recommended in conditions associated with a significant risk of bleeding (such as cases of interventions on deep tissues not easily accessible to local hemostatic measures; see Table 17.3) in patients with nonhigh risk of thrombotic complications.

Perioperative Bridging Therapy: This strategy is indicated in patients who are at high risk of thrombotic complications (see Table 17.3). In these patients the goal is to minimize risk by reducing the duration of the bridging therapy to the minimum and by administering bridging therapy for the duration of subtherapeutic INR. If the procedure is elective, no immediate VKAs reversal is required and VKAs can be discontinued 3–4 days before the procedure (in case of therapeutic INR) as the INR is expected to fall to subtherapeutic values in 3–4 days.

The bridging therapy can be commenced 60 hours after the last warfarin dose (third morning after last evening dose). The INR should be measured the day before surgery to determine whether it is below 1.5–1.7. If not, 1 mg vitamin K can be given orally and the INR repeated on the day of surgery.

Bridging therapy can be conducted with unfractionated heparin (IV or SC) when the INR falls below 2.0, bridging therapy can be started with prophylactic unfractionated heparin (5000 U every 8–12 hours subcutaneously). Those at very high risk of thromboembolic complications (previous systemic embolism in atrial fibrillation, prosthetic heart valves, multiple risk factors) can also be given bridging therapy by administering adjusted-dose heparin (subcutaneous in outpatients or by continuous intravenous infusion in case of hospital admission) to maintain an APTT value equal to 1.5–2 times the normal value of control.

Bridging therapy can also be administered with LMWH subcutaneously as an out- or inpatient for 2–3 days preoperatively, using doses recommended for prophylaxis or, in patients at very high risk of thrombosis, therapeutic doses once (150–200 U/kg) or twice (100 U/kg) daily.

Drug administration immediately prior to surgery must be avoided in these cases. Subcutaneous unfractionated heparin should be discontinued 12 hours before surgery. Intravenous heparin should be discontinued 6 hours before surgery.

LMWH should be discontinued no less than 8–10 hours at the prophylaxis dose or 18 hours preoperatively with treatment doses, with an additional 6 hours interval in case of planned neuroaxial anesthesia.

In VTE, the recurrence risk is highest in the first month after the acute event (40%) and invasive procedures should be deferred, if possible, for at least 1 month, and preferably for 3 months after the acute event. If surgery is necessary within 2 weeks of an acute event, a vena cava filter should be inserted preoperatively or intraoperatively after VKA interruption.

Postoperative Management of Anticoagulation

Intravenous heparin should be resumed 12 hours postoperatively at a rate of no more than 18 U/kg/h. If subcutaneous LMWH is preferred, twice-daily doses are recommended, started 24 hours postoperatively and only after hemostasis has been achieved. In patients with a very high bleeding risk (e.g., after neurosurgery or prostatectomy) heparin is resumed only after clinical evaluation and after at least 48–72 hours. VKAs can be resumed postoperatively as soon as the patient can take solid foods.

References

1 Garcia DA, Baglin TP, Weitz JI, *et al.* Parenteral anticoagulants : antithrombotic therapy and prevention of thrombosis, 9th ed: American College of Chest Physicians evidence-based clinical practice guidelines. *Chest* 2012; 141: e24S–e43S.

2 Anderson JL, Adams CD, Antman EM, *et al.* 2012 ACCF/AHA focused update incorporated into the ACCF/AHA 2007 guidelines for the management of patients with unstable angina/non-ST-elevation myocardial infarction: a report of the American College of Cardiology Foundation/American Heart Association Task Force on Practice Guidelines. *J Am Coll Cardiol* 2013; 61: e179–347.

3 Gould MK, Garcia DA, Wren SM, *et al.* American College of Chest Physicians. Prevention of VTE in nonorthopedic surgical patients: antithrombotic therapy and prevention of thrombosis, 9th ed: American College of Chest Physicians evidence-based clinical practice guidelines. *Chest* 2012; 141 (Suppl.): e227S–77S. Erratum in: *Chest* 2012; 141: 1369.

4 Falck-Ytter Y, Francis CW, Johanson NA, *et al.* American College of Chest Physicians. Prevention of VTE in orthopedic surgery patients: antithrombotic therapy and prevention of thrombosis, 9th ed: American College of Chest Physicians evidence-based clinical practice guidelines. *Chest* 2012; 141 (Suppl.): e278S–325S.

5 Kahn SR, Lim W, Dunn AS, *et al.* American College of Chest Physicians. Prevention of VTE in nonsurgical patients: antithrombotic therapy and prevention of thrombosis, 9th ed: American College of Chest Physicians evidence-based clinical practice guidelines. *Chest* 2012; 141 (Suppl.): e195S–226S.

6 Kearon C, Akl EA, Comerota AJ, *et al.* American College of Chest Physicians. Antithrombotic therapy for VTE disease: antithrombotic therapy and prevention of thrombosis, 9th ed: American College of Chest Physicians evidence-based clinical practice guidelines. *Chest* 2012; 141 (Suppl.): e419S–494S.

7 National Institute for Health and Clinical Excellence (NICE). *Venous Thromboembolic Diseases: The Management of Venous Thromboembolic Diseases and the Role of Thrombophilia Testing.* Clinical Guideline 144. London: National Institute for Health and Clinical Excellence, 2012.

8 Ageno W, Gallus AS, Wittkowsky A, *et al.* Oral anticoagulant therapy. antithrombotic therapy and prevention of thrombosis, 9th ed: American College of Chest Physicians evidence-based clinical practice guidelines. *Chest* 2012; 141 (Suppl.): e44S–e88S.

9 Holbrook A, Schulman S, Witt DM, *et al.* Evidence-based management of anticoagulant therapy. Antithrombotic therapy and prevention of thrombosis, 9th ed: American College of Chest Physicians evidence-based clinical practice guidelines. *Chest* 2012; 141 (Suppl.): e152S–e184S.

10 Palareti G, Legnani C, Guazzaloca G, *et al.* Risk factors for highly unstable response to oral anticoagulation: a case-control study. *Br J Haematol* 2005; 129: 72–78.

11 Schulman S, Kearon C on behalf of the Subcommittee on Control of Anticoagulation of the Scientific and Standardization Committee of the International Society on Thrombosis and Haemostasis. Definition of major bleeding in clinical investigations of antihemostatic medicinal products in non-surgical patients. Scientific and Standardization Committee Communication. *J Thromb Haemost* 2005; 3: 692–694.

12 Palareti G, Leali N, Coccheri S, *et al..* Bleeding complications of oral anticoagulant treatment: an inception – cohort, prospective collaborative study (ISCOAT). Italian Study on Complications of Oral Anticoagulant Therapy. *Lancet* 1996; 348: 423–428.

13 Linkins LA, Choi PT, Douketis JD. Clinical impact of bleeding in patients taking oral anticoagulant therapy for venous thromboembolism: a meta-analysis. *Ann Intern Med* 2003; 13: 893–900.

14 Keeling D, Baglin T, Tait C, *et al.* Guidelines on oral anticoagulation with warfarin – fourth edition. *Br J Haematol* 2011; 154: 311–324.

15 Douketis JD, Spyropoulos AC, Spencer FA, *et al.* Perioperative management of antithrombotic therapy. Antithrombotic therapy and prevention of thrombosis, 9th ed: American College of Chest Physicians evidence-based clinical practice guidelines. *Chest* 2012; 141 (Suppl.): e326S–e350S.

18

The Direct Oral Anticoagulants

David A. Garcia, Mark A. Crowther and Walter Ageno

Key Points

- When compared with warfarin and other vitamin K antagonists, the direct oral anticoagulants (DOACs) exhibit different pharmacodynamics and have distinct mechanisms of action.
- Unlike vitamin K antagonists, the DOACs all are cleared, to differing degrees, by the kidneys.
- Large randomized controlled trials indicate the DOACs are at least as safe and effective as well managed warfarin in many clinical settings, including stroke prevention in atrial fibrillation as well as secondary prevention of venous thromboembolism.
- Clinicians caring for patients who take one of the DOACs should familiarize themselves with both the indications for and the pharmacological properties of the specific drug their patient will use.
- More research is needed to define the optimal management of DOAC-treated patients who require an invasive procedure or experience serious bleeding.

Pharmacology (Table 18.1)

Direct Thrombin Inhibitors

Dabigatran is administered as a prodrug (dabigatran etexilate) because the active drug is not orally available. After absorption, ubiquitous esterases in the gut mucosa, plasma, and liver cleave the etexilate moiety and liberate the active drug, dabigatran, a concentration-dependent, competitive, highly selective, and reversible inhibition of thrombin (Ki 4.5 ± 0.2 μM) [1]. Thrombin blockade results in reduced coagulant potential, reduced platelet activation, reduced feedback activation of coagulation, and reduced fibrin clot stabilization due to a diminution in the conversion coagulation factor XIII to factor XIIIa. As a low molecular weight inhibitor, dabigatran binds only to the active site of thrombin, differentiating its mechanism of action from other thrombin inhibitors such as bivalirudin, which bind to both the active site and the substrate recognition site of thrombin. Inhibition of coagulation peaks between 30 and 120 minutes in different models [1]. Dabigatran bioavailability is about 7%. Its absorption requires an acid environment; as a result, it is administered with tartaric acid and its absorption is reduced by coadministration of proton pump inhibitors – this reduction is likely clinically unimportant. About 80% of circulating dabigatran is excreted unchanged by the kidneys; the normal half-life is 8–10 hours after a single dose (14–17 hours at steady state), and is markedly prolonged with reduced renal function (exceeding 24 hours when the creatinine clearance is less than 30 mL/minute). Absorption is delayed by a high fat meal; however, there are no specific concerning food interactions. The risk of bleeding with dabigatran will be increased by coadministration of other antithrombotics such as aspirin or other

Practical Hemostasis and Thrombosis, Third Edition. Edited by Nigel S. Key, Michael Makris and David Lillicrap.
© 2017 John Wiley & Sons, Ltd. Published 2017 by John Wiley & Sons, Ltd.

Table 18.1 Pharmacological properties of the direct oral anticoagulants.

	Dabigatran	Rivaroxaban	Apixaban	Edoxaban
Coagulation factor inhibited	Thrombin	Factor Xa	Factor Xa	Factor Xa
Time to peak plasma levels	0.5–2 hours	1–4 hours	2.5–4 hours	0.5–2.0 hrs
Bioavailability	7%	80%	80%	60%
Half-life with normal renal function	12–17 hours (repeated dosing) – 9 hours after a single dose	7–17 hours	5–9 hours	6–11 hours
Fraction excreted by nonrenal mechanisms	15–20%	33–60% (dose dependent)	75%	40%
Impact of hepatic disease	Minimal	"Avoid use" in patients with moderate or severe impairment	"Not recommended" with severe impairment	Not reported but dependence on hepatic excretion implies that care should be used in patients with impaired hepatic function
Free fraction in circulation	65%	Less than 10%	13%	40–60%

antiplatelet agents. Absorption of dabigatran etexilate through the gastrointestinal mucosa is impacted by strong P-glycoprotein inhibitors (verapamil) or inducers (rifampin); however, once absorbed dabigatran itself has limited drug–drug interactions (Table 18.2). Dabigatran is usually administered twice daily despite its long half-life; thus, at steady state, there are detectable levels of drug present at trough. Dabigatran is not highly protein-bound in the circulation and thus may be removed by hemodialysis in cases of hemorrhage or overdose. Acutely, charcoal administration may reduce gastrointestinal absorption.

Direct Factor Xa Inhibitors

Rivaroxaban, apixaban, edoxaban, and betrixaban are all highly specific, orally available inhibitors of coagulation factor Xa. This chapter will focus on those agents for which at least one large phase III study has been published: rivaroxaban, apixaban, and edoxaban.

Betrixaban is currently in late-phase clinical development.

Rivaroxaban: Rivaroxaban is a high affinity (Ki 0.4 nmol/L) inhibitor of coagulation factor Xa PM [1]. The anticoagulant effect of rivaroxaban and the other factor Xa inhibitors is limited to reducing the proteolytic activity of factor Xa – downstream effects, such as reductions in platelet activation seen with dabigatran occur with factor Xa inhibitor treatment but are an indirect effect being attributable to reduced thrombin generation by the prothrombinase complex. Rivaroxaban reaches its maximal plasma concentration in 2–4 hours after oral administration and its bioavailability is approximately 80%. Unique to rivaroxaban is enhanced oral absorption with food; the time to peak concentration is delayed and the area under the curve (AUC) is increased by 30–40% when rivaroxaban is ingested with a meal. As a result, when used at therapeutic doses (15 or

Table 18.2 Potential drug–drug interactions within the target specific oral anticoagulants. Specific evidence of clinically important changes resulting in thrombosis or bleeding is lacking for almost all of these potential interactions. The reader should consult the prescribing package for updated information on clinically important interactions.

	Dabigatran	Rivaroxaban	Apixaban	Edoxaban
Inhibitors of CYP 3A4 and P-glycoprotein	Clarithromycin	Ketoconazole and other "azole" drugs, lopinavir/ ritonavir, clarithromycin, conivaptan, grapefruit	Ketoconazole and other "azole" drugs, ritonavir, clarithromycin, grapefruit	Not reported
P-glycoprotein inhibitors	Quinidine, amiodarone, verapamil			Quinidine, verapamil, and dronedarone
CYP 3A4 and P-glycoprotein inducers	Rifampin, St. John's wort	Rifampin, St. John's wort, phenytoin carbamazepine, phenobarbitone	Rifampin, carbamazepine, phenytoin, St John's wort	Not reported
Reduced absorption	Proton pump inhibitors			
Enhanced hemorrhagic risk due to coincident anticoagulant effect	NSAIDs, antiplatelet agents, other oral anticoagulants, heparins and related compounds	NSAIDs, antiplatelet agents, other oral anticoagulants, heparins and related compounds	NSAIDs, antiplatelet agents, other oral anticoagulants, heparins and related compounds	NSAIDs, antiplatelet agents, other oral anticoagulants, heparins and related compounds

NSAIDs, nonsteriodal anti-inflammatory drugs.

20 mg once daily) administration with food is recommended. Rivaroxaban has a half-life of 5–9 hours in the young and up to 13 hours in the elderly; it is administered once daily (for example, for long-term secondary prevention of venous thromboembolism (VTE)) or twice daily (for example, in the acute management of VTE). Two-thirds of ingested rivaroxaban is excreted by the kidneys with the majority having undergone metabolism prior to excretion. Administration to patients with renal insufficiency increases inhibition of factor Xa, suggesting a risk for bioaccumulation and associated bleeding, particularly in patients with severe renal impairment. It is highly protein-bound in the circulation and thus not amenable to hemodialysis. In cases of bleeding, oral charcoal may acutely reduce absorption. Charcoal hemoperfusion has been posited as an intervention to remove rivaroxaban from the circulation; however, it has not been tested in clinical practice. Rivaroxaban is metabolized by CYP3A4 and CYP2C8 in addition to other mechanisms. P-glycoprotein mediates its intestinal absorption. Inducers or inhibitors on any of these enzymes may impact rivaroxaban levels. Thus, for example, ketoconazole increased rivaroxaban AUC 2.6-fold, while rifampin reduced rivaroxaban AUC by about 50%. Other drugs that induce CYP3A4 – and thus may reduce rivaroxaban levels – include phenytoin, carbamazepine, phenobarbital, and St John's Wort (Table 18.2).

Apixaban: Apixaban is a low molecular weight, orally available and highly selective inhibitor of coagulation factor Xa (Kd 0.008 nmol/L) [1]. The time-to-effect of apixaban on coagulation is identical to that of rivaroxaban. It reaches its maximum plasma concentration approximately 3 hours after dosing in healthy volunteers and bioavailability is approximately 50%. As with rivaroxaban, apixaban is highly protein-bound, suggesting it will not be removed by dialysis. Food has little impact on apixaban pharmacokinetics. After administration, apixaban is metabolized through multiple routes – of the four direct oral anticoagulants (DOACs) discussed in this chapter, apixaban is the least dependent on kidney function for clearance. Apixaban is generally thought to be free of interactions with drugs, but caution is warranted in patients being treated with strong inhibitors or inducers of both CYP3A4 and P-glycoprotein. The US package insert for apixaban recommends avoiding concomitant use of apixaban in patients treated with strong dual inducers of CYP3A4 and P-glycoprotein, and recommends dose reductions in patients treated with strong inhibitors of CYP3A4 and P-glycoprotein. Given its dependence on hepatic function for clearance, apixaban should not be used in patients with severe renal impairment.

Edoxaban: Edoxaban is also a low molecular weight, high affinity (Ki 0.561 nmol/L) inhibitor of factor Xa. The effect of edoxaban on coagulation is identical to the other direct Xa inhibitors. After a single oral dose, maximal plasma concentrations are seen between 30 minutes and 2 hours after administration and the terminal elimination half-life is 8–10 hours. About 60% of an orally administered dose is absorbed, with the remainder being eliminated unchanged in the feces. About 40% of an absorbed dose of the drug is eliminated unchanged in the urine, with the remainder being metabolized and/or excreted by the liver. Food does not alter the absorption of edoxaban. Edoxaban markedly prolongs the activated partial thromboplastin time (APTT) except at very low doses. It also prolongs the prothrombin time/International Normalized Ratio (PT/INR) in a dose-dependent fashion. Forty to 60% of edoxaban is bound to plasma proteins; the rest is unbound in the circulation. Drug interactions

with edoxaban remain incompletely explored; however, coadministration of P-glycoprotein inhibitors (such as quinidine, verapamil, and dronedarone) increase edoxaban exposure. Less prominent effects were seen with amiodarone, atorvastatin, and digoxin. Coadministration with 325 mg aspirin increased edoxaban exposure by about 30%; lower dose aspirin or naproxen did not increase exposure but all of these drugs had an additive effect on prolongation of the bleeding time seen with edoxaban alone. Neither digoxin nor enoxaparin has an impact on the pharmacokinetics of edoxaban.

Evidence-Based Clinical Indications

The DOACs have been extensively studied in different settings, including: the prevention of VTE in high-risk patient groups; the treatment of deep vein thrombosis (DVT) and pulmonary embolism (PE); stroke prevention in patients with atrial fibrillation; the treatment of acute coronary syndromes; and stroke prevention in patients with mechanical heart valves. The results of phase III clinical trials have currently led to approval for clinical use of four agents: dabigatran, rivaroxaban, apixaban, and edoxaban.

VTE Prevention in Joint Replacement Surgery (Tables 18.3 and 18.4)

Elective major orthopedic surgery is associated with a high risk of VTE. The benefits of thromboprophylaxis are well established and antithrombotic drugs are recommended for a minimum of 10–14 days, and possibly for up to 35 days. A large development program was carried out for dabigatran, rivaroxaban, and apixaban in the setting of total hip and total knee arthroplasty. In all phase III trials, the DOACs were compared to the low molecular weight heparin (LMWH) enoxaparin. Four randomized controlled trials (RCTs) were carried out with two doses of dabigatran, 220 mg and 150 mg administered once daily (except for RE-NOVATE

Table 18.3 Phase III randomized controlled trials comparing the novel oral anticoagulants versus conventional treatment after elective total hip replacement.

Study, year of publication	Drug	Dosage	Timing	Duration of treatment	Primary efficacy outcome,[a] n/N (%)	Major bleeding events, n/N (%)
RE-NOVATE, 2007 [3]	Dabigatran	150 mg o.d.	half-dose 1–4 h after surgery	28–35 days	75/874 (8.6%)	15/1163 (1.3%)
	Dabigatran	220 mg o.d.	half-dose 1–4 h after surgery		53/880 (6.0%)	23/1146 (2.0%)
	Enoxaparin	40 mg o.d.	the evening before surgery		60/897 (6.7%)	18/1154 (1.6%)
RE-NOVATE II, 2011 [5]	Dabigatran	220 mg o.d.	half-dose 1–4 h after surgery	28–35 days	61/792 (7.7%)	14/1010 (1.4%)
	Enoxaparin	40 mg o.d.	the evening before surgery		69/785 (8.8%)	9/1003 (0.9%)
RECORD 1, 2008 [6]	Rivaroxaban	10 mg o.d.	6–8 h after surgery	31–39 days	18/1595 (1.1%)	6/2209 (0.3%)
	Enoxaparin	40 mg o.d.	12 h before surgery		58/1558 (3.7%)	2/2224 (0.1%)
RECORD 2, 2008 [7]	Rivaroxaban	10 mg o.d.	6–8 h after surgery	31–39 days	17/864 (2.0%)	1/1228 (<0.1%)
	Enoxaparin	40 mg o.d.	12 h before surgery	10–14 days	81/869 (9.3%)	1/1229 (<0.1%)
ADVANCE-3, 2010 [11]	Apixaban	2.5 mg b.i.d.	12–24 h after surgery	32–38 days	27/1949 (1.4%)	22/2673 (0.8%)
	Enoxaparin	40 mg o.d.	12 h before surgery		74/1917 (3.9%)	18/2659 (0.7%)

a) In all studies the primary efficacy outcome was the composite of asymptomatic and symptomatic deep vein thrombosis, nonfatal pulmonary embolism, and all-cause mortality.

II, where only one dose, 220 mg, was used) [2–5]. The results of these trials have shown that both doses of dabigatran are as effective as the "European Regimen" of enoxaparin (i.e., 40 mg daily started the evening before surgery) in reducing the risk of VTE and VTE-related mortality and have a similar bleeding profile. However, in a study of patients undergoing total knee replacement, both doses of dabigatran (220 and 150 mg daily) were less effective than the "North American Regimen" of enoxaparin (i.e., 30 mg twice daily, started postoperatively).

Rivaroxaban, administered at a fixed 10 mg once-daily dose, has been evaluated in four phase III RCTs in the RECORD program [6–9]. In all four trials, rivaroxaban resulted superior to enoxaparin, in both the European and the North American regimens, with regards to the primary composite outcome of any DVT, nonfatal PE, and all-cause mortality. No significant difference in major bleeding events was detected.

The ADVANCE program tested apixaban administered at the twice-daily dose of 2.5 mg [10–12]. In the ADVANCE-1 study [10] apixaban failed to meet prespecified criteria for noninferiority compared to twice-daily enoxaparin 30 mg. In the ADVANCE-2 and ADVANCE-3 studies [11,12], treatment with apixaban

Table 18.4 Phase III randomized controlled trials comparing the novel oral anticoagulants versus conventional treatment after elective total knee replacement.

Study, year of publication	Drug	Dosage	Timing	Duration of treatment	Primary efficacy outcome,[a] n/N (%)	Major bleeding events, n/N (%)
RE-MODEL, 2007 [2]	Dabigatran	150 mg o.d.	half-dose 1–4 h after surgery	6–10 days	213/526 (40.5%)	9/703 (1.3%)
	Dabigatran	220 mg o.d.	half-dose 1–4 h after surgery		183/503 (36.4%)	10/679 (1.5%)
	Enoxaparin	40 mg o.d.	the evening before surgery		193/512 (37.7%)	9/694 (1.3%)
RE-MOBILIZE, 2009 [37]	Dabigatran	150 mg o.d.	half-dose 6–12 h after surgery	12–15 days	219/649 (33.7%)	5/871 (0.6%)
	Dabigatran	220 mg o.d.	half-dose 6–12 h after surgery		188/604 (31.1%)	5/857 (0.6%)
	Enoxaparin	30 mg b.i.d.	12–24 h after surgery		163/643 (25.3%)	12/868 (1.4%)
RECORD3, 2008 [8]	Rivaroxaban	10 mg o.d.	6–8 h after surgery	10–14 days	79 / 824 (9.6%)	7/1220 (0.6%)
	Enoxaparin	40 mg o.d.	12 h before surgery		166 / 878 (18.9%)	6/1239 (0.5%)
RECORD4, 2009 [9]	Rivaroxaban	10 mg o.d.	6–8 h after surgery	10–14 days	67/965 (6.9%)	10/1526 (0.7%)
	Enoxaparin	30 mg b.i.d.	12–24 h after surgery		97/959 (10.1%)	4/1508 (0.3%)
ADVANCE-1, 2009 [10]	Apixaban	2.5 mg b.i.d.	12–24 h after surgery	10–14 days	104/1157 (9.0%)	11/1596 (0.7%)
	Enoxaparin	30 mg b.i.d.	12–24 h after surgery		100/1130 (8.8%)	22/1588 (1.4%)
ADVANCE-2, 2010 [12]	Apixaban	2.5 mg b.i.d.	12–24 h after surgery	10–14 days	147/976 (15.1%)	9/1501 (0.6%)
	Enoxaparin	40 mg o.d.	12 h before surgery		243/997 (24.4%)	14/1508 (0.9%)

a) In all studies the primary efficacy outcome was the composite of asymptomatic and symptomatic deep vein thrombosis, nonfatal pulmonary embolism and all-cause mortality.

resulted in a statistically significant reduction in the primary efficacy endpoint, and in a similar safety profile when compared to the European regimen of enoxaparin.

There was considerable variation in the absolute rates of efficacy and safety outcomes for rivaroxaban, apixaban, dabigatran, and enoxa-parin across the studies described, reflecting differences in patient populations, treatment regimens, and outcome definitions. Definitions of efficacy endpoints were similar for all studies, whereas definitions of major bleeding varied across studies of rivaroxaban, apixaban, and dabigatran. This variation in the definition of safety endpoints makes cross-trial comparisons among these agents especially challenging. That notwithstanding, the rates of major bleeding were generally low across all studies; the rates of major bleeding within a category of operation (knee or hip) were comparable.

Based on the results of the studies, dabigatran, rivaroxaban, and apixaban have received approval in several countries for the prevention of VTE in patients undergoing total hip and total knee arthroplasty. The recommended dose of dabigatran is 220 mg once daily, to be reduced to 150 mg once daily in patients with moderate renal insufficiency and in patients older than 75 years. Dabigatran should be started 1–4 hours after completed surgery with half of the recommended dose. Rivaroxaban 10 mg once daily should be started within 6–10 hours of completed surgery and no dose adjustments are recommended. Finally, the approved dose for apixaban is 2.5 mg twice daily, with the first dose to be administered 12–24 hours postoperatively.

VTE Prevention in Medically Ill Patients

Acutely ill medical patients with reduced mobility are at increased risk of VTE. Clinical trials have shown that pharmacological prophylaxis administered for up to 14 days may reduce the risk of VTE in high-risk medical patients without significantly increasing the risk for major bleeding, and low-dose anticoagulants are therefore recommended by international guidelines.

Rivaroxaban has been evaluated for the prevention of VTE in medical patients in the MAGELLAN study [13]. Patients were randomized to receive either subcutaneous enoxaparin 40 mg daily for 10 ± 4 days followed by placebo, or oral rivaroxaban 10 mg daily for 35 ± 4 days. Rivaroxaban was noninferior for the composite of symptomatic VTE or asymptomatic proximal DVT in the head-to-head comparison with enoxaparin at day 10 (2.7% vs. 2.7%, $P = 0.0025$), and was superior at day 35 when compared with enoxaparin followed by placebo (4.4% and 5.7% respectively; $P = 0.0211$). However, much of the efficacy difference stemmed from asymptomatic events and the

primary safety outcome, a composite of major and nonmajor clinically relevant bleeding, was reached more often by patients receiving rivaroxaban (4.1% vs. 1.7%, $P < 0.0001$ for events between day 1 and day 35).

Extended-duration (30 days) apixaban 2.5 mg twice daily was compared with standard-duration (6–14 days) enoxaparin 40 mg daily in the ADOPT study [14]. The primary efficacy outcome, a composite of symptomatic VTE and asymptomatic thrombosis detected by lower extremity ultrasonography, occurred in 2.7% of patients in the apixaban group and in 3.0% of patients in the enoxaparin group ($P = 0.44$). The primary safety outcome major bleeding occurred in 0.5% of patients receiving apixaban and in 0.2% of patients receiving enoxaparin ($P = 0.04$).

The results of the MAGELLAN and ADOPT studies have not led to approval of DOACs as a primary VTE prevention strategy in medical patients. The findings of these trials also raise doubts about the benefits of postdischarge VTE prophylaxis in medical patients.

Treatment of Acute VTE (Table 18.5)

The majority of patients with DVT or PE usually receive a dual-drug approach with LMWH and VKAs. These agents are typically started on the same day, and the LMWH is administered for a minimum of 5 days until the INR is above 2.0. The DOACs have been recently tested in this setting to offer simplified alternatives to the standard of care. Two different approaches have been evaluated: a dual-drug approach requiring lead-in LMWH treatment for a minimum of 5 days before switching to the DOAC (dabigatran or edoxaban), or a single-drug approach with the DOAC as a stand-alone therapy from the beginning (rivaroxaban or apixaban).

In the RE-COVER study, dabigatran was noninferior to warfarin in preventing recurrent VTE, with similar rates of major bleeding events [15].

In the Hokusai-VTE study, also edoxaban was noninferior to warfarin for the primary efficacy outcome of recurrent VTE or VTE-related death; edoxaban was superior to warfarin in the reduction of the primary safety outcome of

Table 18.5 Phase III randomized controlled trials comparing the novel oral anticoagulants versus standard of care for acute venous thromboembolism.

Study, year of publication	Drug	Dosage	Timing	Duration of treatment	Primary efficacy outcome, n/N (%)	Major bleeding events, n/N (%)
RE-COVER I, 2009 [15]	Dabigatran	150 mg b.i.d.	After ≥5 days of UFH or LMWH	6 months	30/1274 (2.4%)	20/1274 (1.6%)
	Warfarin	INR 2.0–3.0	Overlapped with ≥5 days of UFH or LMWH		27/1265 (2.1%)	24/1265 (1.9%)
EINSTEIN DVT, 2010 [17]	Rivaroxaban	15 mg b.i.d. for 21 days, followed by 20 mg o.d.	From first day of treatment	3, 6, or 12 months	36/1731 (2.1%)	14/1718 (0.8%)
	Enoxaparin/ VKA	1 mg/kg b.i.d. for ≥5 days overlapped with a VKA until INR ≥2.0 for 2 days	From first day of treatment		51/1718 (3.0%)	20/1711 (1.2%)
EINSTEIN PE, 2012 [18]	Rivaroxaban	15 mg b.i.d. for 21 days, followed by 20 mg o.d.	From first day of treatment	3, 6, or 12 months	50/2419 (2.1%)	26/2412 (1.1%)
	Enoxaparin/ VKA	1 mg/kg b.i.d. for ≥5 days overlapped with a VKA until INR ≥2.0 for 2 days	From first day of treatment		44/2413 (1.8%)	52/2405 (2.2%)
AMPLIFY, 2013 [19]	Apixaban	10 mg b.i.d. for 7 days followed by 5 mg b.i.d.	From first day of treatment	6 months	59/2609 (2.3%)	15/2676 (0.6%)
	Enoxaparin/ VKA	1 mg/kg b.i.d. for ≥5 days overlapped with a VKA until INR ≥2.0 for 2 days	From first day of treatment	6 months	71/2635 (2.7%)	49/2689 (1.8%)
HOKUSAI, 2013 [16]	Edoxaban	60 mg o.d. or 30 mg o.d.[a]	After ≥5 days of UFH or LMWH	3, 6, or 12 months	130/4118 (3.2%)	56/4118 (1.4%)
	Warfarin	INR 2.0–3.0	Overlapped with ≥5 days of UFH or LMWH		146/4122 (3.5%)	66/4122 (1.6%)

a) In patients with creatinine clearance 30–50 mL/min, weighing ≤60 kg or those receiving concomitant treatment with potent P-glycoprotein inhibitors.
   DVT, deep vein thrombosis; PE, pulmonary embolism; VKA, vitamin K antagonists; UFH, unfractionated heparin; LMWH, low molecular weight heparin.

major or nonmajor clinically relevant bleeding, although no significant difference was observed in the rate of major bleeding events [16].

In the EINSTEIN DVT trial, both symptomatic VTE as well as bleeding were similar between rivaroxaban and LMWH/VKAs [17]. In the EINSTEIN PE study, rivaroxaban was noninferior to enoxaparin/warfarin for primary efficacy outcome, recurrent VTE. The primary safety outcome (major and nonmajor clinically relevant bleeding) occurred with similar frequency in the two treatment groups, rivaroxaban caused less major bleeding than standard therapy with LMWH/VKA [18].

In the AMPLIFY trial, apixaban was noninferior to enoxaparin/warfarin for the reduction of recurrent symptomatic VTE and was associated with a significant reduction in the primary safety outcome, major bleeding [19].

As with studies of VTE prevention, differences in study design make direct comparisons between the DOACs difficult. RE-COVER, AMPLIFY, and Hokusai-VTE were double-blind studies, whereas the EINSTEIN trials were open label. Studies assessing the single-drug approach used different durations for the "loading" dose of the study drug, with high-dose apixaban given for 7 days and high-dose rivaroxaban for 21 days. Parenteral anticoagulation with LMWH, heparin, or fondaparinux prior to randomization was allowed in these studies, but it was usually administered for less than 2 days. In the dabigatran and edoxaban studies, initial parenteral anticoagulation was administered not only to the patients who received warfarin, but also to the patients who received a DOAC (median time of parenteral therapy was 9 days and 7 days, respectively).

Rivaroxaban is currently approved in a number of jurisdictions for the treatment of DVT and PE at the initial 15 mg twice-daily dose for 3 weeks followed by a maintenance dose of 20 mg daily.

Extended Treatment of VTE (Table 18.6)

VKAs are the standard of treatment for the long-term secondary prevention of VTE. It is generally accepted that patients with a major reversible risk factor at the time of their index event can safely withhold anticoagulant therapy after 3 months. For the remaining patients, in particular those with unprovoked events, optimal treatment duration remains uncertain because of a nonnegligible residual risk of recurrence over time. Indefinite treatment duration is currently suggested for these patients, at least as long as the benefit–risk balance remains favorable. Because there is often clinical equipoise associated with the decision to stop or continue anticoagulation after a first unprovoked VTE, most studies of extended treatment with the DOAC have used placebo as a comparator (Figure 18.1).

Dabigatran was compared with placebo in the RE-SONATE trial, and resulted in a 92% relative risk reduction in the incidence of recurrent VTE, with a similar incidence of major bleeding events between the two groups [20]. The composite of major or clinically relevant bleeding was significantly higher with dabigatran compared to placebo. In the RE-MEDY study, carried out in patients at higher risk of recurrence, dabigatran was noninferior to warfarin in the reduction of recurrent VTE, with a significant reduction in the composite of major or clinically relevant bleeding [20].

In the EINSTEIN-Extension study, symptomatic recurrent VTE events were significantly reduced by rivaroxaban and the primary safety outcome of major bleeding was not statistically different between the two groups [17].

In AMPLIFY-EXT, both apixaban doses significantly reduced the risk of recurrent VTE without increasing the incidence of the primary safety outcome major bleeding compared to placebo [21].

The results of these studies indicate that the DOACs are treatment alternatives for those patients who require extended secondary prevention of VTE. While these studies of the DOACs do not offer additional insights about how the patients at highest risk for recurrence might be identified, the low rate of bleeding in all of these "extension" studies may, if resources permit, lower the threshold at which many physicians and patients consider extended anticoagulant therapy.

Table 18.6 Phase III randomized controlled trials comparing the novel oral anticoagulants versus placebo or warfarin for extended treatment of venous thromboembolism.

Study, year of publication	Drug	Dosage	Timing	Duration of treatment	Primary efficacy outcome, n/N (%)	Major bleeding events, n/N (%)
AMPLIFY-EXT, 2012 [21]	Apixaban	2.5 mg b.i.d.	After completion of 6–12 months of anticoagulant therapy	12 months	32/840 (3.8%)	2/840 (0.2%)
	Apixaban	5 mg b.i.d.	After completion of 6–12 months of anticoagulant therapy		34/813 (4.2%)	1/813 (0.1%)
	Placebo	–	After completion of 6–12 months of anticoagulant therapy		96/829 (11.6%)	4/829 (0.5%)
RE-MEDY, 2013 [20]	Dabigatran	150 mg b.i.d.	After completion of 3 months of anticoagulant therapy	6–36 months	26/1430 (1.8%)	13/1430 (0.9%)
	Warfarin	INR 2.0–3.0	After completion of 3 months of anticoagulant therapy		18/1426 (1.3%)	25/1426 (1.8%)
RE-SONATE, 2013 [20]	Dabigatran	150 mg b.i.d.	After completion of 3 months of anticoagulant therapy	12 months	3/681 (0.4%)	2/681 (0.3%)
	Placebo	–	After completion of 3 months of anticoagulant therapy		37/662 (5.6%)	0/662
EINSTEIN EXT, 2010 [17]	Rivaroxaban	20 mg o.d.	After completion of 6–12 months of anticoagulant therapy	6 or 12 months	8/602 (1.3%)	4/598 (0.7%)
	Placebo	–	After completion of 6–12 months of anticoagulant therapy	6 or 12 months	42/594 (7.1%)	0/590

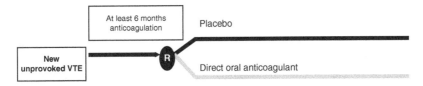

Figure 18.1 Scheme for secondary venous thromboembolism (VTE) prevention (extended treatment) studies. R, randomization.

Stroke Prevention in Atrial Fibrillation (Table 18.7)

Atrial fibrillation (AF) is the most common cardiac arrhythmia and one of the major risk factors for ischemic stroke. VKAs are highly effective in preventing stroke in AF patients, with a 65% relative risk reduction when compared to placebo and a 50% relative risk reduction when compared with aspirin. The DOACs have been compared with warfarin in four large phase III RCTs in AF patients.

The RE-LY trial compared two dabigatran doses with warfarin in patients with nonvalvular AF and at least one risk factor for stroke [22].

The primary outcome of stroke (including hemorrhagic stroke) or systemic embolism was significantly reduced with the higher dose (150 mg b.i.d.) of dabigatran, while the lower dose (110 mg b.i.d.) was noninferior to warfarin. Major bleeding was significantly less common at the lower dabigatran dose, and no difference in major bleeding was observed between the higher dabigatran dose and warfarin. Both dabigatran doses significantly reduced the rates of intracranial bleeding; the higher dose of dabigatran was associated with a statistically significant increase in gastrointestinal bleeding as compared to warfarin.

Table 18.7 Phase III randomized controlled trials comparing the novel oral anticoagulants versus warfarin for stroke prevention in atrial fibrillation patients.

Study, year of publication	Drug	Dosage	Duration of treatment	Primary efficacy outcome, (%/year)	Major bleeding events, (%/year)
RE-LY, 2009 [22]	Dabigatran	110 mg b.i.d.	Median follow-up 24 months	1.5	2.7
	Dabigatran	150 mg b.i.d.		1.1	3.1
	Warfarin	INR 2.0–3.0		1.7	3.4
ROCKET AF, 2011 [23]	Rivaroxaban	20 mg o.d. or 15 mg o.d.[b]	Median follow-up 707 days	2.1[a]	3.6
	Warfarin	INR 2.0–3.0		2.4[a]	3.4
ARISTOTLE, 2011 [24]	Apixaban	5 mg b.i.d. or 2.5 mg b.i.d.[c]	Median follow-up 1.8 years	1.3	2.1
	Warfarin	INR 2.0–3.0		1.6	3.1
ENGAGE TIMI 48, 2013 [25]	Edoxaban	60 mg o.d.	Median follow-up, 2.8 years	1.18	2.75
	Edoxaban	30 mg o.d.		1.61	1.61
	Warfarin	INR 2.0–3.0		1.50	3.43

a) Intention to treat analysis:
b) in patients with a creatinine clearance of 30 to 49 mL/minute
c) in the presence of 2 or more of: age ≥80 years, body weight ≤60 kg, serum creatinine ≥1.5 mg per deciliter.

The ROCKET-AF study compared rivaroxaban with warfarin in patients with AF and at least two additional risk factors for stroke [23]. The incidence of the primary outcome stroke or systemic embolism as well as of major bleeding events was similar between the two groups, while the incidence of intracranial hemorrhage was significantly lower in the rivaroxaban group. Gastrointestinal bleeding occurred more frequently in rivaroxaban-treated patients.

The ARISTOTLE trial compared apixaban and warfarin in patients with AF and at least one additional risk factor for stroke [24]. The incidence of stroke or systemic embolism was significantly reduced by apixaban; major bleeding, intracranial bleeding, and all-cause mortality were all statistically significantly less frequent in the apixaban arm.

Finally, ENGAGE AF TIMI 48 was a three-arm (edoxaban 60 mg daily, edoxaban 30 mg daily, and warfarin) RCT of stroke prevention in AF patients with a CHADS$_2$ score ≥ 2. In both edoxaban groups, the dose was halved if any of the following characteristics was present: estimated creatinine clearance of 30–50 mL per minute, a body weight of 60 kg or less, or use of verapamil or quinidine (potent P-glycoprotein inhibitors). For stroke and systemic embolism, both doses of edoxaban were statistically noninferior to warfarin. Both overall major bleeding and intracranial bleeding were statistically less common at both doses of edoxaban; the benefit was greater for the low-dose edoxaban strategy [25].

In the AVERROES study, patients with AF who were deemed ineligible for VKA treatment were randomized to receive apixaban 5 mg twice daily or aspirin 81–324 mg o.d. [26]. The study was prematurely stopped because of the clear superiority in efficacy of apixaban over aspirin, with a similar safety profile. The primary efficacy outcome (stroke or systemic embolism) was reduced from 3.6% in the group treated with aspirin to 1.6% in the group treated with apixaban. The rate of major bleeding was similar between the two groups, but the power to detect a difference was limited because the early termination of this trial resulted in a lower than anticipated number of bleeding events in both groups.

Following the results of the phase III RCTs, dabigatran, rivaroxaban, apixaban, and edoxaban are approved for stroke prevention in AF patients without significant valvular heart disease (e.g., mechanical valve, significant mitral stenosis). Dabigatran is approved at the 150 mg twice-daily dose, with the 110 mg twice-daily dose proposed for patients aged 80 years or above, patients receiving concomitant verapamil, or, in selected cases, patients between 75 and 80 years. In the United States, 75 mg dabigatran twice daily has been labeled for patients with a creatinine clearance between 15 and 30 mL/min. Rivaroxaban is approved at the 20 mg daily dose, to be reduced to 15 mg daily in patients with creatinine clearance between 15 and 49 mL/minute. Apixaban is approved at the 5 mg twice-daily dose, to be reduced to 2.5 mg twice daily in patients with at least two of the following characteristics: age of 80 years or older, body weight of equal to or less than 60 kg, or serum creatinine of 1.5 mg/dL or above. Edoxaban is approved in two doses: 60 mg once daily for patients with creatinine clearance between 50 and 95 mL/min, and 30 mg once daily in patients with creatinine clearance 15–50 mL/min. Because edoxaban was had inferior efficacy versus warfarin among the subgroup of patients with especially good renal function, the manufacturer recommends it not be used for prevention of stroke in AF patients who have creatinine clearance > 95 mL/min.

Acute Coronary Syndromes

Patients with acute coronary syndromes (ACS) remain at increased long-term risk of recurrent cardiovascular events. Secondary prevention is based on the administration of dual antiplatelet therapy, and the potential benefit of additional anticoagulant remains uncertain. Rivaroxaban and apixaban have been tested in phase III clinical trials to address this issue.

In the ATLAS ACS 2-TIMI 51 trial, patients with a recent ACS were randomized to rivaroxaban 2.5 mg twice daily, rivaroxaban 5 mg twice daily, or placebo, on top of standard antithrombotic treatment for a mean of 13 months [27]. The primary efficacy end-point of cardiovascular mortality, myocardial infarction, or stroke was significantly reduced from 10.7% in the placebo arm to 9.1% and 8.8% in the two rivaroxaban arms, respectively (P = 0.008). Major bleeding (2.1% vs. 0.6%, P <0.001) and intracranial bleeding events (0.6% vs. 0.2%, P = 0.009) were significantly increased with rivaroxaban, but fatal bleeding was not (0.3% vs. 0.2%, P = 0.66). Significantly fewer fatal bleeding events occurred with the 2.5 mg twice-daily dose of rivaroxaban as compared to the 5 mg twice-daily dose (0.1% vs. 0.4%, P = 0.04).

APPRAISE-2 randomized patients with recent acute coronary syndrome and at least two additional risk factors for recurrent ischemic events to apixaban 5 mg twice daily or placebo on top of standard antithrombotic therapy [28]. The study was prematurely stopped after a median follow-up of 241 days because major bleeding rates were significantly higher in the apixaban than in the placebo group (1.3% vs. 0.5%, P = 0.001), with also a great number of intracranial and fatal bleeding events, with no signs of benefit in efficacy (primary efficacy outcome of cardiovascular mortality, myocardial infarction, or ischemic stroke 7.5% vs. 7.9%, P = 0.51).

Practical Considerations

Laboratory Assessment

Although the direct oral anticoagulants have been developed and approved without the need

Table 18.8 Clinical scenarios in which measurement of anticoagulant effect may be desired.

To distinguish between noncompliance and treatment failure in a patient with thrombosis
To allow for risk–benefit calculations in a patient for whom urgent surgery or systemic thrombolysis is being contemplated
To determine the extent to which drug effect (vs. an anatomic cause) is responsible for bleeding
To quantify accumulation (or clearance), such as in a patient with impaired renal function

Source: adapted from Garcia, *et al.* 2013 [38].

for routine monitoring of their effect, clinical scenarios will arise where it may be valuable to determine whether (and to what extent) the coagulant potential of the blood has been impaired (Table 18.8). In such situations, traditional clotting times may reveal the presence or absence of a clinically significant anticoagulant effect (Table 18.9) [29], but must be interpreted with caution. Unlike the effect of vitamin K antagonists, the anticoagulant effect of the DOACs begins to dissipate rapidly within 3–4 hours after the most recent dose. Thus, the expected plasma concentration (and the expected drug effect) will depend heavily on the time elapsed since the last dose was ingested. Although expected peak and trough concentrations have been published [29], there is no evidence with which one could define a "target range" or a cut-off at which the risk of undesirable outcomes such as bleeding or thrombosis would abruptly increase.

Table 18.9 Anticipated effect of direct oral anticoagulants on several laboratory assays. See also Cuker *et al.* 2014 [29].

Novel oral anticoagulant	Prothrombin time (PT)	Activated partial thromboplastin time (aPTT)	Thrombin clotting time (TCT)	Ecarin clotting time	Dilute thrombin time	Anti-Factor Xa activity	
						Clot-based	Chromogenic
Dabigatran	↑ or ↔	↑	↑↑[b]	↑	↑[a]	–	–
Rivaroxaban	↑ or ↔	↑ or ↔	–	–	–	↑	↑[a]
Apixaban	↑ or ↔	↑ or ↔	–	–	–	↑[a]	↑[a]

a) Indicates a preferred test.
b) May be very prolonged even in the presence of clinically unimportant drug concentrations.

Interruption for Elective Procedures

Most chronically anticoagulated patients will, on occasion, need to interrupt their treatment in order to undergo an elective procedure. Data from the three large atrial fibrillation trials suggest that brief (<7-day) interruptions of the DOACs pose very little risk of stroke or other arterial embolism [30–32]. The relatively short half-lives and the rapid onset of the DOACs should simplify the management of patients who require a procedure; for most patients, "bridging" with a parenteral anticoagulant would be unnecessary. For each DOAC, specific information about treatment interruption can be found in the package insert, but generally, the precise timing of periprocedural doses will depend on the bleeding risk inherent to the procedure, the patient's renal function, and the risk of thromboembolism.

Reversal for Surgery or Major Bleeding

There is no high-quality evidence on which to base recommendations for emergent DOAC reversal. That notwithstanding, preclinical evidence from animal models and *in vitro* testing of healthy volunteers suggesting that prothrombin complex concentrates (PCC) or recombinant factor VIIa may be of some benefit has been summarized elsewhere [33]. More targeted interventions (e.g., a monoclonal antibody fragment directed at dabigatran [34]) are expected soon; until such antidotes are available, powerful nonspecific prohemostatic treatments should be reserved for patients with life-threatening hemorrhage. Despite the lack of an antidote for DOACs, a pooled analysis of safety outcomes among the more than 100 000 patients enrolled in phase III clinical trials found that – compared to warfarin – the risk of fatal bleeding was 50% lower among DOAC-treated patients [35]. When possible, surgical intervention should be postponed because, in a patient with normal renal function, a delay of even several hours will significantly improve the patient's hemostatic potential at the time the procedure begins.

Future Directions

Taken together, the clinical trial data establishing the efficacy and safety of the DOACs in AF and VTE are quite convincing. However, there are clinical situations where anticoagulant therapy is indicated but the safety and efficacy of the DOACs are unproven. For example, pending further evidence, the DOACs should not be used in patients with a prosthetic mechanical heart valve [36]. Further, although a small number of patients with cancer-associated VTE were included in the phase III VTE treatment studies, the DOACs have not been compared to LMWH, the current standard of care for venous thrombosis in the setting of active malignancy. Whether the DOACs would provide effective anticoagulation for a patient with a left ventricular assist device is also unknown. Finally, the DOACs have not been examined in dedicated studies of patients with heparin-induced thrombocytopenia or antiphospholipid syndrome, clinical conditions known to be associated with an unusually prothrombotic tendency.

References

1 Scaglione F. New oral anticoagulants: comparative pharmacology with vitamin K antagonists. *Clin Pharmacokinet* 2013; 52: 69–82.

2 Eriksson BI, Dahl OE, Rosencher N, *et al*. Oral dabigatran etexilate vs. subcutaneous enoxaparin for the prevention of venous thromboembolism after total knee replacement: the RE-MODEL randomized trial. *J Thromb Haemost* 2007; 5: 2178–2185.

3 Eriksson BI, Dahl OE, Rosencher N, *et al*. Dabigatran etexilate versus enoxaparin for prevention of venous thromboembolism after total hip replacement: a randomised, double-blind, non-inferiority trial. *Lancet* 2007; 370: 949–956.

4 Committee R-MW, Ginsberg JS, Davidson BL, *et al*. Oral thrombin inhibitor dabigatran etexilate vs North American enoxaparin regimen for prevention of venous

thromboembolism after knee arthroplasty surgery. *J Arthroplasty* 2009; 24: 1–9.

5 Eriksson BI, Dahl OE, Huo MH, *et al*. Oral dabigatran versus enoxaparin for thromboprophylaxis after primary total hip arthroplasty (RE-NOVATE II*). A randomised, double-blind, non-inferiority trial. *Thromb Haemost* 2011; 105: 721–729.

6 Eriksson BI, Borris LC, Friedman RJ, *et al*. Rivaroxaban versus enoxaparin for thromboprophylaxis after hip arthroplasty. *N Engl J Med* 2008; 358: 2765–2775.

7 Kakkar AK, Brenner B, Dahl OE, *et al*. Extended duration rivaroxaban versus short-term enoxaparin for the prevention of venous thromboembolism after total hip arthroplasty: a double-blind, randomised controlled trial. *Lancet* 2008; 372: 31–39.

8 Lassen MR, Ageno W, Borris LC, *et al*. Rivaroxaban versus enoxaparin for thromboprophylaxis after total knee arthroplasty. *N Engl J Med* 2008; 358: 2776–2786.

9 Turpie AG, Lassen MR, Davidson BL, *et al*. Rivaroxaban versus enoxaparin for thromboprophylaxis after total knee arthroplasty (RECORD4): a randomised trial. *Lancet* 2009; 373: 1673–1680.

10 Lassen MR, Raskob GE, Gallus A, *et al*. Apixaban or enoxaparin for thromboprophylaxis after knee replacement. *N Engl J Med* 2009; 361: 594–604.

11 Lassen MR, Gallus A, Raskob GE, *et al*. Apixaban versus enoxaparin for thromboprophylaxis after hip replacement. *N Engl J Med* 2010; 363: 2487–2498.

12 Lassen MR, Raskob GE, Gallus A, *et al*. Apixaban versus enoxaparin for thromboprophylaxis after knee replacement (ADVANCE-2): a randomised double-blind trial. *Lancet* 2010; 375: 807–815.

13 Cohen AT, Spiro TE, Buller HR, *et al*. Rivaroxaban for thromboprophylaxis in acutely ill medical patients. *N Engl J Med* 2013; 368: 513–523.

14 Goldhaber SZ, Leizorovicz A, Kakkar AK, *et al*. Apixaban versus enoxaparin for thromboprophylaxis in medically ill patients. *N Engl J Med* 2011; 365: 2167–2177.

15 Schulman S, Kearon C, Kakkar AK, *et al*. Dabigatran versus warfarin in the treatment of acute venous thromboembolism. *N Engl J Med* 2009; 361: 2342–2352.

16 Hokusai VTEI, Buller HR, Decousus H, *et al*. Edoxaban versus warfarin for the treatment of symptomatic venous thromboembolism. *N Engl J Med* 2013; 369: 1406–1415.

17 Investigators E, Bauersachs R, Berkowitz SD, *et al*. Oral rivaroxaban for symptomatic venous thromboembolism. *N Engl J Med* 2010; 363: 2499–2510.

18 Investigators E-P, Buller HR, Prins MH, *et al*. Oral rivaroxaban for the treatment of symptomatic pulmonary embolism. *N Engl J Med* 2012; 366: 1287–1297.

19 Agnelli G, Buller HR, Cohen A, *et al*. Oral apixaban for the treatment of acute venous thromboembolism. *N Engl J Med* 2013; 369: 799–808.

20 Schulman S, Kearon C, Kakkar AK, *et al*. Extended use of dabigatran, warfarin, or placebo in venous thromboembolism. *N Engl J Med* 2013; 368: 709–718.

21 Agnelli G, Buller HR, Cohen A, *et al*. Apixaban for extended treatment of venous thromboembolism. *N Engl J Med* 2013; 368: 699–708.

22 Connolly SJ, Ezekowitz MD, Yusuf S, *et al*. Dabigatran versus warfarin in patients with atrial fibrillation. *N Engl J Med* 2009; 361: 1139–1151.

23 Patel MR, Mahaffey KW, Garg J, *et al*. Rivaroxaban versus warfarin in nonvalvular atrial fibrillation. *N Engl J Med* 2011; 365: 883–891.

24 Granger CB, Alexander JH, McMurray JJ, *et al*. Apixaban versus warfarin in patients with atrial fibrillation. *N Engl J Med* 2011; 365: 981–992.

25 Giugliano RP, Ruff CT, Braunwald E, *et al*. Edoxaban versus warfarin in patients with atrial fibrillation. *N Engl J Med* 2013; 369: 2093–2104.

26 Connolly SJ, Eikelboom J, Joyner C, *et al.* Apixaban in patients with atrial fibrillation. *N Engl J Med* 2011; 364: 806–817.

27 Mega JL, Braunwald E, Wiviott SD, *et al.* Rivaroxaban in patients with a recent acute coronary syndrome. *N Engl J Med* 2012; 366: 9–19.

28 Alexander JH, Lopes RD, James S, *et al.* Apixaban with antiplatelet therapy after acute coronary syndrome. *N Engl J Med* 2011; 365: 699–708.

29 Cuker A, Siegal DM, Crowther MA, *et al.* Laboratory measurement of the anticoagulant activity of the non-vitamin K oral anticoagulants. *J Am Coll Cardiol* 2014; 64: 1128–1139.

30 Healey JS, Eikelboom J, Douketis J, *et al.* Periprocedural bleeding and thromboembolic events with dabigatran compared with warfarin: results from the Randomized Evaluation of Long-Term Anticoagulation Therapy (RE-LY) randomized trial. *Circulation* 2012; 126: 343–348.

31 Patel MR, Hellkamp AS, Lokhnygina Y, *et al.* Outcomes of discontinuing rivaroxaban compared with warfarin in patients with nonvalvular atrial fibrillation: analysis from the ROCKET AF trial (Rivaroxaban Once-Daily, Oral, Direct Factor Xa Inhibition Compared With Vitamin K Antagonism for Prevention of Stroke and Embolism Trial in Atrial Fibrillation). *J Am Coll Cardiol* 2013; 61: 651–658.

32 Garcia D, Alexander JH, Wallentin L, *et al.* Management and clinical outcomes in patients treated with apixaban vs warfarin undergoing procedures. *Blood* 2014; 124: 3692–3698.

33 Siegal DM, Garcia DA, Crowther MA. How I treat target-specific oral anticoagulant-associated bleeding. *Blood* 2014; 123: 1152–1158.

34 Pollack CV, Jr., Reilly PA, Eikelboom J, *et al.* Idarucizumab for dabigatran reversal. *N Engl J Med* 2015; 373: 511–520.

35 Chai-Adisaksopha C, Crowther M, Isayama T, *et al.* The impact of bleeding complications in patients receiving target-specific oral anticoagulants: a systematic review and meta-analysis. *Blood* 2014; 124: 2450–2458.

36 Eikelboom JW, Connolly SJ, Brueckmann M, *et al.* Dabigatran versus warfarin in patients with mechanical heart valves. *N Engl J Med* 2013; 369: 1206–1214.

37 Ginsberg JS, Davidson BL, Comp PC, *et al.* Oral thrombin inhibitor dabigatran etexilate vs North American enoxaparin regimen for prevention of venous thromboembolism after knee arthroplasty surgery. *J Arthroplasty* 2009; 24: 1–9.

38 Garcia D, Barrett YC, Ramacciotti E, *et al.* Laboratory assessment of the anticoagulant effects of the next generation of oral anticoagulants. *J Thromb Haemost* 2013; 11: 245–252.

19

Antiphospholipid Syndrome

Henry G. Watson and Mark Crowther

Key Points

- The antiphospholipid syndrome (APS) is an acquired autoimmune condition that manifests as thrombosis or adverse pregnancy outcomes.
- The two major subtypes of antiphospholipid antibodies, lupus anticoagulants and anticardiolipin antibodies, are found in a significant number of normal subjects.
- The diagnosis of APS requires that both clinical and laboratory criteria be satisfied.
- There is no consensus as to the mechanism(s) that mediate thrombosis or the described pregnancy-related complications of APS.

Introduction

The antiphospholipid syndrome (APS) is an acquired prothrombotic or thrombophilic state, which is also associated with adverse pregnancy outcomes. An association of antiphospholipid antibodies with a variety of disorders has been made since the first report in patients with systemic lupus erythematosus (SLE), and the clinicopathological criteria for the diagnosis of APS have been agreed internationally [1]. In spite of this, our understanding of the pathogenesis of the condition is limited, particularly with respect to the complications of pregnancy, for which there is no compelling evidence of an ischemic pathogenesis. Because the clinical manifestations of the antiphospholipid syndrome, namely thrombosis and pregnancy failure, are common in the population, differentiation between those individuals with and without the syndrome is heavily dependent on laboratory assays to detect persistent antiphospholipid antibodies. The laboratory-based diagnosis, however, is problematic because of the numerous test and reagent combinations available and disappointing quality assurance data for all tests. This is very important because the diagnosis of antiphospholipid syndrome changes clinical management significantly in those affected. For example, anticoagulation following a first episode of venous thromboembolism should probably be prolonged in those with antiphospholipid syndrome while it is appropriate to consider periods of 3–6 months only in some other patients. Furthermore, while there are good data to inform on the management of venous thromboembolism, the same is not true for arterial thrombosis. Finally, there are conflicting views on the treatment of women with adverse pregnancy outcomes attributable to APS, and asymptomatic patients with "chance findings" of antiphospholipid antibodies.

Definition of Antiphospholipid Syndrome

The antiphospholipid syndrome describes a clinicopathological entity. APS is an acquired prothrombotic state, which probably has an

Practical Hemostasis and Thrombosis, Third Edition. Edited by Nigel S. Key, Michael Makris and David Lillicrap.
© 2017 John Wiley & Sons, Ltd. Published 2017 by John Wiley & Sons, Ltd.

immune-mediated pathogenesis and its diagnosis requires the coexistence of clinical manifestations (thrombosis or adverse pregnancy outcome) with laboratory evidence of antiphospholipid antibodies.

The Sapporo diagnostic criteria for APS were revised in 2005 by an international consensus panel [2] (Table 19.1). A variety of other clinical abnormalities, which are frequently observed in association with antiphospholipid antibodies, are not included in the internationally agreed definition of APS. The most common of these are thrombocytopenia and livedo reticularis/racemosa, which are frequently found in patients who do not otherwise fulfill the criteria for APS (Table 19.2). A controversial possible association is with a neurological condition mimicking multiple sclerosis, which may respond to anticoagulant therapy [3]. Identification of these other associated conditions should lead to consideration of a diagnosis of APS. It is not clear whether thrombosis is implicated in the pathogenesis of these conditions and the role of antithrombotic medicines is even less clear.

Antiphospholipid Antibodies and the Pathology of the Antiphospholipid Syndrome

These are a heterogeneous group of antibodies, which are detected because of their capacity to react with phospholipid either in phospholipid-dependent coagulation assays in the case of a lupus anticoagulant (LA), or bound to enzyme-linked immunosorbent assay (ELISA) plates in the case of anticardiolipin and anti-β_2-glycoprotein 1 antibodies.

The earliest descriptions of antiphospholipid antibodies were in individuals with SLE who had false-positive tests for syphilis. Further investigation of these patients indicated that they had circulating antibodies that were capable of binding to the negatively charged phospholipid, cardiolipin. This gave rise to the nomenclature *anticardiolipin antibodies*.

Table 19.1 Diagnostic criteria for antiphospholipid syndrome.

Clinical criteria

1) Thrombosis
One or more clinical episodes of arterial, venous, or small vessel thrombosis
2) Pregnancy
(a) One or more unexplained deaths of a morphologically normal fetus at or beyond the 10th week of gestation
(b) One or more preterm births of a morphologically normal neonate before the 34th week of gestation because of : (i) eclampsia or severe pre-eclampsia or (ii) recognized features of placental insufficiency
(c) Three or more unexplained consecutive spontaneous miscarriages before the 10th week of gestation, with maternal anatomic or hormonal abnormalities and paternal and maternal chromosomal causes excluded

Laboratory criteria

1) Lupus anticoagulant present in plasma on two or more occasions at least 12 weeks apart
2) Anticardiolipin antibody of immunoglobulin (Ig) G and or IgM isotype in serum or plasma, present in medium or high titer (i.e. >40 GPL units or MPL units or >99th centile) on two or more occasions, at least 12 weeks apart
3) Anti-β_2-glycoprotien I antibody of IgG and/or IgM isotype in serum or plasma (in titer >99th centile), present on two or more occasions at least 12 weeks apart

Antiphospholipid syndrome is present if at least one of the clinical criteria and one of the laboratory criteria are met.

GPL, IgG antiphospholipid units/mL; MPL, IgM antiphospholipid units/mL.

About the same time it was noted that some subjects with SLE had prolonged coagulation times in *in vitro* test systems but had no evidence of a bleeding diathesis. The prolonged clotting times in phospholipid-dependent tests could not be reversed by addition of normal plasma, indicating the presence of an inhibitor, the so-called *lupus anticoagulant*.

Paradoxically, the presence of the LA was associated with an increased risk of thrombosis in patients with SLE, and when it became apparent that the presence of LA or anticardiolipin was associated with an increased thrombosis

Table 19.2 Clinical features of antiphospholipid syndrome (APS), described by a cohort of 1000 European APS patients.

System	Complication (percentage affected)
Obstetric	Early fetal loss (<10 weeks) (35.4 of all pregnancies)
	Late fetal loss (>10 weeks) (16.9 of all pregnancies)
	Premature birth (10.6 of all live births)
	Pre-eclampsia (9.5)
	Eclampsia (4.4)
	Abruptio placentae (2.0)
	Postpartum cardiopulmonary syndrome (0.5)
Peripheral thrombosis	Deep vein thrombosis (38.9)
	Superficial thrombophlebitis (11.7)
	Arterial thrombosis of legs (4.3)
	Venous thrombosis of the arms (3.4)
	Arterial thrombosis of the arms (2.7)
	Subclavian vein thrombosis (1.8)
	Jugular vein thrombosis (0.9)
Hematological	Thrombocytopenia (29.6)
	Hemolytic anemia (9.7)
Skin	Livedo reticularis (24.1)
	Leg ulcers (5.5)
	Pseudovasculitic lesions (3.9)
	Digital gangrene (3.3)
	Cutaneous necrosis (2.1)
	Splinter hemorrhages (0.7)
Neurological	Migraine (20.2)
	Stroke (19.8)
	Transient ischaemic attack (11.1)
	Epilepsy (7.0)
	Multi-infarct dementia (2.5)
	Chorea (1.3)
	Acute encephalopathy (1.1)
	Transient amnesia (0.7)
	Cerebral venous thrombosis (0.7)
Renal	Glomerular thrombosis, renal infarction, renal artery thrombosis, or renal vein thrombosis (2.7)
Cardiac	Valve thickening/ dysfunction (11.6)
	Myocardial infarction (5.5)
	Angina (2.7)
	Myocardiopathy (2.9)

(Continued)

Table 19.2 (Continued)

System	Complication (percentage affected)
	Vegetations (2.7)
	Coronary bypass thrombosis (1.1)
	Intracardiac thrombus (0.4)
Pulmonary	Pulmonary embolism (14.1)
	Pulmonary hypertension (2.2)
	Pulmonary microthrombosis (1.5)
	Fibrosing alveolitis (1.2)
Gastrointestinal	Gut ischaemia (1.5)
	Splenic infarction (1.1)
	Pancreatic infarction (0.5)
	Addison syndrome (0.4)
	Hepatic (Budd–Chiari, small hepatic vein thrombosis) (0.7)
Articular	Arthralgia (38.7)
	Arthritis (27.1)
	Avascular necrosis of the bone (2.4)
Ophthalmological	Amaurosis fugax (5.4)
	Retinal artery thrombosis (1.5)
	Retinal vein thrombosis (0.9)
	Optic neuropathy (1.0)

Source: modified from Cervera *et al.* 2002 [25].

risk, the concept of an acquired prothrombotic or thrombophilic state was proposed.

Although they are called antiphospholipid antibodies, it is now clear that the antigenic targets for most of these antibodies are not phospholipids but proteins that bind to phospholipid (Table 19.3). The most important of these is β_2-glycoprotein 1, an apolipoprotein and member of the complement control protein family, which avidly binds negatively charged phospholipid. The molecule has five domains, and antibodies against a limited epitope on domain 1 (Gly40-Arg43) have been shown to be the most strongly associated with thrombosis [4]. It has also been shown that the binding of β_2-glycoprotein 1 to phospholipid causes a conformational change in the molecule and the exposure of "cryptic epitopes". This may, in part, explain the formation of autoantibodies [5].

Other antigen targets for antiphospholipid antibodies include prothrombin, factor XI, protein C and protein S, and annexin V, all proteins involved in hemostatic pathways that might be relevant in explaining the thrombotic complications associated with these antibodies. In response to these findings, ELISA assays that

Table 19.3 Antigenic targets of antiphospholipid antibodies.

β_2-glycoprotein 1
Prothrombin
Protein C
Protein S
Annexin V
Factors XI and XII

have β_2-glycoprotein 1 and prothrombin as antigen are now commercially available.

Despite this knowledge, the pathogenesis of thrombosis and pregnancy failure in APS remains unclear. Laboratory findings combined with the outcome of clinical studies indicate that the pathological manifestations of APS are caused by a prothrombotic state with little evidence that vascular inflammation contributes significantly to the process. No single mechanism has been shown to underlie the prothrombotic tendency and this is perhaps not surprising given the varied sites of thrombosis and the range of target antigens for antiphospholipid antibodies.

Whether antiphospholipid antibodies are indeed directly pathogenic is debated. IgG from serum of patients with APS has been shown to be pathogenic in animal models of thrombosis and pregnancy loss. Laboratory experiments have assessed the effects of antiphospholipid antibodies on many of the processes involved in hemostasis, thrombosis, inflammation, and fibrinolysis.

There are data to support that antiphospholipid antibodies may induce tissue factor expression by monocytes, inhibit the function of the natural anticoagulants activated protein C and protein S, induce endothelial cell apoptosis and activation, and induce platelet activation following binding to the Fc receptor. All, none, or, more likely, a combination of these mechanisms may contribute to the disease process [5]. Although the criteria for diagnosis of APS state that histological evidence of inflammation excludes the diagnosis, there is increasing experimental evidence that antiphospholipid antibodies may induce an inflammatory state. Upregulation of adhesion molecules such as VCAM-1 and E-selectin and secretion of interleukin-6 has been observed in endothelial cells incubated with antiphospholipid antibodies. Increased leukocyte adhesion to endothelium with associated induction of tissue factor expression could perceivably be involved in the pathogenesis of the condition.

The pathogenesis of pregnancy failure in APS is even more obscure. Knowledge of the possible prothrombotic properties of antiphospholipid antibodies has led to the inference that placental ischemia is the main mechanism resulting in pregnancy failure in APS. The evidence from clinical studies suggesting improved outcome in patients treated with antithrombotic medicines, such as heparin and aspirin, is felt by many to support this hypothesis. However, overt placental ischemia is rare and the observation that the most common manifestation of APS in pregnancy is abortion before 10 weeks (i.e., prior to development of the placental circulation) suggests that other mechanisms must contribute. Complement activation by antiphospholipid antibodies has been linked to early pregnancy loss, and antiphospholipid antibodies have been shown to inhibit trophoblastic proliferation and spiral artery invasion *in vitro*. Interestingly, these effects may also be inhibited by heparin, suggesting that at least part of any benefit for heparin may relate to an anticomplement effect and/or improved implantation.

Other work has suggested that antiphospholipid antibodies may act by displacing the natural anticoagulant annexin V from endothelial cell surfaces, resulting in a procoagulant state. However, as normal expression of annexin V has been demonstrated in affected pregnancies, the importance of these observations remains unclear.

In general, the specificity for thrombosis is higher for LA than it is for anticardiolipin or anti-β_2-glycoprotein 1 and it is higher for high-titer compared with low-titer antibodies. IgM and IgA antibodies have low specificity. In pregnancy, LA have a stronger association with pregnancy loss than other antiphospholipid antibodies. The importance of anti-β_2-glycoprotein 1 in pregnancy is not yet clear.

Clinical Features of APS

Antiphospholipid syndrome affects women more commonly than men. It is a multisystem disorder that may present *de novo* (primary APS) or be associated with an underlying autoimmune condition – most commonly SLE (secondary APS). About half of cases are primary and half secondary.

APS is a multisystem disease with a wide range of clinical symptoms that are summarized in Table 19.2. Clinical features can be broadly split into:

- Thrombotic manifestations that can be either arterial, venous, or microvascular. These include deep vein thrombosis, pulmonary emboli, thrombosis at unusual sites, stroke, and myocardial infarction. The most common presentation of arterial thrombosis is with stroke, while myocardial infarction does not appear common although subclinical myocardial infarction may be under recognized.
- Complications of pregnancy presenting as fetal loss (at any stage of pregnancy), intrauterine growth retardation, and pre-eclampsia.
- Nonthrombotic features including livedo reticularis, Raynaud phenomenon, valvular heart disease, autoimmune cytopenias, psychosis, migraine, and renal disease.
- Catastrophic antiphospholipid syndrome presenting as a microangiopathic process affecting several organs, typically the brain, skin, kidneys and lungs.

Signs and symptoms of the manifestations of APS are quite common from other causes, as are nonclinically significant antiphospholipid antibodies in the normal population. As a result, testing for the condition must be limited to prevent misdiagnosis. The diagnosis should be made after consideration of the clinical features and results of laboratory assays. Testing should be considered in:

- unexplained arterial or venous thrombosis;
- recurrent thrombosis;
- arterial and venous thrombosis in the same patient;
- thrombosis at an unusual site;
- nonrheumatic valve thickening or culture negative vegetations;
- three or more unexplained spontaneous miscarriages (<10 weeks gestation);
- one or more fetal loss (>10 weeks gestation);

- severe or early pre-eclampsia;
- illness with signs of microangiopathic hemolysis;
- unexplained multiorgan failure;
- on diagnosis of SLE.

Diagnosis of Antiphospholipid Syndrome

As already stated, APS is a clinicopathological entity, the diagnosis of which depends upon the identification of a clinical complication combined with demonstration of appropriate antiphospholipid antibodies (Table 19.1). Although criteria for diagnosis have been internationally agreed, the diagnosis of APS is still complicated by two main problems:

- Many antiphospholipid antibodies are not associated with clinical manifestations of APS.
- The standardization of assays for LA and immunologically detectable antiphospholipid antibodies such as anticardiolipin antibodies and anti-β_2-glycoprotein 1 antibodies is very poor.

Transient and Nonpathological Antiphospholipid Antibodies

Both LA and anticardiolipin antibodies, alone or together, are found in a significant number of normal subjects. Like the finding of a positive direct antiglobulin test in approximately 1 in 10 000 blood donors, the finding is of little consequence to the individual but it can generate further investigation and anxiety. One common source of this is the finding of a LA as a consequence of routine coagulation screening in medical and surgical admissions. On some occasions, the antiphospholipid antibody is transient but persistent high-titer anticardiolipin antibodies and strong positive LAs are not uncommon incidental findings. Some series report the finding of antiphospholipid antibodies, more often anticardiolipin, in up to 5% of normal subjects.

Perhaps the most common cause of transient antiphospholipid antibodies is infection (Table 19.4). This is mostly seen following viral infection but may complicate bacterial and parasitic infections also. Although these antibodies are not typically associated with significant disease, purpura fulminans resulting from acquired protein S deficiency is a well-documented complication of varicella infection in children. Some infections such as HIV, hepatitis C, leprosy, syphilis, leptospirosis, leishmaniasis, and malaria are associated with persistent antiphospholipid antibodies. These are rarely linked with the development of clinical features of APS.

The use of certain common drugs is also associated with the development of antiphospholipid antibodies. The association with chlorpromazine is the best documented, and although these antibodies are not typically said to be associated with the development of thrombosis, it may be that this underlies the recently reported association of psychoactive drugs with an increased risk of venous thromboembolism.

Laboratory Assays

The diagnosis of APS is ultimately dependent on the availability of accurate diagnostic assays. A vast amount of work has been carried out to try to standardize assays for anticardiolipin and

Table 19.4 Infections associated with antiphospholipid antibodies.

Viral
Human immunodeficiency virus
Hepatitis C
Varicella
Bacterial
Helicobacter pylori
Syphilis
Leprosy
Leptospirosis
Parasitic
Malaria
Leishmaniasis

LA. Although internationally agreed guidelines have been drawn up to address this, the intricacies of the assays and the plethora of nonstandardized reagents available make this a difficult area. Summarized below are the key features that require attention in detecting antiphospholipid antibodies.

Lupus Anticoagulants

The British Committee for Standards in Haematology (BCSH) guideline on the investigation and management of antiphospholipid syndrome [6] and the updated Scientific Standardization Committee of the International Society of Thrombosis and Hemostasis (ISTH) guidance on detection of LA [7] recommend that the laboratory diagnosis of LA should be carried out following a three-step procedure adhering to the principles:

1) prolongation of a phospholipid-dependent coagulation test;
2) evidence of inhibitory activity on mixing tests;
3) evidence of phospholipid dependence.

In the detection of LA there are many preanalytical issues that need to be attended to. These include appropriate preparation of a platelet-poor plasma (platelet count $<10 \times 10^9/L$). This should be done by double centrifugation rather than filtration, which may generate platelet microparticles.

This process allows the detection of inhibitory activity in the plasma and then facilitates differentiation of LA from specific inhibitors of coagulation, which are less common. As the management of patients with antiphospholipid antibodies often involves antithrombotic medication, while patients with acquired inhibitors of coagulation harbor an often life-threatening bleeding diathesis, differentiation is of paramount importance.

The BCSH and ISTH guidelines both recommend the combined use of a dilute Russell viper venom time and one other assay for the detection of LA [6,7]. Mixing studies are performed to demonstrate inhibitory activity in test plasma.

Errors arising in the mixing procedure relate to the quality of the normal plasma, particularly its platelet content, and to the level of dilution employed. Platelet contamination can result in quenching of the inhibitory effect and therefore to a false-negative result.

Confirmation of the phospholipid dependence of the inhibitor is assessed by adding excess phospholipid to the test system. The rationale for this is that the excess phospholipid neutralizes or bypasses the LA effect. A positive test is suggested by a >50% correction of the clotting time. Platelet membrane particles generated by freeze/thawing of platelet rich plasma or purer forms of phospholipid may be used for this purpose. Platelet membrane preparation suffers from significant batch-to-batch variability, which does not lend itself to standardization.

Specific coagulation factor assays may help to confirm the nature of an inhibitor. They are probably indicated when there is concern about a bleeding diathesis. Simultaneous reduction of more than one coagulation factor may suggest the presence of a LA.

When using this method to detect a LA, factor assays should be performed at numerous plasma dilutions. Unlike the situation where a specific coagulation factor inhibitor is present, the apparent coagulation factor activity rises with greater dilution in the presence of a LA; that is, the assay curves are nonparallel. The results from these assays may vary with different reagents.

Anticardiolipin Assays

A great deal of effort has gone towards producing new more specific assays to measure anti-β_2-glycoprotein 1 and anti-prothrombin activity in the hope that this would improve diagnostic accuracy. Specific anti-β_2-glycoprotein 1 antibody ELISAs are more specific than anticardiolipin assays but they are poorly standardized. Features of the antigen used in the assay such as its purity and oxidation status affect assay performance significantly. Recently, assays that detect only antibodies directed against domain 1 of anti-β_2-glycoprotein 1 have been developed and it is hoped that they may improve sensitivity and specificity for clinical outcomes.

Significant numbers of patients have low-titer anticardiolipin antibodies and in an attempt to address this and to try to more clearly delineate pathological antibodies, the diagnostic criteria state that in order to fulfill a diagnosis of APS, patients should have moderate or high titers of antibody (>40 IgG antiphospholipid units/mL (GPL) or IgM antiphospholipid units/ml (MPL)). However, all tests must be interpreted in conjunction with the relevant clinical information. Furthermore, although assay performance has been improved by these changes, interassay comparability is still poor and it appears that the new specific assays may be no more sensitive for the diagnosis of APS than standard anticardiolipin and LA tests.

Quality Assurance

Quality assurance is a major issue for laboratories attempting to identify and quantify antiphospholipid antibodies. Although national and international standards and guidelines have been prepared (and are adhered to), recent quality assurance exercises still indicate that there are major problems in antiphospholipid antibody testing.

A European Concerted Action on Thrombophilia (ECAT) survey indicated that plasma containing a 10 Bethesda unit inhibitor of factor VIII was wrongly identified as a LA in approximately 20% of 128 participating laboratories.

Likewise, a quality assurance exercise report on detection of anticardiolipin antibodies indicated an interlaboratory coefficient of variation of more than 50% in 74% of tests performed, leaving the authors to conclude that in the majority of cases the laboratories could not decide whether a sample was positive or negative.

Treatment of APS

Primary Prevention of Thrombosis

Asymptomatic Individuals

Asymptomatic individuals with antiphospholipid antibodies may have a higher risk of thrombosis than the general population. This seems especially true for those with a LA [8] and triple positivity [9] but not anticardiolipin alone [10]. In the Leiden thrombophilia study, a population-based study of venous thrombosis, the strongest antiphospholipid associations with thrombosis were for the combination of LA, anti-β_2-glycoprotein 1, and antiprothrombin antibodies [11]. Other studies have questioned the significance of the antiprothrombin antibodies, however. To determine whether primary prophylaxis with aspirin in patients with antiphospholipid antibodies is beneficial in reducing thrombosis, the APLASA study [12] randomized patients to aspirin or placebo. This failed to show any advantage for aspirin as did a further study concentrating on triple-positive patients [9]. Routine treatment of all asymptomatic individuals therefore cannot be recommended although an expert task force [13] recommended the following measures:

- strict control of cardiovascular risk factors in all carriers;
- thromboprophylaxis with low-molecular-weight heparin during high-risk situations (surgery, prolonged immobilization, and the puerperium);
- thromboprophylaxis with low-dose aspirin in those with either a persistent LA, medium high anticardiolipin titers, triple positivity, or other risk factors for thrombosis (including estrogen use).

The BCSH guidance on the same data set is that because there was no benefit for aspirin in these patients, including the subgroup who were triple positive, routine thromboprophylaxis with aspirin should not be offered to these patients [6].

Patients with SLE and Subclinical Antiphospholipid Antibodies

Patients with SLE who have antiphospholipid antibodies have a significantly increased risk of thrombosis, with 20% of patients developing thrombosis over a 10-year period [14]. For SLE patients, regular screening for antiphospholipid antibodies is recommended. For those patients who are positive for either LA or medium–high titers of anticardiolipin, primary prophylaxis with aspirin and hydroxychloroquine has been suggested [13].

Patients with Obstetric APS but no History of Thrombosis

Patients who have purely obstetric APS have been shown to be at increased risk of VTE and possibly also transient ischaemic attack and stroke outside of pregnancy compared with matched populations without persistent antiphospholipid antibodies. The role for thromboprophylaxis in this group is unclear [15].

Treatment of Thrombosis

Treatment of thrombotic events can be grouped as:

- treatment of venous thrombosis;
- treatment of arterial thrombosis which can be further grouped as:
  - treatment of noncardioembolic stroke;
  - treatment of arterial embolism;
  - treatment of myocardial infarction;
  - treatment of other arterial events.

Treatment of Venous Thrombosis

Initial treatment for venous thrombosis in patients with APS is similar to that of those without, that is low–molecular-weight heparin or equivalent followed by dose-adjusted warfarin with an INR target of 2.5. The recent RAPS (rivaroxaban for antiphospholipid syndrome) study failed to demonstrate non-inferiority for rivaroxaban compared to warfarin based on the surrogate endpoint of total thrombin generation [16]. Areas for debate around the management of a first otherwise unprovoked VTE relate to duration and intensity of the anticoagulation.

- Intensity of anticoagulation. Although higher-intensity anticoagulation has been recommended, two randomized controlled trials [17,18] demonstrated no difference in the rate of recurrent thrombosis between those treated with an INR target of 2.5 (range 2–3) and those with an INR target of 3.5 (range 3–4). There was possibly a reduction in the rate of minor bleeding with the lower target INR suggesting that this is the superior regimen.

- Duration of anticoagulation. Patients with APS have a significant risk of recurrent thrombosis on stopping anticoagulation. This led to the consensus that patients with APS should receive indefinite anticoagulation [13,19] following a first unprovoked event. There has been some suggestion that those patients with a first thrombosis and a transient risk factor may only require 3–6 months anticoagulation but this has not been proven in clinical trials. This suggestion does not really fit into routine clinical practice as, in general, most physicians would not routinely look for evidence of antiphospholipid antibodies in provoked episodes of venous thromboembolism. If the circumstances are such that the duration of anticoagulation is going to be determined by the presence or absence of APS, that is if a finite duration is indicated in its absence, then discontinuation of warfarin for a period of around 7 days to facilitate repeat LA testing is reasonable.

Treatment of Arterial Thrombosis

The choice of treatment for arterial events is between antiplatelet agents alone, antiplatelet agents plus warfarin with a target INR 2.5 (range 2.0–3.0), and warfarin alone with an INR 3.5 (range 3.0–4.0). There is no clear consensus [13,19,20] as to which patients should receive what anticoagulants as opposed to antiplatelet drugs. The correct decision will be a balance between:

- The patient's thrombotic risk, highest in those patients with a positive LA, high-titer IgG anticardiolipin, or triple positivity.
- Their bleeding risk on the specific treatment.
- The site of thrombosis. In non-APS patients, nonembolic thrombosis tends to be treated with aspirin while embolism is treated with warfarin. There have been no trials looking at contemporary treatments for myocardial infarction specifically in APS, that is drug eluting stents, but given the improvement in

outcome in non-APS patients it could be argued that in the context of myocardial infarction APS patients should be treated the same as non-APS patients.

Treatment Failures

The rate of treatment failure is higher for APS patients than those without APS. In the event of a treatment failure with warfarin it is usual to increase the intensity of the anticoagulation. This has to be balanced against the increased bleeding risk. Other options include combining antiplatelet agents and anticoagulants and changing to low-molecular-weight heparin.

Prevention of Obstetric Complications

Pregnancy failure is now the most common presentation that results in a diagnosis of APS. This is in part because of the wish (and pressure) to investigate women with this distressing history. Recurrent early fetal loss is the most commonly seen manifestation of APS, although otherwise unexplained fetal death after the first trimester and severe pre-eclampsia before 34 weeks are also recognized features.

The emotive nature of these cases may result in the inappropriate investigation of women with only one or two early abortions, which can result in a chance finding of an innocent antiphospholipid antibody. Having detected antiphospholipid antibodies in women who do not fulfill the APS criteria [21], clinicians find it difficult to withhold treatment, resulting in some women taking aspirin and heparin in subsequent pregnancies, based on very little evidence.

Most proponents of this approach argue that waiting for a third early loss in these women is inappropriate and add that the therapy has so few side-effects that this is not an issue. However, side-effects, although few, are seen and the costs of clinic time and drugs are significant. This practice also converts normal women into patients for the duration of their pregnancy while skewing the perception of benefit for intervention.

The aim of treatment of pregnant patients with APS is to reduce the risk of thrombosis and pregnancy complications. Women who are already anticoagulated with warfarin should be changed to treatment doses of low-molecular-weight heparin for the duration of pregnancy. For those women not on anticoagulants who have previously had an APS-related pregnancy complication, the treatment of choice is aspirin and heparin as demonstrated by a meta-analysis [22]. The addition of heparin to aspirin results in one extra live birth for every 5.6 patients treated. Detailed breakdown of these data have however cast doubt over the degree of benefit for this intervention but this has not affected clinical practice in many settings as yet. Although the largest and best studies were of unfractionated heparin, low molecular weight heparins seem to have become the norm in obstetric practice. There are few data but those that are available seem to show little difference between unfractionated heparin and low-molecular-weight heparin in terms of efficacy. There are fewer long-term complications with low-molecular-weight heparin and the benefits of once-daily dosing may aid compliance. Because of the high risks of complications during pregnancy, these women should preferably be managed in an obstetric unit with expertise in the area.

Catastrophic Antiphospholipid Syndrome

Catastrophic APS is a multisystem disease presenting as microangiopathic hemolysis and multiorgan failure. Commonly affected organs are the brain, kidneys, skin, liver, adrenals, lungs, and heart. There may be an associated coagulopathy. In around half of these cases it is the first presentation of APS. Because of the rarity of the disease there are no treatments of proven efficacy, but high-dose steroids, anticoagulation, plasmapheresis, intravenous immunoglobulin, rituximab, and immunosuppression have all been described [23]. A precipitating cause (e.g., infection) should also be sought and treated.

Antiphospholipid Syndrome with Bleeding

There have been several case reports of patients developing a bleeding diathesis due to a LA, usually secondary to an autoimmune disease. It is thought that the antibody reduces the functional levels of prothrombin. Steroids appear to be effective. Thrombosis remains a risk when the prothrombin levels increase [24].

Practical Approach to Diagnosis

A physician must be aware of the limitations in the assays when making a diagnosis of antiphospholipid syndrome. It has been demonstrated that some antiphospholipid antibodies correlate better with thrombotic risk than others. Lupus anticoagulants are stronger risk factors for thrombosis than anticardiolipin antibodies, IgG anticardiolipin antibodies are more significant than IgM, and high-titer antibodies are more significant than low titer. The correlation between anti-β_2-glycoprotein 1 antibodies and thrombosis and pregnancy morbidity is still debated and the clinical value of testing in this situation has not been clearly established. As a rule, high-titer antibodies have shown a better correlation with thrombosis than low titer and positivity in more than one ELISA (anticardiolipin and anti-β_2-glycoprotein 1) adds to the significance.

Finally, as indicated earlier in the text, testing for APS should be considered only when there is a reasonable clinical suspicion of the diagnosis and when the results will impact on management, for example in a young patient with no risk factors for stroke, or in unprovoked venous thromboembolism. Unselected screening for antiphospholipid antibodies in all patients with thrombotic events is inappropriate and will result in false-positive tests and misdiagnosis. Interpretation of results should always be individualized.

References

1 Wilson WA, Gharavi AE, Koike T, *et al.* International consensus statement on preliminary classification criteria for definite antiphospholipid syndrome: report of an international workshop. *Arthritis Rheum* 1999; 42: 1309–1311.

2 Miyakis S, Lockshin AD, Atsumi T, *et al.* International consensus statement on an update of the classification criteria for definite antiphospholipid syndrome (APS). *J Thromb Haemost* 2006; 4: 295–306.

3 Hughes GR. Migraine, memory loss and "multiple sclerosis". Neurological features of the antiphospholipid (Hughes') syndrome. *Postgrad Med J* 2003; 79: 81–83.

4 De Latt B, Derksen RH, Urbanus RT, *et al.* IgG antibodies that recognise epitope Gly40-Arg43 in domain 1 of beta 2-glycoprotein 1 cause LAC, and their presence correlates strongly with thrombosis. *Blood* 2005; 105: 1540–1545.

5 Urbanus RT, Derksen RHMW, de Groot PG. Current insight into the diagnosis and pathophysiology of the antiphospholipid syndrome. *Blood Rev* 2008; 22: 93–105.

6 Keeling D, Mackie I, Moore GW, *et al.* Guidelines on the investigation and management of antiphospholipid syndrome. *Br J Haematol* 2012; 157: 47–58.

7 Pengo V, Tripodi A, Reber G, *et al.* Update of the guidelines for lupus anticoagulant detection. *J Thromb Haemost* 2009; 7: 1737–1740.

8 Galli M, Luciani D, Bertolini G, *et al.* Lupus anticoagulants are stronger risk factors for thrombosis than anticardiolipin antibodies in the antiphospholipid syndrome: a systematic review of the literature. *Blood* 2003; 101: 1827–1832.

9 Pengo V, Ruffatti A, Legnani C, *et al.* Incidence of a first thromboembolic event in asymptomatic carriers of high risk antiphospholipid antibody profile: a multicenter prospective study. *Blood* 2011; 118: 4714–4718.

10 Naess I, Chritiansen S, Canniegieter S, *et al.* A prospective study of anticardiolipin antibodies as a risk factor for venous thrombosis in a general population (the HUNT study). *J Thromb Haemost* 2005; 4: 44–49.

11 De Groot P, Lutters B, Derksen RH, *et al.* Lupus anticoagulants and the risk of a first episode of deep venous thrombosis. *J Thromb Haemost* 2005; 3: 1993–1997.

12 Erkan D, Harrison M, Levy R, *et al.* Aspirin for primary thrombosis prevention in the antiphospholipid syndrome: A randomized, double-blind, placebo-controlled trial in asymptomatic antiphospholipid antibody–positive individuals. *Arthritis Rheum* 2007; 56: 2382–2391.

13 Ruiz-Irastorza G, Cuadrado MJ, Ruiz-Arruza I, *et al.* Evidence-based recommendations for the prevention and long-term management of thrombosis in antiphospholipid antibody-positive patients: report of a task force at the 13th International Congress on antiphospholipid antibodies. *Lupus* 2011; 20: 206–218.

14 Tektonidou M, Laskari K, Panagiotakos D, *et al.* Risk factors for thrombosis and primary thrombosis prevention in patients with systemic lupus erythematosus with or without antiphospholipid antibodies. *Arthritis Rheum* 2009; 61: 29–32.

15 Gris J, Bouvier S, Molinari N, *et al.* Comparative incidence of a first thrombotic event in purely obstetric antiphospholipid syndrome with pregnancy loss: the NOH-APS observational study. *Blood* 2012; 119: 2624–2632.

16 Cohen H, Hunt BJ, Efthymiou M, *et al.* Rivaroxaban versus warfarin to treat patients with thrombotic antiphospholipid syndrome, with or without systemic lupus erythematosis (RAPS); a randomised controlled, open label, phase2/3, non-inferiority trial. *Lancet Haematology* 2016; 3: e426–436.

17 Crowther MA, Ginsberg JS, Julian J, *et al.* A comparison of two intensities of warfarin for the prevention of recurrent thrombosis in patients with the antiphospholipid antibody syndrome. *N Engl J Med* 2003; 349: 1133–1138.

18 Finazzi G, Marchioli R, Brancaccio V, *et al.* A randomized clinical trial of high-intensity warfarin vs. conventional antithrombotic therapy for the prevention of recurrent thrombosis in patients with the antiphospholipid syndrome (WAPS). *J Thromb Haemost* 2005; 3: 848–852.

19 Giannakopoulos B, Krilis S. How I treat the antiphospholipid syndrome. *Blood* 2009; 114: 2020–2030.

20 Ruiz-Irastorza G, Hunt B, Khamashta MA. A systematic review of secondary thromboprophylaxis in patients with antiphospholipid antibodies. *Arthritis Rheum* 2007; 57: 1487–1491.

21 Creagh MD, Malia RG, Cooper SM, *et al.* Screening for lupus anticoagulant and anticardiolipin antibodies in women with fetal loss. *J Clin Pathol* 1991; 44: 45–47.

22 Mac A, Cheung M, Cheak A, *et al.* Combination of heparin and aspirin is superior to aspirin alone in enhancing liver births in patients with recurrent pregnancy loss and positive antiphospholipid antibodies: a meta-analysis of randomized controlled trials and meta-regression. *Rheumatology* 2010; 49: 281–288.

23 Bucciarelli S, Espinosa G, Cervera R, *et al.* Mortality in the catastrophic antiphospholipid syndrome: causes of death and prognostic factors in a series of 250 patients. *Arthritis Rheum* 2006; 54: 2568–2578.

24 Mazodier K, Arnaud L, Mathian A, *et al.* Lupus anticoagulant-hypoprothrombinemia syndrome: a report of 8 cases and a review of the literature. *Medicine* 2012; 91: 251–260.

25 Cervera R, Pietle JC, Font J, *et al.* Antiphospholipid syndrome: clinical and immunological manifestations and patterns of disease expressions in a cohort of 1000 patients. *Arthritis Rheum* 2002; 46: 1019–1027.

20

Cardiovascular Medicine

Sreekanth Vemulapalli and Richard C. Becker

Key Points

- Coronary artery disease, heart failure, and atrial fibrillation are all cardiac conditions that may be complicated by thrombosis.
- Antiplatelet therapy results in a reduction in myocardial infarction, stroke, and death among a wide range of patients at risk of occlusive vascular events.
- Gastrointestinal bleeding due to arteriovenous malformations occurs in patients with ventricular assist devices.
- Bleeding is the major adverse effect of antiplatelet and anticoagulant drugs and its management in patients with recent thrombosis can be challenging due to the risk of rethrombosis.

Introduction

A balance between thrombosis and excess bleeding is an essential paradigm for practicing physicians in cardiovascular medicine. Although this equilibrium has been fundamental to the understanding of coronary artery disease (CAD), recent work has extended this paradigm to the treatment of atrial fibrillation (AF), heart failure (HF), and the management of cardiac devices. Indeed, therapies for the prevention and treatment of a variety of cardiovascular diseases have been born from decades of collaboration between the cardiology, pathology,

and hematology communities to address several fundamental questions: (i) What is the pathophysiological basis for adverse thrombotic events in CAD, AF, and HF?; (ii) Can pathological thrombosis in CAD, AF, and HF be modulated pharmacologically while minimizing adverse effects on protective hemostasis and patient safety?; (iii) What are the unique thrombotic and hemostatic characteristics of cardiac device management.

The rapid expansion of both pharmacological and device therapies for cardiovascular diseases and an aging population have combined to produce increasing complexity in the management of the hemostatic aspects of cardiac patients. This chapter therefore focuses on the pathobiological mechanisms of coronary atherothrombosis, HF, AF and cardiac devices as a platform for understanding pharmacotherapy and evidence-based treatment strategies in these diseases.

Acute Coronary Syndromes

Epidemiology

Acute coronary syndromes represent coronary emergencies and comprise of three clinical presentations: (i) unstable angina; (ii) non-ST-elevation myocardial infarction (NSTEMI); and (iii) ST-elevation myocardial infarction (STEMI). Together, these three presentations are estimated to account for 1 190 000 hospital discharges in the USA, of which approximately

Practical Hemostasis and Thrombosis, Third Edition. Edited by Nigel S. Key, Michael Makris and David Lillicrap.
© 2017 John Wiley & Sons, Ltd. Published 2017 by John Wiley & Sons, Ltd.

30–40% are due to STEMI. This translated to an inhospital cost of $14 009 per discharge for acute MI [1].

Pathophysiology

Autopsy studies of patients with sudden cardiac death and acute coronary syndromes have indicated a number of pathophysiological mechanisms. Through and through rupture of the fibrous atherosclerotic cap, superficial erosion, intraplaque hemorrhage, and erosion of a calcified nodule are commonly seen in fatal coronary syndromes. The above anatomic mechanisms lead to thrombosis via collagen-mediated platelet activation and tissue factor activation of the coagulation cascade [2]. The dynamic process of plaque rupture may evolve to:

1) A completely occlusive thrombus with ST elevation on the electrocardiogram, known as a STEMI, or new left bundle branch block.
2) Less obstructive thrombi typically produce ST segment depression or T wave changes on the electrocardiogram. If prolonged, this may result in the release of cardiac enzymes and may be diagnosed as non-ST elevation myocardial infarction (NSTEMI).
3) Even less prolonged and/or less flow-limiting thrombi may not cause release of cardiac enzymes and is therefore called unstable angina.

Therapies for Acute Coronary Syndromes

Percutaneous Coronary Intervention

Percutaneous coronary intervention (PCI) refers to invasive, nonsurgical revascularization of the coronary arteries via an endovascular approach. The term encompasses both stent and nonstent procedures, such as balloon angioplasty, and atherectomy. PCI was initially developed in the 1970s and was characterized by balloon inflation within atherosclerotic plaques, resulting in plaque compression and increased luminal diameter. This technique, though occasionally still used today, was often complicated by coronary dissection, acute arterial recoil, and frequent restenosis. Bare metal stents were

therefore developed to prevent arterial recoil and dissection and subsequently became the standard of care in PCI. Bare metal stents require the use of antiplatelet agents to prevent stent thrombosis and are still subject to significant rates of restenosis. The advent of drug-eluting stents has reduced the restenosis rate, but has increased the need for prolonged dual antiplatelet therapy to prevent stent thrombosis. Nevertheless, PCI has become the primary treatment for high-risk patients with acute coronary syndromes (ACS) and for most patients with angina unresponsive to medical therapy.

Fibrinolysis

The goal of fibrinolytic therapy is rapid restoration of flow in an occluded vessel (STEMI) achieved by accelerating fibrinolysis of a coronary arterial thrombus. Mechanistically, fibrinolytic drugs accelerate the conversion of plasminogen to plasmin, a serine protease that degrades the insoluble fibrin clot matrix. Large, placebo-controlled clinical trials have consistently demonstrated improved ventricular function, decreased infarct size, and reduced mortality in patients receiving fibrinolytic therapy *within 6 and potentially up to 12 hours of the onset of STEMI.* Several agents are available and approved for use in STEMI (Table 20.1) [3].

Complications of Fibrinolytic Therapy: The most serious is intracerebral hemorrhage, which occurs in between 0.5% and 1.0% of patients. Major risk factors for intracranial hemorrhage include:

- age greater than 75,
- hypertension,
- low body weight,
- female gender, and
- coagulopathy.

Because of this significant increased risk, primary PCI is preferred when performed in a timely fashion. Nevertheless, the relative advantages and limitations of each therapy should be considered for each individual patient. In comparison, fibrinolytic therapy has not been effective in patients with NSTEMI or unstable angina.

Table 20.1 Fibrinolytic therapy recommendations.

Fibrinolytic agents used in STEMI:
    streptokinase
    alteplase
    tenecteplase
    reteplase

In the absence of contraindications, fibrinolytic therapy should be given to patients with STEMI and onset of ischemic symptoms within the previous 12 hours when it is anticipated that primary PCI cannot be performed within 120 minutes of first medical contact

In patients who are candidates for fibrinolytic therapy, administration as soon as possible (ideally within 30 minutes) is recommended

Fibrinolytic therapy is not recommended in patients with a history of intracranial hemorrhage, or with a history of head trauma, or with ischemic stroke within the past 6 months

MI, myocardial infarction; STEMI, ST-elevation myocardial infarction.

Antiplatelet Therapy in ACS

Therapies aimed at disrupting platelet activity (Figure 20.1) are successful in decreasing cardiovascular morbidity and mortality. In the largest investigation to date, the Antiplatelet Trialists' Collaboration (ATC), a systematic overview of trials of antiplatelet therapy, demonstrated a reduction in myocardial infarction, stroke, and death with antiplatelet therapies among a wide range of patients at risk of occlusive vascular events [4].

Aspirin: Benefits

Aspirin is an irreversible inhibitor of platelet cyclooxygenase (COX)-1, thereby impairing prostaglandin metabolism and thromboxane (TX) A_2 synthesis. In the acute setting of STEMI, aspirin (162.5 mg/day) reduced 5-week mortality by 23%. In addition, aspirin significantly reduced nonfatal reinfarction and nonfatal stroke [5]. In patients presumed to have an ischemic stroke, aspirin therapy reduced the risk of early recurrent ischemic stroke and improved long-term outcomes. Among patients with stable vascular disease, low-dose aspirin was found to significantly reduce the risk of

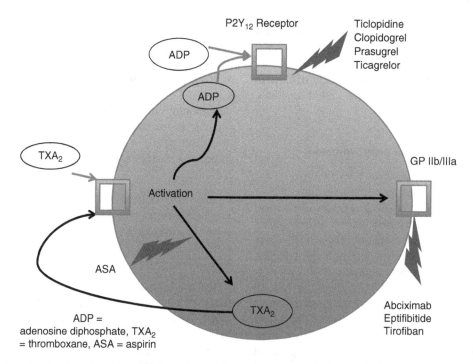

Figure 20.1 Mechanism of action of antiplatelet agents in acute coronary syndromes. ADP, adenosine diphosphate; TXA_2, thromboxane, ASA, aspirin.

cardiovascular events, as well as each individual endpoint of myocardial infarction, stroke, and death [6]. In patients without established vascular disease, based on a meta-analysis of six trials (including more than 90 000 men and women), low-dose aspirin was found to significantly reduce a composite of myocardial infarction, stroke, or cardiovascular death in women and men [7]. Interestingly, women were noted to have their greatest benefit via a reduction in the risk of stroke, whereas men tended to have their greatest benefit in the reduction in the risk of myocardial infarction.

Importantly, the optimal dose of aspirin is controversial. There is evidence to support dosages from 81 to 325 mg (75 to 300 mg in UK). Nevertheless, because of the increased risk of adverse events with increasing dosage, most uses in cardiovascular medicine require 75–81 mg/day, with the exception of acute myocardial infarction or stroke, where 162–325 mg is the preferred dose.

Aspirin: Risks
Aspirin is responsible for minor and major gastrointestinal bleeding as well as gastric ulcers, renal insufficiency, and allergic reactions. Additionally, some studies have suggested an increased risk of hemorrhagic stroke.

Thienopyridines: Clopidogrel, Ticlopidine, and Prasugrel
The thienopyridines ticlopidine and clopidogrel inhibit adenosine diphosphate (ADP) receptor-mediated platelet activation; they are more potent platelet inhibitors than aspirin. Because ticlopidine has been associated with thrombotic thrombocytopenic purpura and neutropenia, it is rarely used. In randomized trials, clopidogrel has been shown to reduce cardiovascular events in patients with cardiovascular disease [8]. Indications include:

- adjunct therapy in acute management of STEMI;
- invasive and conservative management of NSTEMI and unstable angina;
- adjunct therapy following PCI; and

- lone therapy in the secondary prevention of coronary artery disease.

Prasugrel: Prasugrel is a new thienopyridine, a $P2Y_{12}$ inhibiting prodrug, with a faster onset of action and greater potency than clopidogrel. In clinical trials of patients with ACS undergoing PCI, but not in those with ACS treated with medical management, prasugrel was superior to clopidogrel in reducing the combined incidence of MI, stroke, or cardiovascular death as well as stent thrombosis. However, prasugrel did not reduce overall mortality and increased major, life-threatening, and fatal bleeding as compared to clopidogrel. Prasugrel is contraindicated in patients with active bleeding or a history of transient ischemic attack (TIA) or stroke [8]. As a result, prasugrel is indicated as adjunctive therapy in the management of patients with ACS undergoing PCI (Table 20.2).

Ticagrelor: Unlike the thienopyridines, ticagrelor is a *reversible* inhibitor of the $P2Y_{12}$ receptor with a faster onset of action and greater potency than clopidogrel. In the PLATO trial of patients with ACS, the composite endpoint of death from vascular causes, MI, or stroke was reduced with ticagrelor as compared to clopidogrel [9]. Importantly, there was no significant difference in the rates of major bleeding; however, ticagrelor was associated with a significantly higher rate of major bleeding not associated with coronary artery bypass grafting. Also of note, a pre-specified subgroup analysis seemed to indicate an interaction between concomitant aspirin dosing and ticagrelor-associated bleeding. As a result, ticagrelor is most commonly used with aspirin doses ≤100 mg. Ticagrelor is indicated as adjunctive therapy in the management of patients with ACS (Table 20.2).

Intravenous Antiplatelet Therapy in ACS

Glycoprotein IIb/IIIa Inhibitors: Activation of the platelet-surface glycoprotein (GP) IIb/IIIa receptor is the final common pathway in the process leading to platelet aggregation and, eventually, thrombus formation (Figure 20.1).

Table 20.2 Agent-specific characteristics for oral anti-platelet drugs.

Agent	Route of administration	Plasma half-life	Clearance	Indications
Aspirin	Oral and intravenous	15–20 minutes	Reticuloendothelial system	ACS, stroke, PCI, peripheral artery disease, primary prevention, secondary prevention
Clopidogrel	Oral	8 hours	Liver	ACS, stroke, PCI, peripheral artery disease, secondary prevention
Prasugrel	Oral	7 hours	Renal	ACS undergoing PCI
Ticagrelor	Oral	7–9 hours	Renal and Liver	ACS

ACS, acute coronary syndrome; PCI, percutaneous coronary intervention.

The intravenous GPIIb/IIIa receptor inhibitors have been established as effective therapy for the reduction of ischemic events when used in both the management of ACS and as adjunctive therapy during PCI [1]. Because of their increased potency as antiplatelet agents, bleeding is a major side-effect that needs to be considered with their use (Table 20.3).

Anticoagulant Therapy in ACS
In the setting of ACS, anticoagulants are used to suppress the risk of recurrent cardiovascular events and systemic thromboembolism. The heparins (unfractionated heparin, low-molecular-weight heparin, and fondaparinux), direct thrombin inhibitors (bivalirudin), are the most commonly used agents; however, newer agents are being developed and studied in clinical trials [10].

Unfractionated Heparin (UFH): Compared with aspirin alone, UFH (plus aspirin) reduces nonfatal cardiovascular events in the setting of ACS. Major limitations specific to UFH include the need for frequent monitoring and a narrow therapeutic window. Other limitations of UFH include heparin-induced thrombocytopenia (HIT) and a reduced ability to inactivate thrombin bound to fibrin.

Low-Molecular-Weight Heparins (LMWH) enoxaparin: LMWHs have pharmacological and biological advantages over heparin that render them more convenient to administer and less

Table 20.3 Agent-specific characteristics for glycoprotein (GP)-IIB/IIIA receptor antagonists.

Characteristic	Abciximab	Eptifibatide	Tirofiban
Type	Antibody	Peptide	Nonpeptide
Molecular weight, Daltons	≈50 000	≈800	≈500
Platelet-bound half-life	Long	Short	Short
Plasma half-life	Short (minute)	Extended (2 hours)	Extended (2 hours)
Drug/GPIIb/IIIa receptor ratio	1.5–2.0	250–2500	>250
50% return of platelet function	12 hours	≈4 hours	≈4 hours
Route of clearance	RES	Renal/hepatic	Renal
Dose adjustment required with renal insufficiency	No	Yes	Yes

RES, reticuloendothelial system.

likely to cause HIT [11]. They lack the nonspecific binding affinities of UFH and, as a result, have more predictable pharmacokinetic and pharmacodynamic properties (Table 20.4). The most frequently studied LMWH in ACS is enoxaparin. Compared with UFH, enoxaparin provides clinical benefit. In a meta-analysis of 12 randomized trials in the setting of ACS, enoxaparin versus UFH was associated with a significant 16% reduction in the rate of death or myocardial infarction with a small but significant increase in the risk of major bleeding [12].

Fondaparinux: Fondaparinux, a synthetic pentasaccharide selectively inhibiting factor Xa shares all the pharmacological and biological advantages of LMWHs over UFH (Table 20.4). Two large trials have tested the role of fondaparinux in ACS: OASIS (Organization to Assess Strategies in Acute Ischemic Syndromes)-5 Study [13] and OASIS-6 in STEMI [14]. OASIS-5 demonstrated noninferiority of fondaparinux as compared to enoxaparin with respect to efficacy, and a lower rate of major bleeding. Among STEMI patients in OASIS-6, as compared with "usual care," fondaparinux was effective in reducing death and reinfarction. In subsequent analyses almost the entire difference in mortality between fondaparinux and enoxaparin-treated patients at the end of the study could be attributed to the lower rate of bleeding associated with fondaparinux. However, fondaparinux appears to be associated with a small but increased risk of catheter-associated thrombosis, thereby making it an unattractive anticoagulant option during PCI.

Thrombin Inhibitors: Direct thrombin inhibitors bind to thrombin and interrupt its interaction with substrates. Based on several large-scale clinical trials [15], bivalirudin, an intravenously administered direct and reversible inhibitor of thrombin, is FDA approved for use in patients with non-ST segment elevation ACS who are undergoing PCI. Compared with other anticoagulants, bivalirudin's major benefit is a marked reduction in major bleeding. The use of bivalirudin in patients with STEMI was evaluated in the HORIZONS-AMI [16] trial. In addition to the observed decrease in net adverse clinical events, there was a corresponding decrease in major bleeding with bivalirudin.

Bleeding and Outcomes in Acute Coronary Syndromes

Although bleeding has always been considered an important safety concern for patients with ACS or undergoing PCI, only recently have the long-term effects of bleeding on mortality been explored. In a meta-analysis of four multicenter, randomized clinical trials of patients with NSTEMI, Rao *et al.* demonstrated increases in 30-day and 6-month mortality with increasing bleeding severity [17]. Subsequently, a study aggregating data from other ACS trials

Table 20.4 Anticoagulants used in acute coronary syndromes.

Agent	Route of administration	Plasma half-life	Clearance	Indications
UFH	Intravenous or subcutaneous	30–60 minutes	Reticuloendothelial system	Venous thromboembolism; ACS
LMWH	Intravenous or subcutaneous	3–6 hours	Renal	Venous thromboembolism; ACS
Fondaparinux	Subcutaneous	17–21 hours	Renal	Venous thromboembolism; ACS (not in patients undergoing PCI)
Bivalirudin	Intravenous	25 minutes	20% renal	PCI; HIT

ACS, acute coronary syndrome; HIT, heparin induced thrombocytopenia; LMWH, low-molecular-weight heparin; PCI, percutaneous coronary intervention; UFH, unfractionated heparin.

confirmed a dose-related association between bleeding and death in ACS patients [18]. Although the exact contribution of bleeding to overall mortality in ACS remains undefined, fondaparinux is associated with both a reduced bleeding risk and reduced mortality versus enoxaparin in ACS. The authors subsequently concluded that bleeding is an important predictor of outcomes in ACS [19].

Mechanisms by which Bleeding Leads to Increased Cardiac Events in ACS

Although not well understood, several mechanisms have been proposed to explain the association of bleeding with mortality in ACS. Certainly, the hemodynamic effects associated with massive bleeding might result in higher mortality. Even lesser levels of bleeding, however, have been shown to increase levels of neurohormones, such as norepinephrine, angiotensin, endothelin-1, and vasopressin in order to maintain blood pressure. These neurohormones have been associated with cardiac events [17].

In addition to the neurohormonal activation associated with bleeding, measures taken as a result of bleeding, including discontinuation of antiplatelet and anticoagulant therapy, may paradoxically increase mortality. In the GRACE registry of ACS patients, those with bleeding complications more frequently had antithrombotic therapy, including aspirin, thienopyridines, and heparin, discontinued. Discontinuation of aspirin, thienopyridines, or unfractionated heparin in the setting of major bleeding resulted in higher inhospital mortality rates [20]. Given that patients with ACS and those undergoing PCI are in a heightened state of platelet activation and thrombosis, withholding antithrombotic therapy may result in activation of the coagulation system and potential stent thrombosis [21].

Defining Hemorrhagic Risk

Risk of hemorrhage associated with antithrombotic therapy, in addition to its intrinsic effects on primary hemostasis, secondary hemostasis, and intensity of effect, is influenced strongly by patient characteristics. Advanced age, renal insufficiency, presence of hypertension, and combined antiplatelet and anticoagulant therapy contribute to the overall risk of hemorrhagic events, including central nervous bleeding [22]. Table 20.5 suggests several management pathways for hemorrhagic complications associated with these agents.

Gastrointestinal (GI) hemorrhage is second only to mucocutaneous bleeding as a source of major bleeding and as a source of major events among patients receiving platelet-directed therapy. Available evidence suggests that risk is increased when aspirin and clopidogrel are used in combination. Patient and drug-specific factors increasing the risk for GI bleeding in the setting of dual antiplatelet therapy include advanced age, concurrent use of warfarin, steroids, nonsteroidal anti-inflammatory drugs, and *Helicobacter pylori* infection [23].

Peripheral Arterial Disease

Epidemiology

Peripheral arterial disease (PAD) represents atherosclerosis of the aorta, iliac, and lower extremity arteries and is a major source of morbidity and mortality. Epidemiological studies indicate that the disease affects between 4 and 12% of adults in the United States. Clinically, disease manifestations of PAD range from asymptomatic in 20–50% of patients, to atypical leg pain in 40–50%, to typical claudication in 10–35%, and critical limb ischemia in 1–2% [24].

Peripheral Arterial Disease and Cardiovascular Risk

Although PAD is associated with significant lower-extremity symptoms and complications, the majority of patients have coexistent CAD and suffer morbidity and mortality related to MI, stroke, and cardiovascular death. Patients with PAD but no clinical evidence of CAD have the same the same relative risk of CV death as those patients whose primary diagnosis is CAD [25]. As a result, the initial goals of management

Table 20.5 Agent-specific approach to hemorrhagic complications.

Agent	Category	Mechanism of Action	Antidote	Available substrate for attenuating effects
Aspirin	Platelet antagonist	Cyclo-oxygenase inhibition	DDAVP	Platelet transfusion
Clopidogrel	Platelet antagonist	ADP receptor inhibition	None	Platelet transfusion
Prasugrel	Platelet antagonist	ADP receptor inhibition	None	Platelet transfusion
Ticagrelor	Platelet antagonist	ADP receptor inhibition	None	Platelet transfusion
Ticlopidine	Platelet antagonist	ADP receptor inhibition	None	Platelet transfusion, FFP, Cryoprecipitate
Abciximab	Platelet antagonist	GP-IIb/IIIa receptor inhibition	None	Cryoprecipitate, FFP, platelet transfusion
Tirofiban	Platelet antagonist	GP-IIb/IIIa receptor inhibition	None	Cryoprecipitate, FFP, platelet transfusion
Eptifibatide	Platelet antagonist	GP-IIb/IIIa receptor inhibition	None	Cryoprecipitate, FFP, platelet transfusion
UFH	Anticoagulant	Anti-IIa and –Xa via ATIII	Protamine	None
LMWH	Anticoagulant	Anti-IIa and –Xa via ATIII	Protamine (60% effective)	None
Fondaparinux	Anticoagulant	Anti-Xa via ATIII	None	None
Lepirudin	Anticoagulant	Anti-IIa (direct)	None	FFP, plasmapheresis
Argatroban	Anticoagulant	Anti-IIa (direct)	None	FFP, plasmapheresis
Bivalirudin	Anticoagulant	Anti-IIa (direct)	None	FFP, plasmapheresis
Danaparoid	Anticoagulant	Anti-IIa (direct)	None	Plasmapheresis

DDAVP, 1-deamino-8-D-arginine vasopressin; ADP, adenosine diphosphate; GP, glycoprotein; UFH, unfractionated heparin; LMWH, low molecular weight heparin; FFP, fresh frozen plasma.

are twofold: cardiovascular risk reduction and the treatment of leg symptoms with the purpose of improving mobility.

Antiplatelet and Anticoagulant Therapy for Cardiovascular Risk Reduction

Aspirin

Although well proven to reduce cardiovascular mortality in CAD, there are relatively few data evaluating the efficacy of aspirin in patients with PAD. A 2009 meta-analysis of aspirin therapy in patients with PAD showed no significant change in cardiovascular events, all cause mortality, or cardiovascular mortality [26]. This particular meta-analysis did not demonstrate any change in major bleeding associated with aspirin therapy in PAD. Despite the relatively sparse data, aspirin at a dose of 75–325 mg daily is given a class I recommendation (should perform) for the reduction of MI, stroke, and vascular death in patients with symptomatic PAD [27].

Clopidogrel

The thienopyridine, clopidogrel, has also been investigated in patients with peripheral arterial disease. In a secondary analysis of the PAD subset of the Clopidogrel versus Aspirin in Patients at Risk of Ischemic Events (CAPRIE) trial, clopidogrel use was associated with reduction in stroke, MI, and vascular death versus aspirin [28]. Given that there are no randomized trial comparisons of aspirin and clopidogrel for the prevention of cardiovascular events in patients with PAD, clopidogrel (75 mg) is also given a class I recommendation.

Warfarin

Multiple studies have attempted to evaluate the utility of oral anticoagulants in peripheral arterial disease. A meta-analysis of nine trials involving 4889 patients found that, compared to aspirin, oral anticoagulant therapy did not change mortality or graft occlusion, but did increase major bleeding [29]. The subsequent WAVE trial pitted oral anticoagulation with warfarin plus antiplatelet therapy with aspirin against aspirin alone for the prevention of MI, stroke, or cardiovascular death. Though there was no significant difference in ischemic events, oral anticoagulation in addition to aspirin therapy was associated with increased life-threatening bleeding [30]. As a result, oral anticoagulation with warfarin is given a class III (contraindicated) recommendation for PAD patients in the American College of Cardiology Foundation/American Heart Association (ACCF/AHA) guidelines [27].

Drug Therapy after Revascularization

In contrast to the data regarding aspirin use in symptomatic PAD, there is definitive data regarding its use as adjuvant therapy after lower-extremity bypass. In a meta-analysis, the Antiplatelet Trialists' Collaboration demonstrated an odds reduction of 43% for the prevention of vascular occlusion with aspirin therapy as compared to placebo [31].

Percutaneous transluminal angioplasty (PTA) with or without stenting has become popular for the treatment of aortoiliac and superficial femoral artery lesions. PTA, however, induces a prothrombotic condition wherein atherosclerotic plaque is disrupted and platelet adhesion and aggregation ensues. A 2005 Cochrane review of these studies concluded that aspirin, 50–330 mg with or without dipyridamole, started before femoropopliteal endovascular treatment was the most effective and safest strategy to reduce reocclusion at 6 and 12 months as compared to placebo or Vitamin K antagonist [32]. Given its efficacy, the ACCF/AHA guidelines give aspirin therapy a class I indication (should perform) for patients undergoing lower extremity revascularization, either by bypass grafting or by endovascular means [27]. Although not studied in a randomized fashion, a strategy of aspirin plus clopidogrel for 24 hours before and 4 weeks after endovascular procedures has become a common approach to the reduction of acute and subacute thrombotic complications after endovascular procedures [33].

Ventricular Assist Devices

Despite advances in medical therapy, mortality for end-stage heart failure remains high. Although cardiac transplantation remains an option for many endstage heart failure patients, due to a limited supply of donor organs, each year thousands of patients die while waiting for a heart transplant. Left ventricular assist devices (LVADs) are designed to provide either a bridge to transplantation or a "destination" therapy for those who don't qualify for cardiac transplantation.

The first generation of LVADs were "pulsatile flow" devices designed to mimic the pulsatile (systolic and diastolic) output of the native human heart (Figure 20.2) [34]. In the landmark REMATCH trial, these devices significantly improved survival but were large and plagued by thrombotic and mechanical complications related to maintaining pulsatility. Second-generation devices were designed to have continuous flow and mitigate mechanical failures.

The potential advantages of continuous-flow pumps were tested in a randomized trial in 2009, when investigators randomized patients to either the pulsatile-flow HeartMate XVE or the continuous-flow HeartMate II device. Patients randomized to the continuous-flow HeartMate II device had greater survival at 2 years free of disabling stroke or reoperation [35]. In order to

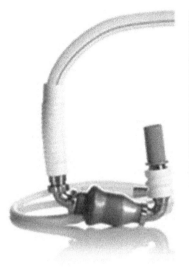
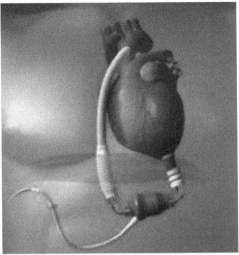

Figure 20.2 Photograph and diagram of HeartMate II device. *Source:* reprinted with permission of Thoratec Corporation.

prevent device thrombosis leading to device failure, death, or stroke, patients randomized to the HeartMate II were treated with aspirin and warfarin with a goal INR of 2.0 to 3.0.

Bleeding in Continuous-Flow Ventricular Assist Devices

Continuous-flow VADs have been associated with bleeding complications. In clinical trials the most common adverse event in the first 30 days after device implantation is nonsurgical bleeding resulting in blood transfusion or surgery [36].

The most common clinical manifestation of this is gastrointestinal bleeding. The potential mechanisms for increased GI bleeding associated with continuous-flow VADs are varied. Combined antiplatelet and anticoagulant therapy, as suggested by guidelines developed from the HeartMate II Pivotal Trial [37] lower the bleeding threshold. Second, LVAD-induced impaired platelet aggregation, acquired von Willebrand disease, and angiodysplasia have all been proposed as possible mechanisms [38]. Because no endoscopic studies yet exist detailing the extent of arteriovenous malformation (AVM) before and after VAD placement, or the rate of AVM formation, it is difficult to prospectively balance the risk of thromboembolism and GI bleeding.

Management of Bleeding in Continuous-flow Ventricular Assist Devices

Given that the incidence of GI and intracranial bleeding in continuous-flow VADs may be as high as 30% and 11%, respectively [35,39], VAD centers have adopted different strategies to mitigate the risk of bleeding. Although the presence of acquired von Willebrand multimer deficiency in continuous flow VAD patients would suggest that bleeding can be managed with 1-deamino-8-d-arginine vasopressin (DDAVP) or Humate-P, there are no data assessing or comparing various management strategies. Therefore, recommendations are made based on clinical experience and expert opinion. At Duke University, an algorithm has been developed to investigate and treat episodes of GI bleeding in continuous-flow VAD patients (Figure 20.3) [40]. Currently, no consensus guidelines exist with regards to the appropriate level of anticoagulation or appropriate changes to anticoagulant regimen as a result of bleeding events.

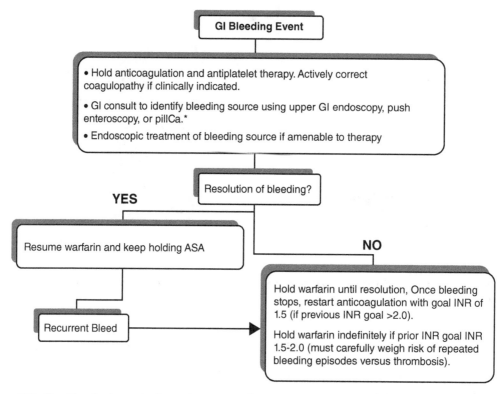

Figure 20.3 Algorithm for the evaluation and treatment of gastrointestinal (GI) tract bleeding (the Duke approach). In the event that a patient supported with an axial-flow device develops GI tract bleeding, consultation from a GI specialist is of benefit to identify the bleeding source through endoscopy or use of the PillCam device. Initially, antiplatelet medication should be discontinued and bleeding should be reassessed. If bleeding continues, warfarin should be discontinued. Once the patient is hemodynamically stable, a target international normalized ratio (INR) of 1.5 to 2.0 is recommended. The medical team should consider alternative therapies to stop bleeding, including cryoprecipitate, platelets, factor VIII, octreotide, and desmopressin (DDAVP) in the event of uncontrolled hemorrhage. *There are no data indicating that endoscopy or the PillCam are beneficial in management of GI bleeding early after left ventricular assist device (LVAD) implantation when pre-LAVD endoscopy showed no bleeding source. *Source:* Suarez J *et al.* 2011 [40]. Reproduced with permission of Wolters Kluwer Health.

Management of Ventricular Assist Device Thrombosis

Device-associated thrombosis is a potentially life-threatening complication of VAD support. In the multicenter trial demonstrating the efficacy of the continuous-flow HeartMate II device, the reported incidence of device-associated thrombosis was 0.02 events per patient year [35]. Multiple factors, including subtherapeutic anticoagulation, retained ventricular or atrial thrombus, low pump speeds, AF, bacteremia, and hypercoagulable states, may predispose patients to VAD thrombosis. Although management strategies may include device replacement, this is associated with high morbidity and mortality. As a result, clinicians have successfully managed VAD thrombosis with both GPIIB-IIIA inhibitors [41] and intracavitary thrombolysis [42].

Balancing Ventricular Assist Device-Related Thromboembolic and Bleeding Risk

In the absence of significant long-term follow up of thrombotic and bleeding events in continuous-flow VADs, the best current evidence suggests that bleeding and thrombotic events are minimized with low-dose aspirin therapy (81 mg daily) in addition to dose-adjusted warfarin with an INR goal of 1.5 to 2.5 [43]. Several caveats exist to this recommendation. First, new oral anticoagulants such as direct thrombin and factor Xa inhibitors have not been evaluated in the setting of VAD usage. Secondly, the optimal INR goal for patients with another indication for anticoagulation (such as AF or mechanical valve) has not been established. In the absence of follow-up data or guidelines, VAD centers have adopted center-specific approaches for patients with multiple indications for anticoagulation. We currently recommend an INR goal of 2.0–3.0 for patients with AF and a $CHADS_2$ risk >1 or previous stroke.

The International Society of Heart and Lung Transplantation (ISHLT) has published guidelines regarding the perioperative, GI bleeding, and long-term management of anticoagulant and antiplatelet therapies in patients with LVADs [44].

Electrophysiological Catheter Ablation

Over the past 20 years, radiofrequency catheter ablation has revolutionized the management of cardiac arrhythmias. In general, the technique of catheter ablation relies on the administration of radiofrequency energy, or cryoablation, to induce selective tissue damage in an area of electrically active myocardium. Focal ablation can be effective in terminating and preventing recurrence of arrhythmias.

Atrial Fibrillation Ablation

All ablation with radiofrequency energy is associated with heat-related denaturation of fibrinogen to fibrin and the formation of char/coagulum at the catheter/tissue interface. Recent studies employing diffusion-weighted MRI of the brain have demonstrated silent cerebral lesions after AF ablation [45,46]. Thus, while atrial fibrillation ablation is often undertaken to restore sinus rhythm, in part to avoid the need for continued anticoagulation, catheter ablation itself induces localized coagulation within the left atrium.

Atrial Fibrillation Ablation and Hemostasis

Given that patients who are eligible for atrial fibrillation ablations are often being treated with systemic anticoagulation due to the associated risk of thromboembolism, the periablation management of anticoagulation for atrial fibrillation ablations is a subject of importance. Conventional practice has dictated the cessation of systemic anticoagulation and institution of a "bridging" regimen periprocedurally, this strategy was associated with an excess of vascular access site complications. However, a retrospective cohort study of 2600 patients who underwent atrial fibrillation ablation with an open irrigation catheter while on uninterrupted therapeutic warfarin found no increase in major or minor bleeding complications [47]. Furthermore, this strategy also prevented any strokes or TIAs. As a result of this study, many centers are moving towards completion of atrial fibrillation ablation without interruption of therapeutic warfarin.

Atrial Fibrillation Ablation and Management of Novel Anticoagulants

Given the increasing use of novel anticoagulants (dabigatran, rivaroxiban, and apixaban) for thromboembolic prophylaxis in atrial fibrillation, periprocedural management of these agents has become a significant aspect of the care of patients with atrial fibrillation. Studies assessing the peri-atrial fibrillation ablation management of novel anticoagulants are few. A recent study examining the use of nearly uninterrupted dabigatran periprocedurally found that it is associated with both bleeding and thrombotic complications as compared to periprocedural warfarin [48]. In contrast, a secondary analysis of the ROCKET-AF trial showed no difference in stroke, systemic embolism, bleeding, or death between periprocedural rivaroxaban and periprocedural warfarin, though the number of events in both arms was low [49]. Although the FDA package inserts of all of the novel anticoagulants suggest regimens for periprocedural management, given the unique prothrombotic properties of catheter ablation, in the absence of major societal guidelines, expert opinion and local regimens are often followed.

Long-Term Management of Oral Anticoagulation after Atrial Fibrillation Ablation

Decision-making regarding cessation of oral anticoagulation after atrial fibrillation ablation is a complex problem chiefly because the standard for demonstrating freedom from arrhythmia is not defined. In the absence of clear societal guidelines for this issue, retrospective studies have suggested that low-risk patients with paroxysmal atrial fibrillation and a $CHADS_2$ score of 0 or 1 may be discharged postablation on aspirin 325 mg/day monotherapy [50].

Transcatheter Aortic Valve Replacement

A percutaneous approach to treating advanced aortic valve disease represents a major advance in the care of patients who are poor candidates for surgical valve repair. This development is particularly relevant with an aging population in whom calcific aortic stenosis is a common occurrence, with an incidence approaching 5.0% in persons greater than 75 years of age and significant associated morbidity, mortality, and health-care expenditures [51].

Clinical Experience

The PARTNER (Placement of Aortic Transcatheter Valves) Study was the first prospective, randomized trial of Transcatheter Aortic valve replacement (TAVR). Among patients with high risk for aortic valve surgery, there was a trend towards reduction of death from any cause via TAVR as compared to surgical valve replacement. This came at a cost of increased stroke rate and vascular complications, but decreased major bleeding [52]. Among patients with prohibitive surgical risk (not surgical candidates),

there was a statistically significant 20% risk reduction in the rate of death with TAVR versus medical therapy. Again, however, TAVR was associated with increased risk of stroke and vascular complications [53].

Stroke in Transcatheter Aortic Valve Replacement

Stroke rates in TAVR are higher than with aortic valve surgery or medical therapy, with 30-day event rates at 5.5% and 6.7% in high-risk patients and inoperable patients, respectively [54]. Approximately half of all strokes occur within 48 hours of the procedure and, accordingly, are considered procedure related. The causes of late neurological events (>48 hours after the procedure) are multifactorial and may include occult atrial fibrillation and thrombogenicity of the implanted valve. Given that TAVR-associated stroke is associated with a threefold increase in 30-day mortality rate, at the present time, aspirin and clopidogrel are used to diminish risk.

Bleeding in Transcatheter Aortic Valve Replacement

Bleeding complications are common among patients undergoing TAVR, with life-threatening and major hemorrhagic events occurring in upward of 15% and 25% of patients, respectively [55]. In a majority of instances, bleeding occurs at arterial access sites owing to vascular trauma from large sheath size and existing vascular disease. Patients undergoing TAVR also carry risk factors for bleeding, including advanced age, renal insufficiency, poor functional class, and, perhaps more often than recognized, an acquired form of von Willebrand disease from flow-associated shear stress across a narrowed aortic valve [56]. Pre- and post-TAVR major or life-threatening hemorrhage is associated with heightened 30-day all-cause and cardiovascular mortality.

Surgical Heart Valve Replacement and Repair

Surgical heart valve replacement and repair represent significant advances in patient care.

The surface of bioprosthetic valves (usually porcine or bovine) is markedly denuded of endothelial cells, exposing collagen and the basement membrane. Upon exposure to circulating blood, the surface is promptly covered by platelets and fibrin. An endothelial cell layer is reconstituted over time. Consequently, American College of Chest Physicians Guidelines suggest aspirin for all patients undergoing bioprosthetic aortic valve replacement and consideration of oral anticoagulant therapy for the initial 3 months after surgery [57].

The materials used most often for constructing mechanical valves include metals and carbon. Given the thrombogenicity associated with these materials and poor endothelialization of their surfaces, indefinite systemic anticoagulation is generally recommended [57]. Although rare in the setting of appropriate anticoagulation for mechanical valves, prosthetic valve thrombosis is a feared complication that can result in stroke, heart failure, or death. Although the conventional therapy has been surgical thrombectomy with or without valve replacement, multiple recent studies have evaluated protocols of transesophageal echocardiography guided systemic thrombolysis as an alternative to surgical therapy for prosthetic valve thrombosis [58,59].

Conclusion

With a rapidly expanding use and number of antiplatelet agents and anticoagulants within an older and complex medical population, antithrombotic therapies in cardiovascular disease have entered a new era. Coupled with a rapidly expanding array of invasive cardiovascular procedures and indwelling devices, the hematologist will be confronted by new drugs used in combination and broadening indications and bleeding complications. Though society guidelines will continue to form the framework for patient care, appropriate clinical decisions will be dependent on a thorough understanding of the pathophysiology of disease and the risks, benefits, and pharmacology of these agents.

References

1 Jneid H, Anderson JL, Wright RS, *et al.* ACCF/AHA focused update of the guideline for the management of patients with unstable angina/non-ST-elevation myocardial infarction (updating the 2007 guideline and replacing the 2011 focused update): A report of the American college of cardiology foundation/American heart association task force on practice guidelines. *J Am Coll Cardiol* 2012; 60: 645–681.
2 Libby P, Theroux P. Pathophysiology of coronary artery disease. *Circulation* 2005; 111: 3481–3488.
3 O'Gara PT, Kushner FG, Ascheim DD, *et al.* ACCF/AHA guideline for the management of ST-elevation myocardial infarction: Executive summary: A report of the American college of cardiology foundation/American heart association task force on practice guidelines. *Circulation* 2013; 127: 529–555.
4 Antithrombotic Trialists. Collaborative meta-analysis of randomised trials of antiplatelet therapy for prevention of death, myocardial infarction, and stroke in high risk patients. *BMJ* 2002; 324: 71–86.
5 Isis-2 (Second International Study Of Infarct Survival) Collaborative Group. Randomized trial of intravenous streptokinase, oral aspirin, both, or neither among 17,187 cases of suspected acute myocardial infarction: *J Am Coll Cardiol* 1988; 12: 3A–13A.
6 Berger JS, Brown DL, Becker RC. Low-dose aspirin in patients with stable cardiovascular disease: A meta-analysis. *Am J Med* 2008; 121: 43–49.
7 Berger JS, Roncaglioni MC, Avanzini F, *et al.* Aspirin for the primary prevention of cardiovascular events in women and men: A sex-specific meta-analysis of randomized controlled trials. *JAMA* 2006; 295: 306–313.
8 Eikelboom JW, Hirsh J, Spencer FA, *et al.* Antiplatelet drugs: Antithrombotic therapy and prevention of thrombosis, 9th ed: American college of chest physicians evidence-based clinical practice guidelines. *Chest* 2012; 141: e89S–119S.

9 Wallentin L, Becker RC, Budaj A, *et al*. Ticagrelor versus clopidogrel in patients with acute coronary syndromes. *N Engl J Med* 2009; 361: 1045–1057.

10 Costopoulos C, Niespialowska-Steuden M, Kukreja N, *et al*. Novel oral anticoagulants in acute coronary syndrome. *Int J Cardiol* 2013; 167: 2449–2455.

11 Weitz JI. Low molecular-weight heparins. *N Engl J Med* 1997; 337: 688–698.

12 Petersen JL, Mahaffey KW, Hasselblad V, *et al*. Efficacy and bleeding complications among patients randomized to enoxaparin or unfractionated heparin for antithrombin therapy in non-ST-segment elevation acute coronary syndromes: A systematic overview. *JAMA* 2004; 292: 89–96.

13 Yusuf S, Mehta SR, Chrolavicius S, *et al*. Comparison of fondaparinux and enoxaparin in acute coronary syndromes. *N Engl J Med* 2006; 354: 1464–1476.

14 Yusuf S, Mehta SR, Chrolavicius S, *et al*. Effects of fondaparinux on mortality and reinfarction in patients with acute ST-segment elevation myocardial infarction: The oasis-6 randomized trial. *JAMA* 2006; 295: 1519–1530.

15 Direct Thrombin Inhibitor Trialists' Collaborative Group. Direct thrombin inhibitors in acute coronary syndromes: Principal results of a meta-analysis based on individual patients' data. *Lancet* 2002; 359: 294–302.

16 Stone GW, Witzenbichler B, Guagliumi G, *et al*. Bivalirudin during primary pci in acute myocardial infarction. *N Engl J Med* 2008; 358: 2218–2230.

17 Rao SV, O'Grady K, Pieper KS, *et al*. Impact of bleeding severity on clinical outcomes among patients with acute coronary syndromes. *Am J Cardiol* 2005; 96: 1200–1206.

18 Eikelboom JW, Mehta SR, Anand SS, *et al*. Adverse impact of bleeding on prognosis in patients with acute coronary syndromes. *Circulation* 2006; 114: 774–782.

19 Budaj A, Eikelboom JW, Mehta SR, *et al*. Improving clinical outcomes by reducing bleeding in patients with non-ST-elevation acute coronary syndromes. *Eur Heart J* 2009; 30: 655–661.

20 Spencer FA, Moscucci M, Granger CB, *et al*. Does comorbidity account for the excess mortality in patients with major bleeding in acute myocardial infarction? *Circulation* 2007; 116: 2793–2801.

21 Manoukian SV, Feit F, Mehran R, *et al*. Impact of major bleeding on 30-day mortality and clinical outcomes in patients with acute coronary syndromes: An analysis from the acuity trial. *J Am Coll Cardiol* 2007; 49: 1362–1368.

22 Hart RG, Tonarelli SB, Pearce LA. Avoiding central nervous system bleeding during antithrombotic therapy: Recent data and ideas. *Stroke* 2005; 36: 1588–1593.

23 Abraham NS, Hlatky MA, Antman EM, *et al*. ACCF/ACG/AHA 2010 expert consensus document on the concomitant use of proton pump inhibitors and thienopyridines: A focused update of the ACCF/ACG/AHA 2008 expert consensus document on reducing the gastrointestinal risks of antiplatelet therapy and NSAID use: A report of the American college of cardiology foundation task force on expert consensus documents. *Circulation* 2010; 122: 2619–2633.

24 Hirsch AT, Haskal ZJ, Hertzer NR, *et al*. ACC/AHA 2005 practice guidelines for the management of patients with peripheral arterial disease (lower extremity, renal, mesenteric, and abdominal aortic): A collaborative report from the American association for vascular surgery/society for vascular surgery, society for cardiovascular angiography and interventions, society for vascular medicine and biology, society of interventional radiology, and the acc/aha task force on practice guidelines (writing committee to develop guidelines for the management of patients with peripheral arterial disease): Endorsed by the American association of cardiovascular and pulmonary rehabilitation; national heart, lung, and blood institute; society for vascular nursing; transatlantic inter-society consensus; and vascular disease foundation. *Circulation* 2006; 113: e463–654.

25 Hirsch AT, Criqui MH, Treat-Jacobson D, *et al.* Peripheral arterial disease detection, awareness, and treatment in primary care. *JAMA* 2001; 286: 1317–1324.

26 Berger JS, Krantz MJ, Kittelson JM, Hiatt WR. Aspirin for the prevention of cardiovascular events in patients with peripheral artery disease: A meta-analysis of randomized trials. *JAMA* 2009; 301: 1909–1919.

27 Rooke TW, Hirsch AT, Misra S, *et al.* 2011 ACCF/AHA focused update of the guideline for the management of patients with peripheral artery disease (updating the 2005 guideline): A report of the American College of Cardiology Foundation/American Heart Association task force on practice guidelines. *J Am Coll Cardiol* 2011; 58: 2020–2045.

28 CAPRIE steering committee. A randomised, blinded, trial of clopidogrel versus aspirin in patients at risk of ischaemic events (CAPRIE). *Lancet* 1996; 348: 1329–1339.

29 The effects of oral anticoagulants in patients with peripheral arterial disease: Rationale, design, and baseline characteristics of the warfarin and antiplatelet vascular evaluation (wave) trial, including a meta-analysis of trials. *Am Heart J* 2006; 151: 1–9.

30 Anand S, Yusuf S, Xie C, *et al.* Oral anticoagulant and antiplatelet therapy and peripheral arterial disease. *N Engl J Med* 2007; 357: 217–227.

31 Antiplatelet Trialists' Collaboration. Collaborative overview of randomised trials of antiplatelet therapy–ii: Maintenance of vascular graft or arterial patency by antiplatelet therapy. *BMJ* 1994; 308: 159–168.

32 Dorffler-Melly J, Koopman MM, Prins MH, *et al.* Antiplatelet and anticoagulant drugs for prevention of restenosis/reocclusion following peripheral endovascular treatment. *Cochrane Database Syst Rev* 2005: CD002071.

33 Visona A, Tonello D, Zalunardo B, *et al.* Antithrombotic treatment before and after peripheral artery percutaneous angioplasty. *Blood Transfus* 2009; 7: 18–23.

34 Rose EA, Gelijns AC, Moskowitz AJ, *et al.* Randomized Evaluation of Mechanical Assistance for the Treatment of Congestive Heart Failure Study G. Long-term use of a left ventricular assist device for end-stage heart failure. *N Engl J Med* 2001; 345: 1435–1443.

35 Slaughter MS, Rogers JG, Milano CA, *et al.* Advanced heart failure treated with continuous-flow left ventricular assist device. *N Engl J Med* 2009; 361: 2241–2251.

36 Pagani FD, Miller LW, Russell SD, *et al.* Extended mechanical circulatory support with a continuous-flow rotary left ventricular assist device. *J Am Coll Cardiol* 2009; 54: 312–321.

37 Bonde P DM, Meyer D, Tallaj JJ, *et al.* National trends in readmission (REA) rates following left ventricular assist device (LVAD) therapy. *J Heart Lung Transplant* 2011; 30: S9.

38 John R, Boyle A, Pagani F, *et al.* Physiologic and pathologic changes in patients with continuous-flow ventricular assist devices. *J Cardiovasc Transl Res* 2009; 2: 154–158.

39 Uriel N, Pak SW, Jorde UP, *et al.* Acquired von willebrand syndrome after continuous-flow mechanical device support contributes to a high prevalence of bleeding during long-term support and at the time of transplantation. *J Am Coll Cardiol* 2010; 56: 1207–1213.

40 Suarez J, Patel CB, Felker GM, *et al.* Mechanisms of bleeding and approach to patients with axial-flow left ventricular assist devices. *Circ Heart Fail* 2011; 4: 779–784.

41 Thomas MD, Wood C, Lovett M, *et al.* Successful treatment of rotary pump thrombus with the glycoprotein IIb/IIIa inhibitor tirofiban. *J Heart Lung Transplant* 2008; 27: 925–927.

42 Kiernan MS, Pham DT, DeNofrio D, *et al.* Management of heartware left ventricular assist device thrombosis using intracavitary thrombolytics. *J Thorac Cardiovasc Surg* 2011; 142: 712–714.

43 Boyle AJ, Russell SD, Teuteberg JJ, *et al.* Low thromboembolism and pump thrombosis with the heartmate ii left ventricular assist device: Analysis of outpatient anti-coagulation. *J Heart Lung Transplant* 2009; 28: 881–887.

44 Feldman D, Pamboukian SV, Teuteberg JJ, *et al.* The 2013 international society for heart and lung transplantation guidelines for mechanical circulatory support: Executive

summary. *J Heart Lung Transplant* 2013; 32: 157–187.

45 Schrickel JW, Lickfett L, Lewalter T, *et al.* Incidence and predictors of silent cerebral embolism during pulmonary vein catheter ablation for atrial fibrillation. *Europace* 2010; 12: 52–57.

46 Sauren LD, van Belle Y, De Roy L, *et al.* Transcranial measurement of cerebral microembolic signals during endocardial pulmonary vein isolation: Comparison of three different ablation techniques. *J Cardiovasc Electrophysiol* 2009; 20: 1102–1107.

47 Di Biase L, Burkhardt JD, Mohanty P, *et al.* Periprocedural stroke and management of major bleeding complications in patients undergoing catheter ablation of atrial fibrillation: The impact of periprocedural therapeutic international normalized ratio. *Circulation* 2010; 121: 2550–2556.

48 Lakkireddy D, Reddy YM, Di Biase L, *et al.* Feasibility and safety of dabigatran versus warfarin for periprocedural anticoagulation in patients undergoing radiofrequency ablation for atrial fibrillation: Results from a multicenter prospective registry. *J Am Coll Cardiol* 2012; 59: 1168–1174.

49 Piccini JP, Stevens SR, Lokhnygina Y, *et al.* Outcomes after cardioversion and atrial fibrillation ablation in patients treated with rivaroxaban and warfarin in the rocket af trial. *J Am Coll Cardiol* 2013; 61: 1998–2006.

50 Bunch TJ, Crandall BG, Weiss JP, *et al.* Warfarin is not needed in low-risk patients following atrial fibrillation ablation procedures. *J Cardiovasc Electrophysiol* 2009; 20: 988–993.

51 Reinohl J, von Zur Muhlen C, Moser M, *et al.* Tavi 2012: State of the art. *J Thromb Thrombolysis* 2013; 35: 419–435.

52 Smith CR, Leon MB, Mack MJ, *et al.* Transcatheter versus surgical aortic-valve replacement in high-risk patients. *N Engl J Med* 2011; 364: 2187–2198.

53 Kodali SK, Williams MR, Smith CR, *et al.* Two-year outcomes after transcatheter or surgical aortic-valve replacement. *N Engl J Med* 2012; 366: 1686–1695.

54 Eggebrecht H, Schmermund A, Voigtlander T, *et al.* Risk of stroke after transcatheter aortic valve implantation (TAVI): A meta-analysis of 10,037 published patients. *EuroIntervention* 2012; 8: 129–138.

55 Pilgrim T, Stortecky S, Luterbacher F, *et al.* Transcatheter aortic valve implantation and bleeding: Incidence, predictors and prognosis. *J Thromb Thrombolysis* 2013; 35: 456–462.

56 Bander J, Elmariah S, Aledort LM, *et al.* Changes in von willebrand factor-cleaving protease (adamts-13) in patients with aortic stenosis undergoing valve replacement or balloon valvuloplasty. *Thromb Haemost* 2012; 108: 86–93.

57 Whitlock RP, Sun JC, Fremes SE, *et al.* Antithrombotic and thrombolytic therapy for valvular disease: Antithrombotic therapy and prevention of thrombosis, 9th ed: American college of chest physicians evidence-based clinical practice guidelines. *Chest* 2012; 141: e576S–600S.

58 Ozkan M, Cakal B, Karakoyun S, *et al.* Thrombolytic therapy for the treatment of prosthetic heart valve thrombosis in pregnancy with low-dose, slow infusion of tissue-type plasminogen activator. *Circulation* 2013; 128: 532–540.

59 Ozkan M, Gunduz S, Biteker M, *et al.* Comparison of different tee-guided thrombolytic regimens for prosthetic valve thrombosis: The TROIA trial. *JACC. Cardiovasc Imaging* 2013; 6: 206–216.

21

Cardiothoracic Surgery

Denise O'Shaughnessy and Ravi Gill

Key Points

- Cardiac surgery using cardiopulmonary bypass (CPB) injures the body's hemostatic mechanism. This may be compromised by preoperative anemia and drug therapy. CPB leads to hemodilution, platelet dysfunction, and fibrinolysis.
- Bleeding in the operating room and ICU is poorly researched, with transfusion and reoperation being used in the literature as surrogates.
- Transfusion and reoperation are both associated with poor outcomes after cardiac surgery.
- Transfusion in the UK is highly variable.
- The use of near patient testing (POC) may reduce transfusion requirements, reduce reoperation rates, and improve patient outcomes.

Introduction

The need for clinicians involved with cardiac surgery to understand the normal hemostatic mechanisms cannot be overemphasized. Hemostasis is a balance protecting the integrity of the vascular system after tissue injury and maintaining the fluidity of blood. Excessive bleeding can be due to surgical causes, a derangement of hemostasis, or, more often, a combination of both, of which cardiothoracic surgery is a prime example [1].

As the incidence of heart disease continues to rise, the consequent demand for cardiac surgery increases, with 400 000 in USA, over 100 000 in Europe, and 36 000 in UK per annum. Most of these procedures, together with major heart surgery on congenital defects, are performed on hearts supported by cardiopulmonary bypass. During surgery on the heart, it is common to stop the heart to make it easier to operate on. During this time, the function of the heart and lungs is taken over by a CPB machine.

The heart can be stopped using several different methods. In general, cold or warm blood cardioplegia is infused into the coronary arteries leading to diastolic arrest of the heart. Cardioplegia contains chemicals that reduce the ischemic burden placed on the heart when it is not perfused, allowing surgery to take place in bloodless environment. The heart can also be stopped electrically, and this is referred to as cardiac arrest with ventricular fibrillation.

In conventional coronary artery bypass grafting (CABG), operations are performed after cardioplegic arrest. The pericardium is usually opened longitudinally to allow unrestricted access to underlying heart and proximal great vessels. The pericardium is may be left open at the end of surgery.

Cardiac Surgery without Cardiopulmonary Bypass

CABG can be performed with or without CPB. These minimally invasive procedures restore

Practical Hemostasis and Thrombosis, Third Edition. Edited by Nigel S. Key, Michael Makris and David Lillicrap.
© 2017 John Wiley & Sons, Ltd. Published 2017 by John Wiley & Sons, Ltd.

healthy blood flow to the heart without having to stop the beating heart [2].

It was thought that off-pump coronary artery bypass (OPCAB) would have a lower risk of complications, such as stroke, acute lung injury, renal dysfunction, neurocognitive outcome, and transfusion rates. Although observational data have supported this, randomized clinical trials have proved disappointing.

Performing surgery on a beating heart is technically more difficult than working on a heart that has been stopped with the help of the CPB machine. In addition, the stress on the heart during the procedure may lead to more heart muscle damage, lower blood pressure, irregular heartbeat, and potentially, brain injury. In some cases (usually <10%), it is necessary to convert to conventional CABG methods on an emergency basis.

Currently there are three methods used, as outlined in the following sections.

Minimally Invasive Direct Coronary Artery Bypass

Minimally invasive direct coronary artery bypass (MIDCAB) is for patients with blockage(s) in the arteries on the front of the heart (the left anterior descending (LAD) artery and its branches). A small incision is made on the patient's left chest to expose the heart. After muscles in the area are pushed apart and a small part of the front of the rib (costal cartilage) is removed, the surgeon temporarily closes off the artery that lies underneath and frees its lower end. An opening is made in the pericardium and a device is attached to the heart to reduce its movement. Finally, the surgeon connects the artery below the blockage to the LAD artery or one of its branches. The procure takes 2–3 hours.

Unfortunately, due to the limited size of the incision, the procedure is limited to only a few patients who have a blockage in one or two coronary arteries located on the front side of the heart, whether healthy or considered too high risk for conventional bypass surgery or balloon angioplasty. However, for younger patients, for those who have small coronary arteries and need

several bypasses, or for those whose heart will not tolerate being manipulated during the procedure, it may be preferable to use the traditional CABG technique.

Off-pump Coronary Artery Bypass

During off-pump coronary artery bypass (OPCAB), the chest is opened and grafts harvested conventionally. Like the MIDCAB procedure, a device is used to restrict movement of parts of the heart so that the surgeon can operate on it while it is still beating. The surgeon can repair four to five vessels on the beating heart during the same procedure.

The number of OPCAB procedures grew significantly because of its potential advantages, such as reduced transfusion requirements, decreased risk of stroke, shorter stay in the hospital, and quicker return to normal activities. OPCAB is suitable for patients with poor heart function (very low ejection fraction), severe lung disease (chronic obstructive pulmonary disease and emphysema), and acute or chronic kidney disease. It is also suitable for those at high risk for stroke or for those who have a calcified aorta. However, the proposed advantages have not been seen in randomized controlled trials. Despite this, there is still a place for OPCAB surgery.

Robot-assisted Coronary Artery Bypass

Robot-assisted coronary artery bypass (RACAB) is the latest advance in heart surgery. Surgeons use a robot to perform the bypass. The breastbone does not need to be split open at all. Surgeons do not have direct contact with the patient, performing the operation while watching a videoscreen. As the technology becomes more advanced, the surgeon may perform coronary bypass from a distant site (i.e., from another room or another geographical location).

Anticoagulation during CPB

Heparin is used as the anticoagulant of choice for surgery requiring CPB. It is given in a dose of

300–400 IU/kg. The response to heparin is monitored by the activated clotting time (ACT), aiming to achieve a time of >400 seconds. The ACT is often checked every 30 minutes, leading to additional heparin being given if the ACT falls. However, the ACT is known to be affected by cold and hemodilution. Whilst heparin reversal is not mandatory, the majority of centers administer 1 mL protamine for 1 mL of heparin given.

CPB technical Aspects

In 2002, 80% of all CABG surgery was performed on CPB; the figure in 2010 is still over 70%. During CPB, blood is drained from the right atrium and returned to the aorta, creating a bloodless field for the cardiothoracic surgeon. This is achieved by administrating high doses of heparin to anticoagulate patients (monitored using the ACT or anti-Xa levels), and residual heparin is reversed by protamine at the end of surgery.

The process of CPB:

- activates fibrinolysis,
- disturbs platelet function,
- often reduces the platelet count, and
- reduces the concentration of clotting factors by both consumption and dilution.

Reduction in volume of the CPB circuit and improvements in operative techniques, together with cell salvage and the use of antifibrinolytic drugs, have reduced the need for transfusion. Recent "near patient" coagulation testing devices have enabled much of this progress and include the Haemonetics TEG5000, ROTEM, and Platelet Function Analyzers.

Bleeding can occur intraoperatively, after protamine reversal of heparin, leading to delayed chest closure or in the postoperative environment with blood being shed into the mediastinal and pleural drains. There are two main causes of perioperative bleeding:

1) surgical, due to failure to secure hemostasis at the operative site;

2) nonsurgical, due to failure of hemostatic pathways, and principally due to:
   a) the procedure itself, in this case CPB (the circuit and its effect on hemostasis);
   b) incomplete reversal of heparin by protamine;
   c) antiplatelet drugs (aspirin, clopidogrel, GPIIb/IIIa inhibitors);
   d) a pre-existing bleeding disorder (e.g., hemophilia, von Willebrand disease); or
   e) oral anticoagulation that has not been reversed completely.

Critical rates of blood loss in the ICU are 400–500 mL in the first hour and thereafter 200–300 mL/hour. Critical levels can also be expressed as mL/kg of blood loss, with 2–3 mL/kg being of concern.

The cardiopulmonary Bypass Circuit

Bigelow showed in dogs that circulatory arrest (CA) was possible, allowing simple operations without circulatory support, but only for 15 minutes. Originally invented by Gibbon in the 1930s, the pump oxygenator did not work successfully until the 1950s. Even then, only one in four cases survived and 14–25 L of fresh blood prime was required. Also at this time, Lillehei connected a patient to a volunteer donor (the parent of the patient). He drained the blood from the superior vena cava (SVC) of the patient, and pumped this blood into the femoral vein of the donor. Blood was then returned from the femoral artery of the donor to the carotid artery of the patient. Forty-five patients (mostly children) had operations. The 63% survival, despite no reliable ventilators, blood gas or electrolyte analysis, pacemakers, or defibrillators, was remarkable. However, this was not a long-term solution.

The Gibbon Mayo pump, introduced in 1955, had bubble oxygenators and high-flow total cardiopulmonary support, but still required 10–14 U fresh blood prime. Adaptations over the next 60 years have reduced adult prime volumes to 1.5–2.5 L crystalloid and pediatric prime volumes to 400–1000 mL, including some blood (depending on the size of the child) such that on bypass the hematocrit will not fall below 20%.

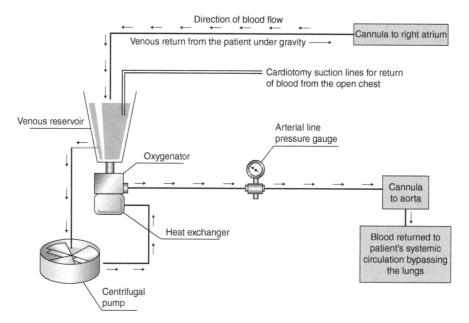

Figure 21.1 Cardiopulmonary bypass circuit.

A representation of current CPB is shown in Figure 21.1.

Hemostasis in Cardiopulmonary Bypass

Hemostasis is a dynamic and extremely complex process, involving many interactive factors. These include coagulation and fibrinolytic proteins, activators, inhibitors, and cellular elements (e.g., platelet cytoskeleton, cytoplasmic granules, and cell surfaces), as described in Chapter 1.

In order to measure any degree of hemostatic imbalance, we need to have the ability to measure the net product of the interactions, which is the three-dimensional clot matrix. Once the coagulation cascade is activated, thrombin is formed.

Thrombin will cleave soluble fibrinogen into fibrin monomers, which polymerize to form protofibril strands and then undergo linear extension, branching, and lateral association, leading to the formation of a three-dimensional matrix of fibrin.

This matrix is given rigidity by the anchoring platelet network, thus allowing resistance to shear. Platelet glycoprotein receptors (GPIIb/IIIa)

bind the polymerized fibrin network to the actin cytoskeleton of the platelet. Actin is a muscle protein that has the ability to transmit contractility force, which is the major contributor to clot strength.

It follows that, in order to adequately treat failures of the hemostatic system, we would need to evaluate and target this interaction of platelet and fibrin in order to assess the basic principles of functional hemostasis: activation, kinetics, contribution, and stability of clotting.

Conventional Tests of Coagulation

Until recently, hemostatic component therapies were guided by the results of conventional laboratory-based testing (see Chapter 2). These tests, which include the prothrombin time (PT), activated partial thromboplastin time (APTT), platelet count, and fibrinogen concentrations, may be unrelated to both postoperative bleeding and the need for blood and component therapies after cardiac surgery.

Inappropriateness of Component Transfusion

The national blood service for England issues approximately 1.7 million units of blood per year (a 16% reduction in the past 4 years), of which 8% are still used in cardiac surgical units. There is a wide unexplained variation in the transfusion practice between different cardiac surgical units.

This was noticed first by Goodenough [3], in a survey of patients undergoing routine heart surgery, who showed that approximately 50% of platelet and 30% of fresh frozen plasma (FFP) transfusions did not conform to the American Association of Blood Banks published guidelines for transfusion practice. Seven years later, Stover and colleagues [4] showed that little improvement had been made in relation to inappropriate ordering and administration of component products.

The findings from the latest UK audit are vey similar to the large US report by Elliott Bennett-Guerrero, who reported findings in 102 470 patients undergoing CABG using CPB in 798 hospitals in the year 2008 [5]. In the total patient population undergoing the surgery, the median percentage of patients receiving red blood cells (RBCs), FFP, and platelets were 60, 22, and 28%, respectively.

The Need for Near-patient Testing

Clinicians have used the traditional tests of coagulation PT/INR for many years; however, the slow turn-around time might explain why they may not be appropriate to be used in such a fluid, rapidly changing environment as cardiac surgery.

Avidan [6] published a randomized study involving 102 patients undergoing coronary artery surgery. Decisions on blood product usage were made either using a laboratory-guided algorithm, or point-of-care thrombelastography (TEG) (Table 21.1). This study demonstrated that using near-patient testing (NPT) or laboratory testing (in appropriate time frames) was better than no test at all. It would seem logical that some form of rapidly available tests of coagulation should be available to help manage patients undergoing cardiac surgery. This might lead to improved patient outcomes and appropriate transfusion of blood and blood component therapy

Early Attempts at Near-patient Testing

A number of suggestions and attempts have been made to develop point-of-care tests to fulfill the need for guiding optimal blood product usage. Early attempts at such devices included the use of machines to produce dedicated heparin/ protamine response curves. Providing an individual solution for a specific patient was shown to be of benefit to reduce both bleeding and the requirement for red cells in patients undergoing heart surgery.

The potential failing in the concept of using a simple coagulation monitor as the only point-of-care test is shown in Figure 21.2.

Table 21.1 Blood components received by the patients. The table shows the number of patients (%) in each group that received transfusions.

Blood component	LAG ($n=51$)	POC ($n=51$)	CD ($n=108$)	$P(X^2)$ test
Red blood cells	35 (69)	34 (68)	92 (85)	0.01
Fresh frozen plasma	0	2 (4)	16 (15)	0.003
Platelets	1 (2)	2 (4)	14 (13)	0.02

LAG, laboratory-guided algorithm;
POC, point of care;
CD, clinical discretion; .

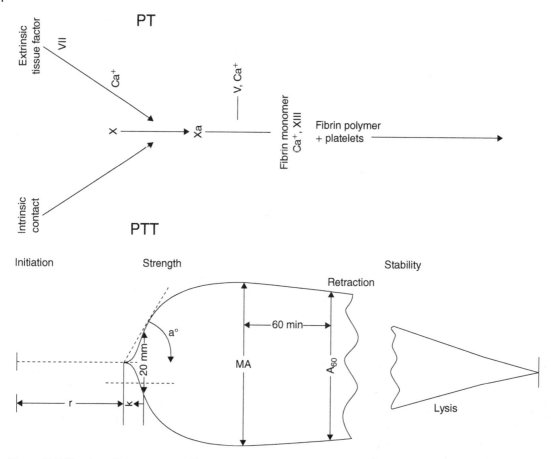

Figure 21.2 The thrombelastogram profile compared with the clotting profile. MA, maximum amplitude; PT, prothrombin time; PTT, partial thromboplastin time.

Standard Laboratory Tests (see chapter 2)

PT and APTT:

These tests use activators to initiate either intrinsic or extrinsic pathways of coagulation. The endpoint for these tests, whether performed in citrated plasma in the laboratory or whole blood in a point-of-care test, is the establishment of fibrin strands.

ACT:

The ACT is a test in which whole blood is added to a tube containing an activator, such as kaolin, and is the test for measuring high doses of heparin (when on bypass). It cannot be used in cases of heparin resistance and is likely to be inaccu-

rate if the patient has an inhibitor (e.g., lupus anticoagulant).

Anti-factor Xa:

Heparin binds to and enhances the activity of antithrombin (AT). Plasma containing heparin is incubated with AT and an excess of factor Xa. It is used primarily to monitor low-molecular-weight heparin (LMWH), which is not detectable by the APTT clotting test. It is a more accurate test for monitoring unfractionated heparin and is the test of choice if there is a lupus anticoagulant present or heparin resistance. There are NPT devices to measure anti-Xa available, but currently, these are used only in the US. When monitoring LMWH, testing should be performed

2–3 hours after the injection with the following targets:

Prophylactic doses of LMWH   0.2–0.4 IU/mL

Therapeutic doses of LMWH   0.4–1.0 IU/mL

CPB (large-dose UFH)   5–8 IU/mL

None of these standard laboratory tests attempt to go further in order to evaluate the kinetics, strength, or relative contribution (platelet to fibrin) of the clot and whether it remains stable over time.

Platelet count:

Normal platelet numbers and function are required for normal hemostasis. A platelet count in patients undergoing surgery gives little information to the clinician. A normal platelet count gives no indication as to the functional capacity of the platelet and therefore is of limited value within the decision-making process, especially as many patients who undergo CPB already present as, or become, thrombocytopenic.

Nonstandard Laboratory Tests

Thrombelastography/ Elastometry

TEM and Haemonetics both produce NPT devices (rotational thrombelastometry (ROTEM) and thrombelastography (TEG)) that measure the viscoelastic properties of a blood clot. It uses a simple premise – that the end result of the process of hemostasis is to create a single product (i.e., the clot) and that the physical properties of the clot (kinetics, strength, and stability) will determine whether the patient will have normal hemostasis, hemorrhage, or develop thrombosis.

The concept of coagulation analysis using the Haemoscope Thrombelastograph was first described in Germany by Professor Hartert, in the 1940s. At this time, the device had two components: the mechanism for measuring clot formation and a mirror-galvanometer recording onto light-sensitive paper. The permanent record of activity was developed on this photographic paper and was available some hours, or days, later.

This somewhat slow, if highly innovative method, no longer takes this amount of time to produce data upon which the clinician can base treatment options. The new software, which can be networked, allows results to be seen anywhere in the hospital in real time and data that is useful to the clinician can be obtained within 10–15 minutes. A rigorous quality assurance program is required to ensure the validity of these results. However, despite these advancements, the principle of producing a trace that identifies a number of variables related to functional disturbances in the hemostatic system is still key to thrombelastographic or elastometric analysis.

Coagulation Analysis: Definitions of Coagulation Parameters using the Thrombelastograph/ Elastometry

Details of normal and abnormal measurement values and suggested therapeutic algorithms for both TEG 5000 and ROTEM can be found on their respective website available at:

TEG 5000: www.haemonetics.com
ROTEM: www.rotem.de/en/

Both devices have their proponents, with TEG being used widely in the USA and UK and ROTEM being used widely in Europe.

Near-patient Testing-based Transfusion Algorithms

The first successful published NPT algorithm came from Mount Sinai Hospital. It was partly TEG-based (celite, with and without heparinase), in conjunction with platelet count and fibrinogen concentration from the laboratory [7]. According to the algorithm:

- If the R-value in the nonheparinase sample was greater than twice that found in the heparinase sample, then the patient was given supplementary protamine.
- If the platelet count was <100 000 and the maximum amplitude was <45 mm, then platelets were administered.

- Fresh frozen plasma (FFP) was given if the celite activated R-value, 10 minutes post protamine administration, was >20 mm.
- Low fibrinogen was treated with cryoprecipitate.
- Episilon-aminocaproic acid (Amicar) was given in the event of excess lysis.

Using this protocol, they showed significant reductions in the use of hemostatic products compared with their more conventional transfusion protocol.

The concept of a TEG-derived algorithm was taken a stage further at Harfield , with measurements taken during the bypass phase in order to predict the need for component products [8]. A study was conducted in 60 patients who were considered to have a higher than average risk of bleeding and thus the need for hemostatic products, but were not given aprotinin or tranexamic acid. They were randomly allocated to have products ordered and administered based on either a TEG-derived decision tree or the clinicians'

discretion after the return of conventional laboratory-based testing results.

Results for the TEG trace were available, on average, 70–90 minutes before conventional tests of coagulation, fibrinogen, and platelet count. This was considered significant in terms of logistical appropriateness. The TEG-guided group also showed a 50% reduction in the number of patients given hemostatic products, with a reduction in the use of FFP from a total of 16 to 5 U in transfused patients. The use of platelet concentrates was reduced, with only one patient receiving a single platelet pool in the TEG-guided group.

The next successful protocol was designed in Southampton (UK) with defined parameters to enable consistent use of blood and components, thus enabling trials comparing nonpharmacological and later different pharmacological agents. It incorporates both static test of coagulation (INR, APTR, platelet count, fibrinogen) and the dynamic results from a TEG (Figure 21.3) [9]. All three of the above algorithms were predominantly TEG driven.

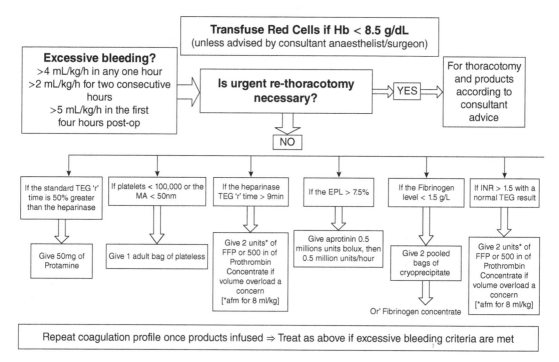

Figure 21.3 The Wessex allogenic blood transfusion protocol. FFP, fresh frozen plasma; MA, maximum amplitude; TEG, thrombelastography. *Source*: Diprose 2005 [9]. Reproduced with permission of Oxford University Press.

More recently there have been two publications looking at the use of ROTEM-driven algorithms. Gorlinger reported the successful reduction of transfusion requirements retrospectively, before and after the implementation of a complex ROTEM and multiplate based transfusion algorithm in 3865 patients [10]. This study described the replacement of FFP with prothrombin complex and fibrinogen concentrates when used in combination with a ROTEM-based algorithm, which resulted in reduced RBC transfusion, postoperative blood loss, reopenings, and adverse events.

Weber has taken this further, using a similar ROTEM and multiplate-based algorithm. In a RCT he randomized patients deemed to be suffering from microvascular bleeding after CPB but still in the operating room, to either transfusion via ROTEM algorithm or standard tests of coagulation. Those patients randomized to therapy guided by the ROTEM machine received less blood and blood products, bleed less in the ICU, and surprisingly had a lower mortality[11].

Extended Uses of ROTEM and TEG

Previously, ROTEM and TEG has been performed on whole blood in many settings, to distinguish between hemostatic and surgical causes of bleeding. Recent new reagents for both systems have allowed it to be used to assess platelet function *ex vivo* as part of the dynamic clot formation in response to certain agonists. Whilst both systems have been validated against flow cytometry and aggregometry, we have yet to see publications of their use in the cardiac surgical setting.

Aspirin and Clopidogrel

The antiplatelet agents exert their affect predominately by inhibiting arachidonic acid and ADP pathways, respectively, with aspirin inhibiting cyclo-oxygenase-mediated production of thromboxane A_2, and clopidogrel selectively inhibiting ADP-induced platelet aggregation, as well as inhibiting conformational change of platelet GPIIb/IIIa such that fibrinogen cannot bind.

It is well established that long-term use of aspirin in patients with vascular disease decreases morbidity and mortality from cardiovascular events by 25% and is a cornerstone of secondary prevention treatment in the setting of coronary artery disease. More recent studies demonstrate the efficacy of clopidogrel, particularly when given with aspirin.

Current guidelines recommend that aspirin and/or clopidogrel be stopped 5 days prior to surgery because of the excessive perioperative bleeding. However, there is marked individual variation in the degree of platelet inhibition [10].

Aspirin and Clopidogrel Resistance

Aspirin resistance is a well-recognized entity, present in 20% of patients with stable coronary artery disease. Patients resistant to aspirin are at greater risk of cardiovascular and neurological events.

Clopidogrel resistance is reported to be 11%, although in one study of patients undergoing percutaneous coronary intervention, the incidence was recorded as 40%.

Platelet Function Analysis

NPT assessment of platelet function may help rationalize the management of patients who continue to take antiplatelet drugs up to the day of surgery as well as identify aspirin or clopidogrel resistance.

Platelet mapping (using a TEG) has been validated in the cardiology setting and could be of use in the cardiac surgical setting [12, 13]. However, it is a technically challenging test to perform. Multiplate is an automated rapid test of platelet function that has been shown to user friendly in both settings [14–16].

Blood and Hemostatic Component Management: Future Development

It is well recognized that postoperative bleeding and the subsequent need for reoperation to control bleeding is associated with an increase in morbidity and mortality following cardiac surgery. Replacement therapy using red cells and plasma-based hemostatic components may themselves be contributors to the morbidity and mortality.

Clinical Indications to Reduce Exposure

The complex relationship between transfusion, mortality, and morbidity is ill defined. There is emerging evidence that blood transfusion is an independent risk factor for death after cardiac surgery. In addition, platelet transfusion is associated with an increased risk of organ dysfunction or death from uncertain causes. Immune modulation may play a role, because leukodepletion of blood may reduce mortality in the critically ill adult and neonate. Given the complexity of these issues, it would seem to be prudent to avoid transfusion unless necessary and to use simple, safe, available methods to reduce the chances of patients needing a transfusion during surgery.

Logistical Indications to Reduce Exposure

The current donor pool is known to be decreasing at 6% per annum, and may well continue to decrease. This trend is probably multifactorial; however, the ongoing public debate concerning variant Creutzfeldt–Jakob disease (vCJD) has to be considered a significant contributory element. Some estimates put the possible overall donor reduction at 50% due to the eventual inclusion of a screening test for vCJD. It remains to be seen whether this trend is capable of being reversed, even with the advent of increased public relations awareness and legislative measures introduced to lower the acceptable donor age limit.

The true role for NPT analysis for an integrated approach to hemostasis management is unknown. Information is the key to this whole process, and any technology that fails to provide relevant information because of scientific or logistical failures only serves to further exacerbate an already complex clinical management task.

Methods to reduce blood loss are:

- preoperative preparation;
- pharmacological strategies[9];
- mechanical strategies [17].

Preoperative Preparation

Anemia is increasingly recognized as a marker of poor outcome after any form of surgery regardless of transfusion. The national surgical quality improvement database from the USA reported the outcomes from 227 445 patients of whom 69 229 were anemic. Mortality increased in a stepwise manner depending upon the level of anemia from 0.78%, to 3.52%, to 10.1% for patients with no, mild, and moderate to severe anemia, respectively [18].

In the cardiac surgical population, Hung and colleagues have shown that 35% of patients presenting for elective cardiac surgery in a large UK centre were anemic and that the length of hospital stay and mortality was increased [19]. Ranucci has published data linking anemia, bleeding, and transfusions in 17 000 patients undergoing cardiac surgery [20]. Anemia was a key component in the poor outcome of patients.

With the availability of rapid, safe intravenous iron therapy, the above data highlights the importance in the identification, diagnosis, and treatment of anemic patients awaiting cardiac operations.

Pharmacological Methods

Pharmacotherapy is a component in minimizing blood loss and transfusion in cardiothoracic surgery. Nothing beats meticulous surgical technique, but some loss is inevitable. Both aprotinin and tranexamic acid are antifibrinolytic agents that have been used widely in this setting to reduce blood loss.

Aprotinin

This is a nonspecific serine protease inhibitor (inhibits plasmin at low dose, kallikrein at high dose, and inhibits activated protein C and thrombin). In addition to its antifibrinolytic properties, it may have effects on preventing platelet activation by blocking the thrombin-activated protease-activated receptor 1 (PAR1) and it appears to affect novel anti-inflammatory targets, preventing trans-migration of leukocytes.

Efficacy is dose-dependent over a wide range of surgery, and high-dose regime reduces blood requirements and perioperative bleeding by two-thirds; however, adverse events have been reported and, as a result of the BART study, its routine use is now precluded [21].

Tranexamic Acid

Tranexamic acid is a synthetically derived antifibrinolytic agent that has its effects by the prevention of the interaction between plasminogen with fibrin via interaction with lysine residues. It is has been shown to reduce blood loss and transfusion but not to the same extent as aprotinin. There is little evidence about the optimal or safe dose.

Studies Comparing Antifibrinolytic Agents

Antifibrinolytic therapy has been extensively studied in cardiac surgical patients, with three major meta-analyses favoring their use in terms of reduction of exposure to allogenic blood and in reduction in postoperative blood loss. The Cochrane Collaboration identified seven studies that compared aprotinin with tranexamic acid. This showed a nonsignificant trend to benefit in the aprotinin group. Only one of these trials reported the use of cell salvage.

In Southampton, UK, 186 patients were randomized to one of three treatment groups in addition to intraoperative cell salvage (ICS). The aprotinin treatment protocol was 2 million kallikrein inhibitor units (m kiu) at the start of surgery, 2 m kiu in the CPB prime, and 0.5 m kiu hourly; the tranexamic acid (TEA) group received 5 g of the agent in the CPB prime followed by 1.25 g/hour infusion throughout the operation (Table 21.2) [9].

Adverse effects were no different between the groups, and the conclusion drawn was that the most effective intraoperative pharmacological regime to use with ICS was aprotinin. A simplified analysis of cost based on the prices of blood

Table 21.2 Results of study comparing blood-saving properties of antifibrinolytics.

Patients	Number of patients transfused according to treatment group		
	Red blood cells	FFP	Platelets
Control (n=61)	27	32	24
TEA (n=62)	20	14	10
Aprotinin (n= 63)	8	4	3

FFP, fresh frozen plasma; TEA, tranexamic acid.

in the UK demonstrated that either of the antifibrinolytic drugs reduced the average cost per patient by approximately £150.

The large-scale Canadian trial, Blood Conservation Using Antifibrinolytics: A Randomized Trial in a Cardiac Surgery Population (BART), suspended enrollment after more patients receiving aprotinin died within the first 30 days of the trial as compared with patients taking the other antifibrinolytics, epsilon-aminocaproic acid or tranexamic acid [21]. This trial lead to the widespread suspension of the use of aprotinin with consequent increase in transfusion of patients undergoing cardiac surgery. Recently, Health Care Canada reviewed the data from this trial and have reinstated its license for use. At present there is still considerable debate about the BART study findings.

Recombinant Factor VIIa

Factor VIIa (Novoseven) is approved for the treatment of hemophilia with inhibitors. In recent years, there has been increasing interest in using factor VIIa in major hemorrhage in nonhemophilia patients.

A total of 89% of patients with complex non-coronary surgery on CPB will have an allogeneic transfusion. FVIIa has been used on a named patient basis to terminate bleeding in patients with serious hemorrhage who already have had numerous units of blood and products [22].

Karkouti designed the Toronto protocol for managing cardiac patients if there was over 2 L postoperative loss of blood or the patient received more than 4 U of red cells, had ongoing blood loss in theatre that precluded sternal closure, blood loss of >100 mL/mL/hour in ICU, or blood loss refractory to conventional therapy [23].

Of 4630 patients who underwent CPB, 655 (14%) met the criteria, and within this group 114 received at least one dose of FVIIa. The study cohort had a higher overall risk profile and more frequently underwent complex surgical procedures and longer bypass times. Those receiving <8 U of blood were classified as the early therapy group. The recorded adverse events were 24% in the untreated group, 30% in the early therapy, and 60% in the late therapy groups. However, there were many confounding effects, which, if taken into account, suggested that FVIIa may be associated with better outcomes if given early.

The conclusion was that definitive multi-center, randomized clinical trials are warranted. Similar audits have been published from Australia, Mount Sinai Hospital (New York), Illinois, and Chicago.

In the UK, Diprose and colleagues [24] describe a pilot study of 20 patients receiving complex surgery and highly likely to bleed excessively (Figure 21.4). These were randomized to receive FVIIa or placebo after CPB and reversal of hepa-

rin. Only 2 of 10 patients in the FVIIa group were exposed to allogeneic transfusion compared with eight in the placebo group (P = 0.037). In the FVIIa group, 13 U of blood or products were given compared with 103 U in the placebo group. Patients with coronary artery disease were excluded from the study. No adverse effects were found, but the cost of the drug would currently limit the use of FVIIa in this manner.

A large-scale, world-wide, multicentre trial randomized 172 patients bleeding in the ICU after cardiac surgery to either recombinant FVIIa (rFVIIa) or placebo. This showed that rFVIIa significantly reduced blood loss, transfusion requirements, and reopening rates. However, there were more critical serious adverse events in the rFVIIa group. Although this did not reach statistical significance, they were deemed to be highly clinically significant [25].

Prothrombin Complex Concentrates (PCCs)

Despotis [26] measured the relationship between hemostatic changes in platelets and clotting factors in patients on CPB (Figure 21.5). Nonbleeders had an average platelet count of over 100×10^9/L, and none of the vitamin K-dependent factors (II, VII, IX, and X) fell below 40%. Those with microvascular bleeding averaged 1 hour longer on CPB than those without microvascular bleeding, and their clotting factors were 10–30% lower.

The Wessex protocol therefore recommends measuring the INR as part of their protocol, advising the use of FFP or prothrombin complex concentrates (PCCs). PCCs are a low-volume concentration of factors II, VII, IX, and X, which is now recommended for the urgent reversal of oral anticoagulation (warfarin) and are increasingly being used as a rapid low-volume replacement of FFP in cardiac surgery [9, 10, 26].

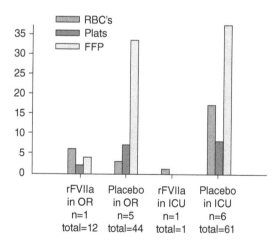

Figure 21.4 Type of product transfused. Total number of units transfused by group in the operating room (OR) and intensive care unit (ICU). FFP, fresh frozen plasma; RBC, red blood cell. *Source*: Diprose, 2005 [24]. Reproduced with permission of Oxford University Press.

Preoperative Assessment Clinics

The prescribing clinician should anticipate and plan ahead for the situation that may necessitate transfusion and aim to reduce the chance that the patient will actually need to be given blood.

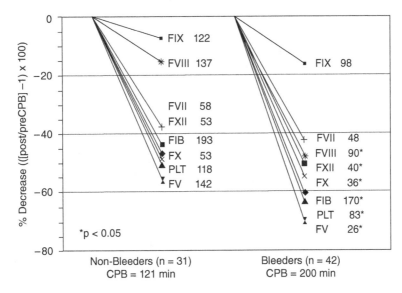

Figure 21.5 Reduction in coagulation proteins in coronary artery bypass grafting. CPB, cardiopulmonary bypass.

Assessment of patients specific to hemostasis should include:

- *Diagnosis of any bleeding disorder*: Previously undiagnosed bleeding disorders are common and can lead to greater use of donor blood if not known about prior to surgery. Consider specific questions about bleeding history in the standard presurgical assessment.
- *Assessment of patient's current medication, its potential for increasing bleeding tendency, and impact on recovery*: Commonly used drugs increase bleeding time (aspirin, NSAIDs, coumarins). Some of these drugs can be stopped prior to surgery; others may need to be continued, but the surgical team needs to be aware.
- *Identification of problems that may require specialist intervention* (immune thrombocytopenic purpura, post-transfusion purpura).
- *Patient beliefs* (e.g., Jehovah's Witnesses).

Diagnosis of a Bleeding Disorder

Although most hemostatic defects in hospitalized patients are acquired, underlying mild hereditary disorders may only manifest in the hospital setting, such as mild hemophilia A (deficient factor VIII), mild hemophilia B (deficient factor IX), and mild hemophilia C (deficient factor XI), all of which prolong the APTT. If patients are found to have hemophilia, it is essential that a hematologist advises on best treatment, which can vary from desmopressin (DDAVP) preoperatively followed by an antifibrinolytic postoperatively to the giving of regular doses of a recombinant or allogeneic replacement factors.

Assessment of Current Medication

Antiplatelet Drugs

Clopidogrel causes platelet inhibition via a different mechanism to that of aspirin, and following coronary stenting the two drugs are increasingly being prescribed together. There is growing evidence that the hemorrhagic risk is increased when the two drugs are taken concurrently. An increasing number of patients take antiplatelet agents. NSAIDs, dipyridamole, aspirin, and clopidogrel are all implicated in increased surgical blood loss. Ideally, these drugs should be stopped prior to surgery, to allow platelet function to return to normal.

The time required off the drug to ensure normal platelet function varies. NSAIDs provide reversible inhibition of cyclo-oxygenase, and their antiplatelet effects are half-life dependent (usually hours). Aspirin and clopidogrel lead to irreversible inhibition of platelet aggregation for the lifespan of the platelet (~10 days). These drugs need to be stopped for 7 days to be confident of adequate platelet function. However, due consideration must be given to the risks associated with stopping these drugs in surgical patients.

Many patients are presenting for emergency coronary revascularization having had failed coronary stenting procedures. These patients have usually received aspirin and clopidogrel. Hemorrhage during the subsequent surgery may be a major problem. Use of platelet function analyzers may be useful here, as 15% of patients have normal platelet function despite therapy, and in others the degree of dysfunction is variable.

Clopidogrel is a prodrug. The active metabolite circulates for approximately 18 hours after the last dose, and may permanently inhibit any platelets present during this time (whether endogenous or transfused). Surgery is best delayed for at least 24 hours after the last dose of clopidogrel.

Surgery in patients who have received clopidogrel in the last 7 days should, where possible, be postponed. If the surgery is a genuine emergency, platelets should be made available for transfusion, and consideration given to using aprotinin. Delaying for 24 hours after the last dose of clopidogrel will improve the response to platelet transfusion.

Warfarin

With a patient on oral anticoagulant therapy, it is sufficient to stop warfarin 3 days before surgery and restart the usual maintenance dose the evening of the surgery. If they have a mechanical heart valve or have had a venous thromboembolism in the past, this period should be covered by heparin. Having stopped warfarin, if the INR preoperatively is over 2.5, small amounts of vitamin K (1–2 mg) may be given.

References

1 Bevan DH. A review of cardiac bypass haemostasis, putting blood through the mill. *Br J Haematol* 1999; 104: 208–219.

2 Van Dijk D, Nierich AP, Jansen EWL. Early outcome after off-pump vs on pump CABG, results from a randomised study. *Circulation* 2001; 104: 1761–1766.

3 Goodenough LT, Johnston MFM, Toy PTCY, and the Medicine Academic Award Group. The variability of transfusion practice in coronary artery bypass surgery. *JAMA* 1991; 265: 86–90.

4 Stover FP, Stegel IC, Parks R, *et al.* Variability in transfusion practice for coronary artery bypass surgery persists despite national consensus guidelines: a 24-institution study. *Anesthesiology* 1998; 88: 327–333.

5 Bennett-Guerrero E, Zhao Y, O'Brien S, *et al.* Variation in use of blood transfusion in coronary artery bypass graft surgery. *JAMA* 2010; 304: 1568–1575.

6 Avidan MS, Alcock EL, Da Fonseca J, *et al.* Comparison of structured use of laboratory tests or near-patient assessment with clinical judgement in the management of bleeding after cardiac surgery. *Br J Anaesth* 2004; 92: 178–186.

7 Shore-Lesserson L, Manspeizer HE, Francis S, *et al.* Intraoperative thrombelastograph analysis (TEG r) reduces transfusion requirements. *Anesthesia Analg* 1998; 86: S104.

8 Von Kier S, Royston D. Reduced hemostatic factor transfusion using heparinase-modified thrombelastograph analysis (TEG) during cardioplumonary bypass. *Anesthesiology* 1998; 89: A911.

9 Diprose P, Herbertson MJ, O'Shaughnessy D, *et al.* A randomised double-blind placebo-controlled trial of antifibrinolytic therapies used in addition to intra-operative cell salvage. *Br J Anaesth* 2005; 94: 271–278.

10 Gorlinger K, Dirkman D, Hanke A, *et al.* First line therapy with coagulation factor concentrates cobined with Point-of-Care coagulation testing is associated with decreased allogeneic blood transfusion in cardiovascular surgery. *Anesthesiology* 2011; 115: 1179–1191.

11 Weber C, Gorlinger K, Meininger D, *et al.* Point-of-care testing. A prospective randomized clinical trial of the efficacy in

coagulopathic cardiac surgery patients. *Anesthesiology* 2012; 117; 531–547.

12 Agarwal S, Coakely M, Reddy K, *et al*. A comparison of the platelet function analyzer and modified TEG with light transmission platelet aggregometry. *Anaesthesiology* 2004; 105: 676–683.

13 Gwozdziewicz M, Nemec P, Zezula R, *et al*. Platelet mapping in postoperative management of acute aortocoronary bypass thrombosis. *Kardiochirurgia I Torakochirurgia Polska* 2006; 3: 214–216.

14 Reece MJ, Klein AA, Salviz EA, *et al*. Near-patient platelet function testing in patients undergoing coronary artery surgery: a pilot study. *Anaesthesia* 2011; 66: 97–103.

15 Velik-Salchner C, Maier S, Innerhofer P, *et al*. Point-of-care whole blood impedance aggregometry versus classical light transmission aggregometry for detecting aspirin and clopidogrel: the results of a pilot study. *Anesth Analg* 2008; 107: 1798–1806.

16 Rahe-Meyer N, Winterhalter M, Froemke C, *et al*. Platelet concentrates transfusion in cardiac surgery and platelet function assessment by multiple electrode aggregometry. *Acta Anaesthesiol Scand* 2009: 53: 168–175.

17 McGill N, O'Shaughnessy D, Pickering R, *et al*. Mechanical methods of reducing blood loss in cardiac surgery. A randomised controlled trial. *BMJ* 2002; 324: 1299.

18 Musallam K, Tamim H, Richards T, *et al*. Pre operative anaemia and postoperative outcomes in non cardiac surgery: A retrospective cohort study. *Lancet* 2011; 378: 1396–1407.

19 Hung M, Besser M, Sharples LD, *et al*. The prevalence and association with transfusion, intensive care unit stay and mortality of preoperative anaemia in a cohort of cardiac surgery patients. *Anaesthesia* 2011; 9: 812–818.

20 Ranucci M, Di Dedda U, Castelvecchio S, *et al*. Impact of preoperative anemia on outcome in adult cardiac surgery: a propensity-matched analysis. *Ann Thorac Surg* 2012; 94: 1134–1142.

21 Fergusson MHA, Hébert PC, Mazer D, *et al*. A comparison of aprotinin and lysine analogues in high-Risk cardiac surgery: the BART Study. *N Engl J Med* 2008; 358: 2319–2331.

22 Despotis G, Avidan M, Lublin DM. Off-label use of recombinant factor VIIa concentrates after cardiac surgery. *Ann Thorac Surg* 2005; 80: 3–5.

23 Karkouti K, Yau TM, Riazi S, *et al*. Determinants of complications with recombinant factor VIIa for refractory blood loss in cardiac surgery. *Can J Anaesth* 2006; 53: 802–809.

24 Diprose P, Herbertson MJ, O'Shaughnessy D, *et al*. Activated recombinant factor VII after CPB reduces al-logeneic transfusion in complex non-coronary cardiac surgery: randomised double-blind placebo-controlled pilot study. *Br J Anaesth* 2005; 95: 596–602.

25 Gill R, Herbertson M, Vuylsteke A *et al*. Safety and efficacy of recombinant activated factor VII: a randomized placebo-controlled trial in the setting of bleeding after cardiac surgery. *Circulation* 2009; 120: 21–27.

26 Despotis GJ, Joist JH, Goodenough LT. Monitoring of haemostasis in cardiac surgical patients: impact of point-of-care testing on blood loss and transfusion outcomes. *Clin Chem* 1997; 43: 1684–1696.

22

Neurology

Michael Wang, Natalie Aucutt-Walter, Valerie L. Jewells and David Y. Huang

Key Points

- Ischemic stroke can be thrombotic or embolic in etiology.
- Acute management of ischemic stroke includes evaluation by a neurovascular specialist for consideration of thrombolytic therapy with intravenous tissue plasminogen activator.
- Secondary stroke prevention for ischemic stroke typically includes antithrombotic therapy. Patients with ischemic stroke or transient ischemic attack and atrial fibrillation should be considered for anticoagulation therapy with warfarin or a novel oral anticoagulant.
- Venous sinus thrombosis (VST) occurs when there is occlusion of one or more of the dural venous sinuses.
- Magnetic resonance venography is usually diagnostic for VST and reveals thrombosis in the major venous structures.
- Acute treatment of VST is generally with intravenous heparin to an activated partial thromboplastin time of 60–80 seconds, followed by anticoagulation therapy with warfarin for 3–6 months.
- There are various conditions that can contribute to intracerebral hemorrhage (ICH), but the predominant risk factor is hypertension.
- ICH management includes control of blood pressure, seizure, infection, fever, glucose, and increased intracranial pressure.

- Hemostasis treatment using recombinant activated factor VII is not recommended for treatment of acute ICH.
- Use of anticoagulation therapy with warfarin or any of the novel oral anticoagulants can increase the risk of ICH.
- Subarachnoid hemorrhage (SAH) is often due to a ruptured aneurysm and is diagnosed by imaging and/or lumbar puncture.
- Initial management of aneurysmal SAH is focused on reducing the likelihood of rebleeding with blood pressure control and surgical or endovascular interventions to secure ruptured aneurysms.
- Vasospasm of the cerebral arteries is common after an aneurysmal SAH and can cause delayed cerebral ischemia.
- Congenital activated protein C resistance is the most common inherited risk factor for venous thrombosis.
- Antiphospholipid syndrome is an acquired hypercoagulable state that is associated with venous and arterial thrombotic events.
- Hyperhomocystinemia is associated with accelerated premature atherosclerosis. The incidence of stroke increases with increased homocysteine levels.
- Sickle cell disease is the most common cause of pediatric ischemic stroke.
- The most devastating and common neurological complication of hemophilia A is ICH.

Practical Hemostasis and Thrombosis, Third Edition. Edited by Nigel S. Key, Michael Makris and David Lillicrap.
© 2017 John Wiley & Sons, Ltd. Published 2017 by John Wiley & Sons, Ltd.

- Three novel oral anticoagulants (dabigatran etexilate, rivaroxaban, and apixaban) have been approved in many countries for primary and secondary stroke prevention in patients with atrial fibrillation. Dabigatran is a direct thrombin inhibitor, while rivaroxaban and apixaban are factor Xa inhibitors.
- The use of the novel oral anticoagulation agents increases the risk of ICH and bleeding at other sites. We outline in this chapter our institution's guidelines for the reversal or management of bleeding with these anticoagulants.

Neurological complications of hematological disease can present in many ways. Examples include seizure triggered by cerebral ischemia or hemorrhage and headache in patients with sickle cell disease. The overwhelming majority of these neurological complications are vascular in nature, owing to the fact that most hematological abnormalities lead to either thrombosis in the cerebral vasculature or brain hemorrhage. Associated cerebrovascular events include both ischemic and hemorrhagic strokes, as well as cerebral venous sinus thromboses.

Ischemic Stroke

Ischemic stroke can be divided into two broad categories: embolic and thrombotic. Classically, acute embolic stroke is associated with sudden onset of a maximal neurological deficit. Emboli typically arise from the heart or from ulcerated and/or fatty unstable carotid or aortic plaques. Atrial fibrillation predisposes patients to formation of cardiac thrombi and is associated with a sixfold increased risk for stroke [1]. Cardiac emboli are highly correlated with large vessel ischemia. Warfarin is strongly recommended for stroke prevention in the presence of atrial fibrillation unless otherwise contraindicated [2].

Thrombotic infarction, including lacunar infarction, is the result of progressive occlusive disease of the cerebral vasculature. Predisposing factors for thrombotic strokes include hypertension, diabetes, hypercholesterolemia with atherosclerotic disease, and tobacco abuse. Such infarcts are often preceded by transient ischemic attacks (TIAs) and may progress over hours or days in a stuttering fashion. TIAs are often seen with carotid stenosis, often present with border zone or "watershed" ischemic injury distal to the area of critical stenosis, and are commonly due to friable plaques that result in distal occlusive infarction. Plaques most likely to result in TIAs have a large plaque burden, small lumen area, and/or a thin fibroatheromatous cap [3]. Up to 33% of patients who experience a TIA will develop a disabling stroke within 5 years, with the incidence of stroke after TIA being 10–20% in the first 12 months and 5% each year thereafter [1]. Small infarcts, often referred to as lacunar infarcts, are most often associated with small vessel occlusive disease. Typically, these lacunes are deep ischemic lesions <10 mm in diameter and account for between 10% and 25% of all ischemic strokes [1]. The pathophysiology of small vessel disease is thought to be multifactorial and includes small vessel lipohyalinosis and fibrinoid degeneration, decreased perfusion of the penetrating arteries, and atheromatous occlusion or embolism. Predisposing risk factors include hypertension, diabetes, hypercholesterolemia with atherosclerotic disease, and tobacco abuse.

Acute management of suspected ischemic stroke involves rapid assessment of the patient's presenting symptoms by a neurovascular specialist or at the nearest emergency department. Patients who present <3 hours from symptom onset may be candidates for thrombolytic therapy with intravenous recombinant tissue plasminogen activator (IV-tPA). Prior to administering IV-tPA, the patient should have noncontrast head CT to rule out intracerebral hemorrhage and determine that the stroke involves less than one-third of the middle cerebral artery (MCA) territory, as well as laboratory tests, including coagulation studies, complete blood count (CBC), and serum glucose. Contraindications and guidelines for IV-tPA administration are widely published and should be reviewed carefully prior to administering the drug [4]. Treatment is associated with a 6% risk of bleeding complications, including intracranial hemorrhage, and patients and/or their families should be counseled about the benefits and risks associated with thrombolytic therapy. In addition, the ECASS-3 trial demonstrated that IV-tPA administered between 3 and 4.5 hours after onset of symptoms significantly improved clinical outcomes in a subset of patients with acute ischemic stroke [5]. Other acute treatments, including intra-arterial thrombolytic therapy and mechanical endovascular clot retrieval using aspiration or evacuation devices, are limited to centers with experienced interventionalists. Currently, there exists some debate with regards to whether thrombectomy improves clinical outcomes.

Beyond the acute interventions, general management of ischemic stroke concentrates on rehabilitation, prevention of complications (e.g., falls, aspiration risk, etc.), and secondary stroke prevention. All patients presenting with stroke or TIA symptoms should undergo a complete stroke evaluation to identify stroke etiology and risk factors. Guidelines for the early management of patients with ischemic stroke were published by the American Stroke Association in 2013 [4]. Patients with ischemic stroke or TIA should be started on an antithrombotic agent. For patients with stroke or TIA and atrial fibrillation, anticoagulation with warfarin or a novel oral anticoagulant should be considered for stroke prevention. We will discuss the new oral anticoagulation drugs in broader depth under the novel anticoagulant agent section of this chapter.

Venous Sinus Thrombosis

Venous sinus thrombosis (VST) describes occlusion of one or more of the dural venous sinuses that drain the brain. VST may present as gradual onset of severe headache. Other presenting symptoms include seizure, somnolence, and cranial nerve palsies. Less frequently, VST may present with gradual neurological deficits when secondary venous infarcts or subarachnoid hemorrhage (SAH) develop. SAH is usually in the region of thrombosed cortical veins, and typically is seen over the cerebral convexities [6]. In one series of 154 cases of VST, the transverse sinus was the most common site of thrombosis followed by the sagittal and sigmoid sinuses. Nearly half of the patients in this series had involvement of multiple sinuses [7]. Additionally, in our practice we see a large percentage of focal cortical vein thrombosis leading to neurological findings including infarction. These thromboses can extend to the major venous sinuses, but if treated promptly can have a good prognosis [8].

Magnetic resonance venography (MRV) is usually diagnostic for VST and readily reveals thrombosis in the major venous structures, including the superior (Figure 22.1), transverse, and sigmoid sinuses as well as the veins of Labbe and Trolard and smaller cortical veins. Asymmetry of the transverse and sigmoid sinuses is frequently encountered and, most commonly, the left sinuses are smaller, but a

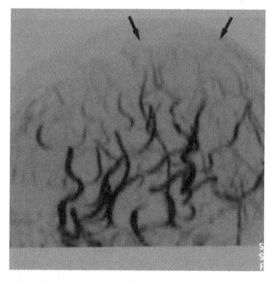

Figure 22.1 A sagittal three-dimensional time-of-flight magnetic resonance venography was obtained in this patient presenting with headache and altered mental status. The superior sagittal sinus is absent due to thrombosis (arrows).

difference of 3 mm or greater would be abnormal [9]. Susceptibility weighted imaging (SWI) has improved the ability to see smaller venous thrombi in the sinuses/cortical veins [10]. Thrombosis of the deep venous system (internal cerebral veins, straight sinus, and vein of Galen) can also be seen. Thrombosis of the deep venous structures typically results in thalamic infarcts. Head CT demonstrates up to 70% of lesions within 7 days, but MRV and SWI are more sensitive in the acute setting, allowing for appropriate therapy initiation. Venous phase angiography is considered the gold standard for diagnosis and will show a contrast filling defect; however, this procedure is seldom performed with the greater availability of MRV/ SWI. Etiologies of VST include:

- trauma,
- infection,
- pregnancy/postpartum period,
- oral contraceptives,
- volume depletion,
- dehydration,
- hyperosmolar states,
- hematological disorders (myeloproliferative, sickle cell disease, disseminated intravascular coagulation, hypercoagulable states),
- carcinoma,
- congestive heart disease,
- chemotherapy,
- mastoiditis,
- systemic lupus erythematosus (SLE).

Acute treatment is generally with intravenous heparin to an activated partial thromboplastin time of 60–80 seconds. This is followed by warfarin therapy for 3–6 months. Anticoagulation with warfarin has been shown to be safe even in patients with secondary intracerebral hemorrhage. The novel oral anticoagulation agents have not been studied in this population of patients, but may be considered for patients who cannot tolerate warfarin therapy. Good results from catheter-infused thrombolytic therapy at the site of thrombosis have been reported in many small series. Catheter-based intravenous thrombolysis is generally reserved for those patients who progress while on intravenous heparin, as the risk of hemorrhagic complications increases with intervention [11]. Such interventions can be used even during pregnancy [12]. Patients who have seizures as a complication of VST should be treated with an anticonvulsant. However, prophylaxis with anticonvulsants in the absence of seizures is not a common practice.

Long-term prognosis of VST is good. In a prospective series of 624 patients followed for 16 months, 80% had minor or no residual deficits, and approximately 10.5% resulted in severe morbidity or mortality [13]. Multivariate predictors of death or dependence were:

- age >37 years,
- male sex,
- coma,
- mental status disorder,
- hemorrhage on admission CT scan,
- thrombosis of the deep cerebral venous system,
- central nervous system infection,
- cancer [13].

Intracerebral Hemorrhage

Intracerebral hemorrhage (ICH) into the brain parenchyma accounts for 10% of all strokes and the majority of hemorrhagic strokes. ICH is typically of sudden onset with a smooth progression of symptoms. Unlike ischemic stroke, patients seldom awaken with symptoms. Nearly 40% of all cases are associated with severe headache, and 50% of patients have a change in mental status. Nausea and vomiting are common. The differential diagnosis for ICH includes:

- amyloid angiopathy (Figure 22.2a,b),
- anticoagulation or bleeding diatheses,
- thrombolysis,
- sympathomimetic drugs,
- vascular malformations,
- brain tumor or metastasis,
- vasculitis,
- venous thrombosis.

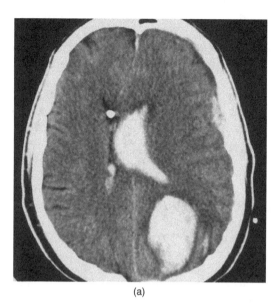

(a)

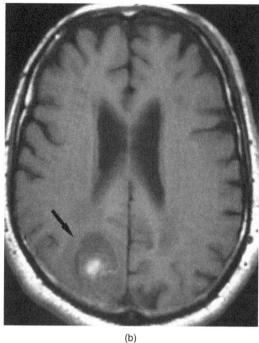

(b)

Figure 22.2 (a) This axial computed tomography image demonstrates a large left parietal–occipital parenchymal hemorrhage in a patient with amyloid angiopathy, which extended into the left lateral ventricle and resulted in the patient's death. (b) An axial T1 noncontrasted image in another patient with amyloid angiopathy demonstrates a mirror image parenchymal hemorrhage with surrounding vasogenic edema (arrow).

Hypertension is the predominant risk factor. Location of ICH in order of frequency is as follows:

- putaminal or basal ganglia (35–50%),
- subcortical white matter (30%),
- cerebellar (15%),
- thalamic (10–15%),
- pontine (5–12%).

The duration of bleeding is usually minutes to hours, although hematoma expansion can continue for up to 24 hours. Use of warfarin or other anticoagulants may increase the time window for hematoma expansion. Clinical deterioration after 24 hours is usually due to secondary ischemia and hemorrhage-induced edema rather than recurrent bleeding. Mortality rates are as high as 30–40% in the first 30 days, with more than half of these deaths occurring within the first 48

hours. Independent predictors of poor prognosis include:

- low Glasgow Coma Scale (GCS),
- depressed level of consciousness,
- age >75,
- bleed volume >30 mL,
- intraventricular hemorrhage,
- concurrent antiplatelet therapy,
- hyperglycemia,
- infratentorial location.

Diagnosis of ICH is often made by emergent head CT. MRI FLAIR, GRE/T2* and SWI are more sensitive for hemorrhage detection but require more time for image acquisition. In addition, GRE T2* and SWI imaging may help identify the numerous microhemorrhages typically seen with amyloidosis and therefore aid diagnosis [14]. CTA/CTV and/or MRA/MRV may also be helpful for identification of an underlying vascular malformation, aneurysm, angioma, tumor, cavernoma, or deep venous anomaly such as a cavernoma. If these studies are negative, angiography may be necessary to evaluate for these etiologies. In addition, SWI may assist in the identification of these lesions, and if initial imaging is unrevealing, it should be repeated in 3–4 months when the intraparenchymal blood has cleared.

Guidelines for the management of ICH were published in *Stroke* in 2010 [15]. ICH management includes control of blood pressure, seizure, infection, fever, glucose, and increased intracranial pressure (ICP). Aggressive blood pressure management remains controversial, and blood pressure guidelines vary. In general, patients are at increased risk for rebleeding and hematoma enlargement with systolic blood pressures >160 mmHg [16]. However, blood pressure reduction should be balanced with the risk of concurrent ischemia, as blood pressures that are dramatically lower than the patient's baseline can lead to decreased cerebral perfusion pressure (CPP). This is of particular concern in patients with a large ICH, cerebral edema, or other factors that increase ICP [16]. When ICP is elevated (>20 mmHg), blood pressure should be titrated to maintain a CPP of 50–70 mmHg (CPP = mean arterial pressure – ICP). In the acute setting, pressures can be lowered with short-acting agents, such as intravenous labetalol or nicardipine, which allow for rapid titration. However, it is worth noting that the INTERACT2 trial demonstrated that intensive lowering of blood pressure within 6 hours of spontaneous ICH onset did not result in a significant reduction in the rate of the primary outcome of death or severe disability [17].

When monitoring and treating increased ICP following ICH, intraventricular pressure monitors should be placed in patients with a GCS <9 or with clinical deterioration in their neurological exam [16]. Approaches such as head-of-bed elevation and head positioning are simple and often effective for quickly lowering ICP. Other interventions should be limited to

situations where herniation is of immediate concern. Patients with significant mass effect from bleeding or intraventricular extension are at risk for obstructive hydrocephalus, and ventricular drain placement may be necessary. Hyperventilation to keep the $P\text{CO}_2$ between 28 and 30 torr is effective to reduce increased ICP, with peak effect within 30 minutes. However, the effect is transient and only lasts until the pH of cerebrospinal fluid equilibrates with systemic pH, usually within a few hours [18]. Osmotic agents such as mannitol and hypertonic saline may be used for short periods, but use for more than a few days can lead to rebound increases in ICP. Steroids should be avoided as they have not been shown to be effective.

There are few indications for surgical intervention in ICH. Indications for surgical intervention are generally limited to patients with:

- cerebellar hemorrhage >3 cm in size and brainstem compression,
- herniation,
- acute hydrocephalus,
- neurological deterioration.

Patients with lobar clots within 1 cm of the cortex may also be considered for surgical resection based on a trend toward a positive effect of surgery over medical management for such patients in the International Surgical Trial for Intracerebral Hemorrhage (STICH) [19].

Hemostasis treatment using recombinant activated factor VII (rFVIIa) for ICH has been investigated in a phase 3 trial [20]. Compared with placebo, treatment with rFVIIa at 20 and 80 µg reduced hematoma growth but did not improve functional outcome. In addition, 80 µg of rFVIIa was associated with a nonsignificant but increased frequency of adverse arterial thromboembolic events compared with placebo. Therefore, rFVIIa is not currently recommended for treatment of acute ICH.

Use of warfarin for anticoagulation to INR 2.5–4.5 increases the risk of ICH by up to 10-fold and doubles the mortality. Patients with ICH who are anticoagulated with warfarin should have their INR corrected as quickly as possible with prothrombin complex concentrate (PCC) or rFVIIa. Intravenous vitamin K should be administered without delay, because peak effect is dependent on protein synthesis, approximately 6–8 hours later. Although fresh frozen plasma (FFP) is commonly used, large volumes need to be given and only partial correction is observed.

Patients on the novel oral anticoagulants are at increased risk of ICH. Currently, there are no specific reversal agents or pharmacological antidotes for the novel anticoagulant agents. Our institution has developed a set of guidelines for the reversal or management of bleeding with these anticoagulants; these guidelines are outlined in the novel anticoagulant agent section of this chapter.

Subarachnoid Hemorrhage

Subarachnoid hemorrhage (SAH) is often the result of a ruptured saccular aneurysm but may also arise from head trauma, extension of ICH into the subarachnoid space, spinal arteriovenous malformation, or idiopathic causes. Aneurysmal ruptures account for 80% of all nontraumatic SAHs and are of greatest concern, given a high mortality rate of approximately 45%. Presenting symptoms include a sudden and severe "thunder clap" headache, with an acute change in mental status, in some cases leading to lethargy and coma. Sudden loss of consciousness occurs in up to 20% of patients. Meningeal signs, papilledema, and seizure are common at presentation. Increased size of the bleed and the presence of intraventricular extension are correlated with increased mortality. Head CT is often diagnostic of SAH, but up to 15% of cases of aneurysmal SAH will have a normal study. MRI with FLAIR/SWI has been shown to be 6.2–7.5% more sensitive than head CT [21] in one study while the use of SWI detected 10% more SAH in another study by Wu *et al.* [22]. Additionally, if imaging is normal but the suspicion for SAH is high, an emergent lumbar puncture should be performed to evaluate for blood or xanthrochromia in the spinal fluid, which is indicative of a sentinel bleed. Patients with sentinel bleeds have a >50% risk of rebleeding in the next 48–72 hours.

Initial management of aneurysmal SAH is focused on reducing the likelihood of rebleeding. Between the time of SAH symptom onset and aneurysm obliteration, blood pressure should be controlled with a titratable agent to balance the risk of stroke, hypertension-related rebleeding, and maintenance of cerebral perfusion pressure. The magnitude of blood pressure control to reduce the risk of rebleeding has not been established, but there is general agreement that a decrease in systolic blood pressure to <160 mmHg is reasonable. Short-term (<72 hours) therapy with antifibrinolytic agents such as aminocaproic acid and tranexamic acid has been shown to decrease the incidence of rebleeding when there is a delay in securing the aneurysm. However, the potential benefits of antifibrinolytic therapy need to be weighed against the potential of increased risk for ischemic stroke. Surgical or endovascular interventions to secure ruptured aneurysms should be performed once patients are stabilized.

Vasospasm of the cerebral arteries is common after an aneurysmal SAH, occurring most frequently 7–10 days after aneurysm rupture and resolving after 21 days. Patients are at increased risk for ischemic stroke from vasospasm and should receive nimodipine, which reduces long-term injury from vasospasm. Maintenance of euvolemia and normal circulating blood volume is also recommended to prevent delayed cerebral ischemia. Patients with extensive bleeding or intraventricular extension may develop obstructive hydrocephalus, and cerebrospinal fluid diversion with a ventricular drain may be necessary to treat elevated ICP. The use of prophylactic anticonvulsants may be considered in the immediate posthemorrhagic period, but routine long-term use of anticonvulsants is not recommended unless the patient has known risk factors for delayed seizure disorder (e.g., prior seizure history) [23].

Diseases Associated with Ischemic Strokes

Hereditary and Acquired HypercoagulableSstates

A number of diseases have been implicated in the development of ischemic stroke. Table 22.1 lists a variety of hypercoagulable states and the strength of their correlation with stroke. Notably, sickle cell disease, antiphospholipid antibody syndrome, and hyperhomocystine-mia have the strongest association with arterial stroke.

Activated Protein C Resistance/ Factor V Leiden

Congenital activated protein C resistance (APC-R) is the most common inherited risk factor for venous thrombosis. A total of 95% of patients with APC-R have the factor V Leiden mutation. The mutation is present in 2–7% of the Caucasian population [24].

With respect to neurological complications, APC-R correlates almost exclusively with venous thrombosis, with only a few reported cases of arterial strokes in young patients. Symptoms of acute cerebral venous thrombosis include headache, seizure, somnolence, and cranial nerve palsies. Patients with suspected venous thrombosis should have neurological imaging with MRI/MRA and MRV. SAH can result from the rupture of congested cerebral veins. If cranial nerve palsies are present on examination (i.e., defects of cranial nerves III, IV, and VI associated with ptosis and facial pain), cavernous sinus thrombosis should be suspected. Treatment for stroke patients with cerebral venous thrombosis is low-molecular-weight heparin or warfarin.

Antiphospholipid Antibody Syndrome

Antiphospholipid syndrome (APS) is an acquired hypercoagulable state that is associated with venous as well as arterial thrombotic events. Arterial events occur most commonly in the cerebrovasculature. Stroke or TIA is the initial clinical manifestation in approximately 20% of patients subsequently diagnosed with APS. Involvement of the cerebral cortex and subadjacent white matter by platelet-fibrin microthrombi is most common [25]. The pathogenesis of thrombosis in APS is uncertain (see Chapter 19).

Antiphospholipid antibodies are found in >10% of patients with acute ischemic stroke, and the vast majority of patients are young (<50 years) [24]. APS should be considered in the work-up of all young patients presenting with an ischemic arterial or venous stroke secondary to thrombosis. APS is suspected in patients with a history of multiple miscarriages, dementia, optic neuropathy, thrombocytopenia, SLE or SLE-like syndromes, or complicated migraine.

Table 22.1 Strength of association of coagulopathy with arterial stroke.

Coagulopathy	Arterial stroke risk
Sickle cell disease	Strong
Antiphospholipid antibody syndrome	Strong
Hyperhomocystinemia	Moderate
Activated protein C resistance	Mild
Prothrombin gene mutation	Mild
Protein S deficiency	Mild
Protein C deficiency	Rare
Antithrombin III deficiency	Rare

Source: modified from Moster et al., 2003 [24].

Testing for APS includes evaluation for IgG antiphospholipids on two separate occasions at least 12 weeks apart. Stroke risk is greatest with IgG antiphospholipids >40 GPL units and may not be clinically significant at lower levels [26]. Treatment is generally with warfarin to prevent recurrent systemic thrombosis. However, in patients with prior stroke and a single positive test result for antiphospholipid antibodies, aspirin (325 mg/day) appears to be as effective as moderate-intensity warfarin (INR 1.4–2.8) for preventing recurrent stroke [25].

Hyperhomocystinemia

Hyperhomocystinemia has a prevalence of 5–10% in the general population and is associated with accelerated premature atherosclerosis. Increased fasting levels of homocysteine have been related to the prevalence of extracranial common carotid artery stenosis of >25% in the Framingham cohort. Fasting homocysteine levels above 15.4 µmol/L significantly increase the patient's risk for stroke, with an odds ratio of 2.5–4.7. Elevated levels increase the odds of carotid intimal thickening more than threefold. Proposed mechanisms of coagulopathy include increased platelet adhesion, activation of the coagulation cascade, conversion of LDL to a proatherogenic form, and endothelial damage.

Most often, hyperhomocystinemia is acquired due to a diet deficient in folate, vitamin B_6, and/or B_{12}. Folate and B_{12} levels should be checked in all patients, especially young patients with unexplained stroke and premature atherosclerosis [27]. Treatment includes vitamin supplementation with folic acid, B_6, and B_{12}. Elevated levels of homocysteine can also be seen with renal insufficiency and concurrent antiepileptic drug use, especially phenytoin.

Hyperhomocystinemia needs to be distinguished from autosomal recessive homocystinuria. Patients who are homozygous for cystathionine beta synthase deficiency can have homocystine concentrations up to 400 µmol/L and present with a marfanoid body habitus, mental retardation, seizure, lenticular dislocations, skeletal abnormalities, and a 20-fold increase in urinary homocysteine excretion over other amino acids [24]. These patients are at high risk for myocardial infarction and ischemic stroke as well as premature death secondary to vascular disease. The incidence of stroke increases with increased homocysteine levels, and heterozygous patients have a milder course and clinical picture.

Sickle Cell Disease

Children with sickle cell disease (SCD) present with a wide variety of chronic neurological syndromes, including:

- ischemic and hemorrhagic stroke,
- dural VST,
- spinal cord infarction,
- transient ischemic attack,
- headache,
- seizure,
- altered mental status,
- cognitive difficulties,
- covert "silent" infarction.

Up to 25% of children with HbSS will have covert or "silent" infarction by adolescence. Silent ischemia can be detected with diffusion-weighted MRI, which reveals ischemic regions, characteristically in the anterior or posterior watershed/border zones. One study enrolled and followed the neuroimaging of 213 HbSS children without a history of overt stroke. In this group, 160 children had normal baseline MRIs and 53 children had MRIs showing silent infarcts. The patients were followed with serial MRIs, and the children with silent infarcts at baseline were significantly more likely to demonstrate new or progressive neurologically silent lesions compared with those whose baseline MRIs were normal. Only 2.5% children with normal baseline MRIs developed silent infarcts on follow-up MRI examination compared with 24.5% who had a baseline silent infarct [28]. These patients may have a normal T2-weighted MRI and a normal neurological examination. Seizure is common in patients with known cerebrovascular disease as well as in patients with covert infarction and should be treated with antiepileptic drug therapy as primary prevention. Interestingly, silent infarction is less common in patients with frequent sickle cell pain and more common in patients with a history of seizure [29].

SCD is the most common cause of pediatric ischemic stroke. The incidence of clinical stroke (i.e., a focal neurological deficit lasting >24 hours) is 250 times more common in a child with SCD than in the general pediatric population [30]. The peak incidence occurs between 2 and 5 years of age [31]. In the longitudinal Cooperative Study of Sickle Cell Disease, 25% of patients with HbSS and 10% of patients with HbSC disease had a stroke by the age of 45 years [30]. This study found that the risk of first ischemic stroke was increased by previous transient ischemic attacks, lower steady-state hemoglobin, previous acute chest syndrome, and systolic hypertension [32]. Neurological deficits are seen most often in the setting of acute infection triggering a sickle cell crisis, but it is not uncommon for overt stroke symptoms to present "out of the blue" in an otherwise well child. High white cell count, low hemoglobin, and oxyhemoglobin desaturation predict neurological complications. Ischemic stroke is often associated with stenosis or occlusion of moderate size vessels (i.e., distal internal carotid or proximal middle cerebral arteries). Sickle cell disease causes a vasculopathy in small arteries, "plugging of the microcirculation" with a resultant progressive segmental narrowing of medium size vessels in the cerebrovasculature (Figure 22.3), leading to occlusion, disease, and eventually the classic "moya moya" appearance on angiography.

In patients presenting with clinical signs of stroke, infarcts in the MCA territory, basal ganglia, or deep white matter usually predict proximal arterial stenosis or occlusion. Infarcts in the parietal–occipital lobes or thalamus associated with complaints of headache often predict VST. SAH and ICH may occur in the setting of acute hypertension or VST [30]. VST often goes undiagnosed, and whenever a sickle cell patient has moderate to severe headache, MRV or CT venography should be performed in addition to conventional neuroimaging.

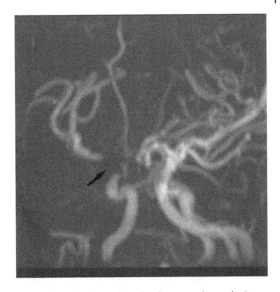

Figure 22.3 Sickle cell can lead to vascular occlusion as seen in this sickle cell patient who has total or near total occlusion of the right supraclinoid internal carotid artery, and M1 segment of the middle cerebral artery with possible reconstitution via the middle meningeal artery. This disease can progress further to a "moya moya" pattern and strokes without transfusion therapy.

Exchange transfusions to keep HbSS <30% are recommended along with adequate hydration, oxygenation, and blood pressure control. Transcranial Doppler (TCD) is a useful screening tool to follow cerebral blood flow in the internal carotid or MCA. TCD velocities over 200 cm/second are associated with a 40% increased stroke risk over the next 3 years [33]. The Stroke Prevention in Sickle Cell Disease Study demonstrated that regular exchange transfusion therapy in patients with transcranial Doppler velocities >200 cm/second led to a 90% reduction in the incidence of stroke for the duration of the study [34]. Unfortunately, widespread patient access to TCD has been limited by both geographical and economic factors. The development of TCD screening programs is patchy in the United States and Europe with only a minority of patients (45% of children ages 2–12 with SCD or thalassemia) being screened annually, primarily due to barriers to care such as long travel distances to the nearest vascular laboratory [35]. Identifying children early on in the disease process and selecting for those who have potential for increased TCD velocities would allow them to be prioritized for routine TCD monitoring, exchange transfusion, and neuroimaging. Rees and colleagues developed a simple index using age and routine blood work (hemoglobin and aspartate transaminase) in order to predict which children are likely to have TCD readings >170 cm/second, placing them at higher risk of developing cerebrovascular disease and resultant ischemic infarcts. This index has been shown to have 100% sensitivity and between 60% and 70% specificity for predicting increased arterial velocities [32].

In addition to the standard therapies (exchange transfusions, hydroxyurea, and blood pressure management), antiplatelet therapy with aspirin has been shown to reduce ischemic stroke risk, as well as prevent silent ischemia and cognitive impairment. A pilot trial using aspirin therapy in sickle cell patients is underway. In the meantime, aspirin therapy should be used with caution in patients with a history of large territory ischemic stroke, subdural, or SAH because of the unknown risk of hemorrhage [1].

Diseases Associated with Hemorrhagic Strokes

Hemophilia A

The most devastating and common neurological complication of hemophilia A is ICH. The incidence of ICH in the general population is around 2%. In contrast, the incidence of ICH in patients with hemophilia A can be as high as 12%. ICH can occur spontaneously or as a result of a minor/ trivial trauma. A review of 170 patients with hemophilia A documented 42 episodes of ICH or spinal hemorrhage in 32 patients. Of those patients presenting with ICH or spinal hemorrhage, 36% were associated with a minor or obvious head trauma, whereas 64% occurred spontaneously. All of the patients presenting with an acute bleed where known to have severe hemophilia A, and nine of the 32 patients (17.6%) presented with recurrent ICH [36].

Sudden onset of headache is the most common presenting symptom of ICH (97.5%) [36]. Other associated symptoms, including nausea, vomiting, and progressive neurological deterioration, are strongly suggestive of intraparenchymal brain hemorrhage and warrant immediate neurological imaging with a CT of the head to assess for intra- or extraparenchymal blood. Patients with brain herniation at presentation have the worst prognosis, as concurrent herniation is near 100% fatal.

Acquired hemophilia A is a rare bleeding disorder caused by the development of autoantibodies that inhibit the action of naturally occurring factor VIII. Patients classically present with prominent extensive subcutaneous hematomas. Unlike classic hemophilia, ICH and hemarthroses are rare with hemophilia A.

In addition to standard management of ICH, treatment of bleeding in a patient with hemophilia consists of administration of coagulation factor concentrates in order to correct the deficiency. If factor VIII concentrate is not available, one should not wait for concentrate but should begin treatment with cryoprecipitate, each unit of which generally contains 80–100 IU of factor VIII, or FFP, which contains all clotting factors.

Novel Anticoagulant Agents

Three novel oral anticoagulants (dabigatran etexilate, rivaroxaban, and apixaban) have been approved in many countries for primary and secondary stroke prevention in atrial fibrillation. The large phase III clinical trials comparing these new agents with warfarin have found that the novel anticoagulants are associated with similar or lower rates of stroke and bleeding risk (particularly intracranial hemorrhage) compared with warfarin. In addition, these agents have the advantage of being administered in fixed doses without routine coagulation monitoring, unlike warfarin. There are no direct comparative studies to date, and the three trials looking at patients with nonvalvular atrial fibrillation are not directly comparable due to differences in study design and patient population enrolled.

Direct Thrombin Inhibitors

Dabigatran is a direct, competitive inhibitor of thrombin. In the RE-LY trial, dabigatran 150 mg twice daily was associated with lower rates of stroke and systemic embolism in patients with atrial fibrillation and risk of stroke compared to warfarin [37]. The usual dosing of this drug in stroke prevention is 150 mg twice daily, though for patients with an impaired creatinine clearance of 15–30 mL/min, the recommended renal-adjusted dose is 75 mg twice daily.

Factor Xa Inhibitors

A number of direct oral factor Xa inhibitors are in development, but thus far only rivaroxaban and apixaban have been licensed for thromboprophylaxis and/or treatment of venous thromboembolism and stroke prevention in atrial fibrillation. The ROCKET-AF trial, which compared rivaroxaban 20 mg once daily with dose-adjusted warfarin in patients with nonvalvular atrial fibrillation and increased risk of stroke, found that rivaroxaban was noninferior to warfarin for the prevention of stroke or systemic embolism. There was no significant between-group difference in the risk of major bleeding, although intracranial and fatal bleeding occurred less frequently in the rivaroxaban group [38].

There have been two clinical trials comparing apixaban with warfarin (ARISTOTLE) and aspirin (AVERROES) for prevention of stroke and other major vascular events in patients with atrial fibrillation. The ARISTOTLE study determined that apixaban 5 mg twice daily was superior to dose-adjusted warfarin (INR 2–3) in preventing stroke or systemic embolism in patients with atrial fibrillation and at least one additional risk factor for stroke [39]. Similarly, the AVERROES study, a double-blind trial comparing apixaban with aspirin for patients with atrial fibrillation who were at increased risk for stroke and for whom vitamin K antagonist therapy was unsuitable, found that apixaban 5 mg twice daily reduced the risk of stroke or systemic embolism without significantly increasing the risk of major bleeding or intracranial hemorrhage [40].

Reversal of Agents

As with warfarin, the use of the novel anticoagulants increases the risk of ICH and bleeding at other sites. However, there are no specific reversal agents or pharmacological antidotes for the novel anticoagulant agents. Thus, management of hemorrhagic complications is primarily supportive. At our institution, guidelines for the reversal or management of bleeding with these anticoagulants have been developed with the input from members of the pharmacy, hematology, and emergency departments. Management of dabigatran-related and factor Xa inhibitor-related bleeding events are summarized below.

For mild bleeding events on dabigatran, it is recommended that the next dose of dabigatran be delayed or discontinued. For moderate bleeding events, supportive care (e.g., symptomatic treatment, mechanical compression, surgical intervention, fluid replacement and hemodynamic support, or blood transfusion) should be considered. If the previous dose of dabigatran was ingested within 2 hours, oral activated charcoal dosed at 1 g/kg (max dose 50 g) can be administered. If hemostasis is not achieved with the aforementioned strategies, administration of 2–4 units of FFP should be considered, along with a hematology/coagulation consult for further recommendations.

When patients present with severe or life-threatening hemorrhagic complications on dabigatran, all of the strategies outlined above should be considered. In addition, nonactivated PCC at 50 units/kg can be given. For refractory bleeding, several treatment options may be considered. Activated prothrombin complex concentrate (aPCC) at 50 units/kg can be administered. Recombinant factor VIIa dosed at 45 µg/kg can be administered intravenously; after several hours, additional doses of 45–90 µg/kg of recombinant factor VIIa may be considered based on bleeding severity and degree of hemostasis achieved. Antifibrinolytic therapy (e.g., tranexamic acid, aminocaproic acid) may be considered to promote hemostasis. Fresh frozen plasma can also be given. A hematology/coagulation consult should be obtained after administration of any of these agents. In the setting of acute renal failure, initiation of hemodialysis may be considered, as hemodialysis is effective at removing approximately 60% of dabigatran.

It should be noted that, unlike dabigatran, rivaroxaban and apixaban are highly protein bound and thus are not dialyzable. Patients with mild bleeding events on apixaban or rivaroxaban should delay or discontinue the next dose of factor Xa inhibitor. For moderate bleeding events, supportive care (e.g., symptomatic treatment, mechanical compression, surgical intervention, fluid replacement and hemodynamic support, or blood transfusion) should be considered. Oral activated charcoal with sorbitol dosed at 50 g can be administered if the previous dose of apixaban or rivaroxaban was ingested within 2 hours.

With regards to management of severe or life-threatening hemorrhagic complications from factor Xa inhibitors, all of the strategies outlined above should be considered. No agent currently available in the United States has been shown to successfully reverse the anticoagulant effects of factor Xa inhibitor-related bleeding events. However, currently available evidence in animal models and healthy volunteers [41] suggests that pharmacological intervention with PCC and recombinant factor VIIa may be considered for severe or life-threatening bleeding. At our institution, we first consider administering nonactivated PCC at 50 units/kg. If adequate hemostasis is not achieved with this strategy, administration of intravenous recombinant factor VIIa dosed at 45–90 µg/kg can be considered. After several hours, treatment with aPCC at 50 units/kg can be considered based on bleeding severity and degree of hemostasis achieved. A hematology/coagulation consult should be obtained with administration of any of these agents.

References

1 Zaidat OO, Lerner AJ. *The Little Black Book of Neurology*, 4th edn. St. Louis: Mosby, 2002.

2 EAFT (European Atrial Fibrillation Trial) Study Group. Secondary prevention in non-rheumatic atrial fibrillation after transient ischaemic attack or minor stroke. *Lancet* 1993; 342: 1255–1262.

3 Fleg JL, Stone GW, Fayad ZA, *et al.* Detection of high-risk atherosclerotic plaque: report of the NHLBI Working Group on current status and future directions. *JACC Cardiovasc Imaging* 2012; 5: 941–955.

4 Jauch EC, Saver JL, Adams HP Jr., *et al.* Guidelines for the early management of patients with acute ischemic stroke. *Stroke* 2013; 44: 870–947.

5 Hacke W, Kaste M, Bluhmki E, *et al.* Thrombolysis with alteplase 3 to 4.5 hours after acute ischemic stroke. *N Engl J Med* 2008; 359: 1317–1329.

6 Verma R, Sahu R, Lalla R. Subarachnoid haemorrhage as the initial manifestation of cortical venous thrombosis. *BMJ Case Reports 2012*; 2012 pii: bcr2012006498.

7 Goske-Bierska I, Wysokinski W, Brown RD Jr., *et al.* Cerebral venous sinus thrombosis: Incidence of venous thrombosis recurrence and survival. *Neurology* 2006; 67: 814–819.

8 Cohen JE, Duck M, Gomori JM, *et al.* Isolated cortical vein thrombosis: a rare cause of venous stroke with good prognosis after timely diagnosis and treatment. *Neurol Res* 2013; 35: 127–130.

9 Manara R, Mardari R, Ermani M, *et al.* Transverse dural sinuses: incidence of anatomical variants and flow artefacts with 2D time-of-flight MR venography at 1 Tesla. *Radiol Med* 2010; 115: 326–338.

10 Hingwala D, Kesavadas C, Thomas B, *et al.* Clinical utility of susceptibility-weighted imaging in vascular diseases of the brain. *Neurol India* 2010; 58: 602–607.

11 Mohr JP, Choi D, Grotter J, *et al. Stroke: Pathophysiology, Diagnosis, and Management*, 4th edn. New York: Churchill Livingstone, 2004.

12 Guo XB, Fu Z, Song LJ, *et al.* Local thrombolysis for patients of severe cerebral venous sinus thrombosis during puerperium. *Eur J Radil* 2013; 82: 165–168.

13 Ferro JM, Canhão P, Stam J, *et al.* Prognosis of cerebral vein and dural sinus thrombosis: results of the International Study on Cerebral

Vein and Dural Sinus Thrombosis (ISCVT). *Stroke* 2004; 35: 664–670.

14 Schrag M, McAuley G, Pomakian J, *et al.* Correlation of hypointensities in susceptibility-weighted images to tissue histology in dementia patients with cerebral amyloid angiopathy: a postmortem MRI study. *Acta Neuropathol* 2010; 119: 291–302.

15 Morgenstern LB, Hemphill JC 3rd, Anderson C, *et al.* Guidelines for the management of spontaneous intracerebral hemorrhage: a guideline for healthcare professionals from the American Heart Association/American Stroke Association. *Stroke* 2010; 41: 2108–2129.

16 Ohwaki K, Yano E, Nagushima H, *et al.* Blood pressure management in acute intracerebral hemorrhage: relationship between elevated blood pressure and hematoma enlargement. *Stroke* 2004; 35: 1364–1367.

17 Anderson CS, Heeley E, Huang Y, *et al.* Rapid blood-pressure lowering in patients with acute intracerebral hemorrhage. *N Engl J Med* 2013; 368: 2355–2365.

18 Broderick JP, Connolly S, Feldmann E, *et al.* Guidelines for the management of spontaneous intracerebral hemorrhage in adults: 2007 update: a guideline from the American Heart Association/American Stroke Association Stroke Council, High Blood Pressure Research Council, and the Quality of Care and Outcomes in Research Interdisciplinary Working Group. *Stroke* 2007; 38: 2001–2023.

19 Mendelow AD, Gregson BA, Fernandes HM, *et al.* Early surgery versus initial conservative treatment in patients with spontaneous supratentorial intracerebral haematomas in the International Surgical Trial in Intracerebral Haemorrhage (STICH): a randomised trial. *Lancet* 2005; 365: 387–397.

20 Mayer SA, Brun NC, Begtrup K, *et al.* Efficacy and safety of recombinant activated factor VII for acute intracerebral hemorrhage. *N Engl J Med* 2008; 358: 2127–2137.

21 Verma RK, Kottke R, Andereggen L, *et al.* Detecting subarachnoid hemorrhage: Comparison of combined FLAIR/SWI versus CT. *Eur J Radiol* 2013; 82: 1539–1545.

22 Wu Z, Li S, Lei J, *et al.* Evaluation of traumatic subarachnoid hemorrhage using susceptibility-weighted imaging. *AJNR* 2010; 31: 1302–1310.

23 Connolly ES Jr, Rabinstein AA, Carhuapoma JR, *et al.* Guidelines for the management of aneurysmal subarachnoid hemorrhage: a guideline for healthcare professionals from the American Heart Association/american Stroke Association. *Stroke* 2012; 43: 1711–1737.

24 Moster ML. Coagulopathies and arterial stroke. *J Neuroophthalmol* 2003; 23: 63–71.

25 Lim W, Crowther MA, Eikelboom JW. Management of antiphospholipid antibody syndrome: a systematic review. *J Am Med Assoc* 2006; 295: 1050–1057.

26 Rand JH. The antiphospholipid syndrome. *Annu Rev Med* 2003; 54: 409–424.

27 Caplan LR. *Caplan's Stroke: A Clinical Approach*, 3rd edn. Boston: Butterworth Heinemann, 2000.

28 Pegelow CH, Macklin EA, Moser FG, *et al.* Longitudinal changes in brain magnetic resonance imaging findings in children with sickle cell disease. *Blood* 2002; 99: 3014–3018.

29 Kinney TR, Sleeper LA, Wang WC, *et al.* Silent cerebral infarcts in sickle cell anemia: a risk factor analysis. *Pediatrics* 1999; 103: 640–645.

30 Kirkham F. Therapy insight: stroke risk and its management in patients with sickle cell disease. *Nat Clin Pract Neurol* 2007; 3: 264–278.

31 Ohene-Frempong K, Weiner SJ, Sleeper LA, *et al.* Cooperative study of sickle cell disease: cerebrovascular accidents in sickle cell disease: rates and risk factors. *Blood* 1998; 91: 288–294.

32 Rees DC, Dick MC, Height SE, *et al.* A simple index using age, hemoglobin, and aspartate transaminase predicts increased intracerebral blood velocity as measured by transcranial doppler scanning in children with sickle cell anemia. *Pediatrics* 2008; 121: 1628–1632.

33 Adams RJ, McKie VC, Carl EM, *et al.* Long-term stroke risk in children with sickle cell disease screened with transcranial doppler. *Ann Neurol* 1997; 42: 699–704.

34 Adams RJ, McKie VC, Hsu L, *et al.* Prevention of a first stroke by transfusions in children with sickle cell anemia and abnormal results on transcranial doppler ultrasonography. *N Engl J Med* 1998; 339: 5–11.

35 Fullerton HJ, Gardner M, Adams RJ, *et al.* Obstacles to primary stroke prevention in children with sickle cell disease. *Neurology* 2006; 67: 1098–1099.

36 Chinthamitr Y, Ruchutrakool T, Suwanawiboon B, *et al.* Intracranial and spinal hemorrhage in adult hemophelia A in siriraj hospital, Thiland. *J Thromb Haemost* 2007; 5 (Suppl. 2): P-S150.

37 Connolly SJ, Ezekowitz MD, Yusuf S, *et al.* Dabigatran versus warfarin in patients with atrial fibrillation. *N Engl J Med* 2009; 361: 1139–1151.

38 Patel MR, Mahaffey KW, Garg J, *et al.* Rivaroxaban versus warfarin in nonvalvular atrial fibrillation. *N Engl J Med* 2011; 365: 883–891.

39 Granger CB, Alexander JH, McMurray JJ, *et al.* Apixaban versus warfarin in patients with atrial fibrillation. *N Engl J Med* 2011; 365: 981–992.

40 Connolly SJ, Eikelboom J, Joyner C, *et al.* Apixaban in patients with atrial fibrillation. *N Engl J Med* 2011; 364: 806–817.

41 Makris M, Van Veen JJ, Tait CR, *et al.* Guideline on the management of bleeding in patients on antithrombotic agents. *Br J Haematol* 2013; 160: 35–46.

portosystemic collaterals (varices) from which blood loss may occur, particularly on a background of thrombocytopenia.

- Ineffective production of platelets secondary to a decrease in liver thrombopoietin synthesis has been reported.

Alcohol-associated liver disease may cause thrombocytopenia by a variety of mechanisms:

- Alcohol is directly toxic to megakaryocytes, leading to inhibition of megakaryopoiesis and decreased platelet production.
- Folate deficiency resulting from poor dietary intake or ineffective hepatic metabolism may result in ineffective megakaryopoiesis.
- Alcohol ingestion is itself associated with decreased platelet survival.

In fulminant viral hepatitis, the marked thrombocytopenia often encountered is caused by both suppression of megakaryopoiesis by virus and increased platelet destruction.

The increase in bleeding time seen in many subjects with severe liver disease is often out of proportion to the associated degree of thrombocytopenia, suggesting the presence of platelet dysfunction. The results of platelet function testing in these patients are inconsistent. Whereas some studies have demonstrated abnormalities in primary and secondary aggregation to adenosine diphosphate (ADP), adrenaline, thrombin, and ristocetin, others have failed to show any functional defect.

The cause of platelet dysfunction in liver disease is unclear. There is an increase in levels of circulating platelet inhibitors, including fibrin degradation products. Ethanol or abnormal high-density lipoproteins may contribute to aggregatory abnormalities in some cases. In others, intrinsic platelet abnormalities have been demonstrated, including acquired storage pool deficiency (platelet nucleotide deficiency), reduced platelet arachidonic acid, and abnormalities of platelet membrane composition and signaling.

Disseminated Intravascular Coagulation

It is generally accepted that many patients with advanced liver disease have activated coagulation and chronic low-grade disseminated intravascular coagulation (DIC). The diagnosis of DIC in subjects with chronic liver disease is complicated by the fact that many of the laboratory abnormalities present are common to both conditions.

Bleeding or thrombosis is usually present in DIC but is not a frequent finding in patients with liver disease coagulopathy alone. Evidence of increased thrombin generation has been demonstrated in chronic liver disease. These effects are at least partially reversible by heparin and include reduced fibrinogen survival and increased markers of thrombin generation (D-dimer, thrombin–antithrombin complexes, fibrinopeptide A, and plasmin–antiplasmin complexes). It may be that liver disease confers a state of increased intravascular coagulation, whereas additional factors such as sepsis or bleeding trigger DIC.

A number of possible causes of chronic DIC in liver disease have been suggested:

- procoagulant factors released from damaged hepatocytes;
- release of intestinal endotoxins into the portal circulation;
- impaired clearance of activated coagulation factors by the damaged failing liver;
- in addition, levels of naturally occurring anticoagulants, including antithrombin, protein C, protein S, and heparin cofactor II, are reduced in proportion to the degree of hepatic dysfunction.

Vitamin K Deficiency

Vitamin K is a fat-soluble vitamin required for the production of a variety of coagulation proteins, including factors II, VII, IX, and X and proteins C and S. Vitamin K deficiency may occur in liver disease as a result of:

- poor dietary intake;
- destruction of vitamin K_2-producing intestinal bacteria by antibiotic therapy;
- bile salts are required for the absorption of vitamin K in the small intestine, so biliary obstruction may therefore lead to vitamin K deficiency; and

- prolonged cholestasis secondary to calculi or neoplasia leads to deficiencies in the vitamin K-dependent coagulation proteins and prolongation of the PT.

Dysfibrinogenemia

One of the earliest coagulation abnormalities seen in chronic liver disease is the production of a dysfibrinogen. This molecule is rich in sialic acid residues and results in abnormal fibrin polymerization. The reduced efficiency in fibrin clot production prolongs both the thrombin time and reptilase time, but has not been shown to contribute to clinical bleeding. Dysfibrinogenemia is most commonly seen in chronic hepatitis and cirrhosis but has also been reported in hepatocellular carcinoma.

Hyperfibrinolysis

Accelerated fibrinolysis is well recognized in hepatic cirrhosis. Forty percent of patients awaiting liver transplant show laboratory evidence of hyperfibrinolysis with short euglobulin lysis times and elevated serum fibrin degradation product concentrations. In addition, low plasminogen levels and elevated fibrinopeptide B, D-dimer and plasmin–α_2-antiplasmin complex concentrations may be demonstrated in subjects with chronic liver disease. Possible mechanisms behind this include decreased hepatic clearance of plasminogen activators (e.g., tissue plasminogen activator, tPA) and a decrease in circulating the fibrinolytic inhibitors plasminogen activator inhibitor type 1 (PAI-1), α_2-antiplasmin, and histidine-rich glycoprotein.

Clinical manifestations of Liver Disease Coagulopathy

Hemorrhage

Bleeding is a common manifestation of chronic liver disease (Table 23.2) and is associated with

Table 23.2 Clinical manifestations of liver disease coagulopathy.

Ecchymoses
Purpura
Oozing from venipuncture or intravenous cannula sites
Dental bleeding
Hematuria
Gastrointestinal and variceal hemorrhage
Epistaxis
Postoperative hemorrhage

substantial morbidity and mortality. Patients may present with both:

- *mucosal bleeding*: resulting from thrombocytopenia and platelet dysfunction leading to failure of primary hemostasis; and
- *soft tissue bleeding*: resulting from the reduction in coagulation proteins with failure of secondary hemostasis.

Once liver disease is diagnosed, it is important to remember that laboratory tests of hemostasis are poorly predictive of bleeding events. This is partly because liver disease bleeding is not only caused by defects in primary and secondary hemostasis, but also is frequently associated with anatomical abnormalities, such as portosystemic varices on a background of raised portal pressure.

Bleeding episodes may also be triggered by operative procedures in previously stable patients. Some patients with advanced chronic liver disease are identified for the first time prior to elective surgery when a coagulation screen is checked. At least 50% of patients with cirrhosis will have varices secondary to portal hypertension at diagnosis, and some will be diagnosed for the first time with liver disease following a variceal bleed.

Thrombosis (Table 23.3)

Abdominal Vein Thrombosis

Thrombosis of the hepatic veins (Budd–Chiari syndrome, BCS), portal, and/or mesenteric veins

Table 23.3 Hypercoagulability and liver disease.

Abdominal vein thrombosis

Deep vein thrombosis and pulmonary embolism

Thrombosis in central venous catheters and extracorporeal circuits

Parenchymal extinction and progressive hepatic fibrosis

are infrequent but significant diseases that frequently occur in younger patients.

Hepatic Vein Thrombosis BCS due to hepatic venous thrombosis has a varied clinical presentation ranging from asymptomatic to fulminant liver failure [5]. A cause can be identified in 75% of these cases (Table 23.4). These include hereditary and acquired prothrombotic states, trauma, and infection. The presence of multiple predisposing factors in BCS is well recognized. Myeloproliferative disorders (MPD) are the most common cause of BCS, with polycythemia vera implicated in 10–40% of cases [6–8]. In 25% of cases, the cause of BCS is not apparent (idiopathic BCS), although the presence of an

Table 23.4 Causes of Budd–Chiari syndrome.

Hereditary prothrombotic disorders:

 Factor V Leiden
 PT 20210 G/A
 Antithrombin deficiency
 Protein C deficiency
 Protein S deficiency

Acquired prothrombotic disorders:

 Myeloproliferative disorders
 Antiphospholipid syndrome
 Paroxysmal nocturnal hemoglobinuria
 Malignancy
 Pregnancy
 Exogenous estrogen

Other:

 Behçet's syndrome
 Caval web
 Dacarbazine
 Aspergillosis
 Inflammatory bowel disease
 Hepatocellular/ renal/ adrenal carcinoma

underlying "latent" MPD is often suspected [9]. The diagnosis of MPD has been greatly improved by the discovery of a point mutation in the Janus kinase 2 (JAK2) gene on the short arm of chromosome 9. JAK2 is a tyrosine kinase that transduces signals triggered by hemopoietic growth factors. In 2005, an acquired mutation in JAK2 (V617F) was reported in MPDs [10–13]. The presence of JAK2V617F in 90% of subjects with polycythemia vera and 50% of those with primary thrombocythemia and myelofibrosis provides us with a new diagnostic test of clonality in these diseases. JAK2V617F has been shown to be present in up to 58.5% of cases of "idiopathic" BCS, indicating the presence of an underlying latent MPD [14].

Portal Vein Thrombosis Portal vein thrombosis (PVT) is often silent and may not be discovered until variceal hemorrhage occurs. Clinical features include abdominal pain, ascites, and rectal bleeding. Thrombosis extending to the mesenteric vessels may lead to mesenteric infarction. Common causes of PVT include hepatic cirrhosis, abdominal sepsis, tumors, and pancreatitis. As in BCS, the role of multiple etiological factors is well recognvized, including hereditary and acquired prothrombotic disorders and estrogen therapy. JAK2V617F has been reported to occur in 17–36% of patients with PVT [15–18]. Anticoagulation therapy with vitamin K antagonists may be hazardous in patients with esophageal varices and, consequently, decisions on treatment are based on extent/ age of thrombosis, presence of varices, history of bleeding, and the presence of an underlying prothrombotic disorder. In acute PVT, anticoagulation is frequently given for a period of 6 months; a longer duration of anticoagulation may be beneficial in chronic PVT or in patients with underlying prothrombotic disorders [19].

Venous Thromboembolism
Deep vein thrombosis and pulmonary embolism occur frequently in hospitalized medical patients, and routine risk assessment and thromboprophylaxis with heparin is now widely

recommended [20]. Despite the hemorrhagic tendency of chronic liver disease, venous thromboembolism (VTE) occurs not infrequently in these patients. Prothrombotic coagulation disturbances in liver disease include reduced levels of anticoagulant proteins (antithrombin, protein C, protein S), antiphospholipid antibodies, and hyperfibrinolysis. The incidence of VTE in chronic liver disease may well be underestimated, as lower limb edema and dyspnea are nonspecific and commonly present in these patients. In one retrospective case–control study of patients with cirrhosis, new VTE was present in 0.5% of inpatients with cirrhosis [21].

Progression of Fibrosis due to Parenchymal Extinction

It is clear that in patients with chronic liver disease (particularly cirrhosis) the prothrombotic state can lead to further hepatic injury ("parenchymal extinction") and progression of fibrosis. This may be due to thrombosis in small intrahepatic vessels. There is some evidence that the prothrombotic state predisposes to accelerated fibrogenesis, for example, the observed association between factor V Leiden mutation and accelerated fibrosis in patients with hepatitis C infection. There is no good evidence to support the use of standard anticoagulation to prevent progression of hepatic fibrosis, but the advent of newer antithrombotics may kindle new interest in this area.

Extracorporeal Circuits

Continuous venovenous hemodialysis and artificial liver support machines both require the exposure of blood to artificial surfaces, inevitably leading to coagulation activation and clotting in the extracorporeal circuit. A variety of anticoagulant strategies have been advocated, often depending on local expertise and the perceived bleeding risk in individual cases.

Laboratory Investigation of Hemostasis in Liver Disease

Clotting Screen

The PT and activated partial thromboplastin time (APTT) are commonly prolonged in chronic liver disease, reflecting a reduction in coagulation factor production by the failing liver (Table 23.5). Patients with abnormal laboratory tests only

Table 23.5 Laboratory abnormalities in liver disease.

Laboratory abnormality	Likely etiology
Isolated ↑ PT	Factor VII deficiency
	Vitamin K deficiency (cholestasis, dietary)
↑ PT + ↑ APTT	Coagulation factor deficiencies
↑ Thrombin time + ↑ Reptilase time	Dysfibrinogenemia, hypofibrinogenemia
Thrombocytopenia	Hypersplenism, DIC
	Suppressed megakaryopoiesis
Abnormal platelet aggregometry	Acquired platelet function defect
↓ Euglobulin clot lysis time	Hyperfibrinolysis: ↓PA I ↓ α_2-antiplasmin

APTT, activated partial thromboplastin time; DIC, disseminated intravascular coagulation; PAI, plasminogen activator inhibitor; PT, prothrombin time.

require treatment to correct coagulopathy when there is evidence of active bleeding or prior to surgery.

Chronic Liver Disease

No single coagulation test is predictive of hemorrhage or thrombosis in patients with chronic liver disease.

- Factor VII has a short half-life and levels fall early in subjects with hepatic impairment. An isolated prolongation of the PT may be the only demonstrable laboratory abnormality in those with mild disease.
- A prolonged PT or international normalized ratio (INR) is a key indicator of hepatic dysfunction and commonly used as a trigger for liver transplantation; however, it is vitamin K-dependent. Although a prolonged PT is often used as a marker of hepatic dysfunction, it is most sensitive to low coagulation factor VII levels and does not accurately reflect the levels of other coagulation factors (e.g., factors II, VIII, X, and VWF).
- Factor V concentration is a sensitive indicator of hepatic disease as this protein is predominantly synthesized by hepatocytes and is not vitamin K dependent.
- Thrombophilia tests: levels of the naturally occurring anticoagulants (antithrombin, protein C, protein S) may all be reduced as a consequence of liver disease. Combined antithrombin and protein C deficiency are usually due to liver disease rather than due to combined inheritance.

Cholestasis

Patients with early vitamin K deficiency secondary to cholestasis have isolated prolongation of the PT, which is correctable by administration of intravenous vitamin K.

Factor VII has the shortest half-life of all the vitamin K-dependent factors and is therefore the first coagulation factor to decrease, hence isolated prolonged PT. With severe prolonged vitamin K deficiency there is reduction in factors II, IX, and X with prolongation of both PT and APTT.

Advanced Hepatocellular Disease

These patients tend to have a more severe derangement of laboratory tests reflecting:

- high incidence of multiple coagulation factor deficiencies;
- hyperfibrinolysis; and
- DIC.

Fibrinogen Level

Fibrinogen levels vary according to the type and severity of liver dysfunction. When measuring fibrinogen concentration, results may vary markedly depending on the methods used. Assays based on the rate of clot formation (e.g., Clauss fibrinogen) result in low levels of fibrinogen more often than assays based on final clot weight. This is because dysfibrinogens and circulating proteins that impair fibrin clot formation may (e.g., fibrinogen degradation products, FDPs) influence rate-dependent assays.

Dysfibrinogenemia

This may prolong thrombin time and reptilase time but is not usually associated with bleeding.

Hyperfibrinolysis

This may lead to hypofibrinogenemia with prolongation of the PT, APTT, thrombin time, and reptilase times. Other laboratory findings include a prolongation of the euglobulin clot lysis time, raised FDP levels, and decreased plasminogen concentration.

Thromboelastography (TEG®) is an investigation measuring the dynamics of clot formation and has been shown to be a more superior predictor of intraoperative bleeding in liver transplantation than standard coagulation tests.

Emerging Evidence for Rebalanced Coagulation in Liver Disease

There is increasing evidence to support a rebalanced hemostatic system associated with acute liver failure and chronic liver disease [22]. The decrease in hepatic synthesis of procoagulant proteins is countered by the concomitant reduction in production of anticoagulant proteins and increased factor VIII. Similarly, impaired primary hemostasis mediated by thrombocytopenia is rebalanced by increased VWF and reduced ADAMTS13. Finally, whilst cirrhosis results in increased t-PA and reduced TAFI, favoring hyperfibrinolysis, the reduction in plasminogen promotes hypofibrinolysis restoring the balance.

Global coagulation assays, such as thrombin generation, thromboelastography/metry and clot lysis assays have been utilized to demonstrate this rebalance *in vitro*. The variable clinical phenotype, with respect to bleeding and thrombotic tendency in patients with liver disease, further supports a model of rebalanced hemostasis. Underlying conditions such as portal hypertension, endothelial dysfunction, infection, and renal impairment contribute to the bleeding risk [4].

Invasive Procedures and Liver Disease

Liver Biopsy

The risk of bleeding after liver biopsy is a small but significant one and has been estimated to occur in 0.4% of cases. In view of this risk, each case should be carefully reviewed to ensure that the procedure is only performed when absolutely necessary.

Percutaneous liver biopsy is relatively safe when the INR is below 1.5 and the platelet count is above 50×10^9/L. In subjects who do not fulfill these criteria, administration of vitamin K, plasma, and platelets should be considered prior to the procedure. Subjects with prolonged bleeding time and history of bleeding may be given desmopressin (DDAVP). Alternative strategies include laparoscopic liver biopsy and biopsy via the transjugular approach.

A high mortality rate has been reported in patients with sickle cell disease undergoing percutaneous liver biopsy and extreme caution is

recommended, particularly in the setting of acute liver failure.

Shunt Insertion in Liver Disease

Portocaval and mesocaval shunts may be inserted to alleviate portal hypertension in decompensated liver disease. These procedures are frequently associated with increased fibrinolysis and DIC. Peritoneal–venous shunt insertion in patients with chronic ascites may trigger significant bleeding. This is thought to be because of the flow of procoagulant and platelet-activating molecules from ascitic fluid into the systemic circulation triggering DIC. Clinically significant bleeding may be avoided by draining ascites prior to opening the shunt or by short-term occlusion of the shunt.

Liver Transplantation

Liver transplantation is being increasingly offered to patients with endstage decompensated liver disease. Marked hemostatic failure with substantial blood loss is frequently seen during liver transplant [23,24], with a strong association between blood loss and mortality rate. Research into the causes of liver transplant coagulopathy have led to improved intraoperative management strategies and decreased mortality rates.

The First Operative (Preimplantation) Stage
There is mild deterioration in the baseline liver disease coagulopathy. This coincides with surgical dissection and mobilization of the diseased liver and is not usually associated with major blood loss.

The Next Three Operative Stages
The coagulation disturbance increases (Table 23.6) and is maximal during the anhepatic stage (because of loss of coagulation factor turnover) and early reimplantation (hyperfibrinolytic) stage. Consumptive thrombocytopenia with DIC often occurs, requiring massive blood product replacement. This is followed by gradual resolution of hemostatic dysfunction

Table 23.6 Coagulation abnormalities during liver transplantation.

Stage of transplant	Hemostatic abnormality
Stage 1: Preimplantation	Mild deterioration of baseline liver disease coagulopathy
Stage 2: Anhepatic	Loss of coagulation factor synthesis and clearance Accelerated fibrinolysis and DIC Consumptive thrombocytopenia tPA released from graft on reperfusion
Stage 3: Reimplantation	Restoration of coagulation factor synthesis and clearance Resolution of hyperfibrinolysis

DIC, disseminated intravascular coagulation; tPA, tissue plasminogen activator.

in the third (reimplantation) stage and postoperative period.

Treatment of Liver Transplant Coagulopathy

This varies according to stage of operation:

- Stage 1 is associated with mild surgical bleeding, not usually requiring aggressive hemostatic support.
- In the anhepatic and reperfusion stages, transfusion with blood, platelets, plasma, and cryoprecipitate may be required to correct profound coagulopathy and prevent major blood loss.
- The reperfusion stage is associated with tPA and endogenous heparin-like substance release from the graft, and antifibrinolytic therapy with aprotinin or tranexamic acid has been shown to be effective in reducing transfusion requirements in this setting.
- Stage 3 is usually associated with resolution of coagulopathy. However, if successful engraftment of the donor liver does not occur, tissue ischemia and necrosis may trigger DIC and further bleeding.

Treatment of Liver Disease Coagulopathy

Treatment of coagulopathy in liver disease is required during episodes of bleeding or prior to invasive procedures. The type of treatment required will depend on the specific hemostatic abnormalities present and the nature of the bleeding event. It is important to remember that most patients with coagulopathy are stable and do not require specific therapy. When bleeding does occur, the associated triggers (e.g., esophageal varices secondary to portal hypertension) need to be addressed in conjunction with strategies to correct coagulopathy.

Vitamin K

Deficiency of vitamin K may occur in liver disease, resulting from poor diet or secondary to malabsorption. Administration of 10 mg vitamin K_1 will correct the PT, at least partially, in most patients within 48 hours. The PT will not fully correct if there is a coexisting defect in hepatic synthetic function.

Plasma

Fresh frozen plasma (FFP) or solvent detergent plasma (SDP) contains all the coagulation factors synthesized by the healthy liver. It may be used to correct multiple coagulation factor deficiencies in bleeding patients or prior to invasive procedures. A significant problem with FFP is the large volume of transfusion required to correct the PT and APTT in severe liver disease, particularly in volume-overloaded patients with ascites and peripheral edema. In addition, repeated transfusions are required to maintain circulating coagulation factor levels. Prothrombin complex concentrates should be used with caution in liver disease, as their use has been associated with thromboembolism and DIC. Cryoprecipitate or fibrinogen concentrate should be used to correct hypofibrinogenemia associated with hyperfibrinolysis or DIC.

Platelets

Platelet transfusions are indicated in bleeding patients with platelet counts of $<10 \times 10^9$/L, or in patients undergoing invasive procedures. Platelet increments are generally poor in subjects with portal hypertension because of sequestration of transfused platelets in the spleen. DDAVP (0.3 µg/kg) may be of value in patients with acquired platelet dysfunction and prolonged bleeding time, but its value in bleeding patients is uncertain.

Antifibrinolytics

Aprotinin, tranexamic acid, and ε-aminocaproic acid have all been shown to reduce operative blood loss and transfusion requirements in liver transplantation. The use of these agents to reduce fibrinolysis associated with chronic liver disease is of uncertain value, and their use in DIC is not recommended.

Other Agents

Heparin and Antithrombin Their use in DIC has not led to significant improvements in blood loss or mortality and is therefore not recommended.

Estrogens There are some reports on efficacy in bleeding related to chronic liver disease, but further data from clinical trials are required before their use can be recommended.

Fibrin glue Local endoscopic applications have been shown to be effective in the treatment of bleeding gastric varices.

Recombinant Factor VIIa Small studies have demonstrated reduced clotting times in chronic liver disease and a reduction in transfusion requirements in liver transplantation. The optimal role for recombinant factor VIIa in the treatment of liver coagulopathy has yet to be defined.

Recombinant Thrombopoietin Receptor Agonists Use of eltrombopag, an oral thrombopoietin receptor agonist, has been shown to successfully improve thrombocytopenia in patients with chronic liver disease with subsequent reduction in the need for platelet transfusion prior to elective procedures. However, its use was associated with a significant increased risk of portal vein thrombosis [25].

References

1 Amirano L, Guardascione MA, Brancaccio V, *et al*. Coagulation disorders in liver disease. *Semin Liver Dis* 2002; 22: 83–96.

2 Ratnoff OD. Hemostatic defects in liver and biliary tract disease. In: Ratoff OD, Forbes CD, eds. *Disorders of Hemostasis*. Philadelphia: WB Saunders, 1996: 422.

3 Northup PG, Sundaram V, Fallon MB, *et al*. Hypercoagulation and thrombophilia in liver disease. *J Thromb Haemost* 2007; 6: 2–9.

4 Tripodi A, Mannucci PM. The coagulopathy of chronic liver disease. *N Engl J Med* 2011; 365: 147–156.

5 Narayanan KV, Shah V, Kamath PS. The Budd–Chiari syndrome. *N Eng J Med* 2004; 350: 578–585.

6 Denninger MH, Chait Y, Casadevall N, *et al*. Cause of portal or hepatic vein thrombosis in adults: the role of multiple concurrent factors. *Hepatology* 2000; 31: 587–591.

7 Valla D, Casadevall N, Lacombe C, *et al*. Primary myeloproliferative disorder and hepatic vein thrombosis: a prospective study of erythroid colony formation in vitro in 20 patients with Budd-Chiari Syndrome. *Ann Intern Med* 1985; 103: 329–334.

8 Primignani M, Martinelli I, Bucciarelli P. Risk factors for thrombophilia in extrahepatic portal vein obstruction. *Hepatology* 2005; 41: 603–608.

9 Pagliuca A, Mufti GJ, Janossa-Tahernia M, *et al*. In vitro colony culture and chromosomal studies in hepatic and portal vein thrombosis: possible evidence of an occult myeloproliferative state. *Q J Med* 1990; 76: 981–989.

10 Baxter EJ, Scott LM, Campbell PJ, *et al*. Acquired mutation of the tyrosine kinase *JAK2* in human myeloproliferative diseases. *Lancet* 2005; 365: 1054–1061.

11 Levine RL, Wadleigh M, Cools J, *et al.* Activating mutation in the tyrosine kinase *JAK2* in polycythemia vera, essential thrombocythemia, and myeloid metaplasia with myelofibrosis. *Cancer Cell* 2005; 7: 387–397.

12 James C, Ugo V, Le Couedic JP, *et al.* A unique clonal *JAK2* mutation leading to constitutive signaling causes polycythemia vera. *Nature* 2005; 434: 1144–1148.

13 Kralovics R, Passamonti F, Buser AS, *et al.* A gain-of-function mutation of *JAK2* in myeloproliferative disorders. *N Engl J Med* 2005; 352: 1779–1790.

14 Patel RK, Lea NC, Heneghan MA, *et al.* Prevalence of the activating JAK2 tyrosine kinase mutation V617F in the Budd-Chiari Syndrome. *Gastroenterology* 2006; 130: 2031–2038.

15 Primigani M, Barosi G, Bergamaschi G, *et al.* Role of the JAK2 mutation in the diagnosis of chronic myeloproliferative disorders in splanchnic vein thrombosis. *Hepatology* 2006; 44: 1528–1534.

16 Kiladjian J, Cervantes F, Leebeek F, *et al.* Role of JAK2 mutation detection in Budd-Chiari Syndrome (BCS) and portal vein thrombosis (PVT) associated to MPD. *Blood* 2006; 108: Abstract 377.

17 Colaizzo D, Amitrano L, Tiscia GL, *et al.* The JAK2 V617F mutation frequently occurs in patients with portal and mesenteric venous thrombosis. *J Thromb Haemost* 2006; 5: 55–61.

18 Regina S, Herault O, D'Iteroche L, *et al.* The JAK2 mutation V617F is specifically associated with idiopathic splanchnic vein thrombosis. *J Thromb Haemost* 2007; 5: 859–861.

19 Condat B, Pessione F, Helene Denninger M, *et al.* Recent portal or mesenteric venous thrombosis: increased recognition and frequent recanalization on anticoagulant therapy. *Hepatology* 2000; 32: 466–470.

20 Hirsh J, Dalen JE, Master MPM, *et al.* American College of Chest Physicians The sixth (2000) ACCP guidelines for antithrombotic therapy for prevention and treatment of thrombosis. *Chest* 2001; 119: 1S–2S.

21 Northup PG, McMahon MM, Ruhl AP, *et al.* Coagulopathy does not fully protect hospitalized cirrhosis patients from peripheral venous thromboembolism. *Am J Gastroenterol* 2006; 101: 1524–1528.

22 Lisman T, Porte RJ. Rebalanced hemostasis in patients with liver disease: evidence and clinical consequences. *Blood* 2010; 116: 878–885.

23 Porte RJ, Knot EA, Bontempo FA. Hemostasis in liver transplantation. *Gastroenterology* 1989; 97: 488–501.

24 Starzl TE, Demertris A, van Thiel DH. Liver transplantation. *N Engl J Med* 1989; 321: 1014–22, 1092–99.

25 Afdhal NH, Giannini EG, Tayyab G, *et al.* Eltrombopag before procedures in patients with cirrhosis and thrombocytopenia. *N Eng J Med* 2012; 367: 716–724.

24

Nephrology

Vimal K. Derebail and Thomas L. Ortel

Key Points

- Chronic kidney disease and uremia are associated with an increase in both bleeding risk and thrombotic risk.
- Patients with the nephrotic syndrome, particularly those with membranous nephropathy, are at higher risk for venous thromboembolic events.
- Venous thromboembolism is more common among patients with antineutrophil cytoplasmic antibody (ANCA) associated vasculitis, particularly during times of active disease.
- Kidney transplantation can lead to relatively hypercoagulable state; patients with renal transplants may be higher risk for thrombotic events that can lead to allograft loss.
- Anticoagulants often require dose adjustment and should be used with consideration in patients with kidney disease because of the higher risk of bleeding in these patients and because some of these agents are renally excreted.

Bleeding in Renal Disease

Clinical Presentation

The association between renal disease and bleeding has been recognized for many years, first being chronicled in 1764 in Morgagni's *Opera Omnia* [1]. Episodes of bleeding may vary widely in their severity and in presentation. Most commonly, patients with renal failure may develop contusions, epistaxis, bleeding at venipuncture or catheter insertion sites, and menorrhagia. Retroperitoneal bleeding may occur spontaneously or after procedures. This population, in particular, is more likely to undergo renal biopsy after which clinically evident bleeding may occur [2].

Gastrointestinal (GI) bleeding is more common in patients with chronic kidney disease (CKD) and endstage renal disease (ESRD). Bleeding from the GI tract is related to a multitude of factors including more commonly peptic ulcer disease and gastritis as well as telangiectasias and angiodysplasia found in the stomach and intestine [2]. Gastrointestinal blood loss can contribute to the chronic anemia of ESRD and is associated with a need for higher doses of erythropoiesis-stimulating agents typically used to treat anemia. Upper GI bleeding in ESRD patients may occur at rates nearly two orders of magnitude greater than the general population [3]. Thirty-day mortality in the outpatient setting following these episodes approaches 7.3% and is twice as high in the inpatient setting at 13.6% [3]. Intracranial hemorrhage in ESRD patients is greater than in the general population, occurring at an estimate of 4.1–6.7 times more commonly [4].

Etiology

Bleeding in patients with renal disease is often multifactorial, as with many other disease states.

Practical Hemostasis and Thrombosis, Third Edition. Edited by Nigel S. Key, Michael Makris and David Lillicrap.

Characteristics that may increase the risk of bleeding include the relatively frequent use of antiplatelet agents or anticoagulant drugs. Anemia, a common manifestation of chronic kidney disease, may also predispose to bleeding by a number of mechanisms. Altered rheology from a paucity of red blood cells leads platelets to travel closer to the center of the blood vessels, disrupting the usual interaction with endothelium that promotes thrombosis. Adenine diphosphate (ADP) and thromboxane A_2, which promote platelet aggregation, are released by red blood cells and are reduced in the setting of anemia [2, 5, 6]. Hemoglobin also scavenges nitric oxide [2, 5, 6] and with reduced hemoglobin, nitric oxide is more abundant, inhibiting platelet activation and causing vasodilation.

Platelet dysfunction associated with uremia is often described as a predominant cause of bleeding in patients. While uremic platelets are often normal in quantity, typical platelet–platelet interactions and platelet interactions with blood vessel walls are diminished. Impaired platelet function occurs due to a number of abnormalities found in uremic patients. Glycoprotein Ib (GPIb) receptor expression is reduced, as is the binding affinity to von Willebrand factor (VWF) [2,6,7]. Platelet cGMP and cAMP are increased and leading to increased NO and prostacyclins. Vascular tone is thereby relaxed, reducing platelet adhesion and platelet–platelet interaction [2]. Platelet fibrinogen binding is altered, as is arachidonic acid metabolism [2,5,7]. Uremic platelets also demonstrate an acquired storage pool defect with reduced ADP and serotonin [2,5–7]. Accumulation of particular uremic substances, including urea, guanidine succinate, phenol, and tryptophan products, inhibit platelet function [1,6]. Small peptides that accumulate in uremia may compete with VWF and fibrinogen and prevent binding of these substances to platelet GPIIb–IIIa receptors [1]. Skin bleeding time and, more recently, the platelet closure test (PFA-100), has been used to detect uremic platelet dysfunction, although it remains unclear if these predict clinical bleeding outcomes [2].

Certain drugs that may reach higher levels in patients with renal disease, such as penicillin G, carbenicillin, ticarcillin, ampicillin, and moxalactam, can also increase the risk of bleeding by binding to platelets and blocking platelet-membrane agonist receptors.

Prevention and Treatment

Interventions to manage bleeding in patients with renal disease are often determined by the location, severity, and acuity of the bleeding event. When limited to external sites, mechanical maneuvers such as applying pressure over the area of bleeding and, if an extremity is involved, elevating the area above the level of the heart can help control or alleviate bleeding [7]. Use of topical hemostatic agents such as absorbable collagen (bovine collagen) provides a scaffold for platelet aggregation [6,8].

To prevent bleeding complications (Table 24.1), antiplatelet drugs, such as aspirin and nonsteroidal anti-inflammatory drugs (NSAIDs), should be held for at least 1 week prior to invasive procedures or surgery [7]. Dialysis can be useful in prevention as well in the actively bleeding uremic patient if it can be performed safely. Removal of uremic toxins that contribute to platelet dysfunction reduces bleeding tendencies and may be particularly effective with peritoneal dialysis [2,8]. Intradialysis heparin should be held for patients with active bleeding or at risk for continued bleeding [6,7]. While removal of uremic toxins may attenuate platelet dysfunction, factors such as contact with the artificial surface of dialyzer membranes, high shear stress, and turbulent blood flow may actually promote platelet activation and coagulation [2,6,7].

Management of anemia is another method for both prevention and treatment of bleeding in renal disease. In acutely bleeding patients, transfusion of packed red blood cells is usually necessary [2,6,7]. Raising the hematocrit to 30% is thought to improve platelet margination and interaction with the vessel wall [2,6,7]. As a preventative measure in the stable CKD or ESRD patient with hematocrit <30%, treatment with erythropoiesis-stimulating agents (ESA) not only improves hematocrit but may also enhance platelet signaling and increase metabolically active

Table 24.1 Prevention and treatment of bleeding in patients with renal failure.

Avoidance of antiplatelet and anticoagulant drugs
Correction of anemia
Red blood cell transfusion
Erythropoiesis-stimulating agents
Dialysis
Pharmacological therapy:
Desmopressin (DDAVP)
Conjugated estrogens
Antifibrinolytics
Cryoprecipitate
Platelet transfusion

reticulated platelets [2,5]. These agents should be started at a dose of 35–50 U/kg three times weekly to achieve hematocrit of 30% [2,6,8]. However, the use of ESAs is not without risks and may contribute to poorly controlled blood pressure and arteriovenous access thrombosis as well as potential thrombotic events and stroke, particularly if anemia is "overcorrected" [9–12].

Desmopressin (1-deamino-8-D-arginine vasopressin; DDAVP) is often used in uremic patients [5,7]. DDAVP interacts with endothelial cells leading to release of stored VWF from Weibel–Palade bodies [2]. Increases in VWF and factor VIII levels occur within 30 minutes to 1 hour of administration [2,5,6]. Because of its relatively rapid onset of action, DDAVP is considered first-line treatment for uremic bleeding. Typically, an intravenous dose of DDAVP at 0.3–0.4 µg/kg is administered over 20–30 minutes. Subcutaneous (0.3 µg/kg) and intranasal (2 µg/kg) routes are also effective, although less so than the intravenous route [8]. The half-life of the agent is roughly 10 hours with bleeding time returning to pretreatment doses after 24 hours [2]. Repeat doses are often unnecessary prior to 24 hours because its mechanism of action is dependent on platelet stores. Adverse reactions to DDAVP include headache, facial flushing, rare thrombotic events, hypotension, and hyponatremia [7,8].

Conjugated estrogens increase VWF and factor VIII synthesis and reduce protein S levels.

When administered at 0.6 mg/kg daily, infused over 30 minutes, for 5 days, estrogens exhibit their maximum effect in 6–7 days and continue to produce a reduction in bleeding time up to 4 days after discontinuation. The duration of effect may be as long as 14–21 days. Side-effects of conjugated estrogen include hot flashes [2,6–8]. Preferably, these agents should be used in the prophylactic setting [2].

Antifibrinolytic agents such as aminocaproic acid and tranexamic acid have been used for tooth extractions and minor oral surgery. Topical aminocaproic acid has been particularly useful for abating mucosal bleeding. Systemic dosing of aminocaproic acid has been reported to cause upper urinary tract obstruction as well as intra-renal microangiopathic thrombosis, renal artery or vein thrombosis, and renal failure, and should be administered with caution [13]. Tranexamic acid is excreted renally and dosing is usually reduced to 5 mg/kg daily with avoidance of prolonged administration [2].

Cryoprecipitate has been suggested for those uremic patients with active bleeding who are nonresponsive to DDAVP [2,6]. Cryoprecipitate is rich in factor VIII, VWF, fibrinogen, fibronectin, and factor XIII, begins to work within minutes, and has a duration of 4–12 hours [2]. However, cryoprecipitate has a variable effect in uremic patients and up to half will have no improvement in bleeding tendency [7]. Severe reactions to cryoprecipitate include rarely anaphylaxis, pulmonary edema, and intravascular hemolysis, and the other potential risks of transfusion of a blood product [2].

Kidney Biopsy

Bleeding Risk

In patients with acute kidney injury of uncertain etiology, renal biopsy is often needed to establish a diagnosis and treatment plan. Particularly in patients with severe renal injury and uremia, this procedure carries a pertinent risk of bleeding. The kidney is a highly vascular organ, receiving a substantial portion of the cardiac output. Bleeding rates of 11–22% have been reported and this varies by biopsy technique. Up to 90% of patients may demonstrate a perirenal hematoma after biopsy by CT scan [2]. Most institutions have now adopted the use of real-time ultrasound guidance and spring-loaded biopsy needles. A meta-analysis of over 9000 patients from studies using these techniques, and published from 1991 to 2011, demonstrated relatively low complication rates [14]. Approximately 3.5% of patients had macroscopic hematuria following biopsy. Transfusions of red blood cells were required in only 0.9% of total patients and ranged from 0% to 7.4% across the studies. When routine postbiopsy imaging was performed, 17% demonstrated a hematoma. Serious complications were very rare; angiographic intervention was needed in only 0.6% of patients; urinary tract obstruction occurred in only 0.3%. Only one patient (0.01%) in the series required nephrectomy for management of life-threatening hemorrhage. Death was attributed to complications from biopsy in 0.02%, or two patients [14]. Risk factors for transfusion included use of larger-gauge needle (14 gauge vs. 16 or 18 gauge), female sex, higher serum creatinine levels (≥2.0 mg/dL), and acute kidney injury (AKI). Also, those with lower prebiopsy hemoglobin levels (<12 g/dL) were more likely to receive a transfusion [14].

Prevention of Bleeding

In addition to the routine assessment of risk factors (such as coagulation studies, hematocrit, and platelet count), prior to any procedure, the patient's personal and family bleeding history should be assessed. Aspirin and other NSAIDs should be discontinued well in advance of the procedure by at least 7 days and some would suggest up to 14 days [2,14]. Warfarin, if a routine drug, should be discontinued 5 days prior to the procedure with low-molecular-weight heparin or unfractionated heparin used a bridge if needed. If heparin is administered as bridging agent, it should be held on the day of the procedure [2]. Those with AKI and markedly reduced renal function should be observed particularly closely. Hypertension should be controlled as

well as possible prior to the procedure. Use of smaller-gauge needles (16 gauge or 18 gauge) is preferable over larger-gauge needles. Patients should be observed for a minimum of 8 hours after the procedure, during which time almost two-thirds of complications are observed [2].

Chronic Kidney Disease and Thrombosis

Clinical Presentation

Despite the bleeding risks associated with renal failure, many patients with chronic kidney disease are hypercoagulable as well. The risk of venous thromboembolism (VTE) is increased among patients with kidney disease. Data from several epidemiological cohorts have demonstrated an increase in the risk of VTE, reaching a 60–70% increase in risk among those with stage 3 and 4 CKD (estimated glomerular filtration rate (eGFR) <60 mL/min/1.73 m^2) when compared to those with normal renal function [15–17]. Hospitalized patients with renal impairment have nearly a fourfold increase in VTE risk compared to those with normal renal function [2]. Even in those with early kidney disease manifested only by albuminuria (urinary albumin excretion (UAE) ≥30 mg/24 hours), the increase in risk of VTE is similar and recurrence of VTE is more likely [17–19]. The risk of cardiovascular disease is also markedly elevated in the CKD population. Mortality from cardiovascular disease is 10 to 20-fold greater in the CKD population [2].

Etiology

As with bleeding, the prothombotic state of CKD is related to a variety of mechanisms that lead to increased coagulation and atherogenesis. CKD patients demonstrate higher fibrinogen levels and enhanced thrombin generation. Factors VII, VIII, and VWF are also elevated. Antithrombin inhibitor activity and the fibrinolytic system are also impaired. Elevations in C-reactive protein (CRP) increase endothelial cell and monocyte interactions, leading to enhanced tissue factor expression and complement and platelet activation. Tissue factor is also increased by a variety of other inflammatory cytokines. Endothelial dysfunction is worsened by uremic toxins and hypertension. Altered lipid metabolism leads to impaired fibrinolysis and accelerated atherosclerosis [2].

Prevention and Treatment

No data exist to provide specific recommendations for modifying VTE risk in patients with CKD. Rather, the clinician should be aware of the heightened risk of thrombosis in this population. Prophylaxis should be considered in the setting of heightened VTE risk such as hospitalization or postsurgically. Treatment of VTE is complicated by the metabolism of some of the usual agents and the bleeding risk in these patients and is discussed in more detail below. While interventions for management of cardiovascular disease parallel the general population, their efficacy in this population is less certain.

Thrombosis in Nephrotic Syndrome

Nephrotic syndrome is defined as the presence of heavy proteinuria (protein loss in the urine greater than 3.5 g/24 hours), hypoalbuminemia (serum albumin less than 3.0 g/dL), and peripheral edema. Hyperlipidemia is also a frequent feature of this syndrome. The association of thrombotic events and hypercoagulability with nephrotic syndrome has been recognized since the mid-nineteenth century [20]. While potentially caused by a number of primary and secondary causes, those associated with thrombotic events include membranous nephropathy, focal segmental glomerulosclerosis (FSGS), minimal change disease, and membranoproliferative glomerulonephritis (MPGN) [21,22].

The most common thrombotic events in patients with nephrotic syndrome are those affecting the deep veins of the lower extremities (DVT). Renal vein thromboses (RVT) have also been reported in patients that have nephrotic

syndrome and seem to be more common in membranous nephropathy. These latter events may occur acutely and present with flank pain and potentially acute renal failure if bilateral. However, RVT may be clinically silent, and found incidentally or only when systematic screening is performed [21]. Arterial thrombotic events are also reported in patients with nephrotic syndrome, but with a much lower frequency.

The heightened risk of venous thromboembolism in patients with nephrotic syndrome among hospitalized patients was noted in a study of nearly 900 000 patients using hospital discharge data. Patients with nephrotic syndrome had a 39% increase in risk of pulmonary embolism (PE) and a 72% increase in DVT. The increase in risk was most marked among patients aged 18–39 years, approaching nearly a sevenfold increase in DVT [23]. Venous thromboembolic events are generally reported to occur in approximately 25% of nephrotic patients, but the frequency varies depending on the cause of nephrotic syndrome as well as the method by which VTE was ascertained. The studies of clinically evident events report much lower incidence of VTE than those which employed systematic screening for these events [21,22,24,25].

Data from a large inception cohort of 1313 patients with nephrotic syndrome demonstrated clinically evident VTE in 3.4% of patients overall during a median follow-up of over 5 years. Membranous patients demonstrated the greatest frequency (7.9%), followed by FSGS patients (3%). The referent population of patients with IgA nephropathy demonstrated VTE in only 0.4% [22].

Hypoalbuminemia, proteinuria, and the ratio of proteinuria to serum albumin have been identified as independent risk factors for VTE in nephrotic syndrome [24–26]. In the aforementioned large inception cohort, histological diagnosis, male sex, hypoalbuminemia (<2.9 g/dL) at presentation, and a diagnosis of cancer were independently associated with increased VTE risk [22]. Proteinuria at presentation, even at extreme values, was not identified in these analyses. In analyses adjusted for sex, cancer, proteinuria, and severity of albuminuria, VTE risk was still found to be the highest in patients with membranous nephropathy followed by FSGS, with adjusted hazard ratios of 10.8 and 5.9, when compared to patients with IgA nephropathy. The reason for the relatively higher frequency of VTE in membranous nephropathy compared to forms of nephrotic syndrome is not known but is consistent with prior reports [22,27].

Another study, evaluating only patients with membranous nephropathy, demonstrated clinically evident VTE in 7.2%, the majority of which occurred within 2 years of diagnosis and during periods of hypoalbuminemia. After adjustment for various confounders, hypoalbuminemia at diagnosis was the only independent predictor of VTE, and VTE was 2.5 times greater among those with a serum albumin level <2.8 g/dL [28]. Several studies have attempted to evaluate whether genetic predispositions to VTE including factor V Leiden, prothrombin G20210A, and methylene tetrahydrofolate reductase (MTHFR) [29–31]. These have largely been small underpowered studies, although case reports have reported instances of VTE in patients with these concomitant conditions.

In a large cohort of pediatric patients with various forms of primary and secondary nephrotic syndrome, thromboembolic events were reported in 9.2% of patients. From this study, age ≥12 years, severity of proteinuria, and prior history of VTE were found to be risk factors associated with VTE [32]. The spectrum of nephrotic syndrome in children is different from that of adults; membranous nephropathy is uncommon in children. These differences in form of nephrotic syndrome may account for differences in identifiable risk factors.

Etiology

The thrombophilia found in patients with nephrotic syndrome is likely multifactorial and complex. Environmental risk factors that may predispose to VTE include hospitalization, immobilization, procedures, and obesity as well as those more specific to nephrotic syndrome, including intravascular volume depletion, and diuretic and steroid use [21,24].

Several potential mechanisms for hypercoagulability have been described in the nephrotic syndrome (Table 24.2). Loss of anticoagulant proteins in the urine seems to be related to alternations in the selective permeability of the glomeruli. Decreased antithrombin III have been reported in 40–80% of nephrotic patients; protein C and S have also been reported to be decreased although less consistently [20]. In addition to the loss of anticoagulants, procoagulant proteins are also increased. Factor V, VIII, VWF, fibrinogen, and α2-macroglobulin may be increased as acute phase reactants. Hypoalbuminemia promotes hepatic fibrinogen synthesis that may promote fibrin formation, increase blood viscosity, and promote platelet and erythrocyte aggregation [33]. The low serum albumin may also directly enhance platelet aggregation by increasing the bioavailability of arachadonic acid [1,20]. LDL cholesterol, commonly elevated in patients with nephrotic syndrome, impairs NO production, and may increase platelet–vessel wall interactions [33].

Treatment

Anticoagulation once a thromboembolic event has occurred in patients with nephrotic syndrome is generally recommended for the duration of the

Table 24.2 Potential mechanisms of thrombophilia in the nephrotic syndrome.

Loss of anticoagulants in the urine
Antithrombin III
Protein C and protein S (possible)
Production of factors that promote thrombosis
Factor V and factor VIII
von Willebrand factor
Plasminogen activator inhibitor 1
Fibrinogen
α_2-plasmin inhibitor
Platelet abnormalities
Mild thrombocytosis
Enhanced platelet aggregation

Source: modified from Loscalzo *et al.* 2013 [20].

nephrotic state [21,34]. Two previous decision analysis studies have attempted to address whether prophylactic anticoagulation should be administered to patients with nephrotic syndrome [26,35]. While both of these concluded that patients should be offered anticoagulation, relatively high estimates of VTE risk were used, and the benefit of anticoagulation was not evaluated in terms of personal variability in disease severity. Generally speaking, warfarin anticoagulation is recommended for those at low risk of bleeding events who have severe nephrotic syndrome from membranous nephropathy (serum albumin <2.0–2.5 g/dL) [34]. However, these recommendations should be tailored to the individual patient. In those with high potential for bleeding complications, anticoagulation may not be desirable at any level of nephrosis. Conversely, in those with higher risks of VTE (family history, immobilization, hospitalization), prophylactic anticoagulation may be particularly desirable. Warfarin remains the typical agent for these patients. Newer anticoagulants have not been assessed in patients with nephrotic syndrome. The use of hydroxymethylglutaryl-CoA (HMG-CoA) reductase inhibitors, or "statins," may also have a role in VTE prevention in nephrotic patients. A single retrospective single-center cohort study of adults with nephrotic syndrome demonstrated a significant reduction in VTE risk among those using statins [36].

ANCA Vasculitis and Venous Thromboembolism

Clinical Presentation

Approximately 10% of patients with antineutrophil cytoplasmic antibody (ANCA) associated small vessel vasculitides develop VTE [37–39]. These system vasculitides include granulomatosis with polyangiitis (GPA, formerly Wegener granulomatosis), microscopic polyangiitis (MPA), and eosinophilic granulomatosis with polyangiitis (EGPA, formerly Churg–Strauss disease). While many organs may be involved in these diseases, renal disease is common and often presents as a pauci-immune crescentic glomerulonephritis. Pulmonary disease, particularly pulmonary hemorrhage, may also occur.

VTE in these patients typically occurs during the times of highest disease activity, more commonly reported in the 3 months preceding and the 6 months following initial diagnosis or relapse [39]. Risk factors in these patients include older age, male sex, and prior history of VTE or stroke [40]. Initial reports suggested a higher frequency in those patients with GPA, but a larger cohort study did not detect an association with ANCA phenotype or with the ANCA serotype (PR-3 or MPO).

Etiology

The mechanisms of the hypercoagulability in ANCA vasculitis are not presently known. One study has evaluated the occurrence of genetic risk factors, factor V Leiden, prothrombin G20210A, and MTHFR, and failed to detect an association [41]. Antiplasminogen antibodies, which delay conversion of plasminogen to plasmin and increase fibrin clot dissolution time, have been reported in ANCA patients [42,43]. These may occur in up to 25% of ANCA patients and seem to correlate with the severity of glomerular lesions [43]. However, at present, it remains unclear if these are associated with an increase in VTE risk. Hypercoagulability in ANCA vasculitis may be mediated by direct injury to endothelial cells, as suggested by the increased numbers of circulating endothelial cells [44]. In one series of pediatric patients with various forms of systemic vasculitis including ANCA, thromboembolic events were associated with microparticle-driven thrombin generation [45]. In patients with EGPA, eosinophils may also release tissue factor and activate factor X [46].

Treatment

Treatment in of VTE in ANCA disease is nonspecific other than accounting for renal function in choosing anticoagulants. Prophylactic anticoagulation is not recommended in ANCA vasculitis due to the potential risk of alveolar hemorrhage in these patients. VTE may occur concurrently or in close proximity to alveolar hemorrhage, and in these cases, an inferior vena cava filter placement is recommended for the prevention of pulmonary embolus. While therapeutic options may be challenging and not easily preventable, the clinician should recognize the increased risk of VTE in ANCA patients with active disease.

Renal Vein Thrombosis

Clinical Presentation

Renal vein occlusion caused by thrombosis was first described by Rayer in 1840 [21,47,48]. Patients may present acutely with main renal vein thrombosis and sudden onset of flank pain and tenderness to percussion, pleuritic chest pain, macroscopic hematuria, unilateral radiographic abnormalities by intravenous pyelogram, and worsening renal function. However, patients with nephrotic syndrome may present subacutely with no symptoms except peripheral edema [24]. Neonates and infants more often have an acute presentation and are found to have abdominal distension, a flank mass from increase in kidney size, hematuria, and proteinuria and may also present with bilateral renal vein thrombosis. Neonates and infants are often diagnosed in the setting of severe dehydration and present with dry mouth, decreased urine output, and decreased skin turgidity. In cases of gradual onset, patients may have no symptoms or nonspecific chronic complaints of nausea, apathy, weakness, and generalized edema and may have symptoms of upper abdominal or flank pain [24].

Etiology

Renal vein thrombosis is a complication of nephrotic syndrome and has been found in patients with primary glomerular diseases, as described above, as well as in other diseases with nephrosis, including rapidly progressive glomerulonephritis, lupus erythematosus, diabetes mellitus, primary amyloidosis, familial Mediterranean fever with amyloidosis, sickle cell disease, sarcoidosis, and vasculitis.

However, several other potential settings are associated with renal vein thrombosis including the following:

- thrombosis of the inferior vena cava with secondary renal vein involvement;
- systemic disease with hypercoagulable states, such as sickle cell disease, primary antiphospholipid syndrome, and advanced malignancy;
- direct extension of tumor into the lumen of the renal veins causing occlusion with thrombosis proximal to the tumor;
- alteration in renal blood flow (i.e., volume loss, diarrhea, sepsis, adrenal hemorrhage, hypoglycemia, seizure disorders or hypoxia in cyanotic congenital heart disease, tricuspid insufficiency, constrictive pericarditis);
- surgically induced renal vein occlusion with thrombosis beyond the ligature [47].

Diagnosis, Treatment, and Prognosis

With acute renal vein thrombosis, kidney size increases within the first week with ultrasonography demonstrating the enlarged kidney and hypoechoic renal cortex [49]. Subsequently, the injured kidney will decrease in size over a couple of weeks and atrophy, with ultrasound demonstrating increased echogenicity [49]. Color Doppler ultrasound improves the ability to detect flow in the renal artery and the renal vein, and its sensitivity is particularly high in detecting renal vein thrombosis in postrenal transplant patients. In chronic renal vein thrombosis, renal venous occlusion leads to development of varicosities, which produce a notching appearance in the ureter and collateral venous drainage around the kidney by intravenous urography [50].

While selective renal venography remains the standard referent, this modality is invasive and potentially associated with complications, including bleeding and inferior vena cava perforation [49]. Doppler ultrasonography is often the primary modality used for identifying renal vein thrombosis. However, this modality may vary from center to center, has a great degree of operator dependence, and is of limited utility in obese patients [49].

Renal computed tomography (CT) enhanced by contrast is the best modality to visualize renal vein thrombosis [49,50]. Indirect CT venography findings consistent with RVT include enlarged kidneys, as seen in ultrasonography, and delayed enhancement of the renal parenchyma [49]. Findings of chronic RVT include attenuation of the affected renal vein due to retraction of the clot and collateral vessels along the ureter and around the kidney. Magnetic resonance imaging (MRI), particularly when utilizing contrast enhancement, has utility similar to that of CT imaging, and has the advantage of avoiding nephrotoxic intravenous contrast [21,49].

Treatment consists of correcting the underlying problem when RVT is related to secondary causes of decreased renal blood flow. Dialysis may be needed in causes of severe renal failure from renal vein thrombosis [47]. The mortality rate can be high, and often patients with renal vein thrombosis are at risk of death from other thromboembolic events, such as pulmonary emboli. Overall survival may be poor with mortality predicted by underlying cancer or infection [51]. In patients with untreated renal vein thrombosis, the incidence of pulmonary embolus has been found to range from 20% to 40% [34]. In a series of neonates with renal vein thrombosis, 70.6% demonstrated irreversible damage, and treatment with unfractionated heparin or low-molecular-weight heparin did not change outcomes. Mortality was reported at 3.3%; approximately 20% had persistent hypertension and 3% required chronic dialysis or renal transplantation [52].

For patients with nephrotic syndrome and renal vein thrombosis, chronic anticoagulation therapy is warranted to prevent further extension of the thrombus and to prevent other thromboembolic events [21,24,48]. Thrombolytic agents have been used for acute RVT, but are associated with high frequency of death due to bleeding complications [48]. Surgical thrombectomy has also been attempted but is only rarely indicated for patients not responding to medical therapy. Percutaneous mechanical thrombectomy has also been used with success [48].

Renal Transplant and Thrombosis

Incidence and Clinical Presentation of Thromboembolic Events

Renal allograft thrombosis has been reported to occur in approximately 1–8% of recipients, with thrombosis accounting for 25–37% of graft loss in the first year after transplantation and up to 45% of transplants lost in the first 90 days [2, 53, 54]. Thrombosis of the renal vein graft is more common than arterial thrombosis and often presents with pain and swelling of the graft, potentially leading to allograft rupture [53,54]. Thrombosis of the renal artery may be asymptomatic, and both renal vein and artery thrombosis can occur at the same time. In one study, risk factors associated with graft thrombosis included use of the donor's right kidney, prior history of any VTE, diabetic nephropathy in the recipient, technical surgical problems, and hemodynamic status of the recipient in the perioperative period. Thrombosis of the renal allograft can lead to delayed graft function and may be associated with extrarenal VTE events [2]. DVT and PE may also occur in up to 8% patients following transplantation; VTE events are more common in the first month after transplantation [2].

Etiology

Following transplantation, localized activation of coagulation occurs in graft vessels with fibrinolysis impaired both on graft endothelium and systemically. Within the allograft, antithrombin, thrombomodulin, and tissue plasminogen activator are all reduced [2]. The systemic circulation is similarly hypercoagulable with increased thrombin–antithrombin and reduced thrombomodulin, antithrombin, and protein C noted immediately postimplantation [2].

Other factors contributing to the risk of graft thrombosis include those associated with the surgical procedure. These include abnormalities of donor vessels such as vessel diameter, multiple renal arteries, and donor artery stenosis. Atherosclerosis of donor or recipient vessels, surgical trauma from repeated attempts at anastomosis, lymphoceles post-transplant, and prolonged ischemia time also contribute to the likelihood of allograft thrombosis [54].

Inherited thrombophilia has been associated with allograft thrombosis. Factor V Leiden in one series was reported to occur in 6% of transplant recipients, conferring a fourfold increase in risk of allograft thrombosis, and accounting for 20% of graft loss in that cohort [30]. Prothrombin G20210A also confers a greater risk of vessel thrombosis and may lead to shorter allograft survival [55]. Acquired thrombophilias have also been associated with allograft thrombosis. Allograft recipients with SLE and antiphospholipid antibodies were found to have a 40% risk of thrombosis, graft loss, or death caused by thromboembolism versus 8% of SLE patients without antiphospholipid antibodies [55].

Diagnosis and Prevention

Color Doppler ultrasonography has become the standard procedure for evaluating renal allograft flow. Complete allograft vein thrombosis can be reliably detected by the presence of reversed diastolic flow in the arteries [56]. Whether or not patients should be screened for thrombophilia prior to transplant has been debated. Some have advocated screening for high-risk patients, such as patients with personal or family history of thrombosis and in children and adolescents who appear to be at higher risk of allograft thrombosis [26,54,55].

The use of anticoagulation at prophylactic or treatment dosing to reduce the risk of allograft thrombosis must be weighed against the risk of bleeding, particularly in the postoperative period. In one study, dalteparin 2500 U daily was given just during the period of hospitalization for low-risk patients and dalteparin 5000 U daily was administered for at least 1 month postoperatively for high-risk patients. In this group of 120 transplant recipients, no events of allograft thrombosis or major hemorrhagic events occurred. These data must be interpreted with caution, as there was also no control group for comparison [57]. However, in those patients felt to be high risk for VTE or allograft thrombosis, particularly those with a personal history of VTE, such an approach is reasonable.

Anticoagulant Use in Kidney Disease

Anticoagulants

As previously noted, patients with renal disease may have bleeding tendencies as well as a predilection for thrombosis. Additionally, many anticoagulants used in practice are excreted by the kidneys. Treating patients with kidney disease with anticoagulants offers a greater challenge in determining dosing and requires closer monitoring for signs of bleeding.

Unfractionated heparin (UFH) is primarily metabolized by the reticulendothelial system with less than 10% excreted in the urine unchanged. For this reason, UFH remains the anticoagulant of choice for patients with severe renal impairment. In unstable patients or at increased bleeding risk or with a need for a procedure, UFH if preferable due to its short half-life and reversibility. Low-molecular-weight heparins (LMWH), in contrast, are excreted by the kidneys. Concerns for bleeding largely apply to those who receive therapeutic doses rather than prophylactic doses. Enoxaparin demonstrates accumulation but tinzaparin does not appear to accumulate even at therapeutic doses. Dalteparin also appears to be safe in CKD patients and has been used at prophylactic doses even in patients with severe renal disease [2].

Guidelines for Mild to Moderate Renal Insufficiency

For the LMWHs, including enoxaparin, dalteparin, and tinzaparin, no dosage adjustments are needed for mild renal insufficiency (creatinine clearance (CL_{cr}) of 50–80 mL/min) and moderate renal insufficiency (CL_{cr} of 30–50 mL/min) [58]. For enoxaparin, it has been reported that the clearance is reduced by 30% in patients with moderate renal insufficiency. Because of concern for drug accumulation in moderate renal insufficiency, reducing the dose is advisable and following antifactor

Xa levels may help guide therapy in patients with moderate renal insufficiency. Also, for the factor Xa inhibitor fondaparinux, there are no dosage adjustments given for mild and moderate renal insufficiency. Patients should be monitored closely for signs of hemorrhage and consideration of following antifactor Xa levels, especially if therapy is anticipated to be prolonged.

Among IV direct thrombin inhibitors, only argatroban does not require dosage adjustments for renal insufficiency. For acute coronary syndrome patients undergoing percutaneous intervention, bivalirudin is not dose reduced. However, for use in patients with heparin-induced thrombocytopenia, we would recommend reducing the dose from 0.15 mg/kg/hour to 0.05 mg/kg/hour. Patients should be monitored closely with checking activated partial thromboplastin time (APTT) 2–3 hours after initiation of drug and after dosage changes. For lepirudin, the manufacturer recommends dosage reduction for patients with $CL_{cr} < 60$. For CL_{cr} between 30 and 60 mL/minute, a reduced bolus dose of 0.2 mg/kg is recommended. For Cl_{cr} 45– 60 mL / minute, the infusion rate should be reduced to 0.075 mg/kg/hour, and for Cl_{cr} 30–44 mL / minute, the infusion rate should be reduced to 0.045 mg/kg/hour. Others have advocated even lower doses of lepirudin infusion as follows: (i) normal renal function, 0.1 mg/kg/hour; (ii) CL_{cr} 45– 60 mL / minute, 0.05 mg/kg/hour; and (iii) CL_{cr} 30– 44 mL / minute, 0.03 mg/kg/hour [58]. Monitoring APTT 4 hours after initiating the infusion and after any dosage changes is required.

Guidelines for Severe Renal Insufficiency

For patients with severe renal insufficiency, defined as a creatinine clearance les than 30 mL/minute, dose reductions are recommended for LMWHs. For DVT prophylaxis, enoxaparin is reduced to 30 mg once daily for abdominal surgery, hip replacement, knee replacement, and in medical patients. For DVT treatment, enoxaparin is reduced to 1 mg/kg and given once daily. For dalteparin, the manufacturing guidelines

only comment that, for cancer patients being treated for a venous thromboembolic event, anti-Xa levels should be monitored and the dose adjusted accordingly. For tinzaparin, there is a 24% decrease in clearance, and therefore it should be used with caution. Fondaparinux is contraindicated for patients with severe renal insufficiency [58].

For mild and moderate renal insufficiency, argatroban is the only direct thrombin inhibitor that does not require a dose adjustment. Bivalirudin should be reduced to 1 mg/kg/hour and with dialysis-dependent patients on nondialysis days, the dose should be reduced to 0.25 mg/kg/hour. For use in patients with heparin-induced thrombocytopenia, we would recommend reducing the dose to 0.03 mg/kg/hour. Patients should be monitored closely with checking APTT 2–3 hours after initiation of the drug and after dosage changes. For lepirudin, the manufacturer recommends reducing the bolus dose to 0.2 mg/kg and to reduce the infusion rate to 0.0225 mg/kg/hour for Cl_{cr} 15– 29 mL / minute and to not use lepirudin for $Cl_{cr} < 15$ mL / minute. The APTT should be monitored after 4 hours of initiating the infusion and after any dosage changes [58].

Oral Anticoagulants

Warfarin has remained the primary oral anticoagulant used in patients with kidney disease. While treatment of VTE is a clear indication for use of this agent, other uses seem to have less evidence. Warfarin has been employed in attempts to maintain the patency of vascular access in hemodialysis patients, but the evidence for its efficacy for this indication is minimal [2]. Primary prevention of stroke in patients with nonvalvular atrial fibrillation has been another common use of warfarin. Because patients with renal disease are at greater risk for bleeding events, the benefit of warfarin is less clear. In CKD stages 1–4 (eGFR of > 15 mL / min/ $1.73 m^2$), anticoagulation does appear to still confer a benefit over the increased potential risk of bleeding [59]. However, the benefit in dialysis-dependent patients is uncertain, and the individual risk of bleeding should be taken into account when determining anticoagulation administration [59]. Warfarin must be used with some caution in patients with advanced renal disease due its potential to accelerate vascular calcification and its association with calciphylaxis [2,60]. When used in patients with renal disease, the starting dose of warfarin should be no more than 5 mg daily with target INR of 2.0–2.5. The first INR should be determined after the first two doses and then followed thrice weekly in the first month and every 2 weeks thereafter [59].

Several new oral anticoagulants have arrived for use in the last several years. Most of these have some component of renal excretion and have not been studied in patients with severe renal disease (CKD stage 5 or dialysis dependent). The direct thrombin inhibitor, dabigatran, has the highest renal excretion at 80% [61]. A dose reduction to 75 mg b.i.d. is recommended for patients with CKD stage 4 (eGFR $15-29\,\text{mL}/\text{min}/1.73\,\text{m}^2$) based upon pharmacological data, although its efficacy in this population is not yet known. The factor Xa inhibitors apixaban and rivaroxaban have less renal excretion at 25% and 35%, respectively. For apixaban, a dose of 5 mg twice daily may be used in patients with stage 3 CKD. Rivaroxaban may be used at a dose of 20 mg daily in patients with eGFR 50–59 mL/min/1.73 m^2 and reduced to 15 mg daily in those with eGFR $30-49\,\text{mL}/\text{min}/1.73\,\text{m}^2$ [61]. Reversal of these agents in the event of a bleeding event or overdose is more difficult than with warfarin. Hemodialysis may play a role in lowering plasma levels of dabigatran although a rebound drug levels may occur with dialysis discontinuation. Dialysis does carry the risk of bleeding with catheter insertion and must be taken into consideration if used [62].

Acknowledgment

Grant support: NEPTUNE Career Development Award, U54-DK-083912, Nephcure Foundation (VKD).

References

1 Sohal AS, Gangji AS, Crowther MA, *et al.* Uremic bleeding: pathophysiology and clinical risk factors. *Thromb Res* 2006; 118: 417–422.

2 Pavord S, Myers B. Bleeding and thrombotic complications of kidney disease. *Blood Rev* 2011; 25: 271–278.

3 Yang JY, Lee TC, Montez-Rath ME, *et al.* Trends in acute nonvariceal upper gastrointestinal bleeding in dialysis patients. *J Am Soc Nephrol* 2012; 23: 495–506.

4 Seliger SL, Gillen DL, Longstreth WT, Jr., *et al.* Elevated risk of stroke among patients with end-stage renal disease. *Kidney Int* 2003; 64: 603–609.

5 Hedges SJ, Dehoney SB, Hooper JS, *et al.* Evidence-based treatment recommendations for uremic bleeding. *Nat Clin Pract Nephrol* 2007; 3: 138–153.

6 Noris M, Remuzzi G. Uremic bleeding: closing the circle after 30 years of controversies? *Blood* 1999; 94: 2569–2574.

7 Gangji AS, Sohal AS, Treleaven D, *et al.* Bleeding in patients with renal insufficiency: a practical guide to clinical management. *Thromb Res* 2006; 118: 423–428.

8 Kaw D, Malhotra D. Platelet dysfunction and end-stage renal disease. *Semin Dial* 2006; 19: 317–322.

9 Phrommintikul A, Haas SJ, Elsik M, *et al.* Mortality and target haemoglobin concentrations in anaemic patients with chronic kidney disease treated with erythropoietin: a meta-analysis. *Lancet* 2007; 369: 381–388.

10 Pfeffer MA, Burdmann EA, Chen CY, *et al.* A trial of darbepoetin alfa in type 2 diabetes and chronic kidney disease. *N Engl J Med* 2009; 361: 2019–2032.

11 Singh AK, Szczech L, Tang KL, *et al.* Correction of anemia with epoetin alfa in chronic kidney disease. *N Engl J Med* 2006; 355: 2085–2098.

12 Drueke TB, Locatelli F, Clyne N, *et al.* Normalization of hemoglobin level in patients with chronic kidney disease and anemia. *N Engl J Med* 2006; 355: 2071–2084.

13 Kaye JD, Smith EA, Kirsch AJ, *et al.* Preliminary experience with epsilon aminocaproic acid for treatment of intractable upper tract hematuria in children with hematological disorders. *J Urol* 2010; 184: 1152–1157.

14 Corapi KM, Chen JL, Balk EM, *et al.* Bleeding complications of native kidney biopsy: a systematic review and meta-analysis. *Am J Kidney Dis* 2012; 60: 62–73.

15 Folsom AR, Lutsey PL, Astor BC, *et al.* Chronic kidney disease and venous thromboembolism: a prospective study. *Nephrol Dial Transplant* 2010; 25: 3296–3301.

16 Wattanakit K, Cushman M, Stehman-Breen C, *et al.* Chronic kidney disease increases risk for venous thromboembolism. *J Am Soc Nephrol* 2008; 19: 135–140.

17 Mahmoodi BK, Gansevoort RT, Naess IA, *et al.* Association of mild to moderate chronic kidney disease with venous thromboembolism: pooled analysis of five prospective general population cohorts. *Circulation* 2012; 126: 1964–1971.

18 Mahmoodi BK, Gansevoort RT, Veeger NJ, *et al.* Microalbuminuria and risk of venous thromboembolism. *JAMA* 2009; 301: 1790–1797.

19 van Schouwenburg IM, Mahmoodi BK, Veeger NJ, *et al.* Elevated albuminuria associated with increased risk of recurrent venous thromboembolism: results of a population-based cohort study. *Br J Haematol* 2012; 156: 667–671.

20 Loscalzo J. Venous thrombosis in the nephrotic syndrome. *N Engl J Med* 2013; 368: 956–958.

21 Wagoner RD, Stanson AW, Holley KE, *et al.* Renal vein thrombosis in idiopathic membranous glomerulopathy and nephrotic syndrome: incidence and significance. *Kidney Int* 1983; 23: 368–374.

22 Barbour SJ, Greenwald A, Djurdjev O, *et al.* Disease-specific risk of venous thromboembolic events is increased in idiopathic glomerulonephritis. *Kidney Int* 2012; 81: 190–195.

23 Kayali F, Najjar R, Aswad F, *et al.* Venous thromboembolism in patients hospitalized with nephrotic syndrome. *Am J Med* 2008; 121: 226–230.

24 Llach F. Hypercoagulability, renal vein thrombosis, and other thrombotic complications of nephrotic syndrome. *Kidney Int* 1985; 28: 429–439.

25 Li SJ, Guo JZ, Zuo K, *et al.* Thromboembolic complications in membranous nephropathy patients with nephrotic syndrome-a prospective study. *Thromb Res* 2012; 130: 501–505.

26 Bellomo R, Atkins RC. Membranous nephropathy and thromboembolism: is prophylactic anticoagulation warranted? *Nephron* 1993; 63: 249–254.

27 Singhal R, Brimble KS. Thromboembolic complications in the nephrotic syndrome: pathophysiology and clinical management. *Thromb Res* 2006; 118: 397–407.

28 Lionaki S, Derebail VK, Hogan SL, *et al.* Venous thromboembolism in patients with membranous nephropathy. *Clin J Am Soc Nephrol* 2012; 7: 43–51.

29 Fabri D, Belangero VM, Annichino-Bizzacchi JM, *et al.* Inherited risk factors for thrombophilia in children with nephrotic syndrome. *Eur J Pediatr* 1998; 157: 939–942.

30 Irish A. Renal allograft thrombosis: can thrombophilia explain the inexplicable? *Nephrol Dial Transplant* 1999; 14: 2297–2303.

31 Sahin M, Ozkurt S, Degirmenci NA, *et al.* Assessment of genetic risk factors for thromboembolic complications in adults with idiopathic nephrotic syndrome. *Clin Nephrol* 2013; 79: 454–462.

32 Kerlin BA, Blatt NB, Fuh B, *et al.* Epidemiology and risk factors for thromboembolic complications of childhood nephrotic syndrome: a Midwest Pediatric Nephrology Consortium (MWPNC) study. *J Pediatr* 2009; 155: 105–110, 10 e1.

33 Rabelink TJ, Zwaginga JJ, Koomans HA, *et al.* Thrombosis and hemostasis in renal disease. *Kidney Int* 1994; 46: 287–296.

34 Glassock RJ. Prophylactic anticoagulation in nephrotic syndrome: a clinical conundrum. *J Am Soc Nephrol* 2007; 18: 2221–2225.

35 Sarasin FP, Schifferli JA. Prophylactic oral anticoagulation in nephrotic patients with idiopathic membranous nephropathy. *Kidney Int* 1994; 45: 578–585.

36 Resh M, Mahmoodi BK, Navis GJ, *et al.* Statin use in patients with nephrotic syndrome is associated with a lower risk of venous thromboembolism. *Thromb Res* 2011; 127: 395–399.

37 Merkel PA, Lo GH, Holbrook JT, *et al.* Brief communication: high incidence of venous thrombotic events among patients with Wegener granulomatosis: the Wegener's Clinical Occurrence of Thrombosis (WeCLOT) Study. *Ann Intern Med* 2005; 142: 620–626.

38 Weidner S, Hafezi-Rachti S, Rupprecht HD. Thromboembolic events as a complication of antineutrophil cytoplasmic antibody-associated vasculitis. *Arthritis Rheum* 2006; 55: 146–149.

39 Stassen PM, Derks RP, Kallenberg CG, *et al.* Venous thromboembolism in ANCA-associated vasculitis–incidence and risk factors. *Rheumatology* 2008; 47: 530–534.

40 Allenbach Y, Seror R, Pagnoux C, *et al.* High frequency of venous thromboembolic events in Churg-Strauss syndrome, Wegener's granulomatosis and microscopic polyangiitis but not polyarteritis nodosa: a systematic retrospective study on 1130 patients. *Ann Rheum Dis* 2009; 68: 564–567.

41 Sebastian JK, Voetsch B, Stone JH, *et al.* The frequency of anticardiolipin antibodies and genetic mutations associated with hypercoagulability among patients with Wegener's granulomatosis with and without history of a thrombotic event. *J Rheumatol* 2007; 34: 2446–2450.

42 Bautz DJ, Preston GA, Lionaki S, *et al.* Antibodies with dual reactivity to plasminogen and complementary PR3 in PR3-ANCA vasculitis. *J Am Soc Nephrol* 2008; 19: 2421–2429.

43 Berden AE, Nolan SL, Morris HL, *et al.* Anti-plasminogen antibodies compromise fibrinolysis and associate with renal histology in ANCA-associated vasculitis. *J Am Soc Nephrol* 2010; 21: 2169–2179.

44 Woywodt A, Streiber F, de Groot K, *et al.* Circulating endothelial cells as markers for ANCA-associated small-vessel vasculitis. *Lancet* 2003; 361: 206–210.

45 Eleftheriou D, Hong Y, Klein NJ, *et al.* Thromboembolic disease in systemic vasculitis is associated with enhanced microparticle-mediated thrombin generation. *J Thromb Haemost* 2011; 9: 1864–1867.

46 Ames PR, Margaglione M, Mackie S, *et al.* Eosinophilia and thrombophilia in Churg Strauss syndrome: a clinical and pathogenetic overview. *Clin Appl Thromb Hemost* 2010; 16: 628–636.

47 Witz M, Kantarovsky A, Morag B, *et al.* Renal vein occlusion: a review. *J Urol* 1996; 155: 1173–1179.

48 Jaar BG, Kim HS, Samaniego MD, *et al.* Percutaneous mechanical thrombectomy: a new approach in the treatment of acute renal-vein thrombosis. *Nephrol Dial Transplant* 2002; 17: 1122–1125.

49 Yang GF, Schoepf UJ, Zhu H, *et al.* Thromboembolic complications in nephrotic syndrome: imaging spectrum. *Acta Radiol* 2012; 53: 1186–1194.

50 Asghar M, Ahmed K, Shah SS, *et al.* Renal vein thrombosis. *Eur J Vasc Endovasc Sur* 2007; 34: 217–223.

51 Wysokinski WE, Gosk-Bierska I, Greene EL, *et al.* Clinical characteristics and long-term follow-up of patients with renal vein thrombosis. *Am J Kidney Dis* 2008; 51: 224–232.

52 Lau KK, Stoffman JM, Williams S, *et al.* Neonatal renal vein thrombosis: review of the English-language literature between 1992 and 2006. *Pediatrics* 2007; 120: e1278–1284.

53 Matas AJ, Humar A, Gillingham KJ, *et al.* Five preventable causes of kidney graft loss in the 1990s: a single-center analysis. *Kidney Int* 2002; 62: 704–714.

54 Bakir N, Sluiter WJ, Ploeg RJ, *et al*. Primary renal graft thrombosis. *Nephrol Dial Transplant* 1996; 11: 140–147.

55 Andrassy J, Zeier M, Andrassy K. Do we need screening for thrombophilia prior to kidney transplantation? *Nephrol Dial Transplant* 2004; 19 (Suppl. 4): iv64–68.

56 Schwenger V, Hinkel UP, Nahm AM, *et al*. Color doppler ultrasonography in the diagnostic evaluation of renal allografts. *Nephron Clin Pract* 2006; 104: c107–112.

57 Alkhunaizi AM, Olyaei AJ, Barry JM, *et al*. Efficacy and safety of low molecular weight heparin in renal transplantation. *Transplantation* 1998; 66: 533–534.

58 Lobo BL. Use of newer anticoagulants in patients with chronic kidney disease. *Am J Health Syst Pharm* 2007; 64: 2017–2026.

59 Reinecke H, Engelbertz C, Schabitz WR. Preventing stroke in patients with chronic kidney disease and atrial fibrillation: benefit and risks of old and new oral anticoagulants. *Stroke* 2013; 44: 2935–2941.

60 Brandenburg VM, Kramann R, Specht P, *et al*. Calciphylaxis in CKD and beyond. *Nephrol Dial Transplant* 2012; 27: 1314–1318.

61 Hart RG, Eikelboom JW, Ingram AJ, *et al*. Anticoagulants in atrial fibrillation patients with chronic kidney disease. *Nat Rev Nephrol* 2012; 8: 569–578.

62 Knauf F, Chaknos CM, Berns JS, *et al*. Dabigatran and kidney disease: a bad combination. *Clin J Am Soc Nephrol* 2013; 8: 1591–1597.

25

Oncology

Anna Falanga and Marina Marchetti

Key Points

- Venous thromboembolism is a common complication of cancer.
- Cancer patients present with a variety of abnormalities of laboratory hemostatic markers.
- Tumor cells can interact with and activate the host hemostatic system.
- Prothrombotic mechanisms may promote tumor growth and dissemination.
- Predictive risk assessment models to identifying patients at high risk of thrombosis are under development.

Introduction

The association between cancer and thrombosis has been known for more than a century. The occurrence of venous thromboembolism is a common complication of cancer. It can also precede the onset of an occult neoplasia, as first reported by Armand Trousseau in 1865. At almost the same time, the possibility that a relationship between the clotting mechanisms and the development of metastasis may occur was postulated by Billroth in 1878.

In the last three decades remarkable progress has been made in this field, both by basic research and clinical studies. It is now clear that there is a two-way connection between coagulation and cancer [1]:

- malignant disease induces a prothrombotic switch of the host hemostatic system;

- prothrombotic mechanisms may promote tumor growth and dissemination.

Recently, molecular studies have demonstrated that oncogenes responsible for neoplastic transformation also drive programs for hemostatic protein expression and clotting system activation [2–4].

Patients with cancer are exposed to a significant risk of thrombosis [5,6], which can be aggravated by antitumor therapies [7]. Data derived from large randomized controlled trials (RCTs) have been used to determine the true incidence of this complication and to define the major risk factors for thrombosis in cancer [8].

Very commonly, cancer patients present with abnormalities of laboratory tests of blood coagulation, even without clinical manifestations of thromboembolism and/or hemorrhage. These abnormalities reveal different degrees of blood clotting activation and characterize the hypercoagulable state of these subjects [9]. The results of laboratory tests in these patients demonstrate that a process of fibrin formation and removal is continuously ongoing during the development of malignancy.

The pathogenesis of thrombophilia in cancer is multifactorial; however, an important factor the tumor cell's capacity to interact with and activate the host hemostatic system. Experimental studies show that fibrin and other coagulation proteins are involved in multiple steps of tumor growth and dissemination. Therefore, pharmacological interventions to prevent thrombotic phenomena

Practical Hemostasis and Thrombosis, Third Edition. Edited by Nigel S. Key, Michael Makris and David Lillicrap.
© 2017 John Wiley & Sons, Ltd. Published 2017 by John Wiley & Sons, Ltd.

in malignancy may possibly contribute to the control of the malignant disease progression.

The aim of this chapter is to summarize the most recent advances in our knowledge on the thrombophilic state of cancer patients and the pathogenic mechanisms of blood clotting activation in this condition, giving also an overview of the current approaches to the prevention and treatment of venous thromboembolism (VTE) in cancer.

Clinical Aspects: Thrombosis and Bleeding

Thrombosis

Although clinically manifest thrombosis in patients with cancer can involve both the venous and arterial systems, thrombotic occlusions of the venous site have been more extensively studied (Figure 25.1). VTE represents an important cause of morbidity and mortality in these patients

[10–12]. Epidemiological data clearly show that patients with cancer have a significantly increased risk of clinically overt thrombosis upon triggering conditions (e.g., long-term bed rest, trauma, surgery), as compared to patients without malignancy. Medical treatments to cure cancer can worsen the patient's thrombophilic state and increase the thrombotic risk associated with this disease.

Thromboembolic manifestations occurring in cancer include:

- venous thrombosis,
- arterial thrombosis,
- nonbacterial thrombotic endocarditis (NBTE),
- thrombotic microangiopathy (TMA),
- veno-occlusive disease (VOD).

Venous Thrombosis

The most common manifestation of venous thrombotic disease is represented by deep vein thrombosis (DVT) of the lower limbs, followed by upper-limb DVT, pulmonary embolism (PE),

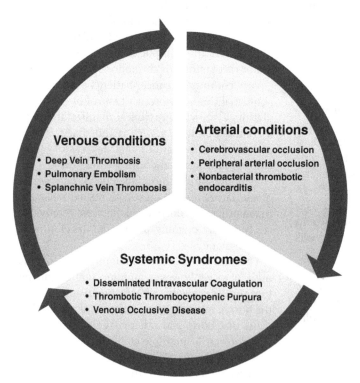

Figure 25.1 Thrombotic disorders associated with cancer. Clinical manifestations of thrombosis in patients with cancer can vary from localized deep venous thrombosis, more frequent in solid tumors, to systemic syndrome, such as disseminated intravascular coagulation (DIC) with consumption of coagulation factors and platelets, which is generally associated to leukemias or widespread metastatic cancer.

Venous conditions
- Deep Vein Thrombosis
- Pulmonary Embolism
- Splanchnic Vein Thrombosis

Arterial conditions
- Cerebrovascular occlusion
- Peripheral arterial occlusion
- Nonbacterial thrombotic endocarditis

Systemic Syndromes
- Disseminated Intravascular Coagulation
- Thrombotic Thrombocytopenic Purpura
- Venous Occlusive Disease

cerebral sinus thrombosis, and migratory superficial thrombophlebitis. Large retrospective and prospective population studies show an overall VTE incidence ranging from 0.6% up to 7.8% [13]. This wide range is due to the presence of many and different factors that contribute to the global VTE risk, the most important being the cancer type [13]. In patients with myeloproliferative neoplasms (MPN), an unusual high prevalence of splanchnic (i.e., Budd–Chiari syndrome and portal vein thrombosis) and cerebral vein thrombosis is reported, and these events are often the presenting feature of the disease, before diagnosis [14].

Arterial Thrombosis

In contrast to VTE, limited data are available on arterial thromboembolic events (ATE) in malignant disease [15,16]. A variety of arterial thrombotic syndromes have been reported in cancer patients and the sites most commonly involved are the peripheral blood circulation of upper and lower extremities and cerebral vessels [17]. The mesenteric vessels, kidney, and liver represent unusual sites of ATE. Nevertheless, ATE incidence in cancer is estimated to be around 2–5%, accounting for 10–30% of total thrombotic complications. According to a retrospective analysis in ambulatory cancer patients receiving chemotherapy, the incidence of symptomatic ATE was 0.27% [16]. In patients with MPN, ATE is a frequent complication, accounting for 60–70% of the thrombotic events, and includes ischemic stroke, acute myocardial infarction, and peripheral arterial occlusion. Typical of MPN, but not exclusive, is the involvement of microcirculation, leading to erythromelalgia, transient ischemic attacks, visual or hearing transitory defects, recurrent headache, and peripheral paresthesia. NBTE is particularly common in MPN but can also be observed in solid tumors. NBTE, detected in 0.9–1.3% of patients dying of cancer, is the cardiac manifestation of systemic hemostatic activation resulting in the formation of platelet and fibrin vegetations on cardiac valves [15]. These vegetations can cause ATE after dislodgement, leading to strokes, splenic infarctions, and acute limb ischemia.

Thrombotic Microangiopathies

TMA in cancer is a rare but severe complication with a short-term life-threatening prognosis, characterized by:

- microangiopathic hemolytic anemia;
- peripheral thrombocytopenia;
- organ failure of variable severity;
- activity of ADAMTS-13 normal or mildly decreased.

TMA may be observed in patients with disseminated adenocarcinomas. Furthermore, it has been described in association with the use of specific chemotherapeutic agents, particularly mitomycin, gemcitabine, and, recently, with some targeted cancer agents, (i.e., immunotoxins, monoclonal antibodies, and tyrosine kinase inhibitors) [18].

The pathogenesis of cancer-associated TMA involves:

- the formation of microscopic tumor embolisms that activate coagulation and intimal proliferation in arterioles, causing severe lumen reduction leading to microangiopathy;
- the production of mucin and tumor necrosis factor-α (TNF-α) by tumor cells that can favor vasoconstriction and endothelial cell apoptosis.

Cancer-associated TMA displays typical features at presentation, which should alert clinicians of the possibility of an underlying malignancy in a patient with a newly diagnosed TMA. [19]. Plasma exchange, the treatment of choice for primary thrombotic thrombocytopenic purpura (TTP), does not have much benefit in cancer-related TMA. The optimal therapy for cancer-associated TMA is unknown but there is evidence that immediate initiation of an effective antineoplastic regimen is important.

Venous Occlusive Disease

VOD is a serious liver disease characterized by obstruction of small intrahepatic central venules by microthrombi and fibrin deposition [20], and is observed in approximately 50–60% of allogeneic hematopoietic stem cell transplanted patients. In the severe form, VOD is associated with a mortality rate close to 85%, as a consequence of multiorgan failure. Risk factors for VOD include hepatic damage, high-dose chemotherapy (i.e., cyclophosphamide, busulfan), abdominal irradiation, female gender, and donor–recipient HLA disparity. The deoxyribonucleic acid derivative defibrotide has proven successfully for the prevention and treatment of VOD [21]; the underlying mechanisms of action include a protective role of this drug on the microvascular endothelium, as suggested by *in vitro* studies [22].

Bleeding

Abnormal bleeding represents an important cause of mortality in cancer, and is observed in about 10% of patients with solid tumors and in a higher proportion of patients with hematological malignancies [23].

Bleeding manifestations include:

- melena,
- hematuria,
- hematemesis,
- hematochezia,
- hemoptysis,
- epistaxis,
- vaginal bleeding,
- ulcerated skin lesions.
- ecchymoses, petechiae, bruising.

Hemorrhage may occur as an acute catastrophic event, episodic major bleeds, or an ongoing low-degree emission.

Potential causes of bleeding are:

- thrombocytopenia,
- decreased synthesis of coagulation factors due to liver dysfunction or vitamin K deficiency,
- oral anticoagulation,
- pre-existing mild coagulation factor deficiencies,
- congenital von Willebrand disease,
- vessel wall erosion,
- DIC,
- acquired inhibitors against blood clotting factors.

Severe DIC is particularly associated with acute leukemia, causing a severe hemorrhage secondary to an excessive consumption of clotting factors and platelets. Intracerebral and pulmonary hemorrhages are relatively common life-threatening complications in acute promyelocytic leukemia (APL), and are the most frequent cause of early death during induction therapy, although they can also occur before APL diagnosis and therapy start. APL patients with concomitant risk factors have a higher risk of developing fatal hemorrhage [24]. Finally, acquired hemophilia is a rare but life-threatening bleeding complication caused by the development of autoantibodies directed against plasma coagulation factors, most frequently factor VIII (i.e., acquired hemophilia A). Because acquired hemophilia can result in significant morbidity and mortality, the differential diagnosis when evaluating the cancer patient with unexplained bleeding should always be considered [23].

Occult Malignancy

Thrombosis can represent the earliest clinical manifestation of an occult cancer [25,26]. Indeed, patients with "idiopathic" VTE have a four- to sevenfold increased risk of being diagnosed with cancer in the first year after thrombosis, as compared to patients with VTE secondary to known causes (e.g., surgery, congenital thrombophilia, oral contraceptives, pregnancy, and immobilization) [27]. In patients with recurrent VTE and in those with bilateral VTE, the risk of cancer is further raised by up to 10-fold. A large population-based study identified the types of cancers most commonly preceded by VTE in the year before diagnosis to be: acute myelogenous leukemia; non-Hodgkin lymphoma; and renal cell, ovarian, pancreatic, stomach, and lung cancers [28]. In spite of this evidence, the question as to whether extensive screening for occult malignancy in patients with idiopathic VTE may lead to improved management of the disease is still standing.

In the prospective multicenter study Screening for Occult Malignancy in patients with venous Thromboembolism (SOMIT), extensive screening was effective in identifying precociously an occult malignancy [29]. Computed tomography (CT) scanning of the abdomen and pelvis was the most effective diagnostic test, and CT scan and a gastrointestinal investigation (such as hemoccult) was the best diagnostic combination. A cost analysis of the different screening strategies of the SOMIT study (in relation to the expected life years gained) showed that some of these approaches may be cost effective [30]. Finally, a prospective cohort follow-up study of 864 consecutive patients with acute VTE [31] suggested that a limited diagnostic work-up (i.e., abdominal and pelvic ultrasound and laboratory markers for malignancy) may have the capacity to identify approximately one-half of the malignancies in patients who were negative on routine clinical evaluation. In most of the cases the malignancies identified by extensive screening are at an early stage, therefore larger clinical trials to establish the impact of this finding on cancer prognosis are warranted.

The hypercoagulable State of Patients with Malignancy

Even in the absence of DIC or manifest thrombosis and before any antitumor therapy, test in cancer patients show several laboratory abnormalities of hemostasis, demonstrating an ongoing hypercoagulable condition [9,32].

Routine Laboratory Tests

The most frequent routine abnormalities reported in cancer are:

- elevated of plasma coagulation factor levels (i.e., fibrinogen, factors V, VIII, IX, and X);
- increased levels of fibrin(ogen) degradation products (FDP, or D-dimers);
- thrombocytosis.

Two large prospective clinical trials evaluating these parameters in cancer patients [11] showed that:

- FDP levels and thrombin time were increased in 8% and 14% of cases, respectively.

- Fibrinogen and platelet count were found more frequently elevated (48% and 36% of the cases, respectively).
- The increase in the levels of these two markers over time directly correlated with the disease progression.

Specialized Tests

More sensitive laboratory tests for the detection of the hypercoagulable state or subclinical DIC (listed in Table 25.1) enable the detection of ongoing activation of blood coagulation *in vivo*. These tests measure the final products of clotting reactions in plasma and include:

- peptides released during the proteolytic activation of proenzymes into active clotting enzymes (i.e., prothrombin fragment 1+2 (F1+2), protein C activation fragment, factor IX and X activation fragments, fibrinopeptide A);
- enzyme–inhibitor complexes produced during the activation of the coagulation and fibrinolytic systems (i.e., thrombin–antithrombin complexes (TAT), plasmin–antiplasmin complexes (PAP));
- cross-linked degradation product (i.e., D-dimer);
- cell membrane-associated markers to study the activation of cellular components of the hemostatic system, including platelets, leukocytes, and endothelial cells.

Studies on the plasma levels of these markers have provided a biochemical definition of the hypercoagulable state in humans.

Although specific assays of coagulation factors are essential for diagnostic purposes, they only give partial information about an individual's hemostatic state. This can be better assessed by various global tests, the most promising being thrombin generation and thromboelastography/thromboelastometry. Standardization of these tests is rapidly progressing, and they are increasingly entering the clinical scene, with the aim of providing additional information on the coagulation process and a meaningful clinical correlation.

Table 25.1 Circulating markers of hemostatic system activation.

Coagulation
   Activated factor VII (FVIIa)
   Thrombin–antithrombin complex (TAT)
   Prothrombin fragment 1+2 (F1+2)
   Fibrinopeptide A and B
Fibrinolysis
   Tissue plasminogen activator (t-PA)
   Plasminogen activator inhibitor-1 (PAI-1)
   Plasminogen
   Plasmin–antiplasmin complex (PAP)
   Fibrin degradation products (FDPs)
   Soluble fibrin
   D-Dimer
Platelets
   β-Thromboglobulin
   Platelet factor 4 (PF4)
   Thromboxane A2 (TxA2)
   Soluble P-selectin
   Membrane P-selectin, CD63
Leukocytes
   Monocytes
      Membrane tissue factor (mTF)
      s-Tissue factor
   Neutrophils
      Membrane CD11b
      ELASTASE
      myeloperoxidase
Endothelium
   Thrombomodulin
   Von Willebrand Factor (VWF)
   t-PA
   PAI-1
   s-E-Selectin
   s-VCAM-1 and s-ICAM-1
   Tissue factor pathway inhibitor (TFPI)

Predictors of Thrombosis

Until recently, only a few prospective studies had evaluated the utility of serial measurements of hemostatic markers for predicting the occurrence of VTE (as confirmed by objective test) in cancer patients. In one of these studies, Falanga *et al.* found that presurgical TAT complex levels were significant predictors of postoperative DVT [33] in patients undergoing surgery for abdominal cancer.

Current research is focusing on a number of biomarkers that may be helpful in identifying cancer patients who are at higher risk of developing DVT and might benefit from primary thromboprophylaxis. Emerging biomarkers are:

- platelet count,
- leukocyte count,
- D-dimer,
- tissue factor (TF),
- P-selectin,
- plasma microparticles.

A prechemotherapy platelet count greater than 350 000 platelet/μL was predictive of subsequent thrombosis during chemotherapy [7]. The inclusion of D-dimer and soluble P-selectin together with clinical parameters in a validated risk assessment model increased the capacity to predict VTE [34,35].

Plasma microparticles are circulating, submicrometric membrane vesicles originating from vascular cells and carrying on their surface TF, adhesive molecules, and procoagulant phospholipids. A study by Toth and colleagues showed that levels of microparticles of platelet origin are elevated in patients with breast cancer compared to patients with benign breast lesions [36]. Patients with essential thrombocythemia, a myeloproliferative neoplasm characterized by high risk of thrombosis, displayed increased levels of circulating microparticles of platelet and endothelial cell origin, particularly in those with additional risk factors for thrombosis [37]. The detection of microparticle levels has been developed recently as a tool to select a high-risk cancer population in a clinical trial to test the efficacy of primary thromboprophylaxis during chemotherapy [38].

Risk Stratification Models

The pretreatment assessment of VTE in cancer is difficult due to the complexity of the interaction and relative effects of each risk factor. In recent years, several demographic, cancer-associated, and treatment-related factors known to increase the risk of thrombosis in cancer have been identified (Figure 25.2). The combination of some of these clinical factors and laboratory biomarkers allowed the development, by Khorana *et al.*, of a VTE risk assessment model specifically for cancer patients undergoing

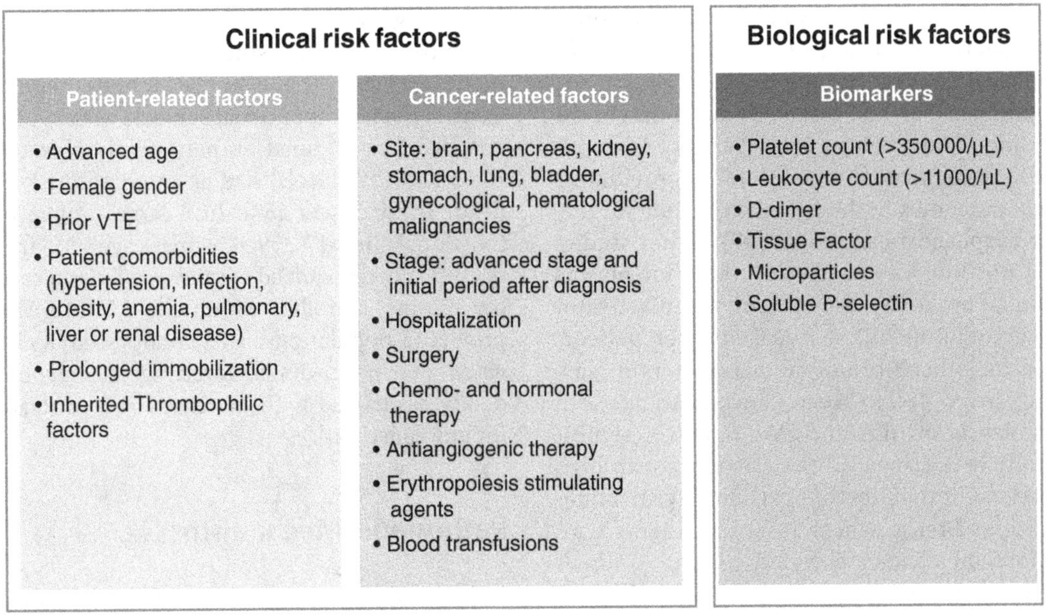

Clinical risk factors		Biological risk factors
Patient-related factors	**Cancer-related factors**	**Biomarkers**
• Advanced age • Female gender • Prior VTE • Patient comorbidities (hypertension, infection, obesity, anemia, pulmonary, liver or renal disease) • Prolonged immobilization • Inherited Thrombophilic factors	• Site: brain, pancreas, kidney, stomach, lung, bladder, gynecological, hematological malignancies • Stage: advanced stage and initial period after diagnosis • Hospitalization • Surgery • Chemo- and hormonal therapy • Antiangiogenic therapy • Erythropoiesis stimulating agents • Blood transfusions	• Platelet count (>350000/μL) • Leukocyte count (>11000/μL) • D-dimer • Tissue Factor • Microparticles • Soluble P-selectin

Figure 25.2 Risk factors for cancer-associated thrombosis. Several clinical and biological factors can contribute to thrombotic risk in cancer patients, these include their demographic characteristics, site and stage of cancer, anti-cancer therapies (including surgery), hospitalization and biomarkers. VTE, venous thromboembolism.

chemotherapy [39]. This risk assessment model is based on five predictive variables:

1) cancer site (very high risk: stomach and pancreas; high risk: lung, lymphoma, gynecological, bladder, and testicular);
2) prechemotherapy platelet count of ≥350 × 10^9/L;
3) hemoglobin levels <100 g/L (or the use of erythropoiesis-stimulating agents);
4) prechemotherapy leukocyte count >11 × 10^9/L;
5) body mass index ≥35 kg/m^2

This model using a simple scoring system, based on readily accessible baseline clinical and laboratory data, and has been shown to accurately predict the short-term risk of symptomatic VTE in patients undergoing chemotherapy-based treatments. The Khorana score has been validated in both prospective and retrospective observational studies [40–43]. In the Vienna Cancer and Thrombosis Study (CATS) the score was expanded by adding two biomarkers (P-selectin and D-dimer), and the prediction

of VTE was considerably improved [40]. A modified Khorana's risk assessment score (the Protecht score) has been designed by adding platinum- or gemcitabine-based chemotherapy to the five predictive variables for identifying high-risk cancer patients in a *post hoc* analysis of the Protecht study [43]. In the setting of multiple myeloma, Palumbo *et al.* published a risk assessment model, based on expert recommendation statements, for the prevention of thalidomide and lenalidomide-associated thrombosis in this disease [44].

The availability of predictive models will allow the possibility of improving outcomes for chemotherapy patients by identifying those who would benefit most from thromboprophylaxis.

Predictors of Survival

A number of studies have been conducted with the aim of defining the predictive value of thrombotic markers for survival of cancer patients. In consecutive outpatients with different types of cancer, baseline TAT, fibrin monomer, and D-dimer levels were predictive for survival at 1 and 3 years [45]. Other small prospective studies have focused on specific types of cancer. Among these, a prognostic significance of TAT and PAP was found in the setting of lung cancer [46]. Plasma PAP levels were recognized to be useful in predicting fatal outcomes in the first 5 days after surgery for esophageal carcinoma [47]. Other studies did not find any predictive value for plasma soluble urokinase-type plasminogen activator receptor (s-uPAR) in breast cancer patients and for other fibrinolytic parameters in gastric cancer [48]. In breast cancer, patients with low levels of uPA and PAI-1 have a significantly better survival than patients with high levels of either factor, particularly in node-negative breast cancer [49]. In patients with colorectal cancer, elevated plasma D-dimer levels before surgery predicted a significantly shorter postoperative survival [50]. Similarly, in the same type of cancer, D-dimer levels were better predictors of overall survival and disease progression than carcinoembryonic antigen [51]. D-dimer measured in preoperative plasma samples from 95 patients with ovarian masses (75 benign, 20 malignant) alone differentiated malignant from benign ovarian tumors and also improved when combined with CA-125 [52].

An attempt has been made to establish whether the presence of persistent biochemical hypercoagulabilty in healthy men may predict death from cancer. A study conducted on 3052 men from the UK National Health Service Central Registry found that subjects with hypercoagulability (defined as persistently elevated F1+2 and FPA levels) had an increased risk of death from cancer [53]. In a large sample of individuals (n = 17 359, 47% men, age ≥35) free of clinically recognized cardiovascular and cancer disease, enrolled within the MOLI-SANI project (a population-based cohort study), elevated plasma D-dimer levels were independently associated with increased risk of death for any cause [54].

Pathogenic Mechanisms

The pathogenesis of the coagulation system imbalance in cancer is complex and involves multiple factors, both clinical and biological [1,9]. General mechanisms related to the host response to the tumor include the acute-phase reaction, paraprotein production, inflammation, necrosis, and hemodynamic disorders, whereas tumor-specific clot-promoting mechanisms include a series of prothrombotic properties expressed by tumor cells. In addition, an important role in cancer-related thrombosis is played by the procoagulant effects triggered by anticancer therapies (Figure 25.3).

Figure 25.3 Mechanisms for activation of blood coagulation and thrombotic diathesis in patients with cancer. Even in the absence of overt clinical symptoms, almost all patients present with laboratory coagulation abnormalities, demonstrating a subclinical activation of blood coagulation, which characterizes a "hypercoagulable state." Multiple factors (i.e., general, tumor-specific and antitumor therapy-related) concur to the activation of blood coagulation and to thrombotic manifestation in cancer patients.

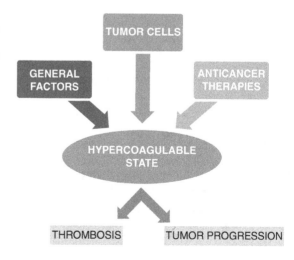

Clinical Factors

Clinical risk factors can be classified in three main categories:

1) patient's characteristics,
2) cancer-related features,
3) type of anticancer therapies.

The first category includes many risk factors that are not exclusive but are frequent amongst cancer patients. These include as advanced age, prolonged immobility, a prior history of thrombosis, high leukocyte and platelet counts, obesity, immobility, and also comorbid conditions such as heart disease, acute infection, and respiratory disease [5,55–57].

Considering the second category, large epidemiological studies have recognized malignant brain tumors, hematological malignancies, and adenocarcinoma of pancreas, stomach, ovary, uterus, lung, and kidney as having the highest VTE risk [58]. Among hematological malignancies, multiple myeloma, non-Hodgkin's lymphoma, and Hodgkin's disease showed the highest VTE incidence [59]. Moreover, advanced, metastatic cancer has been shown to be associated with an increased risk of VTE compared to localized tumors [58].

Last, active anticancer treatments, including chemotherapy, hormonal therapy, antiangiogenic agents, combination regimens, and surgery have a prothrombotic effect [60]. The direct injury of endothelial cells by chemotherapeutic agents, or by tumor-derived products, leading to a loss of antithrombotic properties, is thought to play a role in the increased VTE risk. In addition, an important finding is the elevation in expression of TF and/or phosphatidylserine exposure and the release of microparticles caused by different chemotherapeutic agents [61]. The development of several novel anticancer agents carrying a thrombogenic effect brings this issue to the forefront of cancer medicine.

Biological Factors

Tumor Cell Prothrombotic Mechanisms

In addition to the usual host risk factors for thrombosis, a number of biological pathways

Table 25.2 Tumor cell prothrombotic properties.

Expression of procoagulants that directly activate coagulation:
Tissue factor
Cancer procoagulant
Heparanase
Release of proinflammatory and proangiogenic cytokines that stimulate the prothrombotic potential of endothelial cells:
IL-1β, TNF-α, VEGF, FGF
Expression of fibrinolytic proteins:
t-PA, u-PA, PAI-1, PAI-2, uPAR
Expression of adhesion molecules for host vascular cells:
Integrins, selectins, immunoglobulin family

likely play an important role in the pathogenesis of hemostatic alterations in cancer [9]. Cancer cells can interact with and activate the hemostatic system through (Table 25.2):

- expression of procoagulant proteins,
- production of microparticles,
- release of inflammatory cytokines,
- adhesion to host vascular cells.

In the last decade, molecular studies of experimental models of human cancer have demonstrated the role of oncogene and repressor gene-mediated neoplastic transformation in activating clotting as an integral feature of neoplastic transformation [41] (Figure 25.4). Specifically, targeting activated human MET to the mouse liver, with a lentiviral vector, determined progressive hepatocarcinogenesis, preceded and accompanied by a thrombohemorrhagic syndrome (i.e., venous thrombosis in tail vein and fatal internal hemorrhage) and laboratory signs of DIC. Genome-wide expression profiling of hepatocytes expressing MET showed upregulation of PAI-1 and COX-2 genes with a two- to threefold increase in circulating protein levels [2]. In an *in vitro* model of human glioma cells, the loss of the tumor suppressor gene *PTEN* upregulated the expression TF and increased the levels of plasma clotting proteins [3]. Finally, in human colorectal cancer cells, TF expression was shown to be under the control of two major transforming events

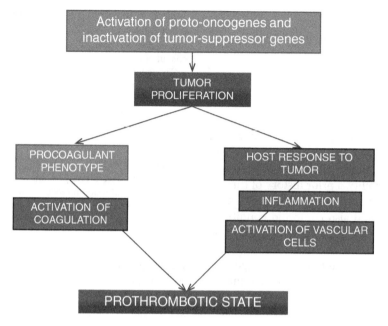

Figure 25.4 Experimental and clinical studies with molecularly well-defined types of cancer cells reveal how oncogenic events may deregulate the hemostatic system. Activated oncogenes (K-ras, EGFR, PML-RARa, and MET) or inactivated tumor suppressors (p53 or PTEN) lead to an induction of procoagulant activity and inhibition of fibrinolysis, which is postulated to promote not only hypercoagulability but tumor aggressiveness and angiogenesis.

driving disease progression: the activation of *K-ras* oncogene and the inactivation of the *p53* tumor suppressor [4].

Procoagulant Activities

Tumor cells may express different types of procoagulants, the best characterized of which are:

- TF,
- cancer procoagulant (CP).

Other tumor cell procoagulant activities are:

- heparanase;
- factor V receptor, which facilitates the assembly of prothrombinase complex; and
- factor XIII-like activity that promotes the cross-linking of fibrin.

The best characterized tumor procoagulant is TF. It is constitutively expressed on malignant cell surface, and can lead to the formation of both localized as well as systemic procoagulant states. TF activity on tumor cells can be potentiated by the expression of anionic phospholipids (i.e., phosphatidylserine) on the outer leaflet of the cell membrane [62,63] and the secretion of heparanase. The main function of heparanase is to degrade heparan sulfates of extracellular matrix, thereby promoting tumor invasion and metastasis. However, heparanase can also interact with TF pathway inhibitor (TFPI) on the cell surface, leading to dissociation of TFPI from the cell membrane of endothelial and tumor cells, which results in an increased cell surface TF activity [64]. Studies suggest an additional role for TF in tumor growth and metastasis, which is not entirely mediated via clotting activation, but may be dependent on signaling through the cytoplasmic domain, suggesting a "noncoagulant" role for TF in cancer disease [65].

Another tumor procoagulant is cancer procoagulant (CP), a cysteine proteinase that, unlike TF, directly activates FX independently of FVII. CP has been detected in various tumor cells and in amnion-chorion tissues but not in normally differentiated cells. In patients with APL, CP, expressed by bone marrow blast cells at the onset of disease, disappears when remission is reached [66]. Similar observations have been reported for breast cancer.

Specific assays for detection of TF, heparanase, and CP have been developed, but which is the most sensitive and accurate method to measure each procoagulant is still matter of standardization. On the other hand, specific assays provide only partial information on the overall cellular procoagulant potential, a problem that can be overcome by the use of global hemostatic assays. Among these, the thrombin generation assay (i.e., Calibrated Automated Thrombogram) seems to be very sensitive in detecting cell-associated TF, as well as other cell-associated procoagulant mechanisms (i.e., contact activation) when performed in the appropriate experimental conditions [67,68].

Microparticles

Microparticles are plasma membrane vesicles, 0.1–1 μm in diameter, produced by active vesiculation of virtually all type of cells, and are characterized by the presence on their surface of a very high concentration of phosphatidylserine [69]. Phosphatidylserine expressed on microparticle surfaces provide a suitable anionic phospholipid surface for assembly of tenase and prothrombinase complexes of blood coagulation, thereby promoting the coagulation cascade. This capacity can be further enhanced by the concomitant expression of TF. Low plasma microparticle levels are present in healthy subjects, the majority being of platelet origin (>80%), but in pathological conditions an overall increment in microparticles occurs and significant amounts of microparticles of other vascular sources, including tumor cells, can be detected. Elevated levels of circulating microparticles (with or without TF) have been described in patients with solid tumors [69]. Microparticles of platelet origin were found to be higher in stage IV versus I and II/III gastric cancer, showing the highest diagnostic accuracy for metastasis prediction [70]. High microparticle levels have been also detected in hematological cancer, including acute leukemia, multiple myeloma [71,72], and essential thrombocythemia [37]. Finally, the pathogenetic role of microparticles in cancer-associated thrombosis has been demonstrated by the development of a DIC-like syndrome in mice after intravenous injection of highly TF-positive microparticles of tumor origin [69].

Fibrinolytic Activities

Tumor cells are also capable of interacting with the host fibrinolytic system, due to the expression of plasminogen activators (uPA and t-PA), their inhibitors (PAI-1 and PAI-2) and receptors such as uPAR [66], and of annexin II, a coreceptor for plasminogen and tissue plasminogen activator (tPA). In APL, the increased expression of annexin II has been linked to an excessive activation of fibrinolysis [73]. It can be hypothesized that, depending on whether pro- or antifibrinolytic prevails, the clinical manifestations of fibrinolysis system alterations may be quite different, from bleeding symptoms as observed in leukemia, to VTE evidenced in solid tumors. Fibrinolysis is also a key component in tumor biology, as it is essential in releasing tumor cells from their primary site of origin, in neoangiogenesis, and in promoting cell mobility and motility.

Inflammatory Cytokines

Tumor cells synthesize and release a variety of proinflammatory cytokines (i.e., TNF-α, IL-1β) and proangiogenic factors (vascular endothelial growth factor (VEGF), basic fibroblast growth factor (bFGF)), which can act on the different hemostatic cells and affect their antithrombotic status.

Downregulation of Anticoagulant Activity: Proinflammatory cytokines can downregulate the expression of thrombomodulin, a potent anticoagulant, expressed by endothelial cell.

Increased Fibrinolysis: The same cytokines stimulate endothelial cells to increase the production of the fibrinolysis inhibitor PAI-1, resulting in a subsequent inhibition of fibrinolysis, which further contributes to the prothrombotic potential of endothelial cells.

Cell–Cell Adhesion: Cytokines contribute to enhance the adhesion potential of the vascular wall, by increasing the expression of surface adhesion molecules of endothelial cells, which become more capable of attracting tumor cells and supporting their extravasation.

Procoagulant Properties: Further, tumor cell cytokines can induce the expression of TF by monocytes and endothelial cells. Tumor-associated macrophages harvested from experimental and human tumors express significantly more TF than control cells. In addition, circulating monocytes from patient with different types of cancer have been shown to express increased TF activity. The upregulation TF together with the downregulation of thrombomodulin lead to a prothrombotic condition of the vascular wall.

Recruitment of White Cells: Tumor cytokines are also mitogenic and/or chemoattractants for polymorphonuclear leukocytes. These cells, upon activation, secrete proteolytic enzymes, which can damage the endothelial monolayer, and produce additional cytokines and chemokines, which support tumor growth, stimulate angiogenesis, and enable metastatic spread via engagement with either venous or lymphatic networks.

Tumor Cell Adhesion Molecules

The tumor cell's capacity to adhere to the endothelium and the underlying matrix is well described and adhesion molecule pathways specific to different tumor cell types have been identified. The relevance of the tight interaction of tumor cells with endothelial cells in the pathogenesis of thrombosis in cancer is related to the localized promotion of clotting activation and thrombus formation. The tumor cell attached to endothelium can release its cytokine content into a protected milieu that favors their prothrombotic and proangiogenic activities. In addition, the adhesion of tumor cells to leukocytes or vascular cells represents the first step in cell migration and extravasation.

Platelets

Similarly to leukocytes, clinical and experimental evidence suggests the importance of platelets in tumor cell dissemination via the bloodstream. Platelets can facilitate tumor cell adhesion and migration through the vessel wall by a variety of mechanisms, including bridging between tumor cells and endothelial cells, and by allowing migration of tumor cells through the endothelial cell matrix by heparanase activity. Tumor cells can activate platelets directly or through the release of proaggregatory mediators including ADP, thrombin, and a cathepsin-like cysteine protease. Upon activation, platelets aggregate and release their granule contents, as shown by the detection of elevated plasma levels of β-thromboglobulin and PF4, and of increased platelet membrane activation markers, such as P-selectin (CD62P) and CD63, in patients with malignancy.

In addition, activated platelets release VEGF and platelet-derived growth factor (PDGF), which play an important part in the tumor neo-angiogenesis process.

Antitumor Therapy Prothrombotic Mechanisms

The pathogenesis of thrombosis during antitumor therapies is not entirely understood, but a number of mechanisms have been identified (Table 25.3) [74]. The first mechanism is caused by the release of procoagulants and cytokines by tumor cells damaged by chemotherapy. The possible role of cytokine release in response to chemotherapy in increasing the thrombotic risk was suggested by experiments showing that plasma samples collected from women with breast cancer after chemotherapy contained higher levels of mediators (likely cytokines) able

Table 25.3 Antitumor therapy prothrombotic mechanisms.

Release of procoagulant activities and cytokines from damaged cells
Direct drug toxicity on vascular endothelium
Induction of monocyte tissue factor
Decrease of physiological anticoagulants (protein C, proteins S, antithrombin)
Apoptosis

to increase the reactivity of endothelial cells to platelets [75]. The direct damage exerted by chemoradiotherapy on vascular endothelium represents another mechanism of drug-induced thrombosis (Figure 25.5) [75]. Radiation therapy can cause endothelial injury, as demonstrated by the release of von Willebrand protein from endothelial cells irradiated with doses up to 40 Gy. In animal studies, bleomycin has been demonstrated to determine morphological damage to the vascular endothelium of the lung, resulting in pulmonary thrombosis and fibrosis [76]. In some experimental models, adriamycin was shown to directly affect glomerular cells, impairing their permeability and leading to a nephrotic syndrome, accompanied by hypercoagulation and increased thrombotic tendency.

Antiangiogenetic drugs, such as thalidomide and lenalidomide, and the anti-VEGF receptor SU5416, represent a new class of substances

with endothelial toxic activity [44,77]. A significant increase in circulating markers of endothelial cell activation has been observed in cancer patients during antiangiogenic therapy with SU5416, particularly in those patients experiencing a thromboembolic event [78]. Direct cause–effect relationship between treatment with L-asparaginase, an enzyme used in the treatment of acute lymphoblastic leukemia, and increased thrombogenic risk have been reported [9,79]. High-dose corticosteroids, which are sometimes given to cancer patients to counteract the nausea associated with chemotherapy, are by themselves associated with a 3.5-fold increase in the odds of developing VTE [80].

Profound changes in the plasma markers of endothelial damage have been reported in patients receiving different types of chemotherapy. Some chemotherapeutic agents can

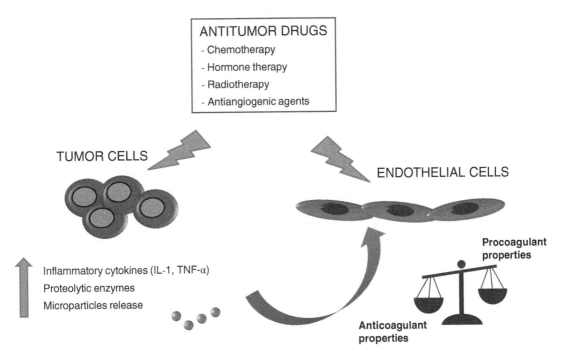

Figure 25.5 Antitumor therapy prothrombotic mechanisms. Tumor cells perturbed by antitumor drugs release a series of soluble mediators (proinflammatoy and proangiogenic cytokines, proteolytic enzymes), which can act on endothelial cells by altering their normal antithrombotic and antiadhesive status or by damaging the endothelial monolayer, with the subsequent exposure of the highly procoagulant endothelial cell matrix. The same antitumor drugs can upregulate the expression of adhesion molecules by tumor cells which become much adhesive towards the endothelium.

directly stimulate the expression of TF procoagulant activity by macrophages and monocytes, thus inducing a procoagulant response from host cells. An elevation in the expression of procoagulant TF and/or phosphatidylserine exposure and the release of microparticles has been observed after treatment with cisplatin or gemcitabine [81], cyclophosphamide [82], doxorubicin and epirubicin [83–85], and daunorubicin [86]. The final mechanism observed involves a reduction in the plasma levels of natural anticoagulant proteins (antithrombin, protein C, and protein S), which is a well-known risk factor for thrombosis, and is likely to be a consequence of a direct hepatotoxicity by radio- and chemotherapy.

Prevention and Treatment of Thrombosis and Bleeding in Cancer

Primary Thromboprophylaxis

In regard to arterial thrombosis, cancer patients share the same general risk factors with noncancer patients (i.e., arterial hypertension, diabetes, dyslipidemia, obesity); additional risk factors are comorbidities including pulmonary and renal disease, infection, blood transfusion, and chemotherapy. Older age (>60 years) and previous thrombosis are well-established cardiovascular risk factors for thrombosis in MPN, which identify the so-called high-risk patients. The impact of newly recognized risk factors, such as leukocytosis and JAK2V617F mutational status and/or mutational burden, are under active investigation [87]. Today, no guidelines or recommendations are available for ATE prophylaxis in the cancer setting. An exception is MPN, in which aspirin, in association or not with hydroxyurea, anagrelide, and/or phlebotomy, has proven to reduce significantly the risk of cardiovascular events [88].

More certainty is available for VTE primary prophylaxis. Thromboprophylaxis with either unfractionated heparin or low molecular weight heparin (LMWH) has been shown to be safe

Table 25.4 Risk of venous thromboembolism in cancer patients undergoing surgery.

Type of surgery	Risk (%)
General	29
Gynecological	20
Urological	41
Orthopedic	50–60
Neurosurgery	28

Source: modified from Clagett and Reisch 1988 [89].

and effective in high-risk settings such as hospitalization for medical illness and the postsurgical period.

Patients with diagnosed malignant disease are at an increased risk of developing "secondary" VTE in specific conditions (e.g., surgery, immobilization) (Table 25.4). These patients have been stratified by the Consensus Conference of the American College of Chest Physicians (ACCP) in their highest risk category for developing "secondary" VTE [90]. In addition, the risk of recurrences is significantly increased in cancer compared with noncancer patients, even during treatments for VTE [56]. There is no evidence that there is a benefit from antithrombotic prophylaxis for all cancer patients; however, there are selected conditions in which prophylaxis has to be considered, such as surgical interventions, acute medical illness, and administration of antitumor therapies [91].

Cancer Surgery

Cancer surgery carries a two- to threefold increased thrombotic risk compared to noncancer surgery of equal intensity. Current European and American guidelines found a high level of consensus on VTE prevention with LMWH in the surgical oncology setting [92–96], particularly in "high-risk" cancer patients undergoing major abdominal or pelvic surgery [97,98].

A higher dose of LMWH has been shown to be more effective than a lower dose in surgical cancer patients, without increasing the hemorrhagic risk [99]. This is of particular relevance as cancer patients are also at high risk of bleeding.

Table 25.5 Prolonged prophylaxis with low molecular weight heparin in surgical cancer patients.

Study	Cancer patients n (%)	Prophylaxis	Major bleeding	Venous thromboembolism incidence
ENOXACAN II Bergqvist *et al.* 2002 [97]	332 (100%)	Enoxaparin vs. placebo for: 19–21 days 6–10 days	0.4% 0%	4.8% 12%
FAME Rasmussen *et al.* 2006 [100]	198 (58%)	Dalteparin vs. no prophylaxis for: 4 weeks 1 week	0% 0%	8.8% 19.6%

A prolonged postoperative prophylaxis up to 1 month after surgery for cancer can add a benefit to reduce the rate of postoperative VTE, as demonstrated by two large clinical trials in cancer patients undergoing abdominal or pelvic surgery [97,100] (Table 25.5).

Medical Conditions

The international consensus is lower in the medical setting, in which two high-risk situations can be identified:

- patients hospitalized or bedridden for prolonged periods of time;
- ambulatory patients receiving chemotherapy or radiation.

Cancer patients hospitalized for an acute medical illness are at risk for thrombosis. They should be considered for thromboprophylaxis with prophylactic doses of LMWH or fondaparinux, but the duration of thromboprophylaxis is undefined.

Although most VTE occurs in the outpatients setting, the guideline panels agree on not recommending routine thromboprophylaxis in ambulatory cancer patients. However, many RCTs have been designed in recent years to evaluate the impact of thromboprophylaxis in ambulatory patients with solid tumors receiving systemic chemotherapy [101–103]. Overall, these studies suggest that outpatient thromboprophylaxis is feasible, safe, and effective. Notably, a low VTE rate is observed in these

studies, which suggests the importance of patient selection by avoiding a wide application of prophylaxis. Thus, the most recent guidelines of the National Comprehensive Cancer Network emphasize the need for VTE risk assessment in ambulatory cancer patients and the need of RCT for patients with a favorable risk–benefit ratio [104]. Other areas of uncertainty include prophylaxis in patients who must receive chemo- radio- or hormone therapy and have a history of VTE, patients with cerebral cancer, patients undergoing surgery other than abdominal or pelvic procedures, or patients undergoing laparoscopy procedures lasting more than 30 minutes [98].

No *ad hoc* studies or guidelines are available to help clinicians with best practices for prophylaxis of VTE in hematological malignancies [105]. For acute leukemia and lymphoma, some information on thromboprophylaxis comes from two studies [106,107], while more data are available for multiple myeloma [108]. Given the higher VTE risk during treatment of multiple myeloma patients with thalidomide or lenalidomide in combination with dexamethasone or multiagent chemotherapy, thromboprophylaxis is recommended. However, the modality (type and dose of antithrombotic drug) is an issue of debate. The prospective randomized trials of GIMEMA, comparing the efficacy of LMWH, warfarin (fixed low-dose or full dose), and aspirin for prophylactic anticoagulation, showed only a trend for a more effective thromboprophylaxis with LMWH [109,110]. The guidelines of ASCO (the American Society of Clinical Oncology), ESMO (the European Society of Medical Oncology), and SISET (the Italian Society for Hemostasis and Thrombosis) recommend prophylaxis with LMWH or adjusted-dose warfarin (INR 2–3) [98,111,112]. The International Myeloma Working Group proposes different thromboprophylactic strategies based on stratification of the patient's risk of VTE [44].

Therefore, thromboprophylaxis in ambulatory cancer patients receiving pharmacological antitumor drugs cannot be recommended until more definite data are available from large randomized clinical trials.

Treatment of Thrombosis

Treatment of ATE in cancer patients relies on antiplatelet and anticoagulant/fibrinolytic agents according to the same protocols recommended for secondary prophylaxis for stroke and myocardial infarction in the noncancer population.

Specific protocols have been developed for acute VTE treatment, which has replaced the traditional regimens based on initial therapy with UFH, LMWH, or fondaparinux followed by long-term therapy with a VKA. Data from various RCTs, comparing LMWH with VKA in long-term VTE therapy in cancer [113–116], show the superiority of LMWH monotherapy, which is now endorsed by international guidelines [111,117]. However, VKA with a target INR of 2–3 are acceptable when LMWH is not available [111]. For patients who develop a recurrence while on LMWH, dose escalation of LMWH is often effective, while for patients who develop a recurrence on VKA therapy, the recommended practice is to switch to LMWH. Raising the intensity of VKA therapy is not recommended because of the potential for increasing bleeding [118,119]. There are limited data on the use, safety, and long-term outcome of vena cava filters. Today, use of these devices can be considered as an alternative to prevent PE (because filters are not effective in reducing DVT risk) only in patients who have a contraindication to anticoagulation [120]. Concerning the duration of VTE treatment, an indefinite anticoagulation is recommended for patients with active malignancy, that is those with metastatic disease or receiving continued chemotherapy, as cancer is a strong continuing risk factor for recurrent VTE [111]. The role of the new oral anticoagulant drugs needs to be tested.

Novel Anticoagulants

Novel oral anticoagulants may rapidly change the therapeutic scenario in cancer patients. These agents, which achieve rapid inhibition of activated factor X (rivaroxaban and apixaban) or thrombin (dabigatran), have no requirement for laboratory monitoring and minimal drug interactions. They are administered orally once or twice a day, making them an easier solution than LMWH, but studies focusing on treatment of cancer-associated thrombosis with these agents are lacking. To date, some of these agents have shown comparable efficacy and safety compared with traditional anticoagulants in RCTs that included primarily patients without cancer [121,122]. Given the higher risk of recurrent thrombosis and bleeding in cancer patients, further research is needed to understand the antithrombotic impact of these new agents in this setting [123].

Prophylaxis and Treatment of Bleeding

The most important issue in bleeding is represented by the prophylaxis and treatment of the fatal hemorrhagic syndrome in APL. Indeed, the management of this syndrome is particularly difficult. When a diagnosis of APL is suspected, three simultaneous actions must be immediately undertaken: the start of all-*trans*-retinoic acid (ATRA) therapy, the administration of supportive care with transfusions of plasma and platelets, and the confirmation of molecular diagnosis [124,125]. Prophylactic platelet transfusion is an essential part of supportive care, in order to maintain a platelet count above 20×10^9/L in nonbleeding patients and above 50×10^9/L in those with active bleeding [87,105]. The role of heparin in the treatment of the coagulopathy is undefined. No systematic studies have evaluated the use of LMWH or any of the newer anticoagulants (i.e., factor Xa and IIa inhibitors, hirudin, fondaparinux) to treat the thrombohemorrhagic syndrome of APL. Other types of therapeutic regimens, including antifibrinolytic agents or protease inhibitors (i.e., aprotinin), have been suggested, but no data from RCTs are available. Interestingly, occurrence of thromboembolic events was reported during antifibrinolytic agent administration in combination with ATRA. A lack of efficacy of tranexamic acid for hemorrhage-associated mortality in APL was shown in the large PETHEMA trial [126].

Anticoagulation and Cancer Survival

An antineoplastic effect of antithrombotic agents in various experimental models (i.e., tumor cell in culture, experimental animals, and cancer patients) has often been suggested [127]. Anticoagulant drugs such as heparins and vitamin K antagonists have both been tested in this context. However, heparins have been more extensively studied. Several reports in animal models demonstrate that heparin can reduce the primary tumor growth or its metastatic spread, while in vitro studies show that LMWH can inhibit neoangiogenesis induced by the tumor cell environment [128,129]. Clinical studies of thrombosis in cancer patients show that, besides their role as antithrombotics, heparins may have beneficial effects on survival in these patients, with a major role for LMWHs compared to UFH. In recent years, a number of prospective randomized clinical trials of LMWH administration to improve survival (as a primary end-point) in cancer patients have been carried out [130–134] (Table 25.6). Altogether, the results of these trials, although not conclusive, look promising in suggesting a benefit of cancer prognosis from LMWH administration, particularly in nonadvanced disease stages [135]. However, the use of anticoagulants as adjuvant therapy for cancer cannot be recommended until additional clinical trials confirm these results [136].

Table 25.6 Randomized clinical trials testing the effect of low molecular weight heparin (LMWH) on survival in cancer patients.

Study	Cancer	Control	LMWH
Altinbas et al. 2004 [130]	Small cell lung cancer	Nil	Dalteparin 5000 IU/day 18 weeks
Kakkar et al. 2004 [131]	Advanced cancer	Placebo	Dalteparin 5000 IU/day 1 year
Klerk et al. 2005 [132]	Metastasized and advanced cancer	Placebo	Nadroparin Therapeutic dose 2 weeks + half dose 4 weeks
Sideras K et al. 2006 [133]	Advanced cancer	Nil	Dalteparin 5000 IU/day
Van Doormaal et al. 2011 [134]	Advanced cancer	Nil	Nadroparin Therapeutic dose 2 weeks + half dose 4 weeks

References

1 Falanga A, Marchetti M, Vignoli A, *et al.* Clotting mechanisms and cancer: implications in thrombus formation and tumor progression. *Clin Adv Hematol Oncol* 2003; 1: 673–678.

2 Boccaccio C, Sabatino G, Medico E, *et al.* The MET oncogene drives a genetic programme linking cancer to haemostasis. *Nature* 2005; 434: 396–400.

3 Rong Y, Post DE, Pieper RO, *et al.* PTEN and hypoxia regulate tissue factor expression and plasma coagulation by glioblastoma. *Cancer Res* 2005; 65: 1406–1413.

4 Yu JL, May L, Lhotak V, *et al.* Oncogenic events regulate tissue factor expression in colorectal cancer cells: implications for tumor progression and angiogenesis. *Blood* 2005; 105: 1734–1741.

5 Heit JA, Silverstein MD, Mohr DN, *et al.* Risk factors for deep vein thrombosis and pulmonary embolism: a population-based case-control study. *Arch Intern Med* 2000; 160: 809–815.

6 Blom JW, Vanderschoot JP, Oostindier MJ, *et al.* Incidence of venous thrombosis in a large cohort of 66,329 cancer patients: results of a record linkage study. *J Thromb Haemost* 2006; 4: 529–535.

7 Khorana AA, Francis CW, Culakova E, *et al.* Risk factors for chemotherapy-associated venous thromboembolism in a prospective observational study. *Cancer* 2005; 104: 2822–2829.

8 White RH, Chew H, Wun T. Targeting patients for anticoagulant prophylaxis trials in patients with cancer: Who is at highest risk? *Thromb Res* 2007; 120: S29–S40.

9 Falanga A. Thrombophilia in cancer. *Semin Thromb Hemost* 2005; 31: 104–110.

10 Levitan N, Dowlati A, Remick SC, *et al.* Rates of initial and recurrent thromboembolic disease among patients with malignancy versus those without malignancy. Risk analysis using Medicare claims data. *Medicine* 1999; 78: 285–291.

11 Sorensen HT, Mellemkjaer L, Olsen JH, *et al.* Prognosis of cancers associated with venous thromboembolism. *N Engl J Med* 2000; 343: 1846–1850.

12 Khorana AA, Francis CW, Culakova E, *et al.* Thromboembolism is a leading cause of death in cancer patients receiving outpatient chemotherapy. *J Thromb Haemost* 2007; 5: 632–634.

13 Khorana AA, Connolly GC. Assessing risk of venous thromboembolism in the patient with cancer. *J Clin Oncol* 2009; 27: 4839–4847.

14 Reikvam H, Tiu RV. Venous thromboembolism in patients with essential thrombocythemia and polycythemia vera. *Leukemia* 2012; 26: 563–571.

15 Sanon S, Lenihan DJ, Mouhayar E. Peripheral arterial ischemic events in cancer patients. *Vasc Med* 2011; 16: 119–130.

16 Di Nisio M, Ferrante N, Feragalli B, *et al.* Arterial thrombosis in ambulatory cancer patients treated with chemotherapy. *Thromb Res* 2011; 127: 382–383.

17 Arboix A. [Cerebrovascular disease in the cancer patient]. *Rev Neurol* 2000; 31: 1250–1252.

18 Blake-Haskins JA, Lechleider RJ, Kreitman RJ. Thrombotic microangiopathy with targeted cancer agents. *Clin Cancer Res* 2011; 17: 5858–5866.

19 Oberic L, Buffet M, Schwarzinger M, *et al.* Cancer awareness in atypical thrombotic microangiopathies. *Oncologist* 2009; 14: 769–779.

20 Kansu E. Thrombosis in stem cell transplantation. *Hematology* 2012; 17 (Suppl. 1): S159–162.

21 Richardson PG, Ho VT, Giralt S, *et al.* Safety and efficacy of defibrotide for the treatment of severe hepatic veno-occlusive disease. *Ther Adv Hematol* 2012; 3: 253–265.

22 Falanga A, Vignoli A, Marchetti M, *et al.* Defibrotide reduces procoagulant activity and increases fibrinolytic properties of endothelial cells. *Leukemia* 2003; 17: 1636–1642.

23 Reeves BN, Key NS. Acquired hemophilia in malignancy. *Thromb Res* 2012; 129 (Suppl. 1): S66–68.

24 Sanz MA, Grimwade D, Tallman MS, *et al.* Management of acute promyelocytic

leukemia: recommendations from an expert panel on behalf of the European Leukemia Net. *Blood* 2009; 113: 1875–1891.

25 Prandoni P, Piccioli A. Thrombosis as a harbinger of cancer. *Curr Opin Hematol* 2006; 13: 362–365.

26 Prandoni P, Falanga A, Piccioli A. Cancer and venous thromboembolism. *Lancet Oncol* 2005; 6: 401–410.

27 Prandoni P, Lensing AW, Buller HR, *et al.* Deep-vein thrombosis and the incidence of subsequent symptomatic cancer. *N Engl J Med* 1992; 327: 1128–1133.

28 White RH, Chew HK, Zhou H, *et al.* Incidence of venous thromboembolism in the year before the diagnosis of cancer in 528,693 adults. *Arch Intern Med* 2005; 165: 1782–1787.

29 Piccioli A, Lensing AW, Prins MH, *et al.* Extensive screening for occult malignant disease in idiopathic venous thromboembolism: a prospective randomized clinical trial. *J Thromb Haemost* 2004; 2: 884–889.

30 Di Nisio M, Otten HM, Piccioli A, *et al.* Decision analysis for cancer screening in idiopathic venous thromboembolism. *J Thromb Haemost* 2005; 3: 2391–2396.

31 Monreal M, Lensing AW, Prins MH, *et al.* Screening for occult cancer in patients with acute deep vein thrombosis or pulmonary embolism. *J Thromb Haemost* 2004; 2: 876–881.

32 Rickles FR, Levine M, Edwards RL. Hemostatic alterations in cancer patients. *Cancer Metastasis Rev* 1992; 11: 237–248.

33 Falanga A, Ofosu FA, Cortelazzo S, *et al.* Preliminary study to identify cancer patients at high risk of venous thrombosis following major surgery. *Br J Haematol* 1993; 85: 745–750.

34 Ay C, Simanek R, Vormittag R, *et al.* High plasma levels of soluble P-selectin are predictive of venous thromboembolism in cancer patients: results from the Vienna Cancer and Thrombosis Study (CATS). *Blood* 2008; 112: 2703–2708.

35 Ay C, Vormittag R, Dunkler D, *et al.* D-dimer and prothrombin fragment 1 + 2 predict

venous thromboembolism in patients with cancer: results from the Vienna Cancer and Thrombosis Study. *J Clin Oncol* 2009; 27: 4124–4129.

36 Toth B, Liebhardt S, Steinig K, *et al.* Platelet-derived microparticles and coagulation activation in breast cancer patients. *Thromb Haemost* 2008; 100: 663–669.

37 Trappenburg MC, van Schilfgaarde M, Marchetti M, *et al.* Elevated procoagulant microparticles expressing endothelial and platelet markers in essential thrombocythemia. *Haematologica* 2009; 94: 911–918.

38 Zwicker JI, Liebman HA, Bauer KA, *et al.* Prediction and prevention of thromboembolic events with enoxaparin in cancer patients with elevated tissue factor-bearing microparticles: a randomized-controlled phase II trial (the Microtec study). *Br J Haematol* 2013; 160: 530–537.

39 Khorana AA, Kuderer NM, Culakova E, *et al.* Development and validation of a predictive model for chemotherapy-associated thrombosis. *Blood* 2008; 111: 4902–4907.

40 Ay C, Dunkler D, Marosi C, *et al.* Prediction of venous thromboembolism in cancer patients. *Blood* 2010; 116: 5377–5382.

41 Moore RA, Adel N, Riedel E, *et al.* High incidence of thromboembolic events in patients treated with cisplatin-based chemotherapy: a large retrospective analysis. *J Clin Oncol* 2011; 29: 3466–3473.

42 Mandala M, Clerici M, Corradino I, *et al.* Incidence, risk factors and clinical implications of venous thromboembolism in cancer patients treated within the context of phase I studies: the 'SENDO experience'. *Ann Oncol* 2012; 23: 1416–1421.

43 Verso M, Agnelli G, Barni S, *et al.* A modified Khorana risk assessment score for venous thromboembolism in cancer patients receiving chemotherapy: the Protecht score. *Intern Emerg Med* 2012; 7: 291–292.

44 Palumbo A, Rajkumar SV, Dimopoulos MA, *et al.* Prevention of thalidomide- and lenalidomide-associated thrombosis in myeloma. *Leukemia* 2008; 22: 414–423.

45 Beer JH, Haeberli A, Vogt A, *et al.* Coagulation markers predict survival in cancer patients. *Thromb Haemost* 2002; 88: 745–749.

46 Taguchi O, Gabazza EC, Yoshida M, *et al.* High plasma level of plasmin-alpha 2-plasmin inhibitor complex is predictor of poor prognosis in patients with lung cancer. *Clin Chim Acta* 1996; 244: 69–81.

47 Nijziel MR, Van Oerle R, Hellenbrand D, *et al.* The prognostic value of the soluble urokinase-type plasminogen activator receptor (s-uPAR) in plasma of breast cancer patients with and without metastatic disease. *J Thromb Haemost* 2003; 1: 982–986.

48 Lotz J, Walgenbach S, Peetz D, *et al.* Postoperative reduction of fibrinolysis as a prognostic factor of fatal outcome. *Clin Appl Thromb Hemost* 2001; 7: 330–334.

49 Annecke K, Schmitt M, Euler U, *et al.* uPA and PAI-1 in breast cancer: review of their clinical utility and current validation in the prospective NNBC-3 trial. *Adv Clin Chem* 2008; 45: 31–45.

50 Kilic M, Yoldas O, Keskek M, *et al.* Prognostic value of plasma D-dimer levels in patients with colorectal cancer. *Colorectal Dis* 2008; 10: 238–241.

51 Blackwell K, Hurwitz H, Lieberman G, *et al.* Circulating D-dimer levels are better predictors of overall survival and disease progression than carcinoembryonic antigen levels in patients with metastatic colorectal carcinoma. *Cancer* 2004; 101: 77–82.

52 Amirkhosravi A, Bigsby GT, Desai H, *et al.* Blood clotting activation analysis for preoperative differentiation of benign versus malignant ovarian masses. *Blood Coagul Fibrinolysis* 2013; 24: 510–517.

53 Miller GJ, Bauer KA, Howarth DJ, *et al.* Increased incidence of neoplasia of the digestive tract in men with persistent activation of the coagulant pathway. *J Thromb Haemost* 2004; 2: 2107–2114.

54 Di Castelnuovo A, de Curtis A, Costanzo S, *et al.* Association of D-dimer levels with all-cause mortality in a healthy adult population: findings from the MOLI-SANI study. *Haematologica* 2013; 98: 1476–1480.

55 Khorana AA, Francis CW, Culakova E, *et al.* Thromboembolism in hospitalized neutropenic cancer patients. *J Clin Oncol* 2006; 24: 484–490.

56 Prandoni P, Lensing AW, Piccioli A, *et al.* Recurrent venous thromboembolism and bleeding complications during anticoagulant treatment in patients with cancer and venous thrombosis. *Blood* 2002; 100: 3484–3488.

57 Semrad TJ, O'Donnell R, Wun T, *et al.* Epidemiology of venous thromboembolism in 9489 patients with malignant glioma. *J Neurosurg* 2007; 106: 601–608.

58 Wun T, White RH. Epidemiology of cancer-related venous thromboembolism. *Best Pract Res Clin Haematol* 2009; 22: 9–23.

59 Khorana AA, Francis CW, Culakova E, *et al.* Frequency, risk factors, and trends for venous thromboembolism among hospitalized cancer patients. *Cancer* 2007; 110: 2339–2346.

60 Falanga A, Marchetti M. Anticancer treatment and thrombosis. *Thromb Res* 2012; 129: 353–359.

61 Lechner D, Weltermann A. Chemotherapy-induced thrombosis: a role for microparticles and tissue factor? *Semin Thromb Hemost* 2008; 34: 199–203.

62 Pickering W, Gray E, Goodall AH, *et al.* Characterization of the cell-surface procoagulant activity of T-lymphoblastoid cell lines. *J Thromb Haemost* 2004; 2: 459–467.

63 Fernandes RS, Kirszberg C, Rumjanek VM, *et al.* On the molecular mechanisms for the highly procoagulant pattern of C6 glioma cells. *J Thromb Haemost* 2006; 4: 1546–1552.

64 Nadir Y, Brenner B, Gingis-Velitski S, *et al.* Heparanase induces tissue factor pathway inhibitor expression and extracellular accumulation in endothelial and tumor cells. *Thromb Haemost* 2008; 99: 133–141.

65 Ruf W. Tissue factor and PAR signaling in tumor progression. *Thromb Res* 2007; 120: S7–S12.

66 Falanga A, Panova-Noeva M, Russo L. Procoagulant mechanisms in tumour cells. *Best Pract Res Clin Haematol* 2009; 22: 49–60.

67 Marchetti M, Diani E, Ten Cate H, *et al.* Characterization of thrombin generation

potential of leukemic and solid tumor cells by the calibrated automated thrombography. *Haematologica* 2012; 97: 1173–1180.

68 Gerotziafas GT, Galea V, Mbemba E, *et al.* Tissue factor over-expression by human pancreatic cancer cells BXPC3 is related to higher prothrombotic potential as compared to breast cancer cells MCF7. *Thromb Res* 2012; 129: 779–786.

69 Falanga A, Tartari CJ, Marchetti M. Microparticles in tumor progression. *Thromb Res* 2012; 129 (Suppl. 1): S132–S136.

70 Kim HK, Song KS, Park YS, *et al.* Elevated levels of circulating platelet microparticles, VEGF, IL-6 and RANTES in patients with gastric cancer: possible role of a metastasis predictor. *Eur J Cancer* 2003; 39: 184–191.

71 Van Aalderen MC, Trappenburg MC, Van Schilfgaarde M, *et al.* Procoagulant myeloblast-derived microparticles in AML patients: changes in numbers and thrombin generation potential during chemotherapy. *J Thromb Haemost* 2011; 9: 223–226.

72 Auwerda JJ, Yuana Y, Osanto S, *et al.* Microparticle-associated tissue factor activity and venous thrombosis in multiple myeloma. *Thromb Haemost* 2011; 105: 14–20.

73 Liu Y, Wang Z, Jiang M, *et al.* The expression of annexin II and its role in the fibrinolytic activity in acute promyelocytic leukemia. *Leuk Res* 2011; 35: 879–884.

74 Lee AY, Levine MN. The thrombophilic state induced by therapeutic agents in the cancer patient. *Semin Thromb Hemost* 1999; 25: 137–145.

75 Bertomeu MC, Gallo S, Lauri D, *et al.* Chemotherapy enhances endothelial cell reactivity to platelets. *Clin Exp Metastasis* 1990; 8: 511–518.

76 Adamson IY, Bowden DH. The pathogenesis of bloemycin-induced pulmonary fibrosis in mice. *Am J Pathol* 1974; 77: 185–197.

77 Kuenen BC, Levi M, Meijers JC, *et al.* Potential role of platelets in endothelial damage observed during treatment with cisplatin, gemcitabine, and the angiogenesis inhibitor SU5416. *J Clin Oncol* 2003; 21: 2192–2198.

78 Kuenen BC, Levi M, Meijers JC, *et al.* Analysis of coagulation cascade and endothelial cell activation during inhibition of vascular endothelial growth factor/vascular endothelial growth factor receptor pathway in cancer patients. *Arterioscler Thromb Vasc Biol* 2002; 22: 1500–1505.

79 Giordano P, Molinari AC, Del Vecchio GC, *et al.* Prospective study of hemostatic alterations in children with acute lymphoblastic leukemia. *Am J Hematol* 2010; 85: 325–330.

80 Weijl NI, Rutten MF, Zwinderman AH, *et al.* Thromboembolic events during chemotherapy for germ cell cancer: a cohort study and review of the literature. *J Clin Oncol* 2000; 18: 2169–2178.

81 Ma L, Francia G, Viloria-Petit A, *et al.* In vitro procoagulant activity induced in endothelial cells by chemotherapy and antiangiogenic drug combinations: modulation by lower-dose chemotherapy. *Cancer Res* 2005; 65: 5365–5373.

82 Swystun LL, Mukherjee S, Levine M, *et al.* The chemotherapy metabolite acrolein upregulates thrombin generation and impairs the protein C anticoagulant pathway in animal-based and cell-based models. *J Thromb Haemost* 2011; 9: 767–775.

83 Swystun LL, Shin LY, Beaudin S, *et al.* Chemotherapeutic agents doxorubicin and epirubicin induce a procoagulant phenotype on endothelial cells and blood monocytes. *J Thromb Haemost* 2009; 7: 619–626.

84 Lechner D, Kollars M, Gleiss A, *et al.* Chemotherapy-induced thrombin generation via procoagulant endothelial microparticles is independent of tissue factor activity. *J Thromb Haemost* 2007; 5: 2445–2452.

85 Boles JC, Williams JC, Hollingsworth RM, *et al.* Anthracycline treatment of the human monocytic leukemia cell line THP-1 increases phosphatidylserine exposure and tissue factor activity. *Thromb Res* 2012; 129: 197–203.

86 Fu Y, Zhou J, Li H, *et al.* Daunorubicin induces procoagulant activity of cultured endothelial cells through phosphatidylserine exposure and microparticles release. *Thromb Haemost* 2010; 104: 1235–1241.

87 Falanga A, Marchetti M. Venous thromboembolism in hematologic malignancies. In: Khorana AA, Francis CW, eds. *Cancer-Associated Thrombosis: New Findings in Translational Science, Prevention, and Treatment*. New York: Informa Healthcare, 2008, pp. 131–149.

88 Landolfi R, Marchioli R, Kutti J, *et al.* Efficacy and safety of low-dose aspirin in polycythemia vera. *N Engl J Med* 2004; 350: 114–124.

89 Clagett GP, Reisch JS. Prevention of venous thromboembolism in general surgical patients. *Results of meta-analysis. Ann Surg* 1988; 208: 227–240.

90 Geerts WH, Pineo GF, Heit JA, *et al.* Prevention of venous thromboembolism: the Seventh ACCP Conference on Antithrombotic and Thrombolytic Therapy. *Chest* 2004; 126 (3 Suppl.): 338S–400S.

91 Lyman GH, Khorana AA, Kuderer NM, *et al.* Venous thromboembolism prophylaxis and treatment in patients with cancer: American Society of Clinical Oncology clinical practice guideline update. *J Clin Oncol* 2013; 31: 2189–2204.

92 Streiff MB. The National Comprehensive Cancer Center Network (NCCN) guidelines on the management of venous thromboembolism in cancer patients. *Thromb Res* 2010; 125 (Suppl. 2): S128–133.

93 Mandala M, Falanga A, Piccioli A, *et al.* Venous thromboembolism and cancer: guidelines of the Italian Association of Medical Oncology (AIOM). *Crit Rev Oncol Hematol* 2006; 59: 194–204.

94 Mandala M, Falanga A, Roila F. Management of venous thromboembolism (VTE) in cancer patients: ESMO Clinical Practice Guidelines. *Ann Oncol* 2011; 22 (Suppl. 6): vi85–92.

95 Lyman GH, Kuderer NM. Prevention and treatment of venous thromboembolism among patients with cancer: the American Society of Clinical Oncology Guidelines. *Thromb Res* 2010; 125 (Suppl. 2): S120–127.

96 Farge D, Debourdeau P, Beckers M, *et al.* International clinical practice guidelines for the treatment and prophylaxis of venous thromboembolism in patients with cancer. *J Thromb Haemost* 2013; 11: 56–70.

97 Bergqvist D, Agnelli G, Cohen AT, *et al.* Duration of prophylaxis against venous thromboembolism with enoxaparin after surgery for cancer. *N Engl J Med* 2002; 346: 975–980.

98 Siragusa S, Armani U, Carpenedo M, *et al.* Prevention of venous thromboembolism in patients with cancer: guidelines of the Italian Society for Haemostasis and Thrombosis (SISET)(1). *Thromb Res* 2012; 129: e171–176.

99 Bergqvist D, Burmark US, Flordal PA, *et al.* Low molecular weight heparin started before surgery as prophylaxis against deep vein thrombosis: 2500 versus 5000 XaI units in 2070 patients. *Br J Surg* 1995; 82: 496–501.

100 Rasmussen MS, Jorgensen LN, Wille-Jorgensen P, *et al.* Prolonged prophylaxis with dalteparin to prevent late thromboembolic complications in patients undergoing major abdominal surgery: a multicenter randomized open-label study. *J Thromb Haemost* 2006; 4: 2384–2390.

101 Agnelli G, George DJ, Kakkar AK, *et al.* Semuloparin for thromboprophylaxis in patients receiving chemotherapy for cancer. *N Engl J Med* 2012; 366: 601–609.

102 Agnelli G, Gussoni G, Bianchini C, *et al.* Nadroparin for the prevention of thromboembolic events in ambulatory patients with metastatic or locally advanced solid cancer receiving chemotherapy: a randomised, placebo-controlled, double-blind study. *Lancet Oncol* 2009; 10: 943–949.

103 Maraveyas A, Waters J, Roy R, *et al.* Gemcitabine versus gemcitabine plus dalteparin thromboprophylaxis in pancreatic cancer. *Eur J Cancer* 2012; 48: 1283–1292.

104 Streiff MB, Bockenstedt PL, Cataland SR, *et al.* Venous thromboembolic disease. *J Natl Compr Canc Netw* 2011; 9: 714–777.

105 Falanga A, Rickles FR. Management of thrombohemorrhagic syndromes (THS) in hematologic malignancies. *Hematology Am Soc Hematol Educ Program* 2007: 165–71.

106 Couban S, Goodyear M, Burnell M, *et al.* Randomized placebo-controlled study of

low-dose warfarin for the prevention of
central venous catheter-associated
thrombosis in patients with cancer. *J Clin
Oncol* 2005; 23: 4063–4069.

107 Cortelezzi A, Moia M, Falanga A, *et al.*
Incidence of thrombotic complications in
patients with haematological malignancies
with central venous catheters: a prospective
multicentre study. *Br J Haematol* 2005; 129:
811–817.

108 Carrier M, Le Gal G, Tay J, *et al.* Rates of
venous thromboembolism in multiple
myeloma patients undergoing
immunomodulatory therapy with
thalidomide or lenalidomide: a systematic
review and meta-analysis. *J Thromb Haemost*
2011; 9: 653–663.

109 Palumbo A, Cavo M, Bringhen S, *et al.*
Aspirin, warfarin, or enoxaparin
thromboprophylaxis in patients with
multiple myeloma treated with thalidomide:
a phase III, open-label, randomized trial.
J Clin Oncol 2011; 29: 986–993.

110 Larocca A, Cavallo F, Bringhen S, *et al.*
Aspirin or enoxaparin thromboprophylaxis
for patients with newly diagnosed multiple
myeloma treated with lenalidomide. *Blood*
2012; 119: 933–939; quiz 1093.

111 Lyman GH, Khorana AA, Falanga A, *et al.*
American Society of Clinical Oncology
guideline: recommendations for venous
thromboembolism prophylaxis and
treatment in patients with cancer. *J Clin
Oncol* 2007; 25: 5490–5505.

112 Mandala M, Falanga A, Roila F. Venous
thromboembolism in cancer patients: ESMO
Clinical Practice Guidelines for the
management. *Ann Oncol* 2010; 21 (Suppl. 5):
v274–276.

113 Meyer G, Marjanovic Z, Valcke J, *et al.*
Comparison of low-molecular-weight heparin
and warfarin for the secondary prevention of
venous thromboembolism in patients with
cancer: a randomized controlled study. *Arch
Intern Med* 2002; 162: 1729–1735.

114 Lee AY, Levine MN, Baker RI, *et al.* Low-
molecular-weight heparin versus a coumarin
for the prevention of recurrent venous

thromboembolism in patients with cancer.
N Engl J Med 2003; 349: 146–153.

115 Deitcher SR, Kessler CM, Merli G, *et al.*
Secondary prevention of venous
thromboembolic events in patients with
active cancer: enoxaparin alone versus initial
enoxaparin followed by warfarin for a
180-day period. *Clin Appl Thromb Hemost*
2006; 12: 389–396.

116 Hull RD, Pineo GF, Brant RF, *et al.* Long-term
low-molecular-weight heparin versus usual
care in proximal-vein thrombosis patients
with cancer. *Am J Med* 2006; 119: 1062–1072.

117 Kearon C, Kahn SR, Agnelli G, *et al.*
Antithrombotic therapy for venous
thromboembolic disease: American College
of Chest Physicians evidence-based clinical
practice guidelines (8th Edition). *Chest* 2008;
133 (6 Suppl.): 454S–545S.

118 Hutten BA, Prins MH, Gent M, *et al.*
Incidence of recurrent thromboembolic and
bleeding complications among patients with
venous thromboembolism in relation to both
malignancy and achieved international
normalized ratio: a retrospective analysis.
J Clin Oncol 2000; 18: 3078–3083.

119 Carrier M, Le Gal G, Cho R, *et al.* Dose
escalation of low molecular weight heparin
to manage recurrent venous
thromboembolic events despite systemic
anticoagulation in cancer patients. *J Thromb
Haemost* 2009; 7: 760–765.

120 Panova-Noeva M, Falanga A. Treatment of
thromboembolism in cancer patients. *Expert
Opin Pharmacother* 2010; 11: 2049–2058.

121 Schulman S, Kearon C, Kakkar AK, *et al.*
Dabigatran versus warfarin in the treatment
of acute venous thromboembolism. *N Engl J
Med* 2009; 361: 2342–2352.

122 EINSTEIN Investigators. Oral rivaroxaban
for symptomatic venous thromboembolism.
N Engl J Med 2010; 363: 2499–2510.

123 Verso M, Agnelli G. New and old
anticoagulants in cancer. *Thromb Res* 2012;
129 (Suppl. 1): S101–105.

124 Falanga A, Russo L, Tartari CJ. Pathogenesis
and treatment of thrombohemorrhagic
diathesis in acute promyelocytic leukemia.

Mediterr J Hematol Infect Dis 2011; 3: e2011068.

125 Falanga A, Marchetti M, Barbui T. All-trans-retinoic acid and bleeding/thrombosis. *Pathophysiol Haemost Thromb* 2003; 33 (Suppl. 1): 19–21.

126 de la Serna J, Montesinos P, Vellenga E, *et al.* Causes and prognostic factors of remission induction failure in patients with acute promyelocytic leukemia treated with all-trans retinoic acid and idarubicin. *Blood* 2008; 111: 3395–3402.

127 Falanga A, Marchetti M. Heparin in tumor progression and metastatic dissemination. *Semin Thromb Hemost* 2007; 33: 688–694.

128 Marchetti M, Vignoli A, Russo L, *et al.* Endothelial capillary tube formation and cell proliferation induced by tumor cells are affected by low molecular weight heparins and unfractionated heparin. *Thromb Res* 2008; 121: 637–645.

129 Norrby K. Low-molecular-weight heparins and angiogenesis. *Apmis* 2006; 114: 79–102.

130 Altinbas M, Coskun HS, Er O, *et al.* A randomized clinical trial of combination chemotherapy with and without low-molecular-weight heparin in small cell lung cancer. *J Thromb Haemost* 2004; 2: 1266–1271.

131 Kakkar AK, Levine MN, Kadziola Z, *et al.* Low molecular weight heparin, therapy with dalteparin, and survival in advanced cancer: the fragmin advanced malignancy outcome study (FAMOUS). *J Clin Oncol* 2004; 22: 1944–1948.

132 Klerk CP, Smorenburg SM, Otten HM, *et al.* The effect of low molecular weight heparin on survival in patients with advanced malignancy. *J Clin Oncol* 2005; 23: 2130–2135.

133 Sideras K, Schaefer PL, Okuno SH, *et al.* Low-molecular-weight heparin in patients with advanced cancer: a phase 3 clinical trial. *Mayo Clin Proc* 2006; 81: 758–767.

134 van Doormaal FF, Di Nisio M, Otten HM, *et al.* Randomized trial of the effect of the low molecular weight heparin nadroparin on survival in patients with cancer. *J Clin Oncol* 2011; 29: 2071–2076.

135 Piccioli A, Falanga A, Prandoni P. Anticoagulants and cancer survival. *Semin Thromb Hemost* 2006; 32: 810–813.

136 Kuderer NM, Khorana AA, Lyman GH, *et al.* A meta-analysis and systematic review of the efficacy and safety of anticoagulants as cancer treatment: impact on survival and bleeding complications. *Cancer* 2007; 110: 1149–1161.

26

Obstetrics, Contraception, and Estrogen Replacement

Amy Webster and Sue Pavord

Key Points

- Pregnancy is associated with a hypercoagulable state and increased risk of venous thromboembolism (VTE), which persists up to 6 weeks postpartum.
- Women should have their risk of VTE assessed throughout pregnancy, taking transient risk factors into account, and receive advice and thromboprophylaxis as appropriate.
- Diagnosis of VTE in pregnancy may be difficult, but objective investigation is essential to ensure appropriate management.
- Anticoagulation in pregnancy is primarily managed with low molecular weight heparin, which can be given at prophylactic or treatment doses depending on requirement. Women should be managed in an appropriate obstetric–hematology unit and management of anticoagulation at the time of delivery should be carefully planned.
- Contraception, hormone replacement therapy, and *in vitro* fertilization are associated with thrombotic risk and women should be counseled appropriately prior to starting treatment.

Physiological Changes in Pregnancy

During pregnancy, there are physiological changes in the levels of coagulation factors and natural anticoagulants, which persist into the early postpartum period and confer a hypercoagulable state. Figure 26.1 shows these changes. The most noticeable are coagulation factors VII, VIII, X, von Willebrand factor, and fibrinogen. Increase in these factors is mediated by the rise in estrogen levels, which leads to increased protein synthesis and enhanced activation by thrombin. The natural anticoagulant, protein S, progressively falls throughout pregnancy, whilst protein C and antithrombin levels remain relatively constant [2]. There is a marked rise in D-dimers and other fibrin degradation products, thought to reflect the increase in fibrinogen, rather than increased fibrinolytic activity. Indeed fibrinolysis is suppressed, by a gradual increase in plasminogen activator inhibitors 1 and 2. It remains low during labor and delivery and returns to normal early after delivery of the placenta [3]. The result of all these changes is a shift towards hypercoagulability, reaching a peak at term and in the early postpartum period, and returning to baseline by 4–6 weeks after delivery.

Venous Thromboembolism

Whilst the hypercoagulability of pregnancy helps to protect against hemorrhage at delivery, it confers an increased venous thrombotic risk of approximately 10 times that of the nonpregnant state. Risk increases as pregnancy advances [4], reaching up to 25-fold shortly after delivery [5]. As such, venous thromboembolism (VTE) is a major cause of pregnancy-related morbidity, with an

Practical Hemostasis and Thrombosis, Third Edition. Edited by Nigel S. Key, Michael Makris and David Lillicrap.
© 2017 John Wiley & Sons, Ltd. Published 2017 by John Wiley & Sons, Ltd.

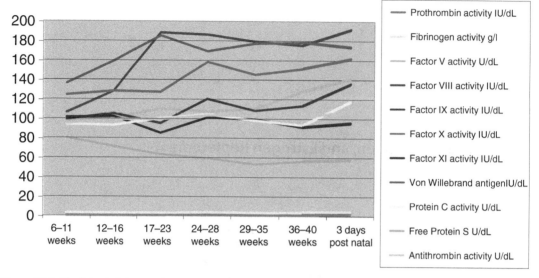

Figure 26.1 Physiological changes in pregnancy. *Source:* modified from Pavord and Hunt, 2010 [1]. *See Plate section for color representation of this figure.*

incidence of 1/1000 pregnancies and is one of the leading causes of maternal death in the UK. Reassuringly, with increased awareness, education, and attention to thromboprophylaxis, maternal death from VTE has fallen from 1.94/100 000 maternities in 2007 to 0.79/100 000 in 2011 [6].

Venous stasis contributes to the risk of VTE and by the third trimester there is up to 50% reduction in lower limb blood flow [7]. Unlike the nonpregnant state, 70% of deep vein thromboses (DVTs) occur in the proximal leg veins, with 90% of these occurring in the left leg, due to compression of the left common iliac vein by the overlying right common iliac artery and gravid uterus (Figure 26.2) [8]. Only 9% of thromboses are confined to distal calf veins and these appear to be equally distributed to either leg [6].

Risk Factors for VTE in Pregnancy

Venous thrombosis is a multihit phenomenon, provoked by congenital and/or acquired risk factors, often acting in synergy with each other. Risk factors may be pre-existing in the patient or develop during pregnancy. These are outlined in Table 26.1.

Table 26.1 Risk factors for venous thromboembolism (VTE) in pregnancy (patient related and pregnancy specific).

Pre-existing

Previous VTE
Family history
Documented thrombophilia
Age >35 years
BMI >30 kg/m²
Parity >3
Smoker
Gross varicose veins
Longstanding immobility such as paraplegia
Medical comorbidities, i.e., systemic lupus erythematous, heart disease, sickle cell disease, nephrotic syndrome

New onset or transient

Immobility, i.e., including prolonged travel
Current systemic infection
Surgical procedure
Dehydration
Hyperemesis gravidarum
Pre-eclampsia
Multiple pregnancy
Ovarian hyperstimulation syndrome
Specific postpartum risks, i.e., prolonged labor, caesarean section, midcavity instrumental delivery

Source: modified from Royal College of Obstetricians and Gynaecologists, 2009 [12].

Figure 26.2 Diagram of iliac vessels.
See Plate section for color representation of this figure.

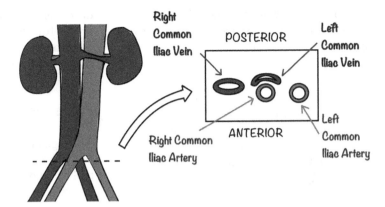

Thrombophilia

Thrombophilias are disorders of hemostasis that predispose to thrombosis. The most common are factor V Leiden and prothrombin G20210A, caused by point mutations in the coagulation factors V and II genes, respectively. Others include deficiencies of the naturally occurring anticoagulants protein C, protein S, and antithrombin, and the acquired thrombophilia, antiphospholipid syndrome. Early studies found the presence of one or more inherited thrombophilias in approximately 50% of women developing VTE during pregnancy or in the postpartum period, although retrospective reporting bias may have led to an overestimation [9]. Whilst different thrombophilias provide a spectrum of relative risk severity, the absolute risk remains modest, given the incidence of VTE in an unselected population of women is 1 : 1000. Antithrombin deficiency, combined thrombophilias, and homozygosity for factor V Leiden or prothrombin gene mutation present the highest risks (Table 26.2).

Previous VTE

Previous history of VTE confers an average increased risk of recurrence in pregnancy of 2–12% [10], being significantly influenced by the circumstances of the previous thrombosis. A history of unprovoked VTE and/or identifiable thrombophilia has been associated with a recurrence rate of 5.9%, whereas no recurrences were seen in women with VTE following a transient risk factor and no underlying thrombophilia [11]. VTE occurring in pregnancy or during treatment with the combined

Table 26.2 Prevalence of inherited thrombophilia and risk of gestational venous thromboembolism (VTE).

Thrombophilia	Prevalence in general population (%)	Odds ratio (95% CI) for gestational VTE
Antithrombin deficiency	0.25–0.55	4.69 (1.30–16.96)
Protein C deficiency	0.20–0.33	4.76 (2.15–10.57)
Protein S deficiency	0.03–0.13	3.19 (0.48–6.88)
Factor V Leiden (heterozygous)	2–7	8.32 (5.44–12.70)
Factor V Leiden (Homozygous)		34.30 (9.86–120.05)
Prothrombin G20210A (heterozygous)	2	6.80 (2.46–18.77)
Prothrombin G20210A (homozygous)		26.36 (1.24–559.29)

oral contraceptive pill confers an increased risk of recurrence in subsequent pregnancies of approximately 9.5% [12].

Obesity

There is increasing focus on the risks of obesity, with the rising incidence in the western world. The national enquiry into maternal obesity, conducted by CMACE in 2010, outlined that 5% of the maternity population in the UK are severely obese (BMI >35 kg/m^2). Within this population, less than 50% of women assessed as intermediate or high risk of VTE were offered antenatal prophylaxis and only 55% offered prophylaxis in the postpartum period. Furthermore, the women that were offered prophylaxis were given doses inadequate for body weight [13]. In a previous case–control study in Denmark, obesity was found to have an adjusted odds ratio (OR) of 14.9 (95% CI: 3.0,74.8) and 4.4 (95% CI: 1.6, 11.9) for pulmonary embolism (PE) and DVT respectively [14]. This study also highlighted the risk of smoking, with an OR of 2.7 and 5.3 for VTE in pregnancy and the puerperium respectively, another risk factor with increasing prevalence.

Superficial Thrombophlebitis

Initially considered to be a benign disease, there is now recognition of the potential thromboembolic complications of superficial thrombophlebitis (SVT). This condition is not infrequent in pregnancy, due to the reduction in vascular tone, hypercoagulability of the blood, and the increased incidence of varicose veins. It most commonly involves the great saphenous vein. Subgroup analysis of the CALISTO double-blind trial comparing fondaparinux 2.5 mg daily with placebo, for 45 days after SVT [15], revealed symptomatic extension in 7.3% of the patients receiving placebo and subsequent DVT or PE in 8.9% and 9.3%, respectively. Thromboembolism was more likely to occur if the SVT was above the knee, within 10 cm of the saphenofemoral junction, or if there was a history of previous VTE. This compared with only 1.1% of those treated with fondaparinux

developing extension and none sustaining DVT or PE [16]. However, as the numbers needed to treat to prevent one VTE was 88, the cost effectiveness is questionable.

Prevention of Gestational VTE

All pregnant women should be assessed for their risk of venous thrombosis, using an evaluation tool based on known risk factors. As clinical circumstances may change, assessment should take place at booking, at each antenatal visit, any admission to hospital, and after delivery. For obviously high-risk women, opportunities for assessment and counseling should be taken prior to pregnancy.

Nonpharmacological measures for preventing thrombosis include ensuring adequate hydration, feet and ankle exercises, and antiembolic stockings. The European Food Safety Authority (EFSA) recommends that water intake for lactating women should compensate the loss of water through milk production, that is an additional amount of 600–700 mL should be added to the 2 L reference daily intake [17]. Ankle exercises involving calf muscle contraction encourage venous return and reduce existing edema.

Unfractionated heparin (UFH) and low molecular weight heparin (LMWH) do not cross the placenta so there is no risk of fetal bleeding or teratogenicity. LMWH is recommended as first-line agent, due to its longer half-life, improved bioavailability, and predictable anticoagulant effect (Table 26.3). It also has less effect on bone demineralization. It is given by subcutaneous injection and women are taught to self-administer treatment. Various preparations are available and each hospital will have its preferred option. One to two percent of women develop local cutaneous allergy at injection sites, necessitating a switch to an alternative LMWH preparation. If allergy occurs to all LMWHs, substitution with the heparan mixture, danaparoid, or the synthetic pentasaccharide, fondaparinux, is necessary. Both are indirect inhibitors of factor Xa, with danaparoid also having some antifactor IIa activity.

Table 26.3 Recommendations for thromboprophylaxis.

Level of risk	Risk factors	Recommendations
High	Single previous VTE with thrombophilia or family history Estrogen-related VTE Recurrent VTE	Require antenatal prophylaxis with LMWH until 6 weeks postpartum
Intermediate	Single previous VTE with no family history Known thrombophilia with no history of VTE Medical comorbidities 3 or more risk factors	Consider antenatal and postnatal prophylaxis with LMWH
Low	<3 risk factors	Mobilize and avoid dehydration

Source: modified from Royal College of Obstetricians and Gynaecologists, 2009 [12].

They have only been studied incidentally in pregnancy but so far have not led to fetal abnormalities or exacerbation of bleeding in the mother or infant. However, until further data are available, the manufacturers' recommendations are to avoid in pregnancy unless the benefits outweigh potential risks. Both have long half-lives that require caution for regional anesthesia and delivery.

Oral direct inhibitors to thrombin and factor Xa are becoming licensed for the prevention of recurrent VTE out with pregnancy but animal models have shown teratogenicity and at present they are considered to be contraindicated in pregnancy [18].

Diagnosis of Acute VTE

The inaccuracy of clinical assessment for VTE is well known, but this is compounded in pregnancy by the frequency of leg swelling, chest pain, and breathlessness unrelated to thrombosis. Objective investigation is essential to avoid under- or overdiagnosis, both of which can lead to serious consequences. Not surprisingly therefore, the percentage of positive scans is reduced to approximately 8% for DVT and <5% of PE [19–21]. Table 26.4 outlines typical signs and symptoms. Any suspected VTE should be treated with therapeutic LMWH whilst awaiting results of imaging, unless there is a contraindication to anticoagulation, such

as active bleeding. There are no data from clinical trials to guide diagnostic strategy in pregnancy and guidelines are extrapolated from nonpregnancy information (Figure 26.3). D-dimers outside of pregnancy are a useful tool for excluding VTE in those with low clinical probability. However, as physiological levels increase throughout pregnancy, due to the rise in fibrinogen, their use for diagnosing gestational VTE is limited and not advised by the Royal College of Obstetrics and Gynaecologists (RCOG). This is not universally accepted, as normal levels may still be present in the first half of pregnancy and could reduce the need for serial imaging.

Table 26.4 Signs and symptoms of venous thromboembolism in pregnancy.

Deep vein thrombosis

Painful leg
Leg swelling
Lower abdominal or buttock pain
Peripheral edema
Raised white cell count, fever

Pulmonary embolism

Chest pain
Shortness of breath
Hemoptysis
Hemodynamic collapse – tachycardia, hypotension
Hypoxia
Right heart failure – raised venous pressure, peripheral edema

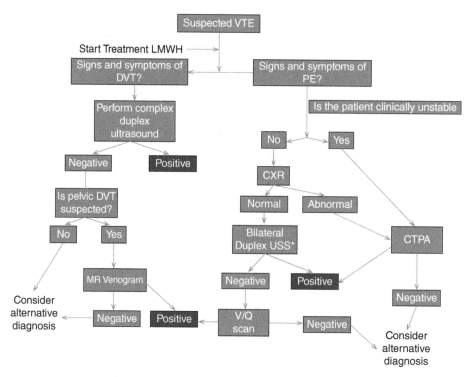

Figure 26.3 A diagnostic algorithm for the investigation of suspected venous thromboembolism. *Yield is low but may be undertaken in some centers to reduce need for imaging. CTPA, computed tomography pulmonary angiogram; CXR, chest X-ray; DVT, deep vein thrombosis; LMWH, low molecular weight heparin; MR, magnetic resonance; PE, pulmonary embolism; USS, ultrasound scan; VTE, venous thromboembolism.

DVT: Compression duplex ultrasound has a sensitivity of 97–100% and specificity 98–99% for diagnosing proximal DVT in pregnancy [22]. If the scan is negative and the clinical suspicion of a DVT is low, anticoagulation can be safely stopped. However, if the calf veins are not visualized and clinical suspicion remains high, anticoagulation should be continued and the scan repeated in 1 week. Compression ultrasound could miss thrombosis in the pelvic veins, where compression is not possible and, if this is suspected, magnetic resonance venography or conventional venography may be required.

PE: In patients without hemodynamic compromise, a chest X-ray should be the first line of investigation. This has a negligible radiation risk. It will be normal in more than half of pregnant women with PE but will help to exclude other pulmonary pathology such as

pneumonia and pneumothorax. If the chest X-ray is abnormal, computed tomography pulmonary angiogram (CTPA) should be performed. This has high sensitivity and specificity for PE and will identify any additional pathology and the presence of right ventricular strain. Some argue that it is oversensitive, identifying subsegmental PEs of questionable significance. Whilst fetal radiation exposure is low, it is associated with potentially significant radiation to the maternal breast tissue, leading to a longer-term increased risk of breast cancer by 14% increase in background risk [23]. Bilateral lower limb compression ultrasound may be considered; the DVT detection rate, in the absence of symptoms and signs in the legs, is extremely low but if positive for DVT, diagnosis of PE can be assumed without the need for further imaging. Perfusion scanning is often the preferred investigation in patients with a normal chest X-ray.

A normal scan excludes PE and an abnormal scan can be followed by ventilation scanning to confirm mismatch. It is associated with higher fetal radiation exposure but the associated increase in childhood cancer risk is negligible, at 1 : 280 000 compared to 1 : 100 000 for CTPA [19]. Although radiation risks of each option are well below the maximum tolerated in pregnancy (50 mSv), effective counseling of the patient is imperative.

Treatment of Acute VTE

Prior to starting therapeutic anticoagulation, all women should have a baseline full blood count, coagulation profile, and renal and liver function testing. LMWH is the treatment of choice. Meta-analysis of LMWH in the treatment of DVT, outside of pregnancy, showed it was more effective and associated with reduced mortality compared to UFH and was equivalent in the treatment of PE. A systematic review of the use of LMWH in pregnancy has confirmed its efficacy and safety [24]. Due to the changes in maternal plasma volume, increased volume of distribution, and increased glomerular filtration, there is suggestion of the shorter half-life of LMWH in pregnancy and need for twice-daily dosing, although recent data confirms efficacy of once-daily dosing, which is likely to have improved compliance [25].

Anti-Xa levels, taken at 3 hours postdose, are useful in this setting, despite their lack of standardization and interlaboratory variation. A target Factor Xa level of 0.5–1.2 IU/mL is considered therapeutic. Repeated factor Xa levels are not routinely recommended, but may be necessary in women at extremes of weight (<50 kg or >90 kg) or in the presence of renal failure where accumulation may occur. Reduction to once-daily dosing can be considered when symptoms and signs have resolved [25].

Treatment should be continued until at least 6 weeks postpartum, with 3–6 months of treatment in total. Regular full blood count monitoring is not required for LMWH in pregnancy as the risk of heparin-induced thrombocytopenia is negligible [26].

Therapeutic anticoagulation should continue throughout pregnancy and for at least 6 weeks postpartum. In line with BCSH and ACCP 9th edition guidelines, treatment for calf veins can be discontinued after 6 weeks, and for proximal DVT/PE treatment should continue for at least 3 months [16,27,28]. Both LMWH and warfarin can be used postpartum and are safe for breast feeding. If there are concerns about ongoing risk for VTE, these should be discussed prior to stopping anticoagulation.

Massive PE: This presents with evidence of hemodynamic compromise (systolic BP <90 mmHg), which cannot be explained by sepsis, arrhythmia, or hypovolaemia. Treatment in these cases should be discussed within the multidisciplinary team, and emergency treatment with oxygen, intravenous fluids, and inotropes if required. Each case will be managed on an individual basis, with UFH titrated to the appropriate activated partial thromboplastin time (APTT) the anticoagulation of choice once PE has been confirmed on CTPA or bedside echocardiography. Successful case reports of thrombolysis in pregnancy are in the literature with a comparable maternal bleeding risk of 6% [19]. UFH, if used, can be associated with heparin-induced thrombocytopenia and therefore the platelet count will need to be monitored every 72 hours until the heparin is stopped. The most at-risk period of this rare immunological complication is day 4 to 14 following first exposure.

Vena Cava (IVC) Filters: The published use of IVC filters in pregnancy is limited to case reports and small case series but may be required in those women who present with an extensive proximal VTE close to delivery (less than 2 weeks), particularly where there is a contraindication to anticoagulation. Retrievable filters should be used and removed once the high-risk period is over, thus avoiding the need for long-term oral anticoagulation [29].

Post-Thrombotic Syndrome

Almost two-thirds of women who have gestational DVT develop objective signs of venous insufficiency in the longer term. The risk is higher in obesity, recurrent VTE, and those with inadequate therapeutic anticoagulation. Counseling about leg care and general measures to prevent post-thrombotic syndrome is a vital part of management of DVT. Class II compression stockings provide graduated external pressure and encourage venous return of blood to the heart. They have been shown to reduce the risk of post-thrombotic syndrome by 50% in non-pregnant patients [30]. Contractions of the calf muscles also help venous blood flow and women should be encouraged to do regular feet and ankle exercises. Elevation of the legs above the level of the heart while lying down makes use of gravitational forces to improve venous drainage.

Warfarin in Pregnancy

Warfarin crosses the placenta and is highly teratogenic. The risk of warfarin embryopathy, which includes chondrodysplasia punctata, nasal hypoplasia, and short proximal limbs, is greatest if taken between 6 and 12 weeks' gestation and in those women on >5 mg warfarin per day. Warfarin may also induce maternal retroplacental bleeding, as well as intracranial hemorrhage and other bleeding in the fetus, leading to neurological abnormalities, microcephaly, miscarriage, and late fetal loss. As a consequence, warfarin should be avoided in the obstetric setting. However, there are occasional circumstances where it becomes necessary, such as in the management of patients with metal heart valves, or where full-dose LMWH has failed to prevent thrombosis. In these situations, LMWH should be used during the highest risk period for warfarin side-effects; these being the first trimester and after 36 weeks' gestation.

Mechanical Heart Valves: Patients with metal heart valves require lifelong warfarin to prevent valve thrombosis with subsequent valve obstruction or systemic embolization. Given the risks of warfarin in pregnancy, the choice of anticoagulation in this setting presents a major challenge. Oral anticoagulants are considered the most efficacious in preventing maternal heart valve thrombosis but the fetal risks are unacceptable to most women, even when substituting LMWH in the first trimester and around the time of delivery. It is therefore increasingly common and accepted practice to offer LMWH throughout pregnancy [27]. Each case needs to be assessed on an individual basis, taking into account previous thrombotic complications and patient preferences, backed up by full counseling and documentation.

For women of child-bearing age who require valve replacement, the use of bioprosthetic valves should be considered to avoid the need for anticoagulation. The disadvantage is the structural deterioration over time, particularly of those in the mitral position. The majority require replacement by 10 years. Choice of valve type therefore requires full information being given to the patient to ensure an informed decision that is understood and mutually agreed.

Management of Delivery on Full Anticoagulation

Labor and delivery are associated with significant bleeding risk and careful management of anticoagulation at this time is crucial. All women on anticoagulants, whether for prophylaxis or treatment, should have a clear labor plan in place. This is most commonly discussed at 34–36 weeks' gestation in a specialized obstetric hematology clinic where the mode of delivery, anesthetic options and management of labor should all be addressed.

Women on full anticoagulants at the time of delivery will be at high risk of complications, due to the nature of the underlying medical condition as well as its required anticoagulation. The delicate balance of risks between bleeding and thrombosis needs to be carefully managed. If warfarin has been used throughout the pregnancy, this should be stopped at 34–36 weeks' gestation and substituted with LMWH to avoid delivery of an anticoagulated baby at significant risk of bleeding. The mode of delivery is determined by obstetric and medical factors, rather than anticoagulation per se. Vaginal delivery is associated with lower risk of complications but may require a planned date to ensure timely omission of LMWH as well as adequate levels of trained staff. Disadvantages of artificially inducing labor are a higher chance of it being prolonged, requiring instrumental intervention or proceeding to Caesarean section. If labor is prolonged, boluses of the shorter-acting UFH may be considered on a 6–8 hourly basis, depending on progress, to avoid long periods without anticoagulation during this high-risk time. After delivery, the third stage of labor should be managed actively with oxytocics to reduce hemorrhagic risk. Any lacerations or episiotomy should be sutured promptly and once hemostasis is considered satisfactory, graduated doses of LMWH may be introduced from 6 hours after delivery.

Regional anesthesia is contraindicated within 12 hours of a prophylactic dose of LMWH and 24 hours after therapeutic doses because of the risk of vertebral canal hematoma. The risk is very small but with potentially grave consequences [1].

Obstetric Antiphospholipid Syndrome

Antiphospholipid syndrome (APS) is an autoimmune condition associated with vascular thrombosis in association with antiphospholipid antibodies (aPL). It may be primary or secondary to an underlying autoimmune disease. This is most commonly systemic lupus erythematous but others, such as inflammatory bowel disease, may be involved. Antiphospholipid antibodies include the lupus anticoagulant, anticardiolipin antibodies, and anti-B2-glycoprotein I antibodies. As transient or incidental antibodies are common, occurring in 3–5% of the general population, positive APS serology is defined by the persistence of aPL antibodies.

Complications of obstetric APS include recurrent fetal loss, intrauterine growth restriction, early-onset pre-eclampsia, prematurity, HELLP syndrome (hemolysis, elevated liver enzymes, low platelets), fetal distress, and fetal death. Approximately 10–20% of women who have a history of recurrent first trimester pregnancy loss are found to have detectable aPL, and have a high risk of further fetal loss if left untreated [31].

Thrombosis may be venous or arterial, with venous events often occurring in unusual sites such as the retinal, cerebral, or axillary veins [32]. Arterial events most commonly involve the central nervous system and patients may present with transient ischemic attacks or stroke. Dermal vessel thrombosis leads to livedo reticularis. Autoimmune cytopenias can develop, most commonly immune thrombocytopenia (ITP), which has been described in up to 30% of cases.

Several pathophysiological mechanisms have been described, perhaps accounting for the different presentations. Histological studies of placentas from these patients demonstrate substantial vasculopathy and placental thrombosis. Placental injury has also been caused by direct damage to trophoblasts by aPL, impairing trophoblastic invasion, and by complement activation through the classical pathway, with influx of inflammatory cells [33].

To avoid inaccurate diagnosis, investigation should only take place in those patients whose clinical features are in keeping with the diagnostic criteria determined by the International Society for Thrombosis and Haemostasis. Persistence of aPL should be demonstrated over at least a 12-week period. The diagnostic criteria are outlined in Table 26.5.

Management of APS depends on the clinical history. This will include the presence of previous thrombotic episodes and other medical conditions. Obstetric management should take place in a specialized center with a multidisciplinary team approach. Prepregnancy counseling should be offered to all women where possible and a clear plan for pregnancy management outlined. LMWH is used to prevent

Table 26.5 Criteria for the diagnosis of antiphospholipid syndrome.

Clinical criteria:

1) Vascular thrombosis – one or more episode of arterial, venous, or small vessel thrombosis
2) Pregnancy morbidity
   a) One or more unexplained pregnancy loss after the 10th week of gestation of a morphologically normal fetus
   b) One or more preterm births before the 34th week of gestation because of eclampsia, pre-eclampsia, or placental insufficiency
   c) Three or more unexplained consecutive spontaneous miscarriages before the 10th week of gestation with exclusion of underlying chromosomal or maternal causes

Laboratory criteria:

1) Positive plasma lupus anticoagulant on 2 or more occasions more than 12 weeks apart
2) Anticardiolipin antibody (IgG and/or IgM) present in medium or high titer on 2 or more occasions more than 12 weeks apart
3) Anti-B2-glycoprotein 1 antibody (IgG and/or IgM) in titer >99th centile present on 2 or more occasions more than 2 weeks apart

Source: modified from Miyakis *et al.*, 2006 [34].

thrombosis, together with low-dose aspirin, to prevent recurrent obstetric morbidity. Monthly fetal growth scans and uterine Doppler studies, to detect notching, help to predict placental dysfunction.

Contraception, HRT, and *in Vitro* Fertilization

Contraception

Meta-analysis shows a 3.5-fold increased risk of VTE associated with the combined oral contraceptive pill (COCP) [35]. The degree of risk depends on the dose of estrogen and type of progesterone [36]. The estrogen compound is ethinylestradiol. Earlier brands contained 150–100 µg of ethinylestradiol, which was reduced to as low as 20 µg for newer brands. The COCPs that contain higher estrogen content have been found to have the highest risk of VTE [35].

Along with the reduction in the estrogen component there was a change in the progesterone component of the COCP in order to minimize side-effects and over time three generations of COCP have been developed. Third-generation pills, containing the progestogens gestodene and desogestrel and the newer agent, drospirenone, have the highest risk, whilst the lowest risks are associated with levonorgestrel, norgestimate, and norethisterone. This has been confirmed by a recent meta-analysis comparing COCPs on a generation by generation basis [35] (Table 26.6). Dianette is also one of the higher-risk preparations. This contains cyproterone acetate 2 mg and ethinylestrodiol 35 µg, and is primarily used for the treatment of acne and hirsutism.

Table 26.6 Risk of venous thromboembolism associated with oral contraceptives.

Generation of contraceptive	Progestogen type	Relative risk of venous thrombosis compared to non-use (95% CI)
1st generation COCP	Norethisterone and lynestrol	3.2 (2.0–5.1)
2nd generation	Norgestrel and levonorgestrel	2.8 (2.0–4.1)
3rd generation	Gestodene, desogestrel, norgestimate	3.8 (2.7–5.4)
Most recent	Drospirenone	3.8 (2.7–5.5)
Antiandrogen	Cyproterone acetate	3.8 (2.7–5.5)

Source: data from Stegeman *et al.* [35].
COCP, combined oral contraceptive pill.

There are no randomized controlled trial data comparing the risk of VTE between different routes of administration of hormones and information about nonoral combined preparations arises from case–control and cohort studies [37]. Transdermal contraceptives and vaginal rings have been shown to increase the risk of VTE by two times when compared to levonorgestrel containing COCP [37]. The estimated risk of DVT with norelgestromin patch was 53 per 100 000 and 149 per 100 000 for etonogestrel ring [38].

Despite the increase in relative risk of thrombosis with combined contraceptives, the absolute risk remains low, given the incidence of VTE in women of child bearing age is about 2/10 000. The greater risk of VTE associated with pregnancy and the puerperium means that the benefit of combined contraceptives, in preventing unwanted pregnancies, outweighs their risks. However, before initiating treatment, women should be assessed for their risk of VTE and counseled appropriately. Risk is maximal during the first year of treatment, falling thereafter but remaining greater than in nonusers.

Progesterone Only Pills

Progesterone only preparations can be administered orally, by subcutaneous implant, intramuscular injection, or by an intrauterine device. Current evidence suggests that there is no increased risk associated with these methods of contraception [39] and they offer a valid alternative for at-risk women. The exception is intramuscular depot injection, which was shown by meta-analysis to be associated with a relative risk of VTE of 2.67 (CI 1.29–5.53) [39]. This may reflect the high dose, with 150 mg medroxyprogesterone administered as a depot, compared with 20 μg of levonorgestrel released daily from the intrauterine device.

Current guidelines from the RCOG advise against combined preparations in women with a personal history of VTE or known thrombophilia but consider the benefits of progesterone-only preparations to outweigh the risks.

Hormone Replacement Therapy

The use of exogenous estrogen in oral hormone replacement therapy (HRT) confers a similarly increased relative risk of VTE as the COCP; however, the absolute risk is higher in HRT than in COCP users, due to their older age (Table 26.7). Meta-analysis confirmed the higher risk in the first year of use, with an odds ratio of 4.0 (2.9–5.7), compared with treatment for more than 1 year 2.1 (1.3 – 3.8) ($P < 0.05$) [40]. There was no significant difference between unopposed oral estrogen and combined estrogen progesterone preparations. In women with inherited thrombophilias, the addition of oral HRT further enhances VTE risk in a synergistic manner. The increased risk associated with oral HRT disappears 4 months after discontinuing.

Transdermal preparations include patches, gels, spray, creams, and the vaginal ring. They bypass first-pass metabolism and avoid hepatic induction of clotting factors, allowing for improved efficacy with fewer side-effects. Doses are reduced and do not appear to increase thrombotic risk [40,41]. This applies to estrogen alone, combined estrogen, and progesterone and also the synthetic steroid, tibolone. More recently, micellar nanoparticle estradiol emulsion has gained FDA approval. It provides an alternative transdermal delivery and avoids irritation and other adverse effects [42].

Before starting HRT, women should be counseled about the associated VTE risk, amongst other deleterious consequences [43,44]. Current

Table 26.7 Risk of venous thromboembolism (VTE) associated with hormone replacement therapy (HRT).

HRT preparation	Absolute risk of VTE per 1000 person years
Combined estrogen progestogen	2.6 (2.0–3.2)
Estrogen alone	2.2 (1.6–3.0)
Transdermal	1.2 (0.9–1.7)
Tibolone	0.9 (0.8–1.1)

RCOG guidelines state that a personal history of VTE is a contraindication to oral HRT and first-degree family history of VTE or known thrombophilia are relative contraindications. Transdermal treatment should be offered as an alternative if the benefits to symptoms and quality of life outweigh the risks [45,46].

In Vitro Fertilization

Infertility affects more than 10% of couples worldwide. IVF involves downregulation of natural hormone production followed by ovarian stimulation. During the stimulatory phase endogenous estrogens increase 10–100 fold. Given the known prothrombotic effect of exogenous estrogen therapy, it is likely to be this aspect that is responsible for the increased thrombotic risk associated with IVF. The older age (median age 33 years) and higher incidence of multiple pregnancies are confounding factors but multivariate analysis confirms an increased risk associated with the procedure itself. Not surprisingly, the greatest relative risk is in the first trimester, with a demonstrated hazard ratio of 4.05 (2.54–6.46). Relative risk was less high in the third trimester than in non-IVF pregnancies and equal in the postpartum period [47].

Ovarian Hyperstimulation

Over stimulation of the ovaries occurs in approximately 5% of stimulated ovarian cycles, most commonly a few days following follicular rupture or egg retrieval for IVF. It is exacerbated if pregnancy is successful. Cardinal features include marked ovarian enlargement, with over production of ovarian hormones and vasoactive substances, causing increased capillary permeability and, in severe cases, large fluid shifts into the extracellular spaces. Around 10% develop VTE but interestingly, in atypical locations. Common sites are the internal jugular vein, subclavian veins, inferior vena cava, iliofemoral veins, and intracerebral veins. The reason for these unusual sites has not been clarified.

References

1 Pavord S, Hunt B. *The Obstetric Hematology Manual*. Cambridge Medicine, 2010.
2 Clark P, Brennand J, Conkie JA, *et al*. Activated protein C sensitivity, protein C, protein S and coagulation in normal pregnancy. *Thromb Haemost* 1998; 79: 1166–1170.
3 Bonnar J, McNicol GP, Douglas AS. Fibrinolytic enzyme system and pregnancy *Br Med J* 1969; iii: 416–420.
4 Voke J, Keidan J, Pavord S, *et al*. The management of antenatal venous thromboembolism in the UK and Ireland: a prospective multicentre observational survey. *Br J Haematol* 2007; 139: 545–558.
5 McColl MD, Ramsay JE, Tait RC, *et al*. Risk factors for pregnancy associated venous thromboembolism. *Thromb Haemost* 1997; 78: 1183–1188.
6 Saving Mothers' Lives: Reviewing maternal deaths to make motherhood safer: 2006–2008. *BJOG* 2011; 18: 1–203.
7 Macklon NS, Greer IA. The deep venous system in the puerperium: an ultrasound study. *Br J Obstet Gynaecol* 1997; 104: 198–200.
8 Ray JG, Chan WS. Deep vein thrombosis during pregnancy and the puerperium: a meta-analysis of the period of risk and the leg of presentation. *Obstet Gynecol Surv* 1999; 54: 265–271.
9 Nelson SM, Greer IA. Thrombophilia and the risk for venous thromboembolism during pregnancy, delivery and puerperium. *Obstet Gynecol Clin N Am* 2006; 33: 413–427.
10 James AH. Prevention and management of venous thromboembolism in pregnancy. *Am J Med* 2007; 120: s26–34.
11 Brill-Edwards P, Ginsberg JS, for the Recurrence Of Clot In This Pregnancy (ROCIT) Study Group. Safety of withholding antepartum heparin in women with a previous episode of venous thromboembolism. *N Engl J Med* 2000; 343: 1439–44.
12 Royal College of Obstetricians and Gynaecologists. Reducing the risk of thrombosis and embolism during pregnancy and the puerperium *RCOG Green Top Guideline*, No 37a, 2009.

13 Modder J, Fitzsimons K. *CMACE/RCOG Joint Guideline: Management of Women with Obesity in Pregnancy*. Royal College of Obstetricians and Gynaecologists, 2010.

14 Larsen TB, Sørensen HT, Gislum M, *et al*. Maternal smoking, obesity and risk of venous thromboembolism: a population based nested case-control study. *Thromb Res* 2007; 120: 505–509.

15 Leizorovicz A, Becker F, Buchmuller A, *et al*. Clinical relevance of symptomatic superficial-vein thrombosis extension: lessons from the CALISTO study. *Blood* 2013; 122: 1724–1729.

16 Decousus H, Prandoni p, Mismeti P, *et al*. Fondaparinux for the treatment of superficial vein thrombosis in the legs. *N Engl J Med* 2010; 363: 1222–1232.

17 EFSA Panel on Dietetic Products, Nutrition, and Allergies (NDA). Scientific opinion on dietary reference values for water. *EFSA J* 2010; 8: 1459.

18 Bates SM, Greer IA, Middeldorp S, *et al*. VTE, thrombophilia, anti-thrombotic therapy and pregnancy: antithrombotic therapy and prevention of thrombosis guidelines 9th edition, American College of Chest Physicians 2012. *Chest* 2012; 141 (2 Suppl.): e737S–e801S.

19 Royal College of Obstetricians and Gynaecologists. Thromboembolic disease in pregnancy and the puerperium: acute management. *RCOG Green Top Guideline*, No 28, 2007.

20 British Thoracic Society Standards of Care Committee Pulmonary Embolism Guideline Development Group. British Thoracic Society guidelines for the management of suspected acute pulmonary embolism. *Thorax* 2003; 58: 470–484.

21 Scarsbrook AF, Evans AL, Owen AL, *et al*. Diagnosis of suspected venous thromboembolic disease in pregnancy. *Clin Radiol* 2006; 61: 1–12.

22 Kyrle PA, Eichinger S. Deep vein thrombosis. *Lancet* 2005; 365: 1163–1174.

23 Remy-Jardin M, Remy. Spiral CT angiography of the pulmonary circulation. *Radiology* 1999; 212: 615–636.

24 Patel RP, Hunt BJ. Where do we go now with low molecular weight heparin use in obstetric care? *J Thromb Haemost* 2008; 6: 1461–1467.

25 Patel JP, Green B, Patel RK, *et al*. Population pharmacokinetics of enoxaparin during the antenatal period. *Circulation* 2013; 128: 1462–1469.

26 Linkins LA, Dans AL, Moores LK, *et al*. Treatment and prevention of Heparin-Induced Thrombocytopenia: Antithrombotic therapy and prevention of thrombosis 9th edition: American college of chest physicians evidence based clinical practice guidelines. *Chest* 2012; 141 (Suppl.): e495S–530S.

27 Bates SM, Greer IA, Pabinger I, *et al*. Venous thromboembolism, thrombophilia, antithrombotic therapy and pregnancy: American College of Chest Physicians Evidence-Based Clinical Practice Guidelines (8th edition). *Chest* 2008; 133: 844S–886S.

28 Keeling D, Baglin T, Tait C, *et al*.: British Committee on Standards in Haematology. Guidelines on oral anticoagulation with warfarin 4th Edition. *Br J Haematol* 2011; 154: 311–324.

29 British Committee for Standards in Haematology Writing Group. Guidelines on use of IVC filters. *Br J Haematol* 2007; 134: 590–595.

30 Musani MH, Matta F, Yaekoub AY, *et al*. Venous compression for prevention of postthrombotic syndrome: a meta-analysis. *Am J Med* 2010; 123: 735–740.

31 Yetman DL, Kutteh WH. Antiphospholipid antibody panels and recurrent pregnancy loss: prevalence of anticardiolipin antibodies compared with other antiphospholipid antibodies *Fertil Steril* 1996; 66: 540–546.

32 Cervera R, Piette JC, Font J, *et al*. Euro-Phospholipids Project Group. Antiphospholipid syndrome: Clinical and immunologic manifestations and patterns of disease expression in a cohort of 1000 patients. *Arthritis Rheum* 2002; 46: 1019–1027.

33 Girardi G, Redecha P, Salmon JE. Heparin prevents antiphospholipid antibody induced

fetal loss by inhibiting complement activation. *Nat Med* 2004; 10: 1222–1226.

34 Miyakis S, Lockshin MD, Atsumi T, *et al.* International consensus statement on an update of the classification criteria for definite antiphospholipid syndrome (APS). *J Thromb Haemost* 2006; 4: 295–306.

35 Stegeman BH, de Bastos M, Rosendaal FR, *et al.* Different combined oral contraceptives and the risk of venous thrombosis: Systematic review and network meta-analysis. *BMJ* 2013; 347: f5298.

36 Hannaford PC. Epidemiology of the contraceptive pill and venous thromboembolism. *Thromb Res* 2011; 127: S30–S34.

37 Allan GM, Koppula S. Risks of venous thromboembolism with various hormonal contraceptives. *Can Fam Physician* 2012; 58: 1097.

38 Lopez LM, Grimes DA, Gallo MF, *et al.* Skin patch and vaginal ring versus combined oral contraceptives for contraception. *Cochrane Database Syst Rev* 2013; (4): CD003552.

39 Mantha S, Karp R, Raghavan V, *et al.* Assessing the risk of venous thromboembolic events in women taking progestin-only contraception: A meta-analysis. *BMJ* 2012; 345: e4944.

40 Canonico M, Plu-Bureau G, Lowe G, *et al.* Hormone replacement therapy and risk of venous thromboembolism in postmenopausal women: systematic review and meta-analysis *BMJ* 2008; 336: 1227–1231.

41 Renoux C, Dell'Aniello S, Suissa S. Hormone replacement therapy and the risk of venous thromboembolism: a population based study. *J Thromb Haemost* 2010; 8: 979–986.

42 Valenzuela P, Simon JA. Nanoparticle delivery for transdermal HRT. *Maturitas* 2012; 73: 74–80.

43 Marjoribanks J, Farquhar C, Roberts H, *et al.* Long term hormone therapy for perimenopausal and postmenopausal women (review). *Cochrane Database Syst Rev* 2012; (7): CD004143.

44 Schierbeck LL, Rejnmark L, Tofteng CL, *et al.* Effect of hormone replacement therapy on cardiovascular events in recently postmenopausal women: Randomised trial. *BMJ* 2012; 345: e6409.

45 Royal College of Obstetricians and Gynaecologists. *Venous thromboembolism and Hormone Replacement Therapy*, guideline No.19. RCOG, 2011.

46 American College of Obstetricians and Gynaecologists. Committee Opinion No. 556. Postmenopausal estrogen therapy: route of administration and risk of venous thromboembolism. *Obstet Gynecol* 2013; 121: 887–890.

47 Henriksson P, Westerlund E, Wallen H, *et al.* Incidence of pulmonary and venous thromboembolism in pregnancies after in vitro fertilisation: cross sectional study. *BMJ* 2013; 346: 1–11.

27

Pediatrics

Mary E. Bauman, Aisha Bruce and M. Patricia Massicotte

Key Points

- There has been a dramatic increase in the incidence of thrombosis in children, with a number of high-risk cohorts.
- Developmental hemostasis plays a major role in the etiology, incidence, and management of thrombosis.
- Sequelae of thrombosis in children are severe, necessitating careful consideration of treatment.
- Current therapies are challenging to use safely. New agents require formal evaluation and studies are underway.
- Extrapolating adult guidelines for treatment to children are not appropriate and may cause harm.

Quaternary Care Pediatrics: Trading One Problem for Another

There has been a dramatic increase in the diagnosis of thrombosis in children over the past decade [1]. As a result, many health professionals are now confronted with diagnosis and management of thrombosis in children. The unique differences in children are important and therefore extrapolating management from adult practice is inappropriate. The differences include normal childhood nutrition, ongoing growth, acquired and developmental

differences in hemostasis, and differences drug metabolism

The intention of this chapter will be to provide a practical guide to diagnosis and management of thrombosis in children. Within this chapter the term "children" will be used to describe infants and children unless otherwise stated.

Hemostasis in Children

The hemostatic differences in children compared to adults affect the incidence, etiology, and management of thrombosis in children [2].

Developmental Hemostasis

Normal physiological hemostasis in children is known as developmental hemostasis. Although the cell-based model of anticoagulation is important to simplify and facilitate understanding of developmental hemostasis, the cascade model will be applied in this discussion (see Chapter 1). As in adults, the cascade model of coagulation and fibrinolysis include two pathways responsible for hemostasis with a number of protein components, which when activated by a stimulus interact with red blood cells and platelets and result in thrombus formation (coagulation) and/or thrombus degradation (fibrinolysis). Procoagulant proteins factors XII, XI, , X, IX, VIII, VII, V, II, high molecular weight kininogen (HMWK), and fibrinogen are activated by a stimulus (e.g., sepsis, trauma, surgery) resulting

Practical Hemostasis and Thrombosis, Third Edition. Edited by Nigel S. Key, Michael Makris and David Lillicrap.
© 2017 John Wiley & Sons, Ltd. Published 2017 by John Wiley & Sons, Ltd.

in production of thrombin (FIIa). Thrombin activates fibrinogen into fibrin, the precursor of a polymerized clot. The fibrinolytic system is subsequently activated to break down the clot. Proteins are present to prevent massive clot formation and facilitate clot lysis. Antithrombin, protein C, protein S, and α2-macroglobulin inhibit clot formation, while plasminogen activator inhibitor 1 inhibits clot lysis.

The Differences in Children

In infants, contact factors XII, X, HMWK, and the vitamin K-dependent factors II, VII, IX, and X are at lower physiological concentrations and reach adult levels at approximately 6 months of age [2]. In contrast, α2-macroglobulin is at 200% of adult levels and declines to adult normal levels during adolescence, which is hypothesized to protect children from thrombosis. In addition, when hemostasis is activated, children

generate 30–50% less thrombin compared to adults [3,4] and have, overall, less activity of the fibrinolytic system [5] (Table 27.1).

Studies suggest that platelet number and function in children are similar to that in adults. However, *in vitro* neonatal platelets are demonstrated to be hyporeactive to thrombin, adenosine diphosphate/ epinephrine, and thromboxane A$_2$ [6].

Despite these differences, hemostatic balance is maintained within the normal neonate and child.

Cohorts of Children at Risk for Thrombosis

There are numerous cohorts of children that are at high risk for venous or arterial thrombosis [7]. These include:

- *Children with chronic medical conditions*: 63% of children diagnosed with thrombosis

Table 27.1 Coagulation inhibitor reference values for neonates and children.

Coagulation inhibitors (%)	Age						
	Day 1	Day 3 adapted from	1 month–1 year	1– 5 years	6–10 years	11–16 years	Adults
Antithrombin	76* (58–90)	74* (60–89)	109* (72–134)	116* (101–131)	114* (95–134)	111* (96–126)	96 (66–124)
	n=18 (9F/12M)	n=22 (10F/12M)	n=41 (8F/33M)	n=49 (26F/23M)	n=59 (25F/34M)	n=26 (8F/18M)	n=43
Protein C chromogenic	36* (24–44)	44* (28–54)	71* (31–112)	96* (65–127)	100 (71–129)	94* (66–118)	104 (74–164)
	n=22 (9F/13M)	n=21 (10F/11M)	n=25 (5F/20M)	n=42 (21F/21M)	n=53 (21F/32M)	n=25 (8F/17M)	n=42
Protein C clotting	32* (24–40)	33* (24–51)	77* (28–124)	94* (50–134)	94* (64–125)	88* (59–112)	103 (54–166)
	n=20 (9F/11M)	n=22 (11F/11M)	n=24 (4F/20M)	n=39 (16F/23M)	n=50 (17F/33M)	n=20 (6F/14M)	n=44
Protein S clotting	36* (28–47)	49* (33–67)	102* (29–162)	101* (67–136)	109* (64–154)	103* (65–140)	75 (54–103)
	n=22 (13F/9M)	n=24 (11F/13M)	n=41 (8F/33M)	n=49 (26F/23M)	n=59 (25F/34M)	n=27 (9F/18M)	n=44

Source: modified from Monagle *et al.* 2006 [2].
For each assay the first row shows the mean and boundaries including 95% of the population. The second row shows the number of individual samples and the ratio of males (M) to females (F) for each group * Denotes values that are significantly different from adult values (*P* <0.05).

had at least one chronic complex medical condition [1].

- *Children with congenital heart disease*: Advances in therapeutic interventions in children with acquired and congenital heart disease have resulted in increased survival. As a result, a large percentage of children requiring long-term anticoagulation have coexisting cardiac conditions with surgical interventions such as tristage Fontan palliation and mechanical valves. Thromboembolic events within Fontan circuits are a major cause of morbidity and mortality, with reported incidences of thrombosis and stroke from 3% to 16% and 3% to 19%, respectively. Studies have demonstrated that children post-Fontan procedure who received thromboprophylaxis, with either well-controlled warfarin (INR 2–3) or aspirin, had a decreased risk of thrombosis compared to children who were poorly controlled on warfarin or received no therapy [8–11].
- *Children with central catheters*: Central venous catheter-related thrombosis is relatively common [11]. There is no reported difference in incidence between tunneled lines compared with peripherally inserted central catheters [12].
- *Acquired heart disease such as cardiomyopathy or Kawasaki disease* [13].
- *Nephrotic syndrome*: Up to 25% of children with nephrotic syndrome develop venous thromboembolism (VTE). VTE etiology in this group is multifactorial, with disease-associated coagulopathy a significant contributor [14].
- *Sepsis*: Emerging data describes the role of neutrophils in activation of thrombosis and subsequent development of VTE in patients with sepsis. Neutrophils are activated by microbial pathogens and release highly charged mixtures of DNA (deoxyribonucleic acid) and nuclear proteins termed neutrophil extracellular traps. In addition to limiting pathogen dispersion and entrapment, these electrostatically charged adhesive networks trigger intrinsic coagulation [15].
- *Klippel–Trenaunay syndrome*: This is a congenital combined vascular (capillary, venous, and lymphatic) malformation with localized disturbed limb growth and results in approximately one-third of children diagnosed with VTE. VTE was often associated with very high D-dimer levels in children [16,17].
- *Liver transplantation*: Hepatic artery thrombosis is a common complication following liver transplantation and is associated with significant mortality and morbidity [18,19].
- *Acute otitis media/ mastoiditis*: Many case studies describe an association with cerebral sinovenous thrombosis and resultant morbidity.
- *Antiphospholipid antibody* (APLA): APLAs include anticardiolipin antibody, lupus anticoagulant, and β_2-glycoprotein 1. APLAs are associated with an increased risk of thrombosis in children [20]. Consideration may be given to evaluation of APLAs in children who present with what appears to be idiopathic thrombosis.
- *Malignancy*: Treatment with *Escherichia coli* asparaginase, concomitant steroids, presence of central venous lines (CVLs), and thrombophilic abnormalities are established risk factors for thromboembolism [21].
- *Children undergoing cardiac catheterization*: Systemic arterial thromboembolic events in children often occur as a result of the placement of an arterial line or following cardiac catheterization. Thromboprophylaxis during cardiac catheterization is recommended [22].

Traumatic injuries in pediatrics are not strongly associated with development of thrombosis and therefore routine thromboprophylaxis is not recommended. The risk of VTE increases >18 years of age and the reported strongest risk factor for VTE in this population was the presence of a central venous line. Given that developmental hemostasis is resolved and the coagulation system of a child postpuberty is similar to that of an adult, adolescents should be individually evaluated for DVT risk in comparison to risk for hemorrhage. If the individual patient risk for thrombosis is considered to be high, enoxaparin 30 mg b.i.d. is commonly used in an adolescent >50 kg and titrated down for children weighing <50 kg [1].

Indications for Anticoagulation

Congenital Heart Disease

Congenital heart disease is one of the most common inborn defects, occurring in 0.8% of newborn infants. Many children with congenital heart disease have extracardiac shunts surgically placed as palliation for their condition, including Blalock Taussig shunts, Norwood Sano, Central Right Ventricle to Pulmonary Artery shunts, Glenn shunts, and Fontan shunts. These shunts vary in diameter and flow characteristics and are often considered at increased risk for thrombosis. Although there are no well-designed studies evaluating the use of anticoagulant or antiplatelet agents in this patient population, they are commonly used as thromboprophylaxis [8–10]. There are a number of other cardiac indications where anticoagulants and/or antiplatelets are used as thromboprophylaxis; however, there are no well-designed studies to provide safety and efficacy data for any therapeutic agent. Children with mechanical heart valves placed are prescribed long-term vitamin K antagonists (VKAs) as thromboprophylaxis as per adult guidelines [20].

Deep venous and Arterial Thrombosis and Pulmonary Embolism

Clinical symptoms of thrombosis vary depending on the location of the thrombus. For example, a deep venous thrombosis in a limb may be associated with pain, swelling, skin discoloration, and altered perfusion, whereas an intracardiac thrombus can range from asymptomatic to congestive heart failure, pulmonary embolism, or sequelae secondary to an embolus, including stroke, and organ or limb compromise.

Pulmonary embolism (PE) is rare in children, and most commonly occurs as a result of deep venous thrombosis [23]. The following radiographic tests may be used to diagnose PE in children: ventilation perfusion scan, spiral computed tomography (CT), magnetic resonance imaging (MRI), magnetic resonance venography (MRV), or pulmonary angiogram.

Long-term Anticoagulation in Children

Children requiring long-term primary thromboprophylaxis, such as children with congenital heart disease, present increased challenges, including life-long monitoring. A child with a mechanical heart valve may initiate anticoagulation at age 5 years, whereas an adult may begin VKAs much later in life; this results in many more patient years of anticoagulation.

Adherence to long-term anticoagulation, particularly during adolescence, is particularly challenging. Empowering these patients to participate actively in their health management is believed to improve adherence and long-term outcomes [24].

Diagnosis of Thrombosis in Children

Both venous and arterial thromboses require rapid diagnosis and treatment to prevent thrombus extension or embolism, which could result in mortality or morbidity.

Clinical studies have determined that the most sensitive diagnostic methods for diagnosing upper system thrombosis are ultrasound for jugular venous thrombosis and venography for intrathoracic vessels [25]. For symptomatic thrombosis of both the upper and lower system, ultrasound may be used; however, if the clinical suspicion for thrombosis is high and ultrasound is negative, further imaging such as MRI, CT, and/or venography of the suspicious venous or arterial system should be considered. There are no studies determining the sensitivity and specificity of these imaging techniques in children; however, they are commonly used. There has been a move towards MRI angio/venography over CT due to concern related to the high radiation dose associated with CT [26].

Intracardiac thromboses are often incidental findings for children with comprised cardiac function and may be identified through echocardiogram (thoracic or transesophageal as it provides better visualization), cardiac catheterization, angiogram, or cardiac MRI or CT.

D-dimers are of limited use in children although normal reference ranges have been reported [27]. They are sensitive yet not specific, which is problematic in the pediatric population as D-dimers are often elevated with any inflammatory condition, including potentially viral infections that are particularly common amongst children. Additionally, children with chronic disease may have elevated D-dimers.

Epidemiology of Thrombosis in Children

Thrombosis in children most commonly associated with more than two risk factors [28]. Idiopathic thrombosis in children is rare.

Outcomes of Thrombosis in Children

Post-thrombotic Syndrome in Children

Post-thrombotic syndrome is characterized by pain, swelling, and alterations in perfusion, which may result in skin ulceration. There is no treatment; however, palliation may include the use of compression stockings. There are a number of tools used to evaluate the severity of post-thrombotic syndrome [27].

Loss of venous access secondary to thrombosis is problematic in this vulnerable population. In children with chronic health conditions, venous access is often required for future procedures and therapies.

Outcomes of Systemic Arterial Thrombosis in Children

Outcomes of systemic arterial thrombosis in children are:

- Loss of life, limb, or organ, dependent on thrombus location, may occur.

- Limb length discrepancy and intermittent claudication secondary to decreased perfusion has been reported.

The Importance of Antithrombotic Therapy

Treatment of thrombosis in children is important due to resultant morbidity and mortality. Unlike adults, even asymptomatic clots result in serious sequelae in children.

- Many children have intracardiac blood shunts (right–left), thus venous thrombi may result in stroke [29].
- There is an association between sepsis and thrombosis [30].
- Pulmonary embolism is often asymptomatic in children due to large cardiopulmonary reserves yet may be life-threatening [31].
- Occlusion of vessels due to thrombosis often results in loss of venous access in children who require intravenous access and therapies to sustain life and optimize treatment [20].
- Post-thrombotic syndrome including pain and swelling often results in limitation of activities, and venous collaterals influence body image and self esteem [32]. These residual symptoms may have a negative impact on the child's quality of life [27].

Therapeutic Agents and Metabolism

Evidence for the safety and efficacy of therapies is established through clinical trials. It is challenging to perform rigorous studies in children [33] and, as a result, the agents that are commonly used for treatment of thrombosis in children are limited to heparin therapy and vitamin K antagonists. Current safety and efficacy data in adults support the premise that, when patients are maintained within their defined therapeutic range, they will be adequately protected from the risk of thrombosis and the risk of a serious adverse event will be minimized [20,34,35]. The risk–benefit ratio of anticoagulation and the impact on patient's health-related quality of life (HRQOL) should be considered in all children and neonates before initiating antithrombotic therapy.

Although the new anticoagulants, such as the direct thrombin inhibitors and direct factor Xa inhibitors, are currently being evaluated in children, it will be a number of years before there is sufficient evidence to support the use of these agents in children (see Section New Agents).

Health-related Quality of Life

Evidence-based medicine requires both patient and health-care provider to systemically assess the quality and strength of the evidence in the context of the patient's HRQOL, which includes the patient's values, preferences, and life experience [36]. HRQOL focuses on dimensions of quality of life specifically related to health and therapeutic management strategies [35]. Traditional measures of safety and efficacy do not consider what the patient considers acceptable or unacceptable, which directly impacts their personal HRQOL. HRQOL is considered the "gold-standard" measurement for patient-relevant outcomes. HRQOL is demonstrated to be impacted by long-term antithrombotic therapy [37,38].

Antithrombotic Therapy in Children

Antithrombotic therapy in children is unique as it is influenced by the dynamically evolving coagulation system (see Section Developmental Hemostasis) in addition to other factors. The risk versus benefit of administering antithrombotic therapy should be carefully considered in all children prior to commencing antithrombotic therapy. Additional factors that influence administration and management of antithrombotic therapy in children include:

- Distribution, binding, and clearance of antithrombotic drugs are age dependent.
- Many children requiring antithrombotic therapy have coexisting medical conditions, which often require concurrent medications that

may interfere with metabolism and clearance of anticoagulant therapies.
- The practical ability to deliver the drug is impacted by difficult venous access, needle phobias, etc.
- Pediatric formulations of antithrombotic drugs are not available, making accurate dose measurement difficult.
- Neonates are at higher risk of intracranial hemorrhage due to immature intravascular development. Strong consideration should be given to obtaining brain-imaging studies in neonates prior to anticoagulation to provide a baseline as part of a risk–benefit assessment. Importantly, brain abnormalities, including intracranial hemorrhage, may be asymptomatic.
- Procedures such as lumbar punctures or spinal anesthesia/ pain management should not be performed while on antithrombotic therapy [39].
- Antithrombotic therapy should be avoided in acute or subacute endocarditis due to the risk of mycotic aneurysms [39].

Heparin

Heparin is a term that encapsulates and describes both unfractionated heparin (UFH) and low-molecular-weight heparins (LMWH).

Unfractionated Heparin in Children

UFH remains a common anticoagulant agent used in hospital settings for children at increased risk of hemorrhage (i.e., postoperatively) or in the intensive care setting. Heparin is not absorbed orally, therefore must be administered intravenously or subcutaneously.

UFH Metabolism in Children
UFH acts via antithrombin-mediated catabolism of thrombin and inhibition of factors IIa, IXa, Xa, XIa, and XIIa. UFH is poorly bioavailable and binds with a number of plasma proteins, endothelial cells, and macrophages and to central lines and IV tubing [40]. Poor bioavailability results in variability in anticoagulant

response. Furthermore, UFH binds to von Willebrand factor and inhibits von Willebrand factor-dependent platelet function, potentially increasing hemorrhage [41].

UFH binds with antithrombin to catabolize thrombin. Antithrombin can be as low as 30% of adult levels in normal infants and as low as 10% of adult levels in infants and children during illness, which further increases the variability in anticoagulant response [42–47]. As a result, the predictability of UFH response is challenging within and between patients and contributes to the high incidence of adverse events related to heparin therapy. Potentiation of the UFH effect by administering antithrombin concentrate may be performed although is controversial [48]. Administering antithrombin is described in infants and children requiring extracorporeal life support [48–51]. However, studies have not been completed to evaluate long-term outcomes and define safety and efficacy of this practice.

UFH Benefits

UFH has a short half-life, therefore clears within 4–6 hours of cessation. It is fully reversible with protamine sulfate.

UFH Limitations

Limitations of UFH are:

- Venous access is required for administration and monitoring of UFH. This is problematic due to limited venous access in children. CVLs are often used for administration and for drawing blood samples, resulting in inaccurate results due to heparin contamination of samples. To minimize heparin contamination of blood samples drawn from CVLs, a large saline flush followed by a large draw of discard blood has been shown to reduce UFH contamination if performed prior to drawing the actual sample to be sent for analysis [40].
- Different formulations are available, including highly concentrated solutions, which have resulted in frequent dosing errors in the pediatric population with consequent fatal hemorrhages [20].

- Poor bioavailability of UFH can result in a variable and unpredictable response [42,43,47].
- UFH is associated with osteopenia, although this may be reversible.
- UHF is associated with heparin-induced thrombocytopenia (HIT), although rare in children this should prompt the discontinuation of heparins and the use of a parenteral nonheparin agent, such as lepirudin, bivalirudin, argatroban, or danaparoid [20].

UFH Dosing in Children

Dosing of UFH in children is age dependent (Table 27.2). The age-dependent dose in children <12 months of age is 28 U/kg/hour and ≥12 months of age is 20 U/kg/hour, IV or SC.

Children will achieve therapeutic UFH (antifactor Xa) levels more quickly if a UFH bolus dose of no greater than 100 U/kg/hour is administered; however, it is important to consider the risk–benefit ratio with regards to hemorrhage.

Heparin doses are subsequently titrated based on laboratory measure of antifactor Xa, or activated partial thromboplastin time (APTT) when an antifactor Xa measure is not available.

Dosing guidelines are provided in Table 27.3.

UFH Subcutaneous Dosing: Therapeutic UFH may be administered subcutaneously. The daily dose in U/kg/hour is divided in two daily doses and is given every 12 hours. Dosing is calculated using the following formula:

SC dose = age-dependent dose (i.e., 20 or 28 U/kg/hour) × patient weight × hours of coverage

SC UFH is monitored by using either the APTT or antifactor Xa level measured at 4–6 hours after the SC dose. The dose is adjusted according to the UFH nomogram (Table 27.3).

UFH Monitoring in Children

Antifactor Xa: The internationally accepted gold standard measure of UFH is the antifactor Xa level, with a target therapeutic range in children of 0.35–0.7 U/mL [20]. Extrapolating the use of the APTT for monitoring from adults to

Table 27.2 Summary of clinical properties of commonly used anticoagulants in children.

Anticoagulant	Properties	Indications	Contraindications	Dose	Monitoring
UFH	Half-life dose dependent (max. 150 minutes)	Immediate postoperative	Thrombocytopenia HIT Known sensitivity to heparin or pork products	Age-dependent dosing	q24h at minimum
	Completely reversible with protamine sulfate	Increased risk of bleeding	Blood monitoring not able to be performed at appropriate intervals	<12 months of age = 28 U/kg/hour	Antifactor Xa level (0.35–0.70 U/mL)
	Poorly bioavailable, requires frequent blood monitoring	Frequent invasive procedures requiring reversal of anticoagulation	Uncontrollable active bleeding	>12 months of age = 20 U/kg/ hour	PTT range must be determined by each hospital to correspond to UFH 0.35–0.7 U/mL
LMWH	Highly bioavailable, "stable drug"	When bleeding risk considered stable	High risk for bleeding		anti-Xa target 0.5–1.0 U/mL
	Not fully reversible	Bridge between heparin and VKA postoperative	Reversal required frequently for interventions		Dose titrated to achieve level
	Antithrombin has less influence	Poor venous access	Hold LMWH for 24 hours before procedure		Minimum monthly levels
	Requires 24 hours to clear anticoagulant effect		Renal or severe hepatic insufficiency		INR or APTT will not be affected
Enoxaparin q12h	Half-life is 3–6 hours	Stable anticoagulant effect required	Hypersensitivity to enoxaparin HIT	Age-dependent dosing, <3 months of age = ~1.5 mg/ kg/ dose; 3 months of age = ~1.0 mg/kg/dose	LMWH level 4–6 hours post dose
Tinzaparin q24h	Half-life is 3–6 hours	Needle-phobic children on long-term therapy		200 mg/kg/dose	Age-dependent LMWH levels <5 years = 2 hours post dose; >5 years = 4 hours post dose
VKA Warfarin	Half-life is 160 hours, oral administration	Long-term anticoagulant therapy	Relative: <1 years of age unless mechanical valve in situ	Load: 0.1–0.2 mg/kg (see text) Maintenance: individualized dosing titrated to INR	INR daily until therapeutic, then decreased frequency when stable with minimum monthly testing Test INR with illness, medication, or diet change

HIT, heparin-induced thrombocytopenia; INR, international normalized ratio; LMWH, low-molecular-weight heparin; PTT, partial thromboplastin time; VKA, vitamin K antagonist.

Table 27.3 Example of a unfractionated heparin (UFH) dosing nomogram using a therapeutic activated partial thromboplastin time (APTT) range of 60–85. Caution: Each institution will have a different therapeutic APTT range and the table should be adjusted accordingly.

PPT(s)	Anti-Xa (U/mL)	Hold UFH (minutes)	Rate change	Repeat antifactor-Xa / APTT
<50	<0.1	0	20%	4 hours
50–59	0.1–0.34	0	10%	4 hours
60–85	0.35–0.70	0	0	24 hours
86–95	0.71–0.89	0	−10%	4 hours
96–120	0.90–1.20	30	−10%	4 hours
>120	>1.20	60	−15%	4 hours

pediatric patients is likely to be invalid, as normal APTTs in infants and children are increased due to developmental hemostasis [20]. Equally, there is a different response to heparin compared with adults; therefore, the use of the APTT to monitor heparin therapy may be invalid. In addition, *in vitro* and *in vivo* data support that the APTT that corresponds to an antifactor Xa level of 0.35–0.7 U/mL varies significantly with age [42,45].

Activated Partial Thromboplastin Time (APTT): Depending on the particular analyzer and reagent used to measure the APTT, a therapeutic APTT can range from 1.5 to 6.2 times baseline [41]. As a result, the therapeutic range for a APTT and its correlation to the antifactor Xa levels must be established by each institution [20].

Activated Clotting Time (ACT): There are no well-designed studies evaluating safety and efficacy ACT in children. Although many healthcare professionals use the ACT to measure anticoagulation, the ACT does not solely reflect the effect of heparin but also reflects changes in the hemostatic system such as coagulation defects, inhibitors, recent infusion of blood products, etc. It is a nonspecific general measure of coagulation and is unable to specifically measure the heparin effect. The accuracy and reliability of the ACT overall is controversial, and is further reduced in children less than 2 years of age [52].

Heparin-induced Thrombocytopenia in Children

HIT is an immune-mediated platelet reaction response to heparin. In adults, HIT is characterized by a sudden drop in platelets by more than 50% after 5 days of first-time heparin exposure or any time after a previous heparin exposure. The incidence among children is <0.1% [53]. The most reliable and accurate test to determine HIT is the serotonin release assay. This assay is performed only in a few laboratories. The enzyme-linked immunosorbent assay (ELISA) is most commonly available; however, the sensitivity is variable compared with the serotonin release assay, as shown by Warkentin [54].

If there is a strong suspicion or a positive diagnosis for HIT, all heparin and LMWH should be discontinued and an alternative agent used (VKA, direct thrombin, or factor Xa inhibitors).

UFH Reversal in Children

Dosing instructions for protamine sulfate are shown in Table 27.4. The maximum dose of protamine sulfate regardless of the amount of UFH received is 50 mg, and should be administered in a concentration of 10 mg/mL at a rate not to exceed 5 mg/minute. The exception to this is for reversal of UFH following cardiopulmonary bypass.

Protamine should not be administered quickly as a rapid infusion may result in cardiovascular collapse. Patients with known hypersensitivity reactions to fish and those who have received

Table 27.4 Unfractionated heparin (UFH) reversal.

Time since end of infusion, or last UFH dose (minutes)	Protamine per 100 U UFH dose (maximum 50 mg/dose) (mg)
<30	1
30–60	0.5–0.75
61–120	0.375–0.5
>120	0.25–0.375

protamine-containing insulin or previous protamine therapy may be at risk of hypersensitivity reactions to protamine sulfate. An APTT 15 minutes after administration will demonstrate the response obtained.

Protamine is cleared from the blood more rapidly than UFH, therefore close monitoring of antifactor Xa or APTT during and following reversal is necessary.

Low Molecular Weight Heparin

LMWHs are often the anticoagulant of choice for pediatric patients when not considered at high risk for hemorrhage. In adults, LMWHs are reported to have equal efficacy to the higher-molecular weight UFH and are associated with a decreased risk for hemorrhage. There are multiple studies evaluating dose requirements required to achieve a therapeutic level that demonstrate that age dependent dosing is required [55–57]. However, there are no well-designed studies evaluating the safety and efficacy of LMWH use in children.

LMWH Metabolism in Children
LMWHs inhibit the activation of the same activated factors as UFH; however, the greatest inhibition occurs for factor Xa. LMWHs have an average molecular weight of 5000 and are synthesized from higher molecular weight heparins (molecular weight 15 000). LMWHs have increased bioavailability, resulting in a more stable anticoagulant effect. There are three commonly used LMWHs (Table 27.2):

- enoxaparin,
- tinzaparin, and
- dalteparin.

LMWH Benefits
The benefits of LMWH include:

- 95% bioavailability making it a more agent;
- requires less frequent blood monitoring (compared to UFH);
- administered subcutaneously, therefore venous access is not required;
- decreased association with HIT (compared to UFH);
- does not interfere with platelet function;
- may be administered at home and caregivers may be taught how to administer LMWH.

LMWH Limitations
The limitations of LMWH are:

- not fully reversible; it is only 80% reversible with protamine sulfate;
- requires daily injections;
- can accumulate the presence of significant renal impairment; in this situation a 50% reduction in LMWH starting dose and more frequent monitoring is required.

LMWH Dosing in Children
Dosing of LMWHs is age dependent (Table 27.2). Recent publications describing enoxaparin dosing have suggested that age-dependent dose requirements [55–57] may be higher than suggested in Table 27.2. Dosing guidelines are provided in Table 27.5.

Whole Milligram Dosing

When enoxaparin doses are <10 mg: if the LMWH level is subtherapeutic, increase the dose by 1 mg and repeat LMWH level [55,58].
Tinzaparin doses <1000 units: if the LMWH level is subtherapeutic, increase the dose by 100 units and repeat LMWH level.

These dose changes have been demonstrated to be effective to achieve target therapeutic ranges, allow for more precise measurement and accurate dosing, and minimize dose measurement errors [58]. Enoxaparin may be administered

Table 27.5 Low-molecular-weight heparin (LMWH) dosing nomogram.

Anti-Xa level (U/mL)	Hold dose?	Dose Δ	Next antifactor Xa level?
<0.35	No	−25%	4 hours post second dose
0.35–0.49	No	−10%	4 hours post second dose
0.5–1.0	No	0	q1–4 weeks
<1.20	Consider	−20%	Consider drawing a trough level 10 hours post dose. If trough <0.5, administer next dose at 20% of previous dose

For doses of enoxaparin <10 mg and for tinzaparin <1000 U, increase or decrease dose by 1 mg or 100 U, respectively.

using an insulin syringe, as 1 U on an insulin syringe is equivalent to 1 mg enoxaparin.

LMWH Monitoring in Children
Only an antifactor Xa level can be used to monitor LMWH effect. LMWH maximally inhibits the activation of procoagulant factor X and minimally inhibits the activation of factor II. Therefore, an APTT will not measure LMWH effect and will only be minimally prolonged (a few seconds). The target antifactor Xa level on blood samples drawn 2–6 hours post-LMWH dose is 0.5–1.0 U/mL [20].

It is recommended that antifactor Xa levels be monitored monthly and dose adjustments be made to maintain an antifactor Xa (LMWH) level (Table 27.5). This is necessary in the pediatric population, as children often outgrow their current dose or there may be some accumulation over time due to insufficient renal clearance.

LMWH Reversal in Children
If anticoagulation with LWMH needs to be terminated for clinical reasons, discontinuation of LMWH injections for 24 hours will usually suffice. If an immediate reversal of effect is required, protamine sulfate reverses 80% of the antifactor Xa activity of LMWHs.

Oral Vitamin K Antagonists

The most commonly prescribed oral VKA is warfarin, with a half-life of 162 hours. Alternatively, in Europe and South America, phenprocoumon is frequently prescribed and has a half-life of 140 hours. VKAs remain the oral anticoagulant of choice in children until studies evaluating the pharmacokinetic, pharmacodynamic, and safety and efficacy studies using alternative agents are completed.

VKA Metabolism in Children
VKAs prevent gamma carboxylation of vitamin K-dependent procoagulant factors II, VII, IX, and X [20]. Pharmacogenomics are currently ongoing to evaluate single nucleotide polymorphisms in cytochrome P450 2C9 (*CYP2C9*) and vitamin K epoxide reductase (*VKORC1*) and their effect on warfarin dose requirements [59].

VKA is challenging to use in children because VKA metabolism can "change on a DIME" as it is altered by entities that are inherent to childhood [60,61]. The components of DIME are:

Diet: changes in eating habits that are normal and common in children.
Illness, such as colds or flu, that are particularly common amongst children.
Medications and dose changes: a large percentage of children have coexisting health conditions necessitating the use of additional medications. Weight-based dosing of most medications administered in childhood results in frequent dose changes, with each influencing VKA metabolism.
Error: missed doses (common in busy families and teenagers).

VKA Benefits in Children
The benefits of VKA for children are:

- oral administration,
- fully reversible.

VKA Limitations in Children

The limitations of VKA for children are:

- a narrow therapeutic index drug;
- VKA therapy in children is difficult (see DIME above);
- no pediatric formulation is available;
- requires frequent monitoring using the international normalized ratio (INR);
- children requiring anticoagulant therapy often have complex underlying health problems that result in frequent reversal for invasive procedures [1];
- drug–drug interactions, including the under reported use of complementary alternative therapies.

VKA and the Challenge of Complementary Alternative Medicines in Children

Complementary alternative medicines (CAMs) include nutritional and dietary supplements. The use of CAMs is highly underreported by children and their families. When children receiving anticoagulation use CAMs, this may influence their level of anticoagulation, resulting in thrombosis or hemorrhage. It is necessary to educate families about CAM use and its potential influence on their child's level of anticoagulation, increasing their risk of thrombosis and/or hemorrhage [62].

VKA Dosing in Children

Points to note in considering VKA dose in children are:

- Children have higher dose requirements compared to adults.
- The usual loading dose is 0.2 mg/kg/day with a maximum loading dose of 5 mg [20].
- Children with Fontan procedures require a decreased loading dose of warfarin (0.1 mg/kg/day) compared to usual loading dose of 0.2 mg/kg/day.
- If the INR reaches 1.6 within the first 3 days of dosing, the loading dose should be decreased by 50%.
- Varied dosing algorithms are available. An example nomogram is provided in Table 27.6.

Table 27.6 Sample warfarin dosing nomogram: maintenance phase for target international normalized ratio (INR) 2.5 (2.0–3.0).

INR	Action
1.1–1.4	Increase dose by 20%
1.5–1.9	Increase dose by 10%
2.0–3.0	No change
3.1–3.5	Decrease dose by 10%
>3.5–4.0	Administer one dose at 50% less than maintenance dose. Then restart at 20% less than previous maintenance dose
4.1–5.0	Hold 1 dose then restart at 20% less than previous maintenance dose
>5.0–<8.0 and no bleeding	Hold dose and repeat INR next day
>5.0 and bleeding OR >8.0	Consider reversal with Vitamin K or with major bleeding use factor concentrate

This nomogram is intended for use once loading phase is completed. Prior to each dose adjustment DIME (see text), as well as patient-specific indications and warfarin response, must be considered.

VKA Monitoring in Children

VKA therapy is monitored using the INR. Time in therapeutic range (TTR) is a commonly used surrogate for safety and efficacy.

Target INRs are in general extrapolated from adult ranges and are as follows.

- systemic thrombosis/ pulmonary embolism INR 2.5 (2–3);
- Fontan target INRs can vary upon individual practice between 1.5 and 3.0;
- mechanical heart valves:
  - aortic valve: target INR 2.5 (2–3);
  - mitral valve: target INR 3.0 (2.5–3.5).

Frequent INR monitoring is important due to the variability of INRs in children. The side-effects associated with oral anticoagulant therapy (bleeding and new or extension of thrombus) increase with poor oral anticoagulant control, as reflected by out-of-range INR. The event rate in children requiring oral antithrombotic therapy for varying etiologies is reported to range from 0% to 0.5% per patient year and 0% to 1.3%

per patient year for bleeding and thrombosis, respectively [20]. The mean INR testing frequency to maintain a stable anticoagulant effect is every 1–2 weeks.

Point-of-care/ Home INR Monitoring: a Solution to VKA Therapy in Children

The use of the point-of-care (POC) INR meter is a solution to improve management of VKA therapy in children. Published pediatric data indicates that TTR with patient self-testing (PST) using a POC INR meter is as high as 83% [63]. Patient self-testing also decreases clinically important events [63], resulting in outcomes equal to or better than those achieved with conventional management by physician or anticoagulation clinics utilizing laboratory INR [63].

The CoaguChek XS® is CE marked and Federal Drug Administration (FDA) approved and its use has been evaluated in children. Each meter has coded test strips that are inserted into the meter and warmed to 37°C. A capillary volume sample of blood (10 μL) is applied onto the test strip. The monitor uses an amperometric (electrochemical) method to monitor blood clotting induced by thromboplastin within the test strip to determine the PT. The PT is then converted to an INR using the International Sensitivity Index (ISI) previously determined and encoded on the chip for each lot of test strips. The CoaguChek XS® uses a recombinant human thromboplastin with an ISI value close to 1.0, consistent with World Health Organization standards. An INR is provided within 1 minute of application of the blood sample to the test strip. The internal quality control is embedded within the test strip and an INR result is not displayed if internal quality control conditions are not met. Regardless of its relative ease of use and minimal invasiveness, the successful implementation of a home POC INR monitoring program requires the generation and standardization of results that are both accurate and reliable [64].

The ease of using a POC INR meter at home facilitates:

- More frequent testing and improved time in therapeutic range as compared to laboratory INR testing in children [63].

- POC INR meters are demonstrated to be both accurate and precise. The INR test uses a capillary blood sample, produces an INR result within 1 minute, enables timely drug dosage adjustment, and allows prompt attention to critical values.
- POC INR test can be performed at the patient's convenience and eliminates the need for the patient to visit the laboratory.
- This convenience facilitates more frequent INR testing, a requirement for children when illness is present or when there is a change in diet or medication.
- POC INR monitoring provides a solution to the problem of pain associated with venipuncture, difficult venous access, and needle phobias.
- POC INR meter use is demonstrated to improve HRQOL [65].

For these reasons, POC INR meters are used for INR measurement in children as an option for improving VKA monitoring [66].

Modalities for POC Home INR Use in Children

Patient self-testing (PST) is where a patient performs and POC INR test at home and reports the INR result to the health-care team to receive further VKA dosing and an INR retest date.

Patient self-management (PSM) is a concept where a patient performing PST takes an active role in managing their treatment and provides potential for improving VKA management. This concept is similar to that accomplished in children with diabetes or asthma. Patients prescribed VKAs (and their families) are educated about VKA management and dosing, and subsequently self-adjust their VKA dose through application of dosing guidelines to the self-tested INR result. PSM is demonstrated to further improve HRQOL and appears to be as safe and effective as PST.

PSM provides the child/ family more investment in managing their health condition. The KIDCLOT PAC QL© is a reliable tool for measuring the impact of VKAs on HRQOL in children [37,38].

HRQOL evaluation demonstrated that in the first year of PSM, HRQOL decreased with subsequent improvement [37]. Focus groups revealed that the parents felt more responsibility, suggesting caregivers have improved awareness and knowledge of warfarin. All patients performing PSM preferred this system to laboratory testing or PST. Families stated it resulted in more independence and confidence in their child's VKA management. Importantly, PSM nurtures awareness and autonomy in teenagers as well as demonstrating increased HRQOL.

VKA Reversal in Children

VKA-induced Coagulopathy: The antidote for warfarin is dependent on whether urgent or nonurgent reversal is necessary [20]. In well, nonbleeding warfarinized children with an INR ≥5 and <8, temporary holding of warfarin alone appears sufficient to reverse warfarin-induced coagulopathy, with 50% returning to their therapeutic range after holding one warfarin dose [67]. For nonurgent reversal, vitamin K is administered at a dose of 0.5–1 mg orally, depending on the patient's size. The administration of vitamin K, either intravenously or intramuscularly, has been shown to be less efficacious than orally, as long as gut absorption is not severely compromised. For urgent reversal (major bleeding [68] or interventional procedure), fresh frozen plasma 20 mL/kg IV or factor concentrate is administered. Prothrombin complex concentrates are available for use and indicated for rapid reversal of VKAs in adults. The available formulations have variable amounts of factor II, VII, IX, X, protein C, protein S, heparin, and may contain antithrombin. In pediatrics there is insufficient evidence available to allow a recommendation for use.

Bridge Anticoagulation in Planned VKA Reversal in Children: Children who are considered to be at high risk for thrombosis (i.e., those with mechanical valves) may require bridge anticoagulant therapy using heparin [20] (see Section UFH dosing in children).

New Agents

The limitations of heparins, including heparin-induced thrombocytopenia, and vitamin K antagonists prompted development of new antithrombotic agents, oral and parenteral. The new agents inhibit thrombin directly (parenteral: argatroban, bivalirudin or lepirudin; oral: dabigatran), inhibit activated factor X (parenteral: fondaparinux; oral: rivaroxaban, apixaban), or have other inhibitory mechanisms (parenteral: danaparoid). All new antithrombotic agents require a formal pediatric investigational program developed by industry, international experts, and the drug regulatory agencies (FDA, EMA) prior to approval to determine pharmacokinetics/ pharmacodynamics (PK/PD), safety, efficacy, and HRQOL.

The direct thrombin inhibitors (DTIs) are not dependent on circulating antithrombin levels, bind both circulating and bound thrombin, do not cause HIT, and have more predictable pharmacokinetics than heparin; however, there are no antidote. Argatroban studies in children have resulted in pediatric dosing guidelines in the prescribing information in the United States [69–71]. Studies are underway in children using bivalirudin. There are ongoing studies in children on the oral DTI, dabigatran (see www.clinicaltrials.gov).

There are studies underway in children on the factor-Xa inhibitors. Although fondaparinux demonstrated safety (efficacy was not assessed), in children it cannot be reversed with protamine [72]. Studies on rivaroxaban are ongoing in children, with initial *in vitro* studies published estimating dosing information [73,74].

Duration and Intensity of Therapy in Children

Duration and intensity of therapy is based on adult recommendations; however, recent pediatric data suggests that this may be in excess of what is required due to earlier thrombus resolution in combination with developmental hemostasis. Until further studies are completed, it is reasonable to base therapy on adult recommendations; however, consideration may be given to the age of child, location of thrombus, risk factors for thrombus, early thrombus resolution, and the impact of antithrombotic therapy on HRQOL.

Current recommendations for prophylaxis/duration of treatment are as follows.

Thromboprophylaxis

There are no data to support the use of routine thromboprophylaxis of CVLs in children [20].

Duration of Treatment

Venous Thrombosis in Children: If the risk factor(s) are resolved then 3 months' duration is reasonable, providing there is no new extension of thrombus on repeated imaging studies. If, however, the risk factor remains (i.e., CVL) ongoing anticoagulation at subtherapeutic levels may be considered [20]. In idiopathic thrombosis a minimum 6–12 months of therapy is suggested. For life-threatening pulmonary embolus, consider thrombectomy or thrombolytic therapy.

Arterial Thrombosis in Children: In catheter-related arterial thrombosis, immediate removal of the catheter should occur with variable duration of therapy as described. Thrombolysis and or thrombectomy may be considered. In idiopathic arterial thrombosis, if life-threatening, thrombectomy or thrombolysis would be recommended as initial treatment. Anticoagulation following thrombus removal has been used in varying doses and duration.

Thrombolytic Therapy

In the presence of thrombosis that threatens the viability of organ, limb, or life, rapid thrombolysis should be strongly considered in the absence of contraindications, such as an elevated APTT and INR, decreased fibrinogen, platelets <100 000, cerebral bleeding, early postoperative, or massive bleeding.

The most common agent used is tissue plasminogen activator (tPa) (activase, alteplase; Genentech, San Francisco, CA). The doses in the literature range from 0.01 to 0.6 mg/kg/hour for varying amounts of time [75].

It is important to ensure that plasminogen levels are sufficient to allow thrombolysis. For this reason, administration of fresh frozen plasma may be considered to provide a plasminogen source with tPa infusion. In children, the risk of major hemorrhage is as high as 54%, requiring transfusion [75].

Streptokinase not recommended in children due to the potential for anaphylactic reaction secondary to antibody development.

Discussion about the risk and benefit of thrombolytic therapy with other health-care professionals and parents or caregivers, followed by documentation of the discussion within the patients' medical records, should occur prior to use.

Antiplatelet Therapy

Antiplatelet therapy has a number of indications in pediatrics, although there are no dose finding, safety, and efficacy studies. Common indications include:

- cardiac indications (extracardiac palliative shunts, intravascular stents, mechanical aortic valves, Kawasaki disease, following heart transplantation, and others);
- following organ transplant (heart, liver).

The most common antiplatelet agents used are aspirin and dipyridamole. There are other agents, with some data currently being investigated. These agents include clopidogrel, ticagrelor, prasugrel, and abciximab.

Antiplatelet Therapy Metabolism in Children

Each agent inhibits platelet function by interrupting different metabolic pathways that are important for optimal platelet shape change, adhesion, and aggregation (Figure 27.1).

Antiplatelet Therapy Benefits in Children

The benefit of antiplatelet therapy in children is the availability of oral administration.

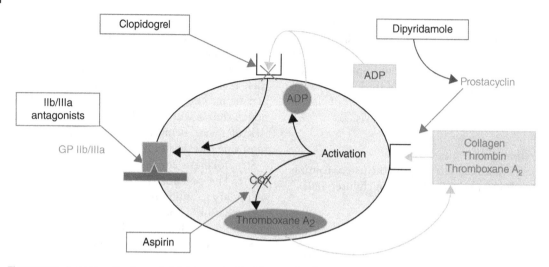

Figure 27.1 Receptor sites for antiplatelet agents. *See Plate section for color representation of this figure.*

Aspirin Limitations in Children

Limitations of aspirin use in children are:

- Aspirin is associated with gastrointestinal bleeding.
- Reye's syndrome is associated aspirin and viral illness, notably varicella or influenza.

Antiplatelet Therapy Dosing in Children

Current dosing recommendations are as follows:

- aspirin 1–5 mg/kg/day;
- dipyridamole 2–5 mg/kg/day;
- clopidogrel 0.2 mg/kg/day.

Antiplatelet Therapy Monitoring in Children

Although not routinely recommended, platelet inhibition may evaluated. There are various methods used to monitor antiplatelet effect (platelet aggregation, PFA100, accumetrics, TEG®); however, none has been demonstrated to be associated with safety and efficacy outcomes. Few studies have examined TEG values in healthy children. Adult comparisons may not be appropriately extrapolated to children [76,77].

Antiplatelet Therapy Reversal in Children

Discontinuation of therapy is sufficient to clear the antiplatelet effect. This may take up to 7 days.

Immunizations and injections may be administered; however, it is imperative to apply 5 minutes of firm pressure on the injection site to minimize bruising. However, special consideration should be given to withholding aspirin with fever or exposure to chickenpox due to the small risk of developing Reye's syndrome. The manufacturer of the varicella vaccine recommends withholding aspirin for 1 week before and 6 weeks following varicella immunization [78].

Thrombophilia Testing in Children

The influence of congenital thrombophilia on childhood thrombosis remains controversial. Congenital thrombophilia refers to alteration in the levels of proteins that facilitate and inhibit clotting. Congenital prothrombotic disorders are relatively rare, but most commonly include factor V Leiden, prothrombin gene G20210A, deficiencies of protein C, protein S, and antithrombin, factor XII deficiency, and increased factor VIII (see Chapter 8). The need to screen for prothrombotic disorders in children with major illnesses, undergoing an invasive procedure or confirmed thrombosis, especially in the presence of clinical risk factors, remains uncertain. Most children with thrombophilic abnormalities without an additional risk factor, such as central lines, prosthetic heart valves, systemic to pulmonary artery shunts, or superior or bicaval pulmonary–arterial anastomosis, do not develop thrombosis until adult life.

Before considering congenital thrombophilia testing in a child due consideration must be given to:

- genetic testing of a child;
- the potential impact on the child and families quality of life;
- will any change in management will result from testing;
- insurance implications for the child and family;
- the ability to educate and inform the child and family of the results [79].

Difficulties in Performing Clinical Trials in Children

The practice of evidence-based medicine is based on the results of properly designed, conducted, and analyzed studies. Evidence for the safety and efficacy of therapies is established through clinical trials. However, there are a number of difficulties in the design and management of clinical trials in children. A significant challenge is that pediatric studies are largely underfunded due to the perception that adult knowledge may be applied to children [33].

Future Perspectives

Increasing data from prospective studies has identified high-risk cohorts of children at risk for thrombosis. Children who develop thrombosis can progress to catastrophic consequences similar to adults. The differences in children, however, preclude the use of adult prophylactic, diagnostic, and treatment guidelines. Consequently, studies in children must be completed to determine "pediatric" evidence-based recommendations incorporating PK/PD and safety and efficacy studies. Presently, these studies are lacking and thus current therapy is recommended for the individual patient based on a crude estimate of risk versus benefit of therapy. Drug regulatory agencies have recognized this and now require pediatric investigational plans using new antithrombotic agents as part of new drug approval. These plans must incorporate PK/PD studies and larger safety and efficacy studies. In addition, quality of life has been recognized as an important outcome measure in these studies. Outcome measures across planned studies must be comparable, thus position documents defining outcomes, including safety and quality of life, have been published by expert groups, including the International Society on Thrombosis and Haemostasis [80].

The completion of these studies is urgently required to provide evidence-based guidance for health-care providers to care for children with or at risk of thrombosis.

References

1 Raffini L, Huang YS, Witmer C, et al. Dramatic increase in venous thromboembolism in children's hospitals in the United States from 2001 to 2007. Pediatrics 2009; 124: 1000–1008.

2 Monagle P, Barnes C, Ignjatovic V, et al. Developmental haemostasis. Impact for clinical haemostasis laboratories. Thromb Haemost 2006; 95: 362–372.

3 Shah JK, Mitchell LG, Paes B, et al. Thrombin inhibition is impaired in plasma of sick neonates. Pediatr Res 1992; 31: 391–395.

4 Andrew M, Mitchell L, Vegh P, et al. Thrombin regulation in children differs from adults in the absence and presence of heparin. Thromb Haemost 1994; 72: 836–842.

5 Andrew M, Vegh P, Johnston M, et al. Maturation of the hemostatic system during childhood. Blood 1992; 80: 1998–2005.

6 Michelson AD. Platelet function in the newborn. Semin Thromb Hemost 1998; 24: 507–512.

7 Tolbert J, Carpenter SL. Common acquired causes of thrombosis in children. Curr Probl Pediatr Adolesc Health Care 2013; 43: 169–177.

8 McCrindle BW, Manlhiot C, Cochrane A, *et al.* Factors associated with thrombotic complications after the Fontan procedure: a secondary analysis of a multicenter, randomized trial of primary thromboprophylaxis for 2 years after the Fontan procedure. *J Am Coll Cardiol* 2013; 61: 346–353.

9 Manlhiot C, Brandao LR, Kwok J, *et al.* Thrombotic complications and thromboprophylaxis across all three stages of single ventricle heart palliation. *J Pediatr* 2012; 161: 513–519 e3.

10 Monagle P, Cochrane A, Roberts R, *et al.* A multicenter, randomized trial comparing heparin/warfarin and acetylsalicylic acid as primary thromboprophylaxis for 2 years after the Fontan procedure in children. *J Am Coll Cardiol* 2011; 58: 645–651.

11 Faustino EV, Spinella PC, Li S, *et al.* Incidence and acute complications of asymptomatic central venous catheter-related deep venous thrombosis in critically ill children. *J Pediatr* 2013; 162: 387–391.

12 Kanin M, Young G. Incidence of thrombosis in children with tunneled central venous access devices versus peripherally inserted central catheters (PICCs). *Thromb Res* 2013; 132: 527–530.

13 Chen K, Williams S, Chan AK, *et al.* Thrombosis and embolism in pediatric cardiomyopathy. *Blood Coagul Fibrinolysis* 2013; 24: 221–230.

14 Kerlin BA, Haworth K, Smoyer WE. Venous thromboembolism in pediatric nephrotic syndrome. *Pediatr Nephrol* 2014; 29: 989–997.

15 Gardiner EE, Andrews RK. Neutrophil extracellular traps (NETs) and infection-related vascular dysfunction. *Blood Rev* 2012; 26: 255–259.

16 Oduber CE, Gerdes VE, van der Horst CM, *et al.* Vascular malformations as underlying cause of chronic thromboembolism and pulmonary hypertension. *J Plast Reconstr Aesthet Surg* 2009; 62: 684–689, 9.

17 Oduber CE, van Beers EJ, Bresser P, *et al.* Venous thromboembolism and prothrombotic parameters in Klippel-Trenaunay syndrome. *Neth J Med* 2013; 71: 246–252.

18 Fan J, Nishida S, Selvaggi G, *et al.* Factor v leiden mutation is a risk factor for hepatic artery thrombosis in liver transplantation. *Transplant Proc* 2013; 45: 1990–1993.

19 Englesbe MJ, Kelly B, Goss J, *et al.* Reducing pediatric liver transplant complications: a potential roadmap for transplant quality improvement initiatives within North America. *Am J Transplant* 2012; 12: 2301–2306.

20 Monagle P, Chan AK, Goldenberg NA, *et al.* Antithrombotic therapy in neonates and children: Antithrombotic Therapy and Prevention of Thrombosis, 9th ed: American College of Chest Physicians Evidence-Based Clinical Practice Guidelines. *Chest* 2012; 141 (2 Suppl.): e737S–801S.

21 Zia AN, Chitlur M. Management of thrombotic complications in acute lymphoblastic leukemia. *Indian J Pediatr* 2013; 80: 853–862.

22 Freed MD, Keane JF, Rosenthal A. The use of heparinization to prevent arterial thrombosis after percutaneous cardiac catheterization in children. *Circulation* 1974; 50: 565–569.

23 Babyn PS, Gahunia HK, Massicotte P. Pulmonary thromboembolism in children. *Pediatric Radiology* 2005; 35: 258–274.

24 Burkhart PV, Sabaté E. Adherence to long-term therapies: evidence for action. *J Nurs Scholarsh* 2003; 35: 207.

25 Male C, Kuhle S, Mitchell L. Diagnosis of venous thromboembolism in children. *Semin Thromb Hemost* 2003; 29: 377–390.

26 Frush DP, Goske MJ, Hernanz-Schulman M. Computed tomography and radiation exposure. *N Engl J Med* 2008; 358: 851.

27 Goldenberg NA, Knapp-Clevenger R, Manco-Johnson MJ, Mountain States Regional Thrombophilia Group. Elevated plasma factor VIII and D-dimer levels as predictors of poor outcomes of thrombosis in children. *N Engl J Med* 2004; 351: 1081–1088.

28 Chan AK, Monagle P. Updates in thrombosis in pediatrics: where are we after 20 years? *Hematology Am Soc Hematol Educ Program* 2012; 2012: 439–443.

29 Barnes C, Newall F, Furmedge J, *et al.* Arterial ischaemic stroke in children. *J Paediatr Child Health* 2004; 40: 384–387.

30 Randolph AG. An evidence-based approach to central venous catheter management to prevent catheter-related infection in critically ill patients. *Critical Care Clinics* 1998; 14: 411–421.

31 Biss TT, Branda LR, Kahr WH, *et al.* Clinical features and outcome of pulmonary embolism in children. *Br J Haematol* 2008; 142: 808–818.

32 Goldenberg NA. Long-term outcomes of venous thrombosis in children. *Curr Opin Hematol* 2005; 12: 370–376.

33 Massicotte MP, Sofronas M, deVeber G. Difficulties in performing clinical trials of antithrombotic therapy in neonates and children. *Thromb Res* 2006; 118: 153–163.

34 Ansell J, Hirsh J, Hylek E, *et al.* Pharmacology and management of the vitamin K antagonists: American College of Chest Physicians Evidence-Based Clinical Practice Guidelines (8th Edition). *Chest* 2008; 133 (Suppl. 6): 160S–198S.

35 Jenney ME, Campbell S. Measuring quality of life. *Arch Dis Child* 1997; 77: 347–350.

36 Terracciano L, Brozek J, Compalati E, *et al.* GRADE system: New paradigm. *Curr Opin Allergy Clin Immunol* 2010; 10: 377–383.

37 Bauman ME, Black K, Bauman ML, *et al.* EMPoWarMENT: Edmonton pediatric warfarin self-management pilot study in children with primarily cardiac disease. *Thromb Res* 2010; 126: e110–e115.

38 Bruce AK, Bauman ME, Jones S, *et al.* Recommendations for measuring health-related quality of life in children on anticoagulation. *J Thromb Haemost* 2012; 10: 2596–2598.

39 Pfizer Canada Inc. *Product monograph: Heparin Sodium Injection USP*. Kirkland, Quebec, 2014. Available at: www.pfizer.ca/sites/g/files/g10017036/f/201505/Heparin-pm_ctl_175554_Dec_16_2014_E.pdf (accessed July 2016).

40 Bauman ME, Belletrutti M, Bauman ML, *et al.* Central venous catheter sampling of low molecular heparin levels: An approach to increasing result reliability. *Pediatr Crit Care Med* 2012; 13: 1–5.

41 Hirsh J, Bauer KA, Donati MB, *et al.* Parenteral anticoagulants: American College of Chest Physicians evidence-based clinical practice guidelines (8th edition). *Chest* 2008; 133 (Suppl. 6): 141S–159S.

42 Ignjatovic V, Furmedge J, Newall F, *et al.* Age-related differences in heparin response. *Thromb Res* 2006; 118: 741–745.

43 Newall F, Johnston L, Ignjatovic V, *et al.* Age-related plasma reference ranges for two heparin-binding proteins--vitronectin and platelet factor 4. *Int J Lab Hematol* 2009; 31: 683–687.

44 Newall F, Ignjatovic V, Johnston L, *et al.* Clinical use of unfractionated heparin therapy in children: Time for change?: Research paper. *Br J Haematol* 2011; 150: 674–678.

45 Newall F, Ignjatovic V, Summerhayes R, *et al.* In vivo age dependency of unfractionated heparin in infants and children. *Thromb Res* 2009; 123: 710–714.

46 Newall F, Chan AK, Ignjatovic V, *et al.* Recommendations for developing uniform laboratory monitoring of heparinoid anticoagulants in children. *J Thromb Haemost* 2012; 10: 145–147.

47 Newall F, Johnston L, Ignjatovic V, *et al.* Unfractionated heparin therapy in infants and children. *Pediatrics* 2009; 123: e510–e518.

48 Kozul C, Newall F, Monagle P, *et al.* A clinical audit of antithrombin concentrate use in a tertiary paediatric centre. *J Paediatr Child Health* 2012; 48: 681–684.

49 Urlesberger B, Zobel G, Zenz W, *et al.* Activation of the clotting system during extracorporeal membrane oxygenation in term newborn infants. *J Pediatr* 1996; 129: 264–268.

50 Niebler RA, Christensen M, Berens R, *et al.* Antithrombin Replacement During Extracorporeal Membrane Oxygenation. *Artif Organs* 2011; 35: 1024–1028.

51 Young G, Yonekawa KE, Nakagawa P, *et al.* Argatroban as an alternative to heparin in extracorporeal membrane oxygenation circuits. *Perfusion* 2004; 19: 283–288.

52 Gruenwald CE, Manlhiot C, Crawford-Lean L, *et al.* Management and monitoring of anticoagulation for children undergoing

cardiopulmonary bypass in cardiac surgery. *J Extra Corpor Technol* 2010; 42: 9–19.

53 Schmugge M, Risch L, Huber AR, *et al.* Heparin-induced thrombocytopenia-associated thrombosis in pediatric intensive care patients. *Pediatrics* 2002; 109: E10.

54 Warkentin TE, Sheppard JI, Moore JC, *et al.* Quantitative interpretation of optical density measurements using PF4-dependent enzyme-immunoassays. *J Thromb Haemost* 2008; 6: 1304–1312.

55 Bauman ME, Belletrutti MJ, Bajzar L, *et al.* Evaluation of enoxaparin dosing requirements in infants and children: Better dosing to achieve therapeutic levels. *Thromb Haemost* 2009; 101: 86–92.

56 Malowany JI, Monagle P, Knoppert DC, *et al.* Enoxaparin for neonatal thrombosis: A call for a higher dose for neonates. *Thromb Res* 2008; 122: 826–830.

57 Malowany JI, Knoppert DC, Chan AKC, *et al.* Enoxaparin use in the neonatal intensive care unit: experience over 8 years. *Pharmacotherapy* 2007; 27: 1263–1271.

58 Bauman ME, Black KL, Bauman ML, *et al.* Novel uses of insulin syringes to reduce dosing errors: a retrospective chart review of enoxaparin whole milligram dosing. *Thromb Res* 2009; 123: 845–847.

59 Lima MV, Ribeiro GS, Mesquita ET, *et al.* CYP2C9 genotypes and the quality of anticoagulation control with warfarin therapy among Brazilian patients. *Eur J Clin Pharmacol* 2008; 64: 9–15.

60 Bauman ME, Black K, Kuhle S, *et al.* KIDCLOT©: The importance of validated educational intervention for optimal long term warfarin management in children. *Thromb Res* 2009; 123: 707–709.

61 Newall F, Johnston L, Monagle P. Optimising anticoagulant education in the paediatric setting using a validated model of education. *Patient Educ Couns* 2008; 73: 384–388.

62 Bauman ME, Mack G, Bruce AK, *et al.* Natural health product utilization in warfarinized children; prevalence and knowledge. *J Pharm Technol* 2012; 28: 100–105.

63 Christensen TD, Larsen TB, Hjortdal VE. Self-testing and self-management of oral anticoagulation therapy in children. *Thromb Haemost* 2011; 106: 391–397.

64 Ansell J, Jacobson A, Levy J, *et al.* International Self-Monitoring Association for Oral Anticoagulation. Guidelines for implementation of patient self-testing and patient self-management of oral anticoagulation. International consensus guidelines prepared by International Self-Monitoring Association for Oral Anticoagulation. *Int J Cardiol* 2005; 99: 37–45.

65 Jones S, Monagle P, Manias E, *et al.* Quality of life assessment in children commencing home INR self-testing. *Thromb Res* 2013; 132: 37–43.

66 Bauman ME, Bruce A, Jones S, *et al.* Recommendations for point-of-care home International Normalized Ratio testing in children on vitamin K antagonist therapy. *J Thromb Haemost* 2013; 11: 366–368.

67 Bauman ME, Black K, Bauman ML, *et al.* Warfarin induced coagulopathy in children: Assessment of a conservative approach. *Arch Dis Child* 2011; 96: 164–167.

68 Mitchell LG, Goldenberg NA, Male C, *et al.* Definition of clinical efficacy and safety outcomes for clinical trials in deep venous thrombosis and pulmonary embolism in children. *J Thromb Haemost* 2011; 9: 1856–1858.

69 Hursting MJ, Dubb J, Verme-Gibboney CN. Argatroban anticoagulation in pediatric patients: a literature analysis. *J Pediatr Hematol Oncol* 2006; 28: 4–10.

70 Potter KE, Raj A, Sullivan JE. Argatroban for anticoagulation in pediatric patients with heparin-induced thrombocytopenia requiring extracorporeal life support. *J Pediatr Hematol Oncol* 2007; 29: 265–268.

71 Dhillon S. Argatroban: a review of its use in the management of heparin-induced thrombocytopenia. *Am J Cardiovasc Drugs* 2009; 9: 261–282.

72 Ignjatovic V, Summerhayes R, Yip YY, *et al.* The in vitro anticoagulant effects of

danaparoid, fondaparinux, and lepirudin in children compared to adults. *Thromb Res* 2008; 122: 709–714.

73 Ignjatovic V, Attard C, Monagle P. Letter to the Editor regarding 'effect of rivaroxaban, in contrast to heparin, is similar in neonatal and adult plasma'. *Blood Coagul Fibrinolysis* 2012; 23: 566.

74 Attard C, Monagle P, Kubitza D, *et al.* The in vitro anticoagulant effect of rivaroxaban in children. *Thromb Res* 2012; 130: 804–807.

75 Manco-Johnson MJ, Grabowski EF, Hellgreen M, *et al.* Recommendations for tPA thrombolysis in children: On behalf of the Scientific Subcommittee on Perinatal and Pediatric Thrombosis of the Scientific and Standardization Committee of the International Society of Thrombosis and Haemostasis. *Thromb Haemost* 2002; 88: 157–158.

76 Alexander DC, Butt WW, Best JD, *et al.* Correlation of thromboelastography with standard tests of anticoagulation in paediatric patients receiving extracorporeal life support. *Thromb Res* 2010; 125: 387–392.

77 Chan KL, Summerhayes RG, Ignjatovic V, *et al.* Reference values for kaolin-activated thromboelastography in healthy children. *Anesth Analg* 2007; 105: 1610–1613.

78 Merck Canada. *Product Monograph. VARIVAX III*, 2016 Available at: www.merck.ca/assets/en/pdf/products/VARIVAX_III-PM_E.pdf (accessed July 2016).

79 Canadian Paediatric Society. Guidelines for genetic testing of healthy children. *Paediatr Child Health* 2003; 8: 42–45.

80 Bruce AK, Bauman M, Jones S, *et al.* Recommendations for measuring health related quality of life in children on anticoagulation. *J Thromb Hemost* 2012; 10: 2596–2598.

28

Intensive and Critical Care

Beverley J. Hunt

Key Points

- Abnormal coagulation screens and thrombocytopenia are common in critically ill patients.
- Blood product usage should be well considered, expeditious and in the bleeding patient guided by coagulation monitoring
- Sepsis and the systemic inflammatory response syndrome are associated with activation of coagulation, but treatment is mainly supportive.
- With few exceptions, thromboprophylaxis should be used in all ICU patients, but reassessed on a daily basis.

Introduction

Thrombosis and coagulopathies are common in Critical Care. Indeed, many patients have multiple haemostatic problems, which may be due to multiple causes. Many coagulopathies produce similar changes in coagulation screen and full blood count (Table 28.1), so any laboratory results need to be looked at in the context of the clinical picture. For example, the changes of hepatic failure produce a similar hemostatic profile to disseminated intravascular coagulation.

Hepatic and renal failure, the thrombotic microangiopathies, and disseminated intravascular coagulation are common in critical care patients but are covered elsewhere in this book.

This chapter covers the residual coagulopathies of critical care, the management of massive pulmonary embolism and prevention of venous thromboembolism, heparin-induced thrombocytopenia, thrombocytosis, sepsis, and the systemic inflammatory response syndrome (SIRS).

As will become evident, there is a dearth of evidence for many aspects of management of critical care hemostasis: this is particularly marked in the management of coagulopathies. Lack of evidence has led to lack of expert consensus on best clinical practice and thus wide variation in management internationally.

Managing Coagulopathies in Critical Care

Many critical care patients have deranged coagulation screens, and it is a first principle of care that these do not require correcting unless they are associated with bleeding. Despite the widespread practice in giving fresh frozen plasma (FFP) to correct coagulopathies prior to invasive procedures, such as inserting large vascular access lines, there is no evidence to support this practice. Indeed, firstly, coagulation screen abnormalities do not predict bleeding and, secondly, the use of FFP does not always correct abnormalities. Studies are required to determine what levels of prolongation of activated partial thromboplastin time/prothrombin time (APTT/PT)

Practical Hemostasis and Thrombosis, Third Edition. Edited by Nigel S. Key, Michael Makris and David Lillicrap.
© 2017 John Wiley & Sons, Ltd. Published 2017 by John Wiley & Sons, Ltd.

Table 28.1 Laboratory findings in various platelet and coagulation disorders in critical care.

Condition	PT	APPT	Fibrinogen levels	D-dimer	Bleeding time	Platelet count	Film comments
Vitamin K deficiency or use of vitamin K antagonist	Prolonged	Normal or mildly prolonged	Normal	Unaffected	Unaffected	Unaffected	
Aspirin and thienopyridines	Unaffected	Unaffected	Unaffected	Unaffected	Prolonged	Unaffected	
Liver failure, early	Prolonged	Unaffected	Unaffected	Unaffected	Unaffected	Unaffected	
Liver failure, end stage	Prolonged	Prolonged	Low	Increased	Prolonged	Decreased	
Uremia	Unaffected	Unaffected	Unaffected	Unaffected	Prolonged	Unaffected	
Disseminated intravascular coagulation	Prolonged	Prolonged	Low	Increased	Prolonged	Decreased	Fragmented red cells
Thrombotic thrombocytopenic purpura	Unaffected	Unaffected	Unaffected	Unaffected	Prolonged	Very low	Fragmented red cells
Hyperfibrinolysis	Prolonged	Prolonged	Low	Very high	Possibly prolonged	Unaffected	

PT, prothrombin time; APTT, activated partial thromboplastin time.

ratios are safe for invasive procedures. Certainly a PT and APTT ratio <1.5 with a platelet count $>75\times10^9/L$ appears safe, and some hemostatic experts consider an APTT and/or PT ratio <2.0 acceptable [1–3].

The lack of good-quality evidence is most marked in the use of blood components to manage major bleeding. The benefits of FFP and platelets were never assessed in randomized clinical trials (RCTs) when they were introduced. Later, concerns about the transmission of transfusion–transmitted infection, and also limitations in the blood supply, led to a more restrictive use of blood components. However, recent retrospective studies of military casualties suggested improved survival with transfusion of one unit of FFP for each unit of red blood cells [4]. These studies were criticized, particularly for methodological flaws including survival bias (those who did not survive were not transfused with FFP) and heterogeneity between studies [5]. Despite the lack of evidence

that bleeding after surgery, gastrointestinal, or obstetric hemorrhage have similar hemostatic changes to acute traumatic coagulopathy, the early use of the 1 : 1 and 1 : 2 ratio has become widespread internationally. This increased use of plasma is not risk free; the incidence of transfusion-related acute lung injury (TRALI) is increased [6], as may be the risk of developing acute respiratory distress syndrome (ARDS) and multiple organ dysfunction syndrome (MODS) [7].

The critical ratio of FFP : red cell transfusion in the management of major bleeding was addressed in the North American Pragmatic, Randomized Optimal Platelets and Plasma Ratios (PROPPR) study ; no difference in mortality at 24 hours or 30 days was seen with early administration of plasma, platelets, and red blood cells in a 1:1:1 ratio compared with a 1:1:2 ratio [8]. Some European centers have abandoned FFP, relying on the exclusive use of factor concentrates using rotational elastometry

(ROTEM®) guided intervention with prothrombin complex concentrate (PCC), factor XIII, and fibrinogen. In contrast, others believe that only fibrinogen supplementation is required, with tranexamic acid, red cells, and intravenous fluid used on an "as needed" basis.

Fibrinogen is a critical hemostatic molecule for forming fibrin, and is also the ligand for platelet aggregation. It is consumed to a larger extent than any other hemostatic protein in those with major bleeding [9], reflecting consumption, loss, dilution, and fibrinogen lysis. Current guidelines for the management of major bleeding now indicate that the trigger level for supplementing fibrinogen should be 1.5–2.0 g/L rather than 1.0 g/L [10]. Whether early fibrinogen supplementation and the use of PCC improves clinical outcomes in patients with major bleeding compared to FFP is unknown and needs to be studied alongside safety, including the rate of hospital-acquired venous thromboembolism [11,12]. Similarly recombinant VIIa, while it has been shown to reduce red cell usage in bleeding but not to reduce mortality, needs further evaluation. Data from placebo-controlled trials show its off license use significantly increases the risk of arterial thrombosis [13,14].

Tranexamic acid is a synthetic derivative of the amino acid lysine, which acts as an antifibrinolytic agent by competitively inhibiting plasminogen, and should be given to all trauma patients bleeding or at risk of bleeding. A large RCT, the Clinical Randomisation of Antifibrinolytics to those with Significant Haemorrhage (CRASH-2), randomized 20 000 trauma patients with bleeding or at risk of significant bleeding to tranexamic acid or placebo. Patients assigned to tranexamic acid had a 1.5% absolute and a 9% relative reduction in mortality [15]; benefit was related to it being given as soon as possible after injury because it ceased to confer benefit and appeared associated with increased mortality if given more than 3 hours after injury [16]. Reassuringly for a hemostatic drug, the incidence of thrombosis post-trauma was not increased. Grade 1 evidence exists to SHO that perioperative intravenous tranexamic acid reduces bleeding and blood transfusion in surgical procedure. There is increasing interest in its use topically, with similar efficacy [17].

Thrombocytopenia

Patients with thrombocytopenia may have petechiae, purpura, and bruising or frank hemorrhage. A full blood count and blood film will confirm a low platelet count and the presence or absence of other diagnostic features, such as red cell fragmentation, platelet morphological abnormalities, or evidence of dysplasia or hematinic deficiency.

Thrombocytopenia may arise because of:

- decreased platelet production,
- increased platelet destruction, and/or
- sequestration in the spleen.

It occurs in up to 20% of medical and 35% of surgical admissions to ICU and may be multifactorial. Table 28.2 lists the differential diagnoses of thrombocytopenia in the ICU setting. There is an inverse relationship between severity of sepsis and platelet count.

Platelet Clumping

Patients with sepsis may develop ethylene diaminetetra acetic acid (EDTA)-dependent antibodies, which cause platelet clumping *ex vivo*, resulting in pseudothrombocytopenia. If platelet clumping is seen on a blood film, a fresh sample should be taken into an alternative anticoagulant, such as citrate.

Patients with Sepsis

Immune Mechanisms

Nonimmune destruction of platelets occurs in sepsis. Immune mechanisms may also contribute, with nonspecific platelet-associated antibodies detected in up to 30% of ICU patients. It is thought that IgG binds to bacterial products on the platelet surface or to an altered platelet

Table 28.2 Differential diagnosis of thrombocytopenia in the ICU setting.

Pseudothrombocytopenia

    Clotted blood sample
    EDTA-dependent antibodies

Drugs

    Heparin, including HAT and HITT
    IIb/IIIa inhibitors (abciximab, eptifibatide, tirofiban)
    Adenosine diphosphate (ADP) receptor antagonists
    (clopidogrel)
    Acute alcohol toxicity

Sepsis

Disseminated intravascular coagulation

Massive blood loss – a dilutional thrombocytopenia

Post cardiopulmonary bypass

    Intra-aortic balloon pump

Renal dialysis

    Immune thrombocytopenic purpura (ITP)

Antiphospholipid syndrome

    Thrombotic thrombocytopenic purpura (TTP)
    Hemolytic uremic syndrome (HUS)
    Hypersplenism
    Hematinic deficiency, particularly acute folate
    deficiency

Pregnancy-associated thrombocytopenia

    Benign gestational thrombocytopenia
    Postpartum HUS
    HELLP
    Preeclampsia

Myelodysplastic syndrome

Carcinoma

Post-transfusion purpura

Hereditary thrombocytopenia

EDTA, ethylene diaminetetra acetic acid; HAT, heparin associated thrombocytopenia; HITT, heparin-induced thrombocytopenic thrombosis.

surface. A subset of patients with platelet-associated antibodies also has autoantibodies directed against glycoprotein IIb/IIIa (i.e., they have idiopathic thrombocytopenic purpura (ITP)). Unfortunately tests for platelet-specific IgG are nonspecific and do not help in the management of septic patients. Bone marrow hemophagocytosis is a common finding in septic thrombocytopenic patients. The marrow is often hypocellular with reduced megakaryocyte numbers.

Nonimmune Mechanisms

Other causes of thrombocytopenia should be sought in a critically ill patient. Thrombocytopenia may occur as:

- A complication of heparin treatment. A mild thrombocytopenia of no clinical significance may be seen in the first few days of heparin therapy – heparin associated thrombocytopenia (HAT).
- This should be differentiated from heparin-induced thrombocytopenic thrombosis (HIT; see below).
- Dilutional thrombocytopenia may occur after trauma or complex surgery.
- Acute folate deficiency has been described in ICU patients.
- Pre-existing disease, such as ITP, cancer, hypersplenism, and myelodysplastic syndrome, may contribute to a low platelet count.

Consumptive coagulopathy is associated with an elevated PT, APTT, thrombin time, D-dimer, and a reduced fibrinogen.

Thresholds for Platelet Transfusion

Guidelines suggest a platelet threshold of 10×10^9/L for platelet transfusion in thrombocytopenic patients without additional risk factors, such as sepsis [18].

Patients with chronic sustained failure of platelet production, such as myelodysplasia or aplastic anemia, may remain free from serious hemorrhage with platelet counts below $5–10 \times 10^9$/L.

As standard platelet counts are produced by cell counters that categorize by size, an immunoplatelet count is occasionally helpful in providing a "true" platelet count by labeling platelet antigens [19]. Long-term prophylactic platelet transfusions may lead to alloimmunization, platelet refractoriness, and other complications of transfusion.

Procedures

For procedures such as lumbar puncture, epidural anesthesia, gastroscopy and biopsy, insertion of indwelling lines, transbronchial biopsy, liver biopsy, and laparotomy, the platelet count should be raised to at least 50×10^9/L. For operations on critical sites, such as the brain or eyes, recommendations are for a platelet count of $75–100 \times 10^9$/L.

Antiplatelet Therapy

In bleeding patients and preprocedure, drugs with antiplatelet activity should ideally be withdrawn. Any underlying disorder associated with platelet dysfunction, such as uremia, should be treated if possible. The hematocrit should be corrected to >0.30 in those with renal failure. The use of desmopressin (DDAVP) may be considered.

Massive Transfusion

In massive blood loss, the platelet count is preserved until relatively late. A platelet count of around 50×10^9/L is expected when red cell concentrates equivalent to two blood volumes have been transfused. The platelet count should be maintained above 50×10^9/L in patients with acute bleeding. A higher target of 100×10^9/L is recommended in some guidelines for those with multiple trauma or central nervous system injury.

Disseminated Intravascular Coagulopathy

Platelet transfusions are indicated in acute disseminated intravascular coagulopathy (DIC) when there is bleeding associated with thrombocytopenia. Management of the underlying disorder and coagulation factor replacement are also required. Frequent full blood count and coagulation screening tests should be carried out, and the platelet count maintained above 50×10^9/L. Platelet transfusions should not be given simply to correct a low platelet count in DIC in the absence of bleeding.

Immune Thrombocytopenia

In patients with ITP, platelet transfusions are reserved for patients with life-threatening gastrointestinal, genitourinary, or central nervous system bleeding or other bleeding associated with severe thrombocytopenia. In ITP, the residual platelets tend to be young and have good hemostatic effect, so patients tend not to bleed unless the platelet count is very low. Platelet transfusions may not produce an incremental rise in patients with ITP due to the effect of the platelet antibodies on the donor platelets. IV methylprednisolone, intravenous gamma globulin, or anti-D (only to be used in the Rhesus-positive patients who have a spleen) can be given to produce platelet increments [20]. The thrombopoietic agents may gain a place in the future management of acute ITP.

Post-Transfusion Purpura

Post-transfusion purpura is due to the presence of a platelet-specific alloantibody (usually antihuman platelet antigen-1a (HPA-1a)) in the recipient, which reacts with donor platelets, destroying them and also the recipient's own platelets. High-dose IVIg (2 g/kg given over 2 or 5 days) is used in the treatment of post-transfusion purpura, with responses in about 85% of patients. Large doses of platelet transfusions may be required to control severe bleeding before there is a response to IVIg. There is limited evidence that HPA-1a-negative platelets are more effective than those from random donors [21].

The Thrombotic Microangiopathies

Profound thrombocytopenia and microangiopathic hemolytic anemia characterize thrombotic microangiopathy, which includes three major disorders: thrombotic thrombocytopenic purpura (TTP), hemolytic uremic syndrome (HUS), and HELLP syndrome (hemolysis, elevated liver function tests and low platelets). These are covered in Chapter 13.

Sepsis and the Systemic Inflammatory Response Syndrome (SIRS)

Sepsis constitutes the systemic inflammatory response to infection. It is the host response rather than the nature of the pathogen that is the major determinant of patient outcome.

Systemic inflammatory response syndrome (SIRS) is manifested by two or more of the following:

- temperature >38°C or <36°C;
- heart rate >90 beats/minute;
- respiratory rate >20 breaths/minute or $Paco_2$ <4.3 kP;, or
- white cell count >12×10⁹/L,<4×10⁹/L, or >10% immature forms.

Sepsis is defined as:
- SIRS resulting from documented infection.

Severe sepsis is associated with:

- organ dysfunction;
- hypoperfusion or hypotension; and
- a mortality rate of 30–50%.

Septic shock is defined as:

- severe sepsis with hypotension (systolic BP <90 mmHg or a reduction of >40 mmHg from baseline);
- in the absence of other causes for hypertension or inotropic or vasopressor treatment; and
- despite adequate fluid resuscitation.

Coagulation is activated in most patients with severe sepsis as evidenced by:

- elevated markers of thrombin turnover, such as thrombin–antithrombin complexes and prothrombin fragment 1 + 2;
- similarly, fibrinolysis is increased with elevated levels of D-dimer;
- decreased protein C and antithrombin levels due to consumption are also common;
- Activation of coagulation may lead to depletion of circulating clotting factors and secondary DIC.

Treatment of SIRS

Pharmacological doses of physiological anticoagulants have been shown to improve survival in DIC in animals. Disappointingly, such trials in humans have failed to show a benefit. Recombinant human activated protein C was initially licensed for adjunctive treatment of severe sepsis with multiorgan failure in 2001. It has anti-inflammatory, antithrombotic, and fibrinolytic properties. The original PROWESS trial [22], showed a decreased absolute mortality of severely septic patients. However, a repeat study failed to show any benefit and there were frequent and serious side-effects from bleeding [23]. Similarly trials of pharmacological doses of antithrombin or tissue factor pathway inhibitor showed no benefit in survival and increased bleeding episodes [24,25].

Sequential Organ Failure Assessment Score

Sequential Organ Failure Assessment (SOFA) is a scoring system to evaluate the severity of critically ill patients in the ICU (Table 28.3). A severity score is needed in clinical research studies to standardize reports, improve the understanding of the course of disease, and allow evaluation of new treatments. Estimates of morbidity serve as a reliable indicator of intensive care performance, allowing comparison between medical centers, cost/benefit analyses, and evaluation of new therapeutic or management modalities.

The SOFA score has been designed to report morbidity and to objectively quantify the degree of dysfunction/failure of each organ daily in critically ill patients.

Heparin Induced Thrombocytopenia

Heparin induced thrombocytopenic thrombosis (HIT) is a transient drug-induced autoimmune prothrombotic disorder initiated by

Table 28.3 The Sequential Organ Failure Assessment (SOFA) score.

System	Description	Score
Respiratory system	<400 ± respiratory support	1
Pao_2/Fio_2 in mmHg	<300 ± respiratory support	2
	<200 and respiratory support	3
	<100 and respiratory support	4
Cardiovascular system	MAP <70 mmHg	1
Vasopressors in gamma/kg/minute	Dopamine ≤5 or dobutamine	2
	Dopamine >5 or epi/norepinephrine ≤0.1	3
	Dopamine >15 or epi/norepinephrine >0.1	4
Liver: Bilirubin µM/L	20–32	1
	33–101	2
	102–204	3
	>204	4
Renal: Creatinine in µM/L or urine output in mL/day	100–170	1
	171–299	2
	300–440 or <500 mL per day	3
	>440 or <200 mL/day	4
Coagulation: Platelets × 10^9/L	101–150	1
	51–100	2
	21–50	3
	<20	4
Glasgow coma score	13–14	1
	10–12	2
	6–9	3
	<6	4

MAP, mean arterial pressure.

heparin. Heparin exposure can induce the formation of pathogenic IgG antibodies that cause platelet activation by recognizing complexes of platelet factor 4 (PF4) and heparin on platelet surfaces. Platelet activation results in thrombocytopenia and thrombin generation, with an increased risk of venous and arterial thrombosis [15].

HIT antibodies are directed against multiple neoepitope sites. Only a minority of PF4/heparin-reactive HIT sera activate platelets *in vitro*. Some HIT-IgG recognize PF4 bound to solid phase even in the absence of heparin. PF4

antibodies usually decline to undetectable levels within a few weeks or months of an episode of HIT, and there is no anamnestic response.

- The frequency of HIT varies widely depending on the type of heparin used and the patient group.
- Unfractionated heparin is associated with a higher incidence of HIT than fractionated heparin.
- Surgical patients have a higher frequency of HIT than either medical or obstetric patients with the same heparin exposure.

- Postoperative orthopedic patients receiving unfractionated heparin have the highest HIT frequency (up to 5%) and require more intense platelet count monitoring than pregnant women receiving low-molecular-weight heparin (LMWH), who have a negligible risk.

Laboratory Diagnosis

HIT antibodies are detected using either:

- commercially available PF4-dependent antigen immunoassays; or
- functional assays of platelet activation and aggregation.

Clinically insignificant HIT antibodies are common in patients that have received heparin 5–100 days earlier. In the ICU setting, HIT is uncommon (0.3–0.5%), whereas thrombocytopenia from other causes is very common (30–50%), as are weakly positive HIT enzyme-linked immunosorbent assay (ELISA) assays in the critical care population.

For laboratory diagnosis of HIT antibodies, both antigen assays and functional (platelet activation) assays are available. Both tests are very sensitive (high negative predictive value) but specificity is poor, especially for the antigen assays, which will also detect nonpathogenic immunoglobulin M and immunoglobulin A class antibodies. Detection of immunoglobulin M or immunoglobulin A antibodies could potentially lead to adverse events, such as bleeding, if a false diagnosis of HIT prompts replacement of heparin by an alternative anticoagulant such as fondaparinux or argatroban, a direct thrombin inhibitor. Assays of platelet activation are technically demanding, time consuming, and not available in all centers. Testing should be performed when HIT is clinically suspected.

Clinical Diagnosis

The initial clinical diagnosis of HIT should be based on the International Society on Thrombosis and Hemostasis (ISTH) scoring system (Figure 28.1) [26,27], and then confirmed by laboratory testing. Isolated HIT is

the occurrence of thrombocytopenia without thrombosis. Retrospective cohort studies indicate that 25–50% of these patients develop clinically overt thrombosis after stopping heparin, usually within the first week. Subclinical thrombosis was found in 8 of 16 patients who underwent routine lower-limb duplex ultrasonography for isolated HIT. Early heparin cessation alone does not reduce the risk of thrombosis in patients with isolated HIT, so alternative anticoagulation is required.

About 25% of HIT patients receiving a heparin bolus develop signs or symptoms, such as fever, chills, respiratory distress, or hypertension. Transient global amnesia and cardiorespiratory arrest have also been reported. About 5–15% of HIT patients develop decompensated DIC.

Thrombocytopenia does not usually develop until day 5–10 of heparin treatment and reaches a median nadir of 55×10^9/L. The platelet count falls below 150×10^9/L in around 90% of HIT cases. Hemorrhage and platelet counts below 10×10^9/L suggest an alternative cause, such as post-transfusion purpura. Patients who have received heparin within the last 100 days may have a fall in platelet count within one day of re-exposure to heparin.

Treatment of HIT

Heparin should be stopped immediately, and not repeated, in those who develop thrombocytopenia or the original platelet count falls by 50% [26,27]. Recent data indicate that, as HIT is strongly associated with thrombosis (odds ratio 12–40), an alternative anticoagulant should be commenced. For treatment of HIT, three alternative anticoagulants are used: the direct thrombin inhibitors, argatroban, the heparinoid, danaparoid (not approved in the United States), and fondaparinux off license. Prophylactic platelet transfusions are relatively contraindicated. Therapeutic doses of anticoagulants are recommended even in the absence of thrombosis.

Figure 28.1 shows one hospital's algorithm for managing HIT.

Argatroban is a direct thrombin inhibitor, has hepatobiliary excretion, and increases the INR.

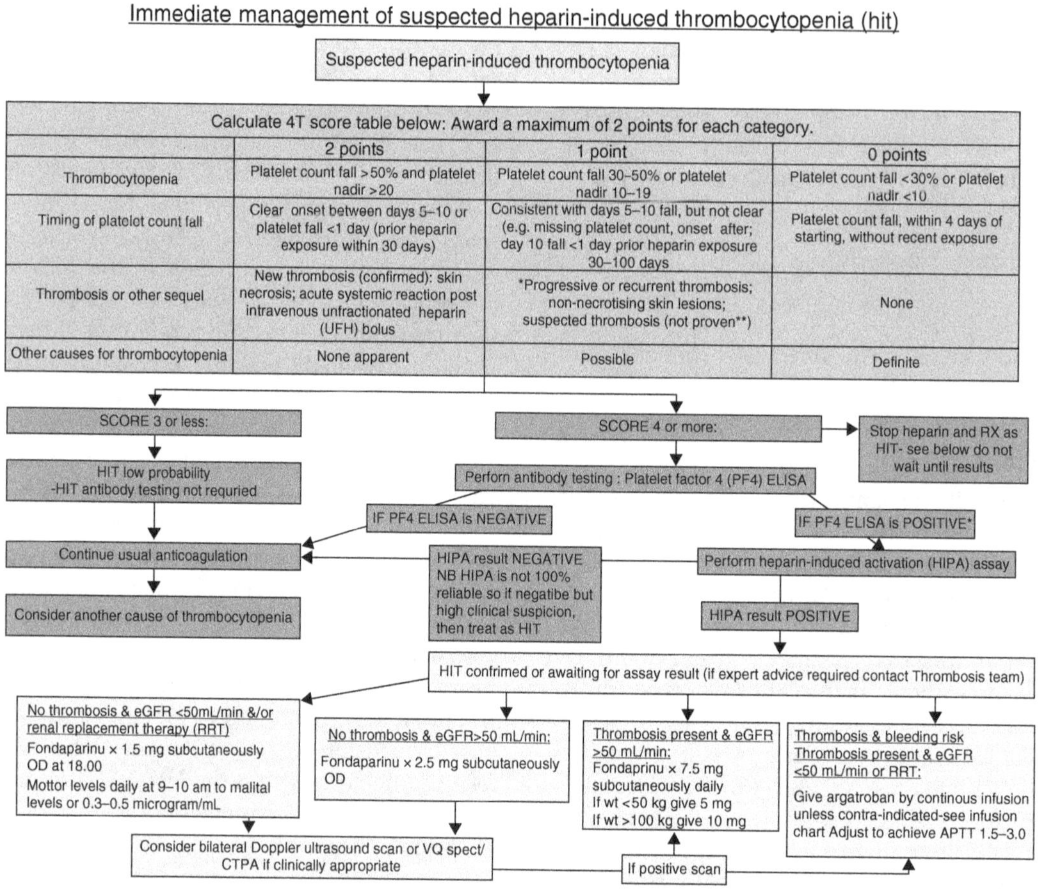

Immediate management of suspected heparin-induced thrombocytopenia (hit)

Figure 28.1 A local management protocol for heparin-induced thrombocytopenia (HIT). APTT, activated partial thromboplastin time; CTPA, computed tomographic pulmonary angiography; eGFR, estimated glomerular filtration rate; ELISA, enzyme-linked immunosorbent assay. *See Plate section for color representation of this figure.*

The dose is 2 mg/kg/minute, without an initial bolus. An APTT target range of 1.5–3.0 times baseline is required. The dose must be reduced in liver failure. As argatroban increases the INR, a higher than usual therapeutic target INR during warfarin cotherapy should be used.

Danaparoid sodium is a heparinoid, which may be used in HIT patients providing there is no evidence of crossreactivity. Danaparoid does not cross the placenta but is renally metabolized. It is given by intravenous injection at a dose of 2500 U (1250 U if body weight <55 kg, 3750 U if >90 kg), followed by an intravenous infusion of 400 U/hour for 2 hours, then 300 U/hour for 2 hours, then 200 U/hour for 5 days. Anti-Xa target range is between 0.5 and 0.8 anti-Xa U/mL and should

be monitored in those with renal impairment or a body weight of over 90 kg. Danaparoid given by subcutaneous injection has 100% bioavailability. The 24-hour intravenous dose can be divided into two or three daily injections.

Fondaparinux is a pentasaccharide that potentiates antithrombin and has only anti-Xa activity. Despite being a synthetic heparin derivative, it does not appear to generate pathological HIT antibodies and has been used safely in those with suspected or confirmed HIT.

There is a 5–20% frequency of new thrombosis despite treatment of HIT patients with an alternative anticoagulant.

The current American College of Chest Physician guidelines [15] recommend that patients who are receiving heparin or have received heparin within the previous 2 weeks should be investigated for a diagnosis of HIT if the platelet count falls by ≥50%, and/or a thrombotic event occurs, between days 5 and 14 (inclusive) following initiation of heparin, even if the patient is no longer receiving heparin therapy when thrombosis or thrombocytopenia has occurred (Grade 1C). For patients with strongly suspected (or confirmed) HIT, whether or not complicated by thrombosis, we recommend use of an alternative, nonheparin anticoagulant (danaparoid (Grade 1B), argatroban (Grade 1C), fondaparinux (Grade 2C), or bivalirudin (Grade 2C)) over the further use of unfractionated heparin (UFH) or LMWH therapy or initiation/continuation of vitamin K antagonists (Grade 1B).

Thrombocytosis

Thrombocytosis is defined as a platelet count of greater than 450×10^9/L. Reactive thrombocytosis is common in ICU patients, particularly in association with surgery or trauma, hemorrhage, acute and chronic infection, malignancy, iron-deficiency anemia, inflammatory disease, and postsplenectomy. The platelet count does not usually exceed 1000×10^9/L in reactive thrombocytosis. Differential diagnoses include myeloproliferative disorders, such as essential thrombocythemia, chronic idiopathic myelofibrosis, and polycythemia vera. A blood film and assessment of JAK-2 status may be helpful in discriminating an underlying malignancy in difficult cases. If a patient is not actively bleeding, thromboprophylaxis with aspirin 75 mg daily is appropriate as there is an increased risk of thrombosis with thrombocytosis [28].

Management of Thromboembolism in ICU

Massive Pulmonary Embolism

Venous thromboembolism (VTE) is an important cause of morbidity and mortality in ICU

patients. Among patients who died in ICU, pulmonary emboli (PE) were reported in 7–27% of postmortem examinations. The mortality rate for PE is <8% when the condition is recognized and treated, but approximately 30% when untreated [29]. A subgroup of patients with nonmassive PE who are hemodynamically stable but with right ventricular dysfunction or hypokinesis confirmed by echocardiography is classified as submassive PE. Their prognosis is different from that of others with nonmassive PE and normal right ventricular function.

Massive PE is characterized by systemic hypotension (defined as a systolic arterial pressure <90 mmHg or a drop in systolic arterial pressure of at least 40 mmHg for at least 15 min which is not caused by new-onset arrhythmias) or shock (manifested by evidence of tissue hypoperfusion and hypoxia, including an altered level of consciousness, oliguria, or cool, clammy extremities). It has a mortality of 18–33% and may present with shock, dyspnea, and confusion. In patients with massive PE and hemodynamic instability, rapid risk assessment is paramount and bedside echocardiography has become the most popular tool. Multislice chest computed tomography (CT) is also useful for identifying patients who may benefit from thrombolysis or embolectomy. Cardiac biomarkers, including troponin and the natriuretic peptides, are sensitive markers of right ventricular function. Low levels of troponin, B-type natriuretic peptide (BNP), and NT-terminal proBNP are all highly sensitive assays for identifying patients with an uneventful clinical course. Multislice chest CT is not only useful to diagnose or exclude PE, it also is useful for risk assessment. A right-to-left ventricular dimension ratio >0.9 on the reconstructed CT four-chamber view identifies patients at increased risk of early death [30].

Treatment of PE

Most DOACs are licensed and available to treat DVT and PE [31], and of equivalent efficacy and safety to LMWH and fondaparinux followed by a vitamin K antagonist [32]. Trials assessing the benefit-to-risk ratio of thrombolysis in DVT are awaited but is recommended for unstable patients with PE, although these patients represent <5% of all patients hospitalized for PE [33].

The streptokinase/urokinase PE thrombolysis trials showed that thrombolytic therapy successfully decreases pulmonary artery pressures acutely with improvements in the lung scan and arteriogram at 12 and 24 hours. There was no overall decrease in mortality in those receiving thrombolysis compared with those receiving heparin therapy. The use of thrombolytic treatment in patients with submassive PE remains controversial although the MOPPETT study suggested benefit of smaller doses of fibrinolytic [34]. Contraindications to thrombolysis include active internal bleeding, a stroke within 2 months, and an intracranial process such as neoplasm or abscess. Relative contraindications include surgery or organ biopsy within 10 days, uncontrolled hypertension, and pregnancy.

The dose of alteplase is 10 mg IV injection over 1–2 minutes followed by an IV infusion of 90 mg over 2 hours (maximum 1.5 mg/kg in patients <65 kg). The dose of streptokinase is 250 000 U by IV infusion over 30 minutes, then 100 000 U every hour for up to 12–72 hours according to clinical condition, with monitoring of clotting parameters. A simplified algorithm for alteplase consisting of 0.6 mg/kg over 15 minutes has been used successfully in many centers, with equivalence to the standard regime demonstrated in two prospective randomized studies. Hemorrhagic complications are higher in patients with a recent invasive procedure, such as pulmonary angiogram or placement of an IVC filter. There is a reported incidence of intracranial hemorrhage of approximately 2%, with higher rates in the elderly and those with poorly controlled hypertension. The major hemorrhage rate ranges from 11% to 20%.

The PREPIC study [35] demonstrated that, at 8 years, vena cava filters reduced the risk of PE but increased that of DVT and had no effect on survival. The authors concluded that, although their use may be beneficial in patients at high risk of PE, systematic use in the general population with VTE is not recommended. A Cochrane review concluded that further trials, especially with retrievable filters, are needed to assess vena caval filter safety and effectiveness [36]. Certainly, current opinion is that, preferably, temporary IVC filters should be used in those with temporary contraindications to anticoagulation in the ITU population and the filter should be removed as soon as possible once anticoagulation has been restarted. There is interest in devices such as the Angel catheter, an IVC device on a central venous catheter, which can be easily inserted and removed.

Surgical intervention should be considered for patients whose condition worsens despite intensive medical treatment. A randomized study of embolectomy versus medical therapy is unavailable. Thrombolytic treatment fails in 15–20% of patients. The mortality after surgical embolectomy is around 30–40%, with a higher mortality in those with a longer duration of hemodynamic instability, a requirement for cardiopulmonary resuscitation and intubation, high doses of catecholamines, metabolic and respiratory acidosis, and poor urine output. Early diagnosis and treatment leads to improved outcomes (Figure 28.2).

Thromboprophylaxis in the ICU

The critically ill are at substantially increased risk of VTE, which contributes significantly to their morbidity and mortality. PE is frequently seen at postmortem in these patients, the incidence being as high as 27%. The incidence of image-proven DVT in critically ill patients ranges from 10% to almost 100%, depending on the screening methods and diagnostic criteria used [37].

Most critically ill patients have multiple risk factors for VTE. Many risk factors predate ICU admission, in particular recent surgery, immobilization, trauma, sepsis, malignancy, increased age, heart or respiratory failure, and previous VTE. These initial VTE risk factors are confounded by others, which are acquired on the

Management of Acute Massive Pulmonary Embolism

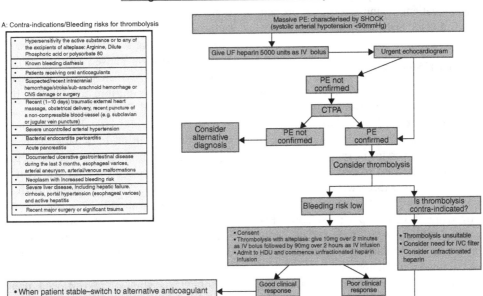

Figure 28.2 A local management algorithm for managing massive pulmonary embolism (PE). CTPA, computed tomographic pulmonary angiography; IVC, inferior vena cava. *See Plate section for color representation of this figure.*

ICU, including immobilization, pharmacological paralysis, central venous catheterization, additional surgical procedures, sepsis, vasopressors, and hemodialysis [38].

Clinically undetected DVT may be present in about 5–25% of patients on admission to a critical care unit. Although the majority of DVTs are clinically silent and often confined to the calf veins, asymptomatic DVT can become symptomatic and lead to embolic complications. There is no way of predicting which at-risk patients will develop symptomatic VTE; it is, however, well recognized that massive PE frequently occurs without warning and is often fatal. PE is found in 15% of critical care patients deaths at postmortem.

Hospitalized patients recovering from major trauma have the highest risk of developing VTE [39]. Without adequate thromboprophylaxis, patients with multisystem failure or major trauma have a DVT risk exceeding 50%, with PE being the third leading cause of mortality after the first day.

Mechanical Measures of Thromboprophylaxis

Immobility increases the risk of DVT tenfold and mechanical methods act by reducing venous stasis in the leg and their advantage is the avoidance of systemic anticoagulation and thus the incumbent risk of bleeding. However, a meta-analysis of only two randomized controlled trials with similar critical care populations showed that neither graduated compression stockings (GECs) nor intermittent pneumatic compression (IPC) devices led to a significant reduction in the risk of VTE [40]. There are no good trials as yet of GECs in medical patients apart from the CLOT study [41], which showed no benefit in stroke patients and the risk of possible harm. CLOT 3 showed, however, that IPC versus no IPC in over 2800 patients did reduce the rate of proximal DVT from 12.1% to 8.5%, and possibly improved survival [42]. In critical care patients the use of IPC but not GECs was associated with a lower VTE incidence regardless of type of pharmacological thromboprophylaxis used, in a study of 798 patients using a multiple propensity scores adjusted analysis [43].

Pharmacological Studies

Both UFH and LMWH have been shown to reduce the risk of VTE in critical care patients. The PROTECT study [44] was a landmark study that randomized 3764 critical care patients to 5000 IU dalteparin versus unfractionated heparin twice daily. The rate of proximal DVT on ultrasound was similar (5.1% with dalteparin vs. 5.8% with UFH), although the rate of PE was significantly lower (1.3% dalteparin vs. 2.3% UFH, hazard ratio 0.51, $P = 00.1$). Rates of major bleeding were also similar but as expected HIT was less common with dalteparin.

A limitation of LMWH in the critical care population is the risk of accumulation in patients with renal impairment leading to an unpredictable and excessive anticoagulation; however, 6.7% of patients receiving dalteparin 5000 IU required renal dialysis during their stay. Renal replacement therapy was cited as a risk factor for bleeding (HR 1.75, 1.2–2.56) in a later publication from the PROTECT group [45]. Paradoxically there is also concern that the use of vasopressors and the metabolic condition of some critically ill patients may reduce the effectiveness of pharmacological prophylaxis. Critically ill patients receiving vasopressor support had significantly lower anti-Xa levels than those patients not on vasopressors. The putative mechanism is decreased absorption of LMWH from the subcutaneous tissues due to reduced perfusion caused by the vasopressor. Multiple organ dysfunction may alter drug metabolism, distribution, and binding to albumen and acute phase proteins.

With few exceptions, thromboprophylaxis should be used in all ICU patients. Decisions regarding the initiation and method of prophylaxis should be based on the balance of bleeding and thrombotic risk. Patients with a high risk of bleeding should be given mechanical prophylaxis, ideally with intermittent pneumatic compression devices, until bleeding risk decreases and prophylaxis with heparin can be commenced.

Prophylaxis should be reviewed daily and altered as necessitated by the patient's clinical status. Prophylaxis should not be interrupted for procedures or surgery unless there is a particularly high bleeding risk. Procedures such as insertion or removal of epidural catheters should be planned to coincide with the nadir of anticoagulant effect. Table 28.4 outlines recommendations for prophylaxis in critically ill patients suggested by Geerts and coworkers [39].

Those that receive either suboptimal or no thromboprophylaxis should have Doppler ultrasound screening. Thromboprophylaxis should be continued until hospital discharge in those at

Table 28.4 Suggested venous thromboembolism prophylaxis in critically ill patients.

Bleeding risk	Thrombosis risk	Prophylaxis
Low	Moderate	Low-dose heparin (LDH) 5000 U SC b.i.d. or LMWH at prophylactic doses
Low	High	LMWH in thromboprophylactic doses
High	Moderate, e.g., medical or postoperative patients	Graduated compression stockings or intermittent pneumatic compression, and LMWH
High	High, e.g., major trauma, orthopedic surgery	Graduated compression stockings or intermittent pneumatic compression, and LMW

LMWH, low-molecular-weight heparin.

high risk, and this period includes inpatient rehabilitation. The ACCP guidelines also recommend that thromboprophylaxis should be continued postdischarge in those with continuing immobility.

Special Situations in Critical Care

Inherited and Acquired Von Willebrand Disease

If unexplained bleeding occurs, consideration should be given to the late presentation of an inherited bleeding disorder and so a personal and family history of easy bruising and bleeding should be sought. Occasionally, conditions such as mild von Willebrand disease (VWD) may present for the first time in adults with persistent oozing postinjury or surgery.

Acquired VWD due to autoantibodies or, more commonly, due to breakdown of high molecular weight von Willebrand factor (VWF) multimers occurs in critical care. The latter is seen in patients with extracorporeal membrane oxygenation [46] and left ventricular assist devices, where high shear stresses induced by the equipment breaks down high molecular weight multimers; the former in patients with aortic valve stenosis, can also lead to gastrointestinal bleeding (Heyde syndrome) due to the removal of the antiangiogenic effect of VWF, resulting in gastrointestinal angiodysplasia [46].

The treatment of acquired VWD is with either desmopressin, which will stimulate endothelial cells to release their residual stores of VWF, or with VWF concentrates; the latter has a much greater chance of success. Antifibrinolytics may be considered to alleviate mucocutaneous bleeding. Acquired VWD due to high shear stresses requires removing the cause wherever possible.

Fibrinolytic Bleeding

Hyperfibrinolysis is the term used when excessive fibrinolysis threatens clot integrity. Abnormal fibrinolytic activity may be overlooked as a cause of bleeding, particularly in liver disease, and it is hard to diagnose due to the absence of a specific routine assay. Clinical suspicion should be high if bleeding continues despite hemostatic replacement therapy, when platelet levels are relatively conserved but fibrinogen levels are disproportionately low and D-dimers are disproportionally high when compared to the picture for DIC. Thrombelastography may help differentiating fibrinolytic activation from coagulation factor deficiency, but is a crude tool, only detecting most marked changes [47]. Fibrinolytic bleeding should be considered, particularly in liver disease and disseminated malignancies. In the authors experience tranexamic acid, either by infusion or orally (depending on the severity of the problem and the state of the patient), is beneficial in controlling bleeding, but needs to be given with thromboprophylaxis in view of the uncertain effect on thrombotic risk.

Renal Failure

For continuous hemofiltration, UFH or LMWH is used commonly, although some units use prostacyclin or regional citrate. Regional citrate anticoagulation has gained popularity as studies have shown it is associated with prolonged filter survival, significantly decreased bleeding risk, and increased completion of scheduled filter life span when compared with heparin [48]. With the use of a heparin, an occasional need for antithrombin replacement is indicated in patients undergoing continuous hemofiltration, or other extracorporeal circulation procedures, if there are low plasma antithrombin levels.

Renal Transplantation and Thrombosis

Some renal transplant recipients have an increased risk of thromboembolism (Table 28.5). The hypercoagulability of these patients persists throughout life, but is most marked in the first 6 months after transplantation. In a large series published by the European Dialysis and Transplantation Association in 1983, 4.4% of deaths occurring in renal transplant recipients were secondary to pulmonary embolus [49,50].

Table 28.5 Possible additional risk factors for venous thromboembolism disease in renal transplant recipients.

Immunosuppressive agents

    Cyclosporine
    Corticosteroids
    Muromonab-CD3 (OKT3)
    Sirolimus
    Mycophenolate mofetil

Antiphospholipid antibodies

Elevated homocysteine levels

Nephrotic syndrome

Pretransplant continuous ambulatory peritoneal dialysis

Post-transplant erythrocytosis

Acute CMV infection

Jehovah's Witnesses

Jehovah's Witnesses do not accept transfusion of blood or its major components, based on the belief that to be transfused with blood is equivalent to eating it and therefore prohibited by scripture. Until 2000, any Jehovah's Witness transfused with a prohibited blood product was expelled from the society and ostracized by other Jehovah's Witnesses. Since 2000, any Jehovah's Witness who "willfully and without regret" accepts blood transfusion is no longer expelled but instead "revokes his own membership by his own actions." Doctors should consider the possibility that individual Jehovah's Witness patients have interpreted this change as allowing them to accept transfusion under certain circumstances. This will require clarification in a one-to-one consultation in absolute medical confidentiality [51].

The Association of Anaesthetists of Great Britain and Ireland (AAGBI) advise that, although it is unlawful to give blood to a patient who has refused it, "for unconscious patients, the doctor will be expected to perform to the best of his/her ability, and this may include giving blood" (AABI, 1999). This would only apply when Jehovah's Witness status is unclear and/or relatives/ associates cannot produce an Advance Directive document.

Before dismissing the use of blood products, there must be a certainty that the patient is a committed Jehovah's Witness, has independently and freely decided to refuse transfusion, and has thought this decision through to the point of death at the time of making an Advance Directive (living will) or additional consent to surgery.

A copy of the Advance Directive should be placed in the patient's notes and the contents respected. If life-threatening bleeding occurs and time allows, a doctor of Consultant status should discuss with the patient, or relative, the implications of withholding blood, and a clear, signed entry should be written in the patient's notes.

The 2000 Watch Tower directive stated that "primary components" of blood must be refused, but that "when it comes to fractions of the primary components, each Christian must conscientiously decide for himself."

Every Jehovah's Witness should decide which products are acceptable to him/her during the consent process. All available blood products should be discussed, as interpretations of a "fraction of the primary component" may hypothetically include products such as leukocyte-depleted red cells and platelets, intravenous immunoglobulin, fibrinogen concentrates, and solvent–detergent treated FFP.

Most Jehovah's Witness patients refuse autologous predonation because blood is separated from the body in storage. Normovolemic hemodilution and some forms of intraoperative cell salvage and hemodialysis may be acceptable because the extracorporeal blood remains in contact with the circulation. Hematological parameters should be optimized preoperatively. Meticulous surgical hemostasis, minimal access surgery, and systemic pre- and perioperative administration of antifibrinolytic agents (tranexamic acid or aprotinin) or desmopressin (DDAVP) should be considered. The use of topical hemostatic plasma fractionation products, such as fibrin glue, may be acceptable to some.

Jehovah's Witness patients accept crystalloids and synthetic colloids, including dextran, hydroxyethyl starch, and gelatins (Haemaccel and Gelofusin) for circulatory support. Most requiring plasma exchange will refuse human albumin but may accept Hetastarch or protein A immunoabsorption as alternatives.

Recombinant blood products are acceptable to many Jehovah's Witnesses. Epoetin beta (NeoRecormin) contains a trace of albumin, whereas Epoetin alpha does not contain albumin and so is more widely accepted. Epoetin alpha (Eprex) is licensed for the treatment of moderate anemia (hemoglobin concentration 10–13 g/100 mL) before elective orthopedic surgery in adults with expected moderate blood loss, to reduce exposure to allogeneic transfusion. It is given by subcutaneous injection (maximum 1 mL per injection site), 600 U/kg every week for 3 weeks before surgery and on the day of surgery or 300 U/kg daily for 15 days starting 10 days before surgery.

Supplementation with folic acid and oral iron, or intravenous folinic acid and iron, should be considered, particularly if the patient is maintained on erythropoietin. Frequency and amount of blood sampling should be minimized.

Granulocyte colony stimulating factor (G-CSF) is acceptable treatment for neutropenia. Recombinant activated factor VII (rFVIIa, NovoSeven) is licensed for the treatment of bleeding episodes in hemophiliacs with inhibitors, and has been used to treat bleeding in platelet disorders as well as those without a pre-existing hemostatic disorder.

Recombinant factor VIII and XI, particularly second-generation products containing no albumin, facilitate therapy of hemophilia A and B in Jehovah's Witness patients. DDAVP is a synthetic product suitable for use in mild hemophilia A and type 1 von Willebrand disease and uremia. Some patients with rare hemorrhagic disorders that currently require plasma-derived therapeutic products (e.g., type 2 or 3 VWD) will accept a purified fractionated product.

Some Jehovah's Witnesses will regard their peripheral blood and bone marrow stem cell as a permissible fraction and consent to collection by leukapheresis or marrow aspiration. Specific treatment of the Jehovah's Witness with other hematological disorders is beyond the scope of this chapter. There should be an open, full, and confidential discussion of all available options. Jehovah's Witnesses exercise the right of any adult with capacity to refuse medical treatment and often carry advance directive cards indicating their incontrovertible refusal of blood.

Despite their belief regarding transfusion, Jehovah's Witnesses do not have a higher mortality rate after traumatic injury or surgery. Transfusion requirements are often overestimated. Increased morbidity and mortality is rarely observed in patients with a hemoglobin concentration >70 g/L, and the acute hemoglobin threshold for cardiovascular collapse may be as low as 30–50 g/L. There are many modalities to treat the Jehovah's Witness patient with acute blood loss. Treatment with recombinant human erythropoietin, albumin, and recombinant activated factor VIIa have all been used with success. Autologous autotransfusion and isovolemic hemodilution can also be used to treat patients who refuse transfusion. Hemoglobin-based oxygen carriers may play a future role as intravascular volume expanders in lieu of transfusion of red blood cell concentrates.

In conclusion, there are many treatment modalities available to assist in the care of Jehovah's Witness patients.

References

1 Desborough M, Stanworth S. Plasma transfusion for bedside, radiologically guided, and operating room invasive procedures. *Transfusion* 2012; 52 (Suppl. 1): 20S–29S.

2 Hall DP, Lone NI, Watson DM, *et al.*; for the Intensive Care Study of Coagulopathy (ISOC) Investigators. Factors associated with prophylactic plasma transfusion before vascular catheterization in non-bleeding critically ill adults with prolonged prothrombin time: a case-control study. *Br J Anaesth* 2012; 109: 919–927.

3 Collins PW, Macchiavello LI, Lewis SJ, *et al.* Global tests of haemostasis in critically ill patients with severe sepsis syndrome compared to controls. *Br J Haematol* 2006; 135: 220–227.

4 Borgman MA, Spinella PC, Perkins JG, *et al.* The ratio of blood products transfused affects mortality in patients receiving massive transfusions at a combat support hospital. *J Trauma* 2007; 63: 805–813.

5 Rajasekhar A, Gowing R, Zarychanski R, *et al.* Survival of trauma patients after massive red blood cell transfusion using a high or low red blood cell to plasma transfusion ratio. *Crit Care Med* 2011; 39: 1507–1513.

6 MacLennan S, Williamson LM. Risks of fresh frozen plasma and platelets. *J Trauma* 2006; 60 (6 Suppl.): S46–50.

7 Inaba K, Branco BC, Rhee P, *et al.* Impact of plasma transfusion in trauma patients who do not require massive transfusion. *J Am Coll Surg* 2010; 210: 957–965.

8 Holcomb JB, Tilley BC, Baranuik S, *et al.* Transfusion of plasma, platelets, and red blood cells in a 1:1:1 vs a 1:1:2 ratio and mortality in patients with severe trauma. The PROPPR Randomized Clinical Trial. *JAMA* 2015: 315; 471–482.

9 Hiippala S. Replacement of massive blood loss. *Vox Sang* 1998; 74 (Suppl. 2): 399–407.

10 Spahn DR, Cerny V, Coats TJ, *et al.*; Task Force for Advanced Bleeding Care in Trauma. Management of bleeding following major trauma: a European guideline. *Crit Care* 2007; 11: R17. Erratum in: *Crit Care* 2007; 11: 414.

11 Rourke C, Curry N, Khan S, *et al.* Fibrinogen levels during trauma hemorrhage, response to replacement therapy, and association with patient outcomes. *J Thromb Haemost* 2012; 10: 1342–1351.

12 Stanworth SJ, Hunt BJ. The desperate need for good-quality clinical trials to evaluate the optimal source and dose of fibrinogen in managing bleeding. *Crit Care* 2011; 15: 1006.

13 Simpson E, Lin Y, Stanworth S, *et al.* Recombinant factor VIIa for the prevention and treatment of bleeding in patients without haemophilia. *Cochrane Database Syst Rev* 2012; (3): CD005011.

14 Levi M, Levy JH, Andersen HF, *et al.* Safety of recombinant activated factor VII in randomized clinical trials. *N Engl J Med* 2010;

363: 1791–1800. Erratum in: *N Engl J Med* 2011; 365: 1944.

15 Shakur H, Roberts I, Bautista R, *et al.*; CRASH-2 Trial Collaborators. Effects of tranexamic acid on death, vascular occlusive events, and blood transfusion in trauma patients with significant haemorrhage (CRASH-2): a randomised, placebo-controlled trial. *Lancet* 2010; 376: 23–32.

16 Roberts I, Shakur H, Afolabi A, *et al.*; CRASH-2 Collaborators. The importance of early treatment with tranexamic acid in bleeding trauma patients: an exploratory analysis of the CRASH-2 randomised controlled trial. *Lancet* 2011; 377: 1096–1101, 1101.e1–2.

17 Hunt BJ, The current place of tranexamic acid in the management of bleeding. *Anaesthesia* 2015; 70 Suppl 1: 50–3.

18 Slichter SJ. Evidence-based platelet transfusion guidelines. *Hematology Am Soc Hematol Educ Program* 2007: 2007: 172–178.

19 Segal HC, Harrison P. Methods for counting platelets in severe thrombocytopenia. *Curr Hematol Rep* 2006; 5: 70–75.

20 Stasi R, Evangelista ML, Stipa E, *et al.* Idiopathic thrombocytopenic purpura: current concepts in pathophysiology and management. *Thromb Haemost* 2008; 99: 4–13.

21 Allen DL, Samol J, Benjamin S, *et al.* Survey of the use and clinical effectiveness of HPA-1a/5b-negative platelet concentrates in proven or suspected platelet alloimmunization. *Transfus Med* 2004; 14: 409–417.

22 Bernard GR, Vincent JL, Laterre PF, *et al.* Recombinant human protein C Worldwide Evaluation in Severe Sepsis (PROWESS) study group. Efficacy and safety of recombinant human activated protein C for severe sepsis. *N Engl J Med* 2001; 344: 699–709.

23 Ranieri VM, Thompson BT, Barie PS, *et al.*; PROWESS-SHOCK Study Group. Drotrecogin alfa (activated) in adults with septic shock. *N Engl J Med* 2012; 366: 2055–2064.

24 Afshari A, Wetterslev J, Brok J, *et al.* Antithrombin III for critically ill patients. *Cochrane Database Syst Rev* 2008; (3): CD005370.

25 Abraham E, Reinhart K, Opal S, *et al.*; OPTIMIST Trial Study Group. Efficacy and safety of tifacogin (recombinant tissue factor pathway inhibitor) in severe sepsis: a randomized controlled trial. *JAMA* 2003; 290: 238–247.

26 Warkentin TE. Hos I diagnose and manage HIT. *Hematol Am Soc Hematol Educ Program* 2011; 2011: 143–149.

27 Linkins LA, Dans AL, Moores LK *et al.* Treatment and prevention of heparin–induced thrombocytopenia: antithrombotic therapy and prevention of thrombosis, 9th ed: American College of Chest Physicians Evidence based Practical Guidelines. *Chest* 2012; 141: e45S–530S.

28 Robinson S, Harrison C. Review: challenges in the management of thrombocytosis in young patients. *Clin Adv Hematol Oncol* 2008; 6: 137–138, 14

29 Geerts WSR. Prevention of venous thromboembolism in the ICU. *Chest* 2003; 124: 357S–363S.

30 Kucher N, Goldhaber SZ. Risk stratification of acute pulmonary embolism. *Semin Thromb Hemost* 2006; 32: 838–844.

31 van Es N, Coppens M, Schulman S, Middeldorp S, Buller HR. Direct oral anticoagulants compared with vitamin K antagonists for acute venous thromboembolism : evidence from phase 3 trials. *Blood* 214; 124: 1968–75

32 EINSTEIN–PE Investigators. Oral rivaroxaban for the treatment of symptomatic pulmonary embolism. *N Engl J Med* 2012; 366: 1287–1297.

33 Sekhri V, Mehta N, Rawat N, *et al.* Management of massive and nonmassive pulmonary embolism. *Arch Med Sci* 2012; 8: 957–969.

34 Sharifi M, Bay C, Skrocki L, *et al.*; "MOPETT" Investigators. Moderate pulmonary embolism treated with thrombolysis (from the "MOPETT" Trial). *Am J Cardiol* 2013; 111: 273–277.

35 PREPIC Study Group. Eight-year follow-up of patients with permanent vena cava filters in the prevention of pulmonary embolism: the PREPIC (Prevention du Risque d'Embolie Pulmonaire par Interruption Cave) randomized study. *Circulation* 2005; 112: 416–422.

36 Young T, Tang H, Aukes J, *et al.* Vena caval filters for the prevention of pulmonary embolism. *Cochrane Database Syst Rev* 2007; (4): CD006212.

37 Attia J, Ray JG, Cook DJ. Deep vein thrombosis and its prevention in critically ill adults. *Arch Intern Med* 2001; 161: 1268–1279.

38 Geerts W, Cook D, Selby R, *et al.* Venous thromboembolism and its prevention in critical care. *J Crit Care* 2002; 17: 93–104.

39 Geerts WH, Bergqvist D, Pineo GF, *et al.* Prevention of venous thromboembolism: American College of Chest Physicians Evidence-Based Clinical Practice Guidelines (8th Edition). *Chest* 2008; 133 (6 Suppl.): 381S–453S.

40 Limpus A, Chaboyer W, McDonald E, *et al.* Mechanical thromboprophylaxis in critically ill patients: a systematic review and meta-analysis *Am J Crit Care* 2006; 15: 402–410.

41 CLOTS Trials Collaboration. Effectiveness of thigh-length graduated compression stockings to reduce the risk of deep vein thrombosis after stroke (CLOTS trial 1): a multicentre, randomised controlled trial. *Lancet* 2009; 373: 1958–1965.

42 CLOTS (Clots in Legs Or sTockings after Stroke) Trials Collaboration. Effectiveness of intermittent pneumatic compression in reduction of risk of deep vein thrombosis in patients who have had a stroke (CLOTS 3): a multicentre randomised controlled trial. *Lancet* 2013; 382; 516–524.

43 Arabi YM, Khedr M, Dara SI, *et al.* Use of intermittent pneumatic compression and not graduated compression stockings is associated with lower incident VTE in critically ill patients: a multiple propensity scores adjusted analysis. *Chest* 2013; 144: 152–159.

44 Cook D, Meade M, Guyatt G, *et al.* PROTECT Investigators for the Canadian Critical Care Trials Group and the Australian and New Zealand Intensive Care Society Clinical Trials Group, Dalteparin versus unfractionated

heparin in critically ill patients. *N Engl J Med* 2011; 364: 1305–1314.

45 Lauzier F, Arnold DM, Rabbat C, *et al.* Risk factors and impact of major bleeding in criticall ill patients receiving hpearin thrombprophylaxis. *Intensive Care Med* 2013; 39: 2135–2143.

46 Heilmann C, Geisen U, Beyersdorf F, *et al.* Acquired von Willebrand syndrome in patients with extracorporeal life support (ECLS). *Intensive Care Med* 2012; 38: 62–68.

47 Raza I, Davenport R, Rourke C, *et al.* The incidence and magnitude of fibrinolytic activation in trauma patients. *J Thromb Haemost* 2013; 11: 307–314.

48 Bagshaw SM, Laupland KB, Boiteau PJ, *et al.* Is regional citrate superior to systemic heparin anticoagulation for continuous renal replacement therapy? A prospective observational study in an adult regional critical care system. *J Crit Care* 2005; 20: 155–161.

49 Kazory A, Ducloux D. Acquired hypercoagulable state in renal transplant recipients. *Thromb Haemost* 2004; 91: 646–651.

50 Irish A. Hypercoagulability in renal transplant recipients. Identifying patients at risk of renal allograft thrombosis and evaluating strategies for prevention. *Am J Cardiovasc Drugs* 2004; 4: 139–149.

51 Hughes DB, Ullery BW, Barie PS. The contemporary approach to the care of Jehovah's witnesses. *J Trauma* 2008; 65: 237–247.

29

Transfusion

Adrian Copplestone

Key Points

- Transfusion of blood products are often used to treat coagulation deficiencies.
- However, because they are live human tissue, they carry risks related to immunization and infection.
- Blood and blood products are also in finite supply from donors and need to be used appropriately.
- This chapter updates recent advice on transfusion therapy, especially in management of trauma.

Introduction

The most common request to hematologists for help in the emergency management of patients in the hospital setting relates to the control of hemorrhage and the use of blood products. Whereas most treatment involves the use of purified drugs, blood and blood products are derived from human blood donors. They are rarely pure; they are subject to biological variation and carry the risk of infection. This chapter discusses some of these issues and describes their use in specialized clinical settings.

Blood Transfusion as a Form of Transplantation

Transfusion with red cells and other blood products is a form of tissue transplantation, which is made easier because the cells lack some or all of the HLA antigens. Because cells lack progenitor capacity, the benefit is temporary but allows time for the body's homeostatic processes to recover. However, the transfused cells contain surface proteins that are foreign to the host and give rise to an immune reaction. The common red cell blood grouping systems are listed in Table 29.1.

The ABO Group

These most important antigens are as a result of the inheritance of enzymes causing alternative glycosylation of the red cell membrane.

- If individuals lack an A or B antigen, they make anti-A or anti-B, respectively, after exposure to these glycopeptides in food.
- Blood group O is due to the lack of A or B antigen and so these people develop anti-A and anti-B antibodies.
- Group AB people have both antigens and lack the anti-A and anti-B antibodies (Table 29.2).

Individuals have naturally occurring circulating immunoglobulin M (IgM) antibodies to the A and B groups they lack. These antibodies are good at fixing complement, have the capacity to cause intravascular hemolysis, and can lead to disseminated intravascular coagulation (DIC). A useful scheme for remembering which ABO groups can be transfused to which patients is shown in Figure 29.1. In allogeneic blood and marrow stem cell transplantation, the picture is more complex because patients take on the blood group of the donor, and hemolysis may occur during the period of changeover.

Practical Hemostasis and Thrombosis, Third Edition. Edited by Nigel S. Key, Michael Makris and David Lillicrap.

Table 29.1 Common red cell blood group systems.

Blood group	Gene location
ABO	9q34.1–q34.2
Rhesus	1p36.11
Lewis	19p13.3
Kell	7q33
Duffy	1q22–23
Kidd	18q11–q12
MN	4q28–31
Ss	4q28–31

Table 29.2 ABO antigen and antibodies.

Blood group	Antigen	Antibody
A	A	anti-B
B	B	anti-A
O	none	anti-A and B
AB	A and B	none

The Rhesus System

The next most important blood group system is the Rhesus (Rh), of which the D antigen is the most immunogenic. The use of Rh D-negative blood for Rh D-negative patients is partly to prevent immunization but also to prevent hemolytic disease of the newborn due to the transplacental passage of anti-D to Rh D-positive children of Rh D-negative mothers.

Red Cell Cross-Matching

Just over 100 years ago, Landsteiner discovered blood groups. Transfusion from donor to patient became feasible when it was possible to determine blood groups and store the blood in an anticoagulated form. In recent years, the speed of matching suitable blood for a patient has been enabled by:

- monoclonal antibodies to achieve more consistent blood grouping results (phenotype);
- knowledge of the genetic basis of blood group to determine the genotype where relevant;
- use of cell panels with wide representation of antigens to enable the exclusion of alloantibodies (antibody screening);
- use of new technologies to enhance the antibody–antigen reaction (low ionic strength saline, gel tubes, microtiter plate capture).

Confidence in the blood group results and the detection of clinically relevant alloantibodies has led to increasing acceptance of electronic cross-matching, where the donor cells and patient serum are not actually tested against each other but a negative result is predicted.

These advances have dramatically reduced the time needed to supply suitable blood, enabling many operations to go ahead on a "blood grouped and screen basis." It also enables blood to be used in a more efficient manner and reduces waste because of expiry. However, the speed of the process may lead clinicians to forget that, when antibodies are present or develop, more steps are necessary to provide compatible blood and this takes longer.

Use of O-Negative Blood

In many emergencies where the blood group is not known, group O, Rh D-negative blood products may be required. If there is a shortage of group O blood, the Rh D-negative blood is reserved for children and women of childbearing age. Men can be given group O Rh D-positive blood and only a proportion will make anti-D.

Figure 29.1 Choice of red cells by ABO group.

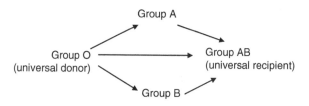

Risks of Transfusion

Donor screening and testing have reduced the risks of transfusion, but it should always be remembered that this process can never be "100% safe." New infections emerge and sometimes the steps taken to improve blood safety adversely affect other blood products.

Infective Risks

Infections can be transmitted by transfusion by a wide variety of organisms. Examples are listed in Table 29.3.

Reducing Risk
Donor screening is designed to select out potential donors who are at higher risk of infection because of lifestyle or travel. All donor blood is tested for:

- HBsAg,
- antibodies to HIV1 and HIV2,

Table 29.3 Examples of transfusion-transmitted infections.

Viruses	Hepatitis A
	Hepatitis B
	Hepatitis C
	HIV
	HTLV 1 and 2
	CMV
	EBV
	Parvovirus
	West Nile virus
Bacteria	*Treponema pallidum* (syphilis)
	Borrelia burgdorferi (Lyme disease)
	Staphylococcus spp.
	Diphtheroids
	Salmonella spp.
	Pseudomonas spp.
	Yersinia spp.
Protozoa	*Plasmodium* spp. (malaria)
	Toxoplasma gondii (toxoplasmosis)
	Trypanosoma cruzi (Chaga disease)

CMV, cytomegalovirus; EBV, Epstein–Barr virus; HTLV, human T-cell leukemia virus.

- syphilis,
- hepatitis C virus,
- human T cell leukemia virus, and
- some donors for cytomegalovirus.

Despite these tests, there exist a small number of donors who are infected but lack antibody; this will be reduced further by nucleic acid testing using polymerase chain reaction technology to look for viral genome.

New agents (e.g., West Nile virus and severe acute respiratory syndrome (SARS)) continue to emerge as pathogens. Steps taken to reduce these risks include:

- donor lifestyle screening,
- antibody testing,
- leukodepletion, and
- DNA/RNA testing.

For plasma products, it is also possible to:

- heat treat,
- nanofilter, or
- disrupt lipid membranes with solvents, methylene blue, or psoralens with ultraviolet light.

Widespread leukodepletion was introduced in the UK in 1998 to reduce the risk of transmission of variant Creutzfeldt–Jakob Disease (vCJD). In addition, there was a major shift of procurement of plasma for plasma products from areas without bovine spongiform encephalopathy (BSE), primarily the USA. No test suitable for donor screening is currently available to detect the abnormal prion. BSE has been transmitted in sheep by transfusion, and in the UK, by 2012, there have been four cases of vCJD transmission by blood transfusion.

Transfusion Reactions

Immediate Hemolytic Reactions

These are likely to be associated with shock, renal failure, and DIC. The most common cause is a patient receiving the wrong blood, in 70% because of the labeling or checking errors at the bedside or in the laboratory. These errors are preventable by the adherence to clear transfusion protocols [1]. The British Committee for Standards in Haematology (BCSH) have produced guidelines for the management of these reactions [2].

Delayed Hemolytic Reactions

These are usually caused by extravascular hemolysis and the boosting of alloantibody levels.

Febrile Transfusion Reactions

Less common now that universal leukodepletion is in place, these are caused by the presence of cytokines and HLA antibodies. Urticarial and allergic reactions can still occur.

Transfusion-Related Acute Lung Injury

Transfusion-related acute lung injury (TRALI) is caused by donor leukocyte antibodies, which cause adult respiratory distress syndrome. The patient becomes acutely short of breath and often requires artificial ventilation and circulatory support. TRALI needs to be distinguished from circulatory fluid overload, which can occur following the transfusion of large volumes, especially in older patients. In the UK, the number of cases of TRALI has fallen after the increased use of male plasma to make fresh frozen plasma (FFP), as males have less immunization by white cell antigens than females (related to pregnancy).

Immunization

Alloimmunization can affect the efficacy of transfusion, especially platelets. It may also affect the subsequent choice of donors for organ transplantation. Immunomodulation can follow transfusion with an increase in infections and increase in relapse of carcinoma following surgery to patients who were transfused.

Post-Transfusion Purpura

Post-transfusion purpura (PTP; Figure 29.2) is a rare complication where severe thrombocytopenia occurs approximately 1 week after transfusion. The recipient is usually HPA1a-negative

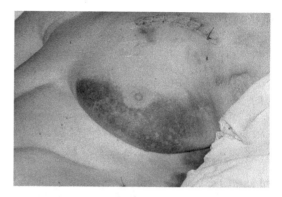

Figure 29.2 Post-transfusion purpura presenting with ecchymosis in a female patient with a platelet count of 10×10^9/L, subsequently shown to be HPA-1a negative with anti-HPA-1a antibodies. Transfusion had been given preoperatively. *Source*: Greaves and Makris, 1997 [3]. Reproduced with permission of Elsevier.

and HLA DR3*1010 and has anti-HPA1a antibodies, although on rare occasions other platelet groups are implicated. Treatment is high-dose intravenous immunoglobulin (IVIg).

Blood Products Available

Red Cells

Whole Blood: Donor blood is anticoagulated in 10% citrate anticoagulant, and during storage, the labile coagulant factors V and VIII and platelets are lost within a few days. Little whole blood is used in the UK because transfusion practice has adopted a component approach.

Leukodepleted Red Cells in Additive Solution: These donor cells are collected in citrate anticoagulant, the white cells are removed by filtration, and the red cells are stored in saline, adenine, mannitol, and glucose (SAG-M). With storage at 4°C, the red cells have a 35-day shelf-life.

Washed Red Cells: For patients who have severe reactions to leukodepleted blood, or who have IgA deficiency, red cells washed in saline can remove plasma proteins that cause the reactions.

Frozen Red Cells: These are used for patients with rare blood groups. The red cells are frozen in glycerol as cryoprotectant and washed before use.

Platelets

Platelet concentrates are prepared from either:

- plateletpheresis of donors using a cell separator machine; or
- combining platelet-rich plasma from buffy coats and packed in four-donor pools.

The shelf-life of platelet concentrates is only 5 days (with testing taking up the first 24–48 hours), but the use of additive solution and microbiological testing may extend this to 7 days.

Platelets are used to correct bleeding resulting from thrombocytopenia or abnormal platelet function, with the exception of immune thrombocytopenia purpura (ITP), thrombotic thrombocytopenia (TTP), and heparin-induced thrombocytopenia (HIT). The latter two conditions are associated with thrombosis, and platelet transfusions can exacerbate the disease [4].

Of the platelet concentrates made from blood donation or plateletpheresis, a significant quantity is given to patients with bone marrow failure. In recent years, the trigger level of platelet count at which platelet transfusion is given has been falling and is usually $10 \times 10^9/L$. Counting platelets accurately at this level is difficult, even using modern automated blood counters. Giving larger doses of platelets less frequently or only treating if the patient has bleeding results in less platelet transfusions but more days of bleeding [5]. Patients may become refractory to repeated platelet transfusion and need more expensive HLA-matched platelets. Another area where large quantities of platelets are used is cardiac surgery. The combined problem is the use of antiplatelet drugs and cardiac–pulmonary bypass circuits. This is discussed in more detail in Chapter 21.

Fresh Frozen Plasma

FFP is used to correct coagulation deficiencies, and there has been considerable debate on the relative merits of different products.

In the ideal world, FFP would provide high concentrations of the relevant factor, be from a low number of screened regular donors, have a viral inactivation step in the production that does not adversely affect the coagulation factors, be procured in a country where BSE is not endemic, come from male donors (to reduce the risk of TRALI), and have appropriate ABO group.

The following are available:

- Single-donor FFP.
- Methylene blue-treated FFP for pediatric use is a single-donor product, procured in the USA. In the UK, it is used primarily for children born after January 1, 1996 when the risk of vCJD from meat was minimized, but its use will extend to other age groups as it becomes more available.
- Solvent detergent FFP (Octaplas®) is a pooled product that is solvent treated to reduce the infective risks. It is used in large quantities in TTP because it is low in high-molecular-weight multimers of von Willebrand factor (VWF), but it has been associated with thrombosis because of protein S deficiency.

The British Committee for Standards in Haematology (BCSH) guidelines [6] suggest that:

- FFP should only be used to replace single inherited clotting factor deficiencies for which no virus-safe fractionated product is available. Currently, this applies mainly to factor V.
- FFP is indicated when there are demonstrable multifactor deficiencies associated with severe bleeding and/or DIC. However, FFP is not indicated in DIC with no evidence of bleeding.
- FFP should not be used to reverse warfarin effect in the absence of bleeding as it has an incomplete effect and is not an ideal product as large quantities are required. Vitamin K and prothrombin complex concentrate should be used when reversing coumarin anticoagulants in patients who are bleeding or at high risk of bleeding.
- Large quantities of FFP are used for correction of abnormal coagulation tests prior to invasive procedures, but the evidence base that this reduces bleeding is weak.

Cryoprecipitate and Methylene Blue-Treated Cryosupernatant

Cryoprecipitate forms when FFP is thawed slowly, and the product, which is refrozen, is rich in fibrinogen and factors VIII and XIII. It is commonly used in the treatment of DIC to replace fibrinogen. Methylene blue-treated Cryo is available for children in the UK.

Cyrosupernatant and Methylene Blue-Treated Cryosupernatant

The complementary product cryosupernatant has been used in conjunction with plasmapheresis in TTP as it lacks high-molecular-weight multimers of VWF; however, solvent detergent is the recommended product in the UK.

Human Albumin Solution

The final product of the plasma fractionation process, human albumin solution (HAS), comes in two strengths: 45 g/L and 20 g/L (salt-poor albumin). It is an important colloid for maintaining the oncotic pressure in the intravascular compartment, and its main indication relates to replacing albumin in severe edematous states. Its use as plasma expander has largely been superseded by crystalloids and gelatin solutions.

Intravenous Immunoglobulin

IVIg solutions are pooled normal human donor immunoglobulins. In the coagulation disorders, they are used as an immunomodulator for the treatment of ITP and PTP. Because supply cannot meet demand, most countries have adopted national clinical guidelines together with a demand management plan.

Coagulation Factor Concentrates

Concentrates are prepared from large pools of donor plasma. They all have steps to reduce viral contamination and most have steps to remove impure proteins. Increasing use of recombinant coagulation factors as these become available is being encouraged:

- Factor VIII for hemophilia A. Some of the intermediate purity products contain useful amounts of VWF as well.
- Factor IX for hemophilia B.
- VWF concentrates are now available for von Willebrand disease (VWD).
- Prothrombin complex concentrate (combined factors II, VII, IX, and X concentrate) is primarily used in the correction of life-threatening hemorrhage in patients on oral vitamin K antagonist anticoagulants.
- Individual concentrates for factors VII, X, and XIII and fibrinogen are available for patients with hereditary deficiencies.

Fibrin Sealants

Mixing thrombin and fibrinogen forms "fibrin glue," which is applied to the site of bleeding and is a popular treatment in neurosurgery.

Autologous Blood

In many situations, it is possible to use the patient's own blood and thereby avoid exposure to the risks of donor blood. However, there are still risks with using autologous blood, mainly related to bacterial infection and the blood being transfused to the wrong patient. A number of approaches are possible.

Predeposit Donation: Blood is venesected prior to elective surgery and retained for up to 4 weeks. By retransfusing older blood during the collection process, up to 4 U of blood can be stored. Surgery must take place on the planned date or the blood may expire. In the UK, the use of predeposit donation has fallen as patients can be more anemic at the time of surgery, and if anemia can be corrected preadmission, the patient can often withstand the loss of volume of blood that would have been transfused.

Cell Salvage: Blood can be aspirated during an operation and washed red cells returned to the patient. This is useful in vascular surgery and is also finding a place in cardiac surgery, trauma, and obstetric patients.

Intraoperative Hemodilution: Blood is venesected at the time of anesthesia, and crystalloid is used as fluid replacement. If bleeding occurs, less red cells are lost because of the lower hematocrit. At the end of the operation, the blood, which also contains coagulation factors and platelets, is retransfused.

Cell Salvage from Wound Drains: Blood is drawn into a sterile container by suction and transfused. This application has been used extensively in orthopedic surgery and has reduced the need for blood in joint-replacement operations.

Drugs that Reduce the Need for Transfusion

A number of drugs are used to either boost the hemostatic system or reduce fibrinolysis. Drugs that can increase the red cells mass are also important.

Desmopressin

Desmopressin (DDAVP), an analogue of antidiuretic hormone, is used in mild hemophilia, VWD, and some platelet disorders. Endothelial stores of VWF are released. Repeated administration is subject to tachyphylaxis.

Tranexamic Acid and Other Fibrinolytic Inhibitors

These are useful in major surgery, but their use needs to be balanced against the risk of venous thromboembolism (VTE). They may also be used in patients with marrow failure who have mucosal bleeding from chronic thrombocytopenia but are refractory to platelet transfusions.
- Aprotinin (Trasylol®) is a bovine protease inhibitor that inactivates plasmin and kallikrein. It has been used in cardiac surgery in patients on cardiopulmonary bypass, with a reduction in the need for transfusion, reoperation for bleeding,

and length of stay in ICU and hospital admission. In 2006, concerns of increased frequency of renal failure and multiorgan failure led to considerable discussion of its role and its use has been largely discontinued since 2007.

Iron

There are many patients who have low iron stores or frank deficiency as a consequence of chronic hemorrhage, either through the disease process or the result of treatment (e.g., nonsteroidal anti-inflammatory drugs). Correction with small doses of iron to improve compliance can avoid the need for transfusion. Where anemia has developed slowly, patients can tolerate quite low hemoglobin levels. Treatment with iron and patience are much safer than "top-up transfusions." Intravenous iron preparations can also help overcome functional iron deficiency seen in anemia of chronic disorders.

Vitamins

Other vitamins (such as folic acid) may also be required in anemic patients with poor intake (elderly or malabsorption) or increased turnover (pregnancy).

Erythropoietin

Erythropoietin (rhEPO) can be useful to boost the erythron. Concomitant iron therapy may also be needed to achieve a rapid response. Its cost has restricted its use in clinical practice, but many patients with renal failure no longer require regular transfusion.

Recombinant Activated Factor VII

This recombinant protein (rFVIIa) was originally used in hemophiliacs with inhibitors, but it was increasingly being used in patients with severe bleeding from multiple trauma or major bleeding in a critical care situation. Many of these patients went on to develop arterial thrombosis and with a systemic review showing poor evidence of efficacy, it is no longer recommended [7].

Use of Blood Products

How Much to Give?

The decision of when to transfuse and how much to give can be difficult [8]. In general, the rule should be to try to avoid transfusion if possible, but if it is necessary, to use sufficient quantities of the right product to achieve the desired effect (usually hemostasis).

Guidelines on the use of red cells have previously advised transfusion based on the reduction of red cell mass, but this can be difficult to estimate in clinical practice. As a result, "Hb triggers" have increasingly been used in the management of patients, particularly in the postoperative setting. In a landmark study [9], Hébert and coworkers showed that, in patients in a critical care unit, a restrictive transfusion policy (Hb trigger 70 g/L, aim Hb 70–90 g/L) had a lower mortality than a more liberal policy (Hb trigger 100 g/L, aim Hb 100–120 g/L), with the possible exception of patients with acute myocardial infarction and unstable angina. Similar results have been reported in patients with acute gastrointestinal hemorrhage [10].

Although Hb trigger levels are easy for clinical teams to use, other factors also affect the Hb level, and the Hb trigger level may need to be adjusted for individual patients based on comorbidities. Other measures may usefully aid the decision as to whether to transfuse, such as the rate of postoperative bleeding. Where this has been measured for a cohort of patients (e.g., postcardiac bypass surgery), deviations from the usual course can be spotted more rapidly and appropriate action taken. Similarly, if more attention was paid to improving anemia preoperatively, there would be less need for transfusion.

Assessment of Hemorrhage

In situations where patients are bleeding, the first question is to determine whether this is surgically correctable. Simultaneously, blood should be sent for blood count and coagulation studies. The prothrombin time (PT) and activated partial thromboplastin time (APPT), combined with supplementary tests (fibrinogen level, thrombin time, equal volume mix with normal plasma) usually give an indication as to the type of hemostatic defect. Confirmation with specific factor levels can follow if necessary.

Blood sampling is important as these patients often have multiple cannulae, and it is important that the sample is not taken through a line contaminated with heparin. The drug chart should be examined, especially for anticoagulants, antifibrinolytics, and antiplatelet drugs. Caution must be taken with blood count samples, as patients may be inappropriately transfused if taken from lines running intravenous fluids.

Near Patient Testing

Because coagulation tests take at least 20 minutes to complete (and usually longer, taking sample transport into account), there has been a move to use near patient testing (NPT) with a number of different devices.

- Whole blood clotting time: activated clotting time (ACT) is used in cardiac surgery to monitor heparin effect.
- PT and APTT devices (e.g., Coaguchek®): these are designed mainly for testing patients on oral anticoagulants.
- Thromboelastography: the TEG® and similar ROTEM® are described in more detail in Chapter 21. Thromboelastography is used in liver and cardiac units and increasingly in other major hemorrhagic situations. It gives information relating to platelet function, clot strength, and fibrinolysis within approximately 15 minutes.
- Platelet function analyses (PFA-100®): an *in vitro* bleeding time test whose current role is determining mild VWD and platelet defects.

Although many hematologists dislike NPT equipment as being "uncontrolled" and lacking some of the strict supervision of laboratory procedures, the immediacy of results has lead to their increased use, and both laboratory and clinical teams should work together to define their role in decision making.

Importance of Good Communication

When dealing with complex patients, there needs to be good communication between the clinical team and the transfusion, hematology, and coagulation laboratories. The hematologist is ideally suited to advise on suitable blood products, facilitate testing to minimize delays, ensure that blood products are dispatched rapidly, and anticipate future requirements, especially if the source of supply is off-site.

Special Situations

Disseminated Intravascular Coagulation

DIC often requires transfusion of coagulation factors and platelets (see Chapter 12). Consumption of products may be dramatic, and regular coagulation tests are required to guide therapy, although treatment is based on the degree of bleeding and organ failure rather than abnormalities in the tests. To reverse the process, the underlying cause must be treated.

Massive Transfusion

Massive blood loss is defined as the loss of the blood volume within 24 hours or more than 50% in 3 hours. This can occur in controlled settings (e.g., surgery) but the commonest cause is trauma. The acute traumatic coagulopathy has been associated with shock and caused by systemic anticoagulation and hyperfibrinolysis. The replacement of the blood volume with stored blood (lacking platelets and factors VIII and V) leads to mucosal bleeding and generalized ooze. Hypothermia, acidosis, and dilutional effects add to the coagulopathy. Early administration of tranexamic acid has been shown to be lifesaving [11]. Recognition of the condition and correction with platelet and FFP/cryoprecipitate transfusion, based on laboratory clotting studies, is important. The military use of "shock packs" (red cells, thawed frozen plasma, and platelets) early in the management of patients with multiple injury is being increasingly used in civilian practice, in an attempt to prevent the generalized bleeding syndrome that occurs in these patients.

Cardiac Surgery

Cardiac surgery uses approximately 10% of the blood supply and is a major user of FFP, second only to critical care units (FFP) and oncology (platelets). This is discussed in detail in Chapter 21.

Obstetrics

Major hemorrhage in obstetrics is an emergency. It can occur for a number of reasons (Table 29.4). It can be dramatic and, in rare cases of maternal mortality, the severity of the situation has often not been recognized. It requires immediate resuscitation, using the group O Rhesus D-negative emergency blood if necessary, and ABO-matched blood, FFP, and platelets dispatched without delay. Further hematological support will depend on coagulation studies. DIC may be present.

Every obstetric unit should have a major hemorrhage protocol, agreed with the hematology laboratory. Good communication with the clinical team, laboratory, and hematologist is essential.

Pediatrics

Neonates and young children have a number of considerations with respect to hemostasis and transfusion:

- Their size means that much smaller volumes are used.
- Donor exposure should be kept to a minimum.
- Their relatively immature immune systems mean that they may not make some antibodies (e.g. anti-A and anti-B), so blood grouping will be different from adults (i.e., no reverse grouping available).

Table 29.4 Causes of major hemorrhage in obstetrics.

Ectopic gestation
Abortion
Placental abruption
Placenta previa
Postpartum: atonic uterus, trauma due to childbirth, coagulation disorders

- Often group O red cells are used, but the plasma should not contain high-titer anti-A or anti-B antibodies. Similarly, note should be taken when using large volumes of FFP or platelets as red cell hemolysis resulting from ABO incompatibility has been reported.
- Their blood may contain maternal IgG antibodies (e.g., hemolytic disease of the newborn).
- Neonates who have received transfusion *in utero*, and children with immunodeficiency, require irradiated blood products (to reduce the risk of transfusion-associated graft-versus-host disease).
- Severe coagulation disorders may present in the neonatal period. Coagulation studies can be difficult to perform and repeated tests will lead to institutional anemia.
- Neonatal thrombocytopenia may have an infective or immune basis. Treatment depends on the cause.

Jehovah's Witnesses

Jehovah's Witnesses belong to the Watch Tower Bible and Tract Society. They believe that trans-fusing blood is equivalent to eating it, and this is prohibited by scripture. Although they refuse transfusion, they accept modern medical care and technology. As mentally competent adults, they have a right to refuse treatment. The situa-tion is more complex in unconscious adults and children. Exactly which blood product is refused is an individual decision, although often guided by church elders (Table 29.5).

Surgery should be planned to minimize blood loss, with good consultation between patient, surgeon, anesthetist, and hematologist. The patient should sign an Advance Directive.

Hemovigilance and Regulation of Transfusion

A decade ago, the recognition that sometimes transfusion can harm patients, resulted in the setting up of Serious Hazards of Transfusion (SHOT) scheme in the UK. SHOT is a voluntary confidential reporting scheme that has been

Table 29.5 Acceptance of blood products by Jehovah's Witnesses.

Refused	Accepted	Variable
Red cells	Crystalloids	Albumin
White cells	Synthetic colloids	Immunoglobulin
Platelets	EPO	Vaccines
Plasma	GCSF	Coagulation factors
	rFVIIa	Cell salvage
	Organ transplant	

EPO, erythropoietin; GCSF, granulocyte colony-stimulating factor; rFVIIa, recombinant factor VIIa.

copied in many other countries. Analysis of adverse events has been invaluable in improving the safety of transfusion. The annual reports give details and recommendations to improve transfusion practice [12].

In Europe, Blood Safety Directives have been incorporated into national legislation (Blood Safety and Quality Regulations in the UK). Reporting of adverse events is mandatory. There needs to be full traceability from donor to patient with records retained for 30 years (in view of vCJD risks). Transfusion laboratories have to maintain a quality management system and are subject to inspection.

In the USA, transfusion laboratories are regu-lated by the Food and Drug Agency. All deaths relating to transfusion need to be reported. Hospitals can apply for accreditation from the Joint Commission for Accreditation for Health-care Organizations, the College of American Pathologists, and American Association of Blood Banks.

The 2012 Annual SHOT report [12] high-lights that Hematology has the most frequent reports and the majority are Acute Transfusion Reactions (ATR), whereas in Emergency Medi-cine, General Medicine, Surgery, and Ortho-pedics there are equal numbers of Handling and Storage errors as ATRs, with Right Patient Right Blood errors making a further significant proportion. Most of these errors can be pre-vented by blood sampling and transfusion being performed by trained staff and taking especial care with patient identification at blood sample labeling, collection, and pre-transfusion checks. Human error occurred in 62% of the incidents reported. There were 1645 incidents reported, which resulted in nine deaths and 134 cases of major morbidity.

Conclusions

Good transfusion practice [13,14] in treating coagulation disorders is a combination of thinking ahead to reduce the need for transfusion and using the appropriate product in the right quantity. Clear documentation of the reasons for transfusion and good institutional protocols also help. Safe transfusion practice requires all staff to be trained and apply these policies, especially in regard to patient identification and documentation.

Web Sites of Interest

British Committee for Standards in Hematology guidelines: www.bcshguidelines.com.
Blood Transfusion Toolkit: www.transfusion guidelines.org.uk.
Serious Hazards of Transfusion: www.shotuk.org.

References

1 British Committee for Standards in Hematology. *Guideline for Administration of Blood Components.* Available at: www.bcshguidelines. com/documents/Admin_blood_components_ bcsh_05012010.pdf (accessed July 2016).

2 Tinegate H, Birchall J, Gray A, *et al.*; British Committee for Standards in Hematology. Guideline for the investigation and management of acute transfusion reactions. *Br J Haematol* 2012; 159: 143–153.

3 Greaves M, Makris, M. *Blood in Systemic Disease.* Missouri: Mosby, 1997.

4 British Committee for Standards in Hematology. Guidelines for the use of platelet transfusions. *Br J Haematol* 2003; 122: 10–23.

5 Stanworth SJ, Estcourt LJ, Powter G, *et al.* A no-prophylaxis platelet transfusion strategy for hematologic cancers. *N Engl J Med* 2013; 368: 1771–1780.

6 British Committee for Standards in Hematology. Guidelines for the use of fresh frozen plasma, cryoprecipitate and cryosupernatant. *Br J Haematol* 2004; 126: 11–28. Amendment available at: www. bcshguidelines.com/documents/ FFPAmendment_2_17_Oct_2007.pdf (accessed July 2016).

7 Simpson E, Lin Y, Stanworth S, *et al.* Recombinant factor VIIa for the prevention and treatment of bleeding in patients without haemophilia. *Cochrane Database Syst Rev* 2012; (3): CD005011.

8 Retter A, Wyncoll D, Pearse R, *et al.*; British Committee for Standards in Hematology. Guidelines on the management of anaemia and red cell transfusion in adult critically ill patients. *Br J Haematol* 2013; 160: 445–464.

9 Hébert PC, Wells G, Blajchman MA, *et al.* A multicenter, randomized, controlled clinical trial of transfusion requirements in critical care. *N Engl J Med* 1999; 340: 409–417.

10 Villanueva C, Colomo A, Bosch A, *et al.* Transfusion strategies in acute upper gastrointestinal bleeding. *N Engl J Med* 2013; 368: 11–21.

11 CRASH-2 Trial Collaborators. The importance of early treatment with tranexamic acid in bleeding trauma patients: an exploratory analysis of the CRASH-2 randomized, controlled trial. *Lancet* 2011; 377: 1096–1101.

12 Bolton-Maggs, PHB, Poles D, Watt A, *et al.*; Serious Hazards of Transfusion (SHOT) Steering Group. *The 2012 Annual SHOT Report, 2013.* Available at: www.shotuk.org (accessed July 2016).

13 McClelland DBL. *Handbook of Transfusion Medicine*, 4th edn, 2007. Available at: www. transfusionguidelines.org.uk (accessed July 2016).

14 Murphy MF, Pamphilon DH, Heddle NM. *Practical Transfusion Medicine*, 4th edn. Oxford: Wiley Blackwell, 2013.

Appendix 1

Reference Ranges

Steve Kitchen and Michael Makris

Background

Interpretation of any laboratory result requires its comparison with a reference range or reference interval. There are detailed guidelines making recommendations about establishment of reference intervals in general [1], and the importance of the reference interval is confirmed by its presence in the US Clinical and Laboratory Improvement Amendments (CLIA) legislation, which requires that laboratories verify that any manufacturer's stated reference intervals are appropriate for the laboratory's patient population [2]. This is particularly true for tests of hemostasis, where it is also the case that relatively subtle local differences in relation to sample collection, processing, storage, and testing may have an impact on the results obtained locally. This means that reference ranges for use in hemostasis must be established or at the very least validated locally. The reference range is influenced not just by the biological variability within and between subjects in health, but also includes the variability associated with the analytical process; so even if the population is the same for two centers, local validation is still required to take account of the analytical variability in that particular center so that it fully reflects the local conditions.

There are essentially two types of reference interval, the most common of which is health associated. This is based on the results obtained for a particular test when performed in healthy normal individuals. The second type of reference interval can be described as decision based [3] and describes the specific limits used for making a clinical decision used to diagnose or manage particular patient groups. In the latter case, the intervals are defined using groups other than healthy normal subjects. This chapter will deal mainly with health-associated reference intervals.

The reference interval derived from healthy normal subjects is more commonly referred to as the normal range. The selection of individuals for testing and method of data handling used for construction of reference ranges is important. Health is not well defined, and results of some coagulation tests are influenced by age, sex, hormone replacement therapy, some oral contraceptive pills, blood group, and other variables, which means that, in some instances, a reference range established by analysis of a carefully matched control group might be required.

Selection of Subjects

The reference range should be established by analyzing a representative subset of subjects drawn from the same population as the test samples. This process is not straightforward because of the many factors that influence levels of hemostatic factors and therefore the results of laboratory tests in this area. The most appropriate group of subjects to use for establishment

Practical Hemostasis and Thrombosis, Third Edition. Edited by Nigel S. Key, Michael Makris and David Lillicrap.
© 2017 John Wiley & Sons, Ltd. Published 2017 by John Wiley & Sons, Ltd.

of a reference range is one that has been matched for age, sex, diet, lifestyle, etc. to the patient population. In practice, however, a more pragmatic approach can be successfully taken in most cases provided that the selection criteria are taken into account when making use of the data. A useful practical approach is to select normal subjects and adopt inclusion/exclusion criteria before analysis. A simple questionnaire can be used to identify subjects taking medications, which may influence results, who can then be excluded. Because there is the possibility to identify unexpected abnormalities during testing, apparently normal subjects may have lifestyle or health insurance implications as a result of taking part. The authors recommend the use of written informed consent so that subjects can choose in advance of recruitment whether they wish to be informed of any such findings. Any outlying results identified in this process should be reviewed by a clinician with hemostasis expertise. This process should take account of any relevant local regulations related to ethics and clinical governance, and any documentation should be approved by relevant local authorities prior to introduction. Once this is in place, subjects can be recruited from the general population, from blood donors, or from hospital staff. It is normally unacceptable to use hospital patients even if they are carefully selected because, by definition, they are unlikely to meet the "normal" criteria.

The demographics of the normal subjects used to establish a reference interval need to be considered because, for example, concentrations of factors VII (FVII), FVIII:C, and FIX and fibrinogen increase with age. In the case of FVIII:C and von Willebrand factor (VWF), there are highly significant differences according to the blood group of the subject [4], with levels approximately 25% lower in group O individuals compared with non-O blood groups. However, many/most centers do not take this latter effect into account when screening for von Willebrand disease (VWD) because the clinical management will normally depend on the actual levels of FVIII and VWF in relation to the clinical needs of the patient irrespective of blood group.

For some tests of hemostasis, sex needs to be taken into account. The lower limits of protein S activity in women compared with men are probably sufficiently great (approximately 20% different at age under 45 years) that a sex-specific reference range is warranted, and where this is not done, the sex of the patient should be taken into account when interpreting results obtained by some methods. This is also the case for homocysteine determinations (approximately 25% lower in females). Sex-specific normal ranges are not needed for other hemostasis tests.

The International Society on Thrombosis and Hemostasis (ISTH) SSC subcommittee on Women's Health Issues has published guidelines on the preanalytical conditions related to the patients' physiological state and other exogenous factors that need to taken into account when performing laboratory tests of hemostasis in women [5]. This includes a review of the evidence for the effects of physical stress (up to 10-hour persistence of a 2.5-fold increase in FVIII/VWF, for example), mental stress (increase in FVIII and VWF after acute mental stress), hormone effects [6], circadian variations, and the effects of posture and diet. Some general recommendations were made that were not restricted to investigation of female patients. These were as follows:

- Abstain from intense physical exercise for 24 hours prior to venipuncture.
- Use an environment where physical and mental stress are lessened.
- Abstain from fatty foods and smoking on the morning of venipuncture.
- Obtain samples early in the morning (7–9 am) after sitting in a relaxed position for 20–30 minutes.

As discussed elsewhere in this chapter, such conditions should only be used for blood collection from normal subjects for establishment of reference intervals if the conditions are also used for patient blood sample collection.

Reference intervals may be required for patient groups other than healthy normal subjects to take account of particular physiological or pathological states. Because of considerable variations in the concentration of clotting factors during pregnancy and development, specific normal ranges for neonatal, pediatric, and pregnant subjects should be available. This is a particular problem where, because of ethical and practical reasons, it is virtually impossible for each laboratory to establish their own neonatal normal ranges, so many laboratories use the same published ranges in newborns. Data on the expected results of clotting tests in older children have also been published. For these studies, it is important to note that ranges for screening tests are only appropriate for the particular technique used in the study, whereas the results of clotting factor assays are normally influenced much less by the method employed and may therefore be a useful guide to centers employing other techniques.

In some cases, the effects of drugs on coagulation tests should be taken into account. For example, if attempting to diagnose protein C or protein S deficiency during vitamin K antagonist (VKA) therapy, a reference range constructed from subjects receiving VKA prophylaxis is necessary to take account of the reductions in protein C and protein S induced by the therapy.

In general, establishing these types of group-specific reference ranges may not always be practical and, for many hemostatic parameters, it may be of debatable clinical value.

Number of Subjects Required

The number of normal subjects required for analysis and construction of a normal range depends on a number of issues. From a statistical validity aspect, the International Federation of Clinical Chemistry and International Committee for Standardisation in Haematology have indicated that the number of subjects required is at least 40 but that this should preferably be 120 to obtain reliable estimates [7]. However, for many tests of hemostasis, the effect of increasing numbers of subjects from 25–30 up to much larger numbers leads to entirely minor and clinically irrelevant differences in the calculated ranges, and in these cases, 25–30 is probably adequate.

A Clinical and Laboratory Standards Institute (CLSI) guideline [8] addressing the prothrombin time (PT) and activated partial thromboplastin time (APTT) considered that the full 120 normal values should be tested by manufacturers when they first develop new methods but, for practical purposes, individual laboratories can obtain a close approximation by testing a minimum of 20 individuals encompassing the age range that patient testing will include. The same guideline reminds the reader that the reference intervals are only a guide to be used in conjunction with the patients clinical picture. The World Federation of Haemophilia laboratory manual considers that 30 is an adequate number of normal subjects for construction of reference ranges for hemostasis tests used in the investigation of bleeding disorders [9].

Processing of Samples

When constructing normal ranges, the samples from normal subjects should be collected, processed, and analyzed locally using identical techniques to those used for the analysis of the patient samples. It is particularly important to use the same blood collection tubes since the composition of the tube, the bung/cap, and the anticoagulant strength can all influence results of hemostasis tests, particularly screening tests such as PT and APTT (for review see [10]). If the normal practice is for samples to be stored deep frozen for batch analysis, then this should also be done for normal samples and in this case −20°C freezers are usually inadequate, particularly those that incorporate an automatic defrost cycle. If patient samples are processed after a delay during which samples are transported to the laboratory over several hours, then a similar delay should be used between collection of samples and testing for the samples from normal subjects used to derive reference intervals. The literature and reagent manufacturer's information should only be used as a guide. Adopting a manufacturer's range without local verification can lead to misdiagnosis. In one study of 23 genetically confirmed protein S-deficient subjects, all 23 were successfully identified as abnormal using a locally determined reference range (even though only 20 normal subjects were analyzed to derive this), whereas four deficient subjects would have been misclassified as normal based on the manufacturer's stated reference range for one particular technique [11].

Change in Reagent Lot Numbers

In the case of some APTT reagents, there has been sufficient variation between different production lots or batches of the reagent to affect the results obtained. It is particularly important to check that any change in APTT reagent lot number does not affect results for patients receiving unfractionated heparin, because there are reports that, for some reagents at least, there can be clinically important differences in the therapeutic range for different lots of the same type of reagent [12]. In this case, it is necessary to reassess the therapeutic range before introducing a new lot number. A method to assess whether a small difference between lots is sufficient to require a full establishment of a new therapeutic range has been described [8]. A change in reagent lot number could also affect the reference range for other screening tests, including the PT as well as global tests of hemostasis, such as thrombin generation tests, thrombelastography/ thomboelastometry, and tests that screen the protein C pathway, including activated protein C resistance tests.

Data Analysis

The reference or normal range is usually constructed from individual results in such a way that it contains 95% of the reference population. When the results are normally distributed, the normal range is conventionally calculated to be the mean ±2 standard deviations, which includes 95% of the population. If the results are not normally distributed, other statistical tests, such as log transformation, should be used first to obtain a normally distributed population. In

some cases, nonparametric methods may be used to identify the central 95% of values.

Assessment of distribution can be done with statistical tests for normality or results of normal subjects can be inspected graphically to identify skewedness or particularly to identify outliers amongst the group. Any outliers (i.e., any result that lies unexpectedly far from the majority of others) should then be excluded from calculations. This can be done statistically using a discordancy test, which identifies extreme outliers amongst the set of results using the deviation from the sample mean and taking account of the estimated variance (as described by Barnett and Lewis [13]) but visual inspection of the data in the form of a bar chart showing the number of observations (y axis) against the relevant test result interval (x axis) is often sufficient [8]. For some tests, the exclusion of outliers can have an important impact on the calculated reference range [14], but it may be useful to calculate the reference range with and without the inclusion of potential outliers, because in many areas of hemostasis testing, this frequently shows that the calculated range is largely unaffected either way, provided a large enough group of subjects have been tested. Because of some of these issues, it is important that those who make interpretations of patient results against reference ranges keep in mind that the reference range should only be a guide to use alongside all other available clinical information.

Examples of Locally Determined Reference Ranges

As discussed above, it is important that a full reference range is established when a newly developed method is introduced or if there has been a significant modification, which may require analysis of up to 120 subjects for fully valid data to be obtained. As mentioned above, the CLSI guideline [1] recognizes that an abbreviated version using a minimum of 20 subjects may be used for validating the transfer of reference values among comparable analytical platforms. Furthermore, there are a number of laboratory tests in hemostasis where agreement between ranges derived in different centers by different techniques/ reagents can be expected to be in good agreement. This should be the case, for example, in relation to many clotting factor assays, where data from external quality assessment programs throughout the world demonstrate that different reagents/ methods are associated with the same laboratory results on average. For this reason, we have included some examples of locally determined reference ranges from our own center in Sheffield, UK at the time of publication of this book (Table 1).

Pregnancy Normal Ranges

Few laboratories have specific normal ranges for pregnant subjects. It is rarely necessary to have a precise range, but it is important for clinicians to be aware of the range and type of changes that occur during this period. Table 2, from a published study, indicates some of the hemostatic variables that change during pregnancy. Shown are the mean values and the calculated normal ranges from the mean ±2 standard deviations [15].

Neonatal Normal Ranges

Adult reference intervals should not be used to interpret results obtained in neonates because there are important differences in the results obtained [16–20].

Table 1 Normal ranges in the authors' laboratory in 2014.

Test	Method	Range	No. of subjects
Bleeding disorders			
FVIII : C	One-stage assay	58–184 IU/dL	25–30
VWF : Ag	Latex	46–146 IU/dL	25–30
VWF : Acivity	Latex (Innovance)	48–173 IU/dL	>30
FIX	APTT based	69–157 IU/dL	25–30
FII	PT-based	84–132 IU/dL	25–30
FV	PT-based	66–126 U/dl	25–30
FVII	PT-based	61–157 IU/dL	25–30
FX	PT-based	74–149 IU/dL	25–30
FXI	APTT-based	67–169 U/dL	25–30
FXII	APTT-based	64–196 U/dL	25–30
FXIII	Spectrophotometric ammonia release	59–185 U/dL	20
α_2-Antiplasmin	Chromogenic	67–103 U/dL	20
Thrombotic disorders			
Antithrombin activity	Chromogenic	85–131 IU/dL	80
Antithrombin antigen	ELISA	83–124 IU/dL	30
Protein C activity	Chromogenic	79–142 IU/dL	80
Protein C antigen	ELISA	75–131 IU/dL	25–30
Protein S total	ELISA	71–136 IU/dL	80
Protein S free	Latex	Males 74–143 IU/dL	40
		Females 67–125 IU/dL	40

APTT, activated partial thromboplastin time; ELISA, enzyme-linked immunosorbent assay; PT, prothrombin time.

Table 2 Normal ranges in pregnancy.

Variable		Pregnancy (weeks' gestation)				Post partum	
(Nonpregnant normal range)		10–15	23–25	32–34	38–40	1	8
Classic APCR (>2.3)	mean	2.89	2.74	2.64	2.66	2.87	3.16
	normal range	2.33–3.45	2.18–3.30	2.16–3.12	2.02–3.30	2.09–3.65	2.34–4.00
Modified APCR (V depleted) (>2.0)	mean	2.63	2.59	2.57	2.62	2.68	2.71
	normal range	2.39–2.87	2.35–2.83	2.35–2.79	2.36–2.88	2.40–2.96	2.43–2.99
FVIII : C U/mL (0.50–2.0)	mean	1.41	1.69	2.06	2.31	2.24	1.25
	normal range	0.51–2.31	0.81–2.49	1.02–3.10	1.43–3.19	0.86–3.62	0.49–2.01
Fibrinogen g/dL (2.0–4.0)	mean	3.3	3.5	4.1	4.5	4.6	2.6
	normal range	2.1–4.5	2.3–4.7	2.9–5.3	3.5–5.5	3.2–6.0	1.8–3.4
Protein C U/mL (0.70–1.25)	mean	0.95	1.04	1.02	1.00	1.16	1.02
	normal range	0.65–1.25	0.68–1.40	0.64–1.40	0.62–1.38	0.76–1.56	0.68–1.36
Free Protein S U/mL (0.63–1.12)	mean	0.62	0.53	0.51	0.51	0.59	0.74
	normal range	0.36–0.88	0.35–0.71	0.33–0.69	0.31–0.71	0.27–0.91	0.52–0.96
D-Dimer ng/mL (<120[a])	mean	35	81	130	193	251	11
	normal range	0–93	0–175	0–286	0–417	0–867	0–22

Source: modified from Horn *et al.* 2001 [14].
a)   D-dimer results vary more than fourfold according to the method used for analysis.

Reference values for coagulation tests in the healthy full-term infant during the first 6 months of life are shown in Table 3. Values from this North American study shown are mean with the normal range based on mean ±2 standard deviations [17].

An Australian group reported age-specific reference ranges for FII, FV, FVII, FVIII, FIX, FX, FXI, FXII, plasminogen, protein C, and protein S in healthy term neonates and healthy children attending for minor surgery [19]. The group sizes were between n = 9 and n = 20 and ELISA (antigen) techniques were used. The ranges reported for FVIII and some other parameters were similar to the activity assay data in Table 3. The group included an adult group and reported an average FV antigen of 0.24 U/mL and average

FXI of 0.43 U/mL in adults. These are much lower than would be anticipated from the literature on FV and FXI assays, which would predict an average close to 1.0 U/mL.

Conclusion

In general, the normal range should be used only as a guide and an aid to clinical interpretation in conjunction with all other available relevant clinical information. The most appropriate normal reference range is one that has been established locally using the same system as for patient samples. It is important to use a technique for which such a local range is in broad agreement with the published literature.

Table 3 Normal ranges for neonates and children.

Tests	Day 1	Day 5	Day 30	Day 90	Day 180	Adult
PT (sec)	13.0 (10.1–15.9)*	12.4 (10.0–15.3)*	11.8 (10.0–14.2)*	11.9 (10.0–14.2)*	12.3 (10.7–13.9)*	12.4 (10.8–13.9)
INR	1.00 (0.53–1.62)	0.89 (0.53–1.48)	0.79 (0.53–1.26)	0.81 (0.53–1.26)	0.88 (0.61–1.17)	0.89 (0.64–1.17)
APTT (sec)	42.9 (31.3–54.5)	42.6 (25.4–59.8)	40.4 (32.0–55.2)	37.1 (29.0–50.1)*	35.5 (28.1–42.9)*	33.4 (26.6–40.3)
TCT (sec)	23.5 (19.0–28.3)*	23.1 (18.0–29.2)	24.3 (19.4–29.2)*	25.1 (20.5–29.7)*	25.5 (19.8–31.2)*	25.0 (19.7–30.3)
Fibrinogen (g/L)	2.83 (1.67–3.99)*	3.12 (1.62–4.62)*	2.70 (1.62–3.78)*	2.43 (1.50–3.79)*	2.51 (1.50–3.87)*	2.78 (1.56–4.00)
F II (U/mL)	0.48 (0.26–0.70)	0.63 (0.33–0.93)	0.68 (0.34–1.02)	0.75 (0.45–1.05)	0.88 (0.60–1.16)	1.08 (0.70–1.46)
F V (U/mL)	0.72 (0.34–1.08)	0.95 (0.45–1.45)	0.98 (0.62–1.34)	0.90 (0.48–1.32)	0.91 (0.55–1.27)	1.06 (0.62–1.50)
F VII (U/mL)	0.66 (0.28–1.04)	0.89 (0.35–1.43)	0.90 (0.42–1.38)	0.91 (0.39–1.43)	0.87 (0.47–1.27)	1.05 (0.67–1.43)
F VIII (U/mL)	1.00 (0.50–1.78)*	0.88 (0.50–1.54)*	0.91 (0.50–1.57)*	0.79 (0.50–1.25)*	0.73 (0.50–1.09)	0.99 (0.50–1.49)
VWF (U/mL)	1.53 (0.50–2.87)	1.40 (0.50 (2.54)	1.28 (0.50–2.46)	1.18 (0.50–2.06)	1.07 (0.50–1.97)	0.92 (0.50–1.58)
F IX (U/mL)	0.53 (0.15–0.91)	0.53 (0.15–0.91)	0.51 (0.21–0.81)	0.67 (0.21–1.13)	0.86 (0.36–1.36)	1.09 (0.55–1.63)
F X (U/mL)	0.40 (0.21–0.68)	0.49 (0.19–0.79)	0.59 (0.31–0.87)	0.71 (0.35–1.07)	0.78 (0.38–1.18)	1.06 (0.70–1.52)
FXI (U/mL)	0.38 (0.10–0.66)	0.55 (0.23–0.87)	0.53 (0.27–0.79)	0.69 (0.41–0.97)	0.86 (0.49–1.34)	0.97 (0.67–1.27)
F XII (U/mL)	0.53 (0.13–0.93)	0.47 (0.11–0.83)	0.49 (0.17–0.81)	0.67 (0.25–1.09)	0.77 (0.39–1.15)	1.08 (0.52–1.64)
Antithrombin (U/mL)	0.63 (0.39–0.87)	0.67 (0.41–0.93)	0.78 (0.48–1.08)	0.97 (0.73–1.21)*	1.04 (0.84–1.24)*	1.05 (0.79–1.31)
Protein C (U/mL)	0.35 (0.17–0.53)	0.42 (0.20–0.64)	0.43 (0.21–0.65)	0.54 (0.28–0.80)	0.59 (0.37–0.81)	0.96 (0.64–1.28)
Protein S (U/mL)	0.36 (0.12–0.60)	0.50 (0.22–0.78)	0.63 (0.33–0.93)	0.86 (0.54–1.18)*	0.87 (0.55–1.19)*	0.92 (0.60–1.24)

Source: modified from Andrew *et al.* 1987 [16].
*Values are indistinguishable from those of the adult.
APTT, activated partial thromboplastin time; INR, international normalized ratio; PT, prothrombin time; TCT, thrombin clotting time; VWF, von Willebrand factor.

References

1 Wayne, PA; Clinical and Laboratory Standards Institute. *How to Define and Determine Reference Intervals in the Clinical Laboratory: Approved Guideline*, Document C28-A2, 2nd edn. CLSI, 2000.

2 *Clinical Laboratory Improvement Amendments of 1988* (CLIA) 42 CFR section 493.1253, part (b) (1) (ii) (2003).

3 Freidberg RC, Souers R, Wagar EA, *et al.* The origin of reference intervals: a college of American Pathologists Q-probes study of "normal ranges" used in 163 clinical laboratories. *Arch Pathol Lab Med* 2007; 131: 348–357.

4 Gill JC, Endres-Brooks J, Bauer PJ, *et al.* The effect of ABO blood group on the diagnosis of von Willebrand's disease. *Blood* 1987; 69: 1691–1695.

5 Blomback M, Konkle BA, Manco-Johnson MJ, *et al.* on behalf of the ISTH SSC on Women's Health Issues. Preanalytical conditions that affect coagulation testing, including hormonal status and therapy. *J Thromb Haemost* 2007; 5: 855–858.

6 Lowe GDO, Rumley A, Woodward M, *et al.* Epidemiology of coagulation factors, inhibitors and activation markers: the third Glasgow MONICA survey I. Illustrative reference ranges by age, sex and hormone use. *Br J Haematol* 1997; 97: 775–784.

7 Solberg HE on behalf of International Federation of Clinical Chemistry (IFCC) and International Committee for Standardization in Hematology (ICSH), IFCC Expert Panel on Reference Values. Approved recommendation on the theory of reference values. Part 5 statistical treatment of collected reference values. Determination of reference limits. *J Clin Chem Clin Biochem* 1987; 25: 645–656.

8 Wayne, PA: Clinical and Laboratory Standards Institute. *One Stage Prothrombin Time (PT) Test and Activate Partial Thromboplastin Time (APTT) Test: Approved Guideline*, Document H47-A2, 2nd edn. CLSI, 2008.

9 Kitchen S, McCraw. *Diagnosis of Haemophilia and Other Bleeding Disorders: a Laboratory Manual*, 2000. Available at: www.wfh.org/publications (accessed July 2016).

10 Adcock D. Sample integrity and preanalytical variables In: Kitchen S, Olson J, Preston FE, eds. *Quality in Laboratory Hemostasis and Thrombosis*, 2nd edn. Oxford, UK: Wiley-Blackwell, 2013, pp. 45–56.

11 Jennings I, Kitchen S, Cooper P, *et al.* Sensitivity of functional protein S assays to protein S deficiency: a comparative study of 3 commercial kits. *J Thromb Haemost* 2003; 1: 1112–1117.

12 Shojania AM, Tetreault J, Turnbull G. The variations between heparin sensitivity of different lots of APTT reagents produced by the same manufacturer. *Am J Clin Pathol* 1988; 89: 19–23.

13 Barnett V, Lewis T. *Outliers in Statistical Data*. Chicester: John Wiley, 1978, pp. 91–93.

14 Horn PS, Feng L, Yanmei L, *et al.* Effect of outliers and non-healthy individuals on reference interval estimation. *Clin Chem* 2001; 47: 2137–2145.

15 Kjellberg U, Anderssson NE, Rosen S, *et al.* APC resistance and other haemostatic variables during pregnancy and puerperium. *Thromb Haemost* 1999; 81: 527–531.

16 Andrew M, Paes B, Milner R, *et al.* Development of the human coagulation system in the full-term infant. *Blood* 1987; 70: 165–172.

17 Andrew M, Paes B, Johnston M. Development of the hemostatic system in the neonate and young infant. *Am J Pediatr Hematol Oncol* 1990; 12: 95–104.

18 Andrew M, Vegh P, Johnston, *et al.* Maturation of the hemostastic system during childhood. *Blood* 1992; 80: 1998–2005.

19 Attard C, Van der Staaten T, Karlaftis V, *et al.* Developmental hemostasis: age-specific differences in the levels of hemostatic proteins. *J Thromb Haemost* 2013; 11: 1850–1854.

20 Sosothikul D, Kittalalayawong Y, Aungbamnet P, *et al.* Reference ranges for thrombotic markers in children. *Blood Coag Fibrinol* 2012; 23: 208–211.

Index

Practical Hemostasis and Thrombosis, Third Edition. Edited by Nigel S. Key, Michael Makris and David Lillicrap.
© 2017 John Wiley & Sons, Ltd. Published 2017 by John Wiley & Sons, Ltd.

The manufacturer's authorised representative in the EU for product safety is Oxford
University Press España S.A. of El Parque Empresarial San Fernando de Henares,
Avenida de Castilla, 2 – 28830 Madrid (www.oup.es/en or product.safety@oup.com).
OUP España S.A. also acts as importer into Spain of products made by the manufacturer.

Printed in the USA/Agawam, MA
January 13, 2025

880951.007